Board Basics

Editor-in-Chief

Virginia U. Collier, MD, MACP, FRCP[2]
Chair Emeritus, Department of Medicine
Christiana Care Health System
Newark, Delaware
Honorary Professor of Medicine
Sidney Kimmel Medical College at Thomas Jefferson University
Philadelphia, Pennsylvania

Contributors

Victoria E. Burke, MD[1]
Assistant Professor of Clinical Medicine
Infectious Diseases Fellowship Associate Program
Louisiana State University Health Sciences Center
New Orleans, Louisiana

Aaron J. Calderon, MD, FACP[2]
Chair, Department of Medicine
Program Director, Internal Medicine Residency
Saint Joseph Hospital
Professor of Clinical Medicine
University of Colorado SOM
Denver, Colorado

Ana M. Cilursu, MD, FACP[1]
Staff Rheumatologist
Shore Physicians Group
Shore Medical Center
Somers Point, New Jersey

Mark Corriere, MD, FACP[2]
Clinical Endocrinologist
Maryland Endocrine
Assistant Professor of Medicine
Johns Hopkins School of Medicine
Baltimore, Maryland

Anthony A. Donato, MD, MHPE, FACP[1]
Associate Program Director, Internal Medicine
Professor of Medicine
Sidney Kimmel Medical College at Thomas Jefferson University
Tower Health Medical Group
Philadelphia, Pennsylvania

Richard S. Eisenstaedt, MD, MACP[1]
Clinical Professor of Medicine
Thomas Jefferson University
Chair, Department of Medicine
Abington Memorial Hospital
Abington, Pennsylvania

Nasrollah Ghahramani, MD, MS, FACP[1]
Professor of Medicine and Public Health Sciences
Vice Chair for Educational Affairs
Interim Chief, Division of Nephrology
Penn State College of Medicine
Hershey, Pennsylvania

Robert G. Kaniecki, MD[1]
Director, UPMC Headache Center
Chief, Headache Division
Assistant Director, Neurology Residency Training Program
Director, Headache Fellowship Program
Assistant Professor of Neurology
University of Pittsburgh School of Medicine
Pittsburgh, Pennsylvania

Gregory A. Masters, MD, FACP[1]
Principal Investigator, National Cancer Institute Community Oncology Research Program
Helen F. Graham Cancer Center and Research Institute
Associate Professor of Medicine
Sidney Kimmel Medical College at Thomas Jefferson University
Philadelphia, Pennsylvania

Brian S. Porter, MD[2]
Cardiologist
Core Physicians
Exeter, New Hampshire

Benjamin T. Suratt, MD[1]
Professor of Medicine and Cell and Molecular Biology
Vice Chair of Medicine for Academic Affairs
Associate Chief, Pulmonary and Critical Care Medicine
University of Vermont College of Medicine
Burlington, Vermont

Jennifer M. Weiss, MD, MS[1]
Assistant Professor of Medicine
Division of Gastroenterology and Hepatology
Department of Medicine
University of Wisconsin School of Medicine and Public Health
Madison, Wisconsin

Jennifer Wright, MD, FACP[1]
Assistant Professor of Medicine
Division of General Internal Medicine
University of Washington School of Medicine
Seattle, Washington

Consultants

Marta Kokoszynska, MD[1]
Instructor, Pulmonary and Critical Care Medicine
University of Vermont Larner College of Medicine
Burlington, Vermont

Dhaval Shah, MD, MBBS[1]
Hematology/Oncology Physician
Helen F. Graham Cancer Center
Newark, Delaware

Board Basics ACP Editorial Staff

Linnea Donnarumma[1], Staff Editor
Margaret Wells[1], Director, Self-Assessment and Educational Programs[1]
Becky Krumm[1], Managing Editor, Self-Assessment and Educational Programs[1]

ACP Principal Staff

Davoren Chick, MD, FACP[2]
Senior Vice President, Medical Education

Patrick C. Alguire, MD, FACP[2]
Senior Vice President Emeritus, Medical Education
MKSAP 18 Editor-in-Chief

Sean McKinney[1]
Vice President, Medical Education

Margaret Wells[1]
Director, Self-Assessment and Educational Programs

Becky Krumm[1]
Managing Editor

Valerie Dangovetsky[1]
Administrator

Ellen McDonald, PhD[1]
Senior Staff Editor

Megan Zborowski[1]
Senior Staff Editor

Jackie Twomey[1]
Senior Staff Editor

Randy Hendrickson[1]
Production Administrator/Editor

Julia Nawrocki[1]
Digital Content Associate/Editor

Linnea Donnarumma[1]
Staff Editor

Chuck Emig[1]
Staff Editor

Joysa Winter[1]
Staff Editor

Kimberly Kerns[1]
Administrative Coordinator

---

1. Has no relationships with any entity producing, marketing, reselling, or distributing health care goods or services consumed by, or used on, patients.

2. Has disclosed relationship(s) with any entity producing, marketing, reselling, or distributing health care goods or services consumed by, or used on, patients.

Disclosure of Relationships with any entity producing, marketing, reselling, or distributing health care goods or services consumed by, or used on, patients.

Patrick C. Alguire, MD, FACP
Royalties
UpToDate

Aaron J. Calderon, MD, FACP
Speakers Bureau
MedStudy
Stock Options/Holdings
Pfizer Inc., Merck, Abbott

Davoren Chick, MD, FACP
Royalties
Wolters Kluwer Publishing
Consultantship
EBSCO Health's DynaMed Plus
Other: Owner and sole proprietor of Coding 101 LLC; research consultant (spouse) for Vedanta Biosciences Inc.

Virginia U. Collier, MD, MACP, FRCP
Stock Options/Holdings
Celgene, Pfizer Inc., Merck, Abbott, Johnson & Johnson, Medtronic plc, Amgen, Roche, Sanofi, Novartis, AbbVie Inc., Stryker, WellPoint Health Networks

Mark Corriere, MC, USN, FACP
Speakers Bureau
Eli Lilly and Co., Sanofi, AstraZeneca

Brian Porter, MD
Other: Medtronic plc: educational support received to attend two-day course on pacemaker interrogations, programming, and implantation

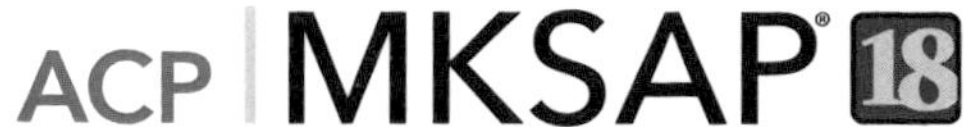

Board Basics®

An Enhancement to MKSAP® 18

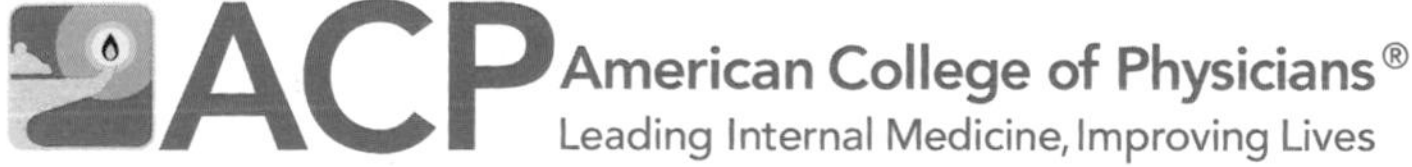

Your Last Stop before the Boards

For the fifth consecutive edition of MKSAP, we bring you Board Basics, the only publication that compiles the essential facts and strategies for passing the Internal Medicine Certification and Maintenance of Certification (MOC) exams into one print book and e-book. We are confident that this volume will continue to meet your needs.

How to Use Board Basics

The goal of Board Basics is to prepare you for the Boards after you have completed a systematic review of MKSAP 18 and its more than 1200 multiple-choice questions. We have combed through the MKSAP 18 content to produce a concise compilation of only the information that you will most likely see in the exam. The sections of Board Basics are organized to mirror those of MKSAP, making it easy for you to locate information within the 11 MKSAP subspecialty sections to further your learning on specific topics as you need. Board Basics is not a concise guide to patient care but, rather, an exam preparation tool to help you quickly recognize the most likely answers on a multiple-choice exam. Drug dosages are not included since they are rarely, if ever, tested. You will also see many sections in which information has been omitted because it is difficult to test or is otherwise unlikely to appear on the exam.

Broad differential diagnoses are not provided for most problems. Instead, Board Basics focuses on the entities that have the highest probability of appearing on the exam as the "correct answers." Critical points that appear on the exam are often presented here in isolation, stripped of context that is not relevant to answering a multiple-choice question. If you review these points shortly before your exam, you will have the best chance of remembering what you need to know to do well. Knowing that most Board questions are prefaced with the words "most likely," we have tried to be very directive, skipping important steps in the patient evaluation. When you see the words "select" or "choose," think in terms of *selecting or choosing a particular answer*, not an intervention in the practice of medicine. Remember that Board Basics is *not* a patient care resource.

Content Organization

Abbreviations, spelled out in a convenient list at the back of the book, are used frequently to increase reading efficiency. Content is organized by topic and in consistent categories, such as Prevention, Screening, Diagnosis, Treatment, and Follow-up. Special components have been designed to enhance learning and recall.

Look for:

- *Don't Be Tricked:* Incorrect answers that may masquerade as correct choices.
- *Test Yourself:* Abbreviated case histories and answers found in Board exam questions.
- *Study Tables:* Key concepts to prepare you for specific types of questions.
- *Yellow highlighting:* We applied our own "marker" to call your attention to important phrases.

Benefits of This Text

For this edition of Board Basics, MKSAP 18 authors reviewed the latest literature and produced 11 concise text sections and 1200 Board-like multiple-choice questions. Next, the content was turned over to 13 carefully selected program directors, instructors, and professors of medicine with expertise in Board preparation and the subspecialties of internal medicine. These physicians culled the essential points from MKSAP 18 and added their insights to update the content of Board Basics. As Editor-in-Chief, I reviewed and distilled the MKSAP 18 text by eliminating overlap and excessive material to focus the text as sharply as possible. The end product is what you have in your hands–the best Board prep tool that you will find anywhere. We hope you enjoy it and benefit from your study. Best wishes on your exam.

Virginia U. Collier, MD, MACP, FRCP
Editor-in-Chief
Board Basics

Acknowledgments

The American College of Physicians (ACP) gratefully acknowledges the special contributions to the development and production of the 18th edition of the Medical Knowledge Self-Assessment Program® (MKSAP® 18) made by the following people:

Graphic Design: Barry Moshinski (Director, Graphic Services), Michael Ripca (Graphics Technical Administrator), and Jennifer Gropper (Graphic Designer).

Production/Systems: Dan Hoffmann (Director, Information Technology), Scott Hurd (Manager, Content Systems), Neil Kohl (Senior Architect), and Chris Patterson (Senior Architect).

MKSAP 18 Digital: Under the direction of Steven Spadt (Senior Vice President, Technology), the digital version of MKSAP 18 was developed within the ACP's Digital Products and Services Department, led by Brian Sweigard (Director, Digital Products and Services). Other members of the team included Dan Barron (Senior Web Application Developer/Architect), Chris Forrest (Senior Software Developer/Design Lead), Kathleen Hoover (Senior Web Developer), Kara Regis (Manager, User Interface Design and Development), Brad Lord (Senior Web Application Developer), and John McKnight (Senior Web Developer).

The College also wishes to acknowledge that many other persons, too numerous to mention, have contributed to the production of this program. Without their dedicated efforts, this program would not have been possible.

MKSAP Resource Site (mksap.acponline.org)

The MKSAP Resource Site (mksap.acponline.org) is a continually updated site that provides links to MKSAP 18 online answer sheets for print subscribers; access to MKSAP 18 Digital; Board Basics® e-book access instructions; information on Continuing Medical Education (CME), Maintenance of Certification (MOC), and international Continuing Professional Development (CPD) and MOC; errata; and other new information.

Disclosure Policy

It is the policy of the American College of Physicians (ACP) to ensure balance, independence, objectivity, and scientific rigor in all of its educational activities. To this end, and consistent with the policies of the ACP and the Accreditation Council for Continuing Medical Education (ACCME), contributors to all ACP continuing medical education activities are required to disclose all relevant financial relationships with any entity producing, marketing, re-selling, or distributing health care goods or services consumed by, or used on, patients. Contributors are required to use generic names in the discussion of therapeutic options and are required to identify any unapproved, off-label, or investigative use of commercial products or devices. Where a trade name is used, all available trade names for the same product type are also included. If trade-name products manufactured by companies with whom contributors have relationships are discussed, contributors are asked to provide evidence-based citations in support of the discussion. The information is reviewed by the committee responsible for producing this text. If necessary, adjustments to topics or contributors' roles in content development are made to balance the discussion. Further, all readers of this text are asked to evaluate the content for evidence of commercial bias and send any relevant comments to mksap_editors@acponline.org so that future decisions about content and contributors can be made in light of this information.

Resolution of Conflicts

To resolve all conflicts of interest and influences of vested interests, ACP's content planners used best evidence and updated clinical care guidelines in developing content, when such evidence and guidelines were available. All content underwent review by peer reviewers not on the committee to ensure that the material was balanced and unbiased. Contributors' disclosure information can be found with the list of contributors' names and those of ACP principal staff listed in the beginning of this book.

Educational Disclaimer

The editors and publisher of MKSAP 18 recognize that the development of new material offers many opportunities for error. Despite our best efforts, some errors may persist in print. Drug dosage schedules are, we believe, accurate and in accordance with current standards. Readers are advised, however, to ensure that the recommended dosages in MKSAP 18 concur with the information provided in the product information material. This is especially important in cases of new, infrequently used, or highly toxic drugs. Application of the information in MKSAP 18 remains the professional responsibility of the practitioner.

The primary purpose of MKSAP 18 is educational. Information presented, as well as publications, technologies, products, and/or services discussed, is intended to inform subscribers about the knowledge, techniques, and experiences of the contributors. A diversity of professional opinion exists, and the views of the contributors are their own and not those of the ACP. Inclusion of any material in the program does not constitute endorsement or recommendation by the ACP. The ACP does not warrant the safety, reliability, accuracy, completeness, or usefulness of and disclaims any and all liability for damages and claims that may result from the use of information, publications, technologies, products, and/or services discussed in this program.

Publisher's Information

Unauthorized Use of This Book Is Against the Law

MKSAP 18 ISBN: 978-1-938245-47-3
(Board Basics) ISBN: 978-1-938245-73-2

Printed in the United States of America.

For order information in the U.S. or Canada call 800-ACP-1915. All other countries call 215-351-2600 (Monday to Friday, 9 AM – 5 PM ET). Fax inquiries to 215-351-2799 or email to custserv@acponline.org.

Errata

Errata for MKSAP 18 will be available through the MKSAP Resource Site at mksap.acponline.org as new information becomes known to the editors.

Table of Contents

Hematology

Infectious Disease

Nephrology

Neurology

Oncology

Pulmonary and Critical Care Medicine

Rheumatology

Cardiovascular Medicine

Acute Chest Pain

Diagnosis

Typical angina includes substernal chest pain with exertion and relief with rest or nitroglycerin. Atypical symptoms are most commonly found in women and in patients with diabetes; these symptoms include exertional dyspnea, fatigue, nausea, and vomiting. Older adult patients may also present atypically.

Signs of cardiac ischemia include new MR murmur and S_3 and S_4 gallops. Patients presenting with ACS may also have signs and symptoms of pulmonary edema, hypotension, confusion, and dysrhythmias.

Several other conditions can also cause acute chest pain:

STUDY TABLE: Other Causes of Acute Chest Pain

Vignette	Consider	Test/Therapy
Young woman with history of migraines, acute chest pain, and ST-segment elevation	Coronary vasospasm (Prinzmetal angina)	Echocardiography; long-acting nitrate, calcium channel blocker
Young person with chest pain following a party	Cocaine	Echocardiography; calcium channel blocker (avoid β-blockers)
A tall, thin person with long arms with acute chest and back pain (especially "tearing" sensation), a normal ECG, and an aortic diastolic murmur	Marfan syndrome and aortic dissection	MRA, CTA, or TEE; immediate surgery for type A dissection
A patient who recently traveled or with immobility, sharp or pleuritic chest pain, and nondiagnostic ECG	PE	CTA; UFH or LMWH
A tall, thin young man who smokes with sudden pleuritic chest pain and dyspnea	Spontaneous pneumothorax	Chest x-ray
A postmenopausal woman with substernal chest pain following severe emotional/physical stress has ST-segment elevation in the anterior precordial leads, troponin elevation, and unremarkable coronary angiography	Stress-induced (takotsubo) cardiomyopathy. Look for characteristic apical ballooning on ventriculogram.	β-blocker, ACE inhibitor
A young man with substernal chest pain, deep T-wave inversions in V_2-V_4, and a harsh systolic murmur that increases with Valsalva maneuver	HCM	Echocardiography, β-blocker

Acute Coronary Syndromes (STEMI, NSTEMI, and Unstable Angina)

Acute coronary syndromes occur when coronary blood flow is disrupted.

Testing

The 12-lead ECG and serum biomarkers distinguish three types of ACS:

STUDY TABLE: Diagnosis of ACS in Patients with Chest Pain

Syndrome	Description
NSTE-ACS	
Unstable angina	**Normal cardiac biomarkers** May have nonspecific ECG changes, ST-segment depression, or T-wave inversion
NSTEMI	**Positive biomarkers** without ST elevations or ST-elevation equivalents May have nonspecific ECG changes, ST-segment depression, and T-wave inversion
STEMI	ST-segment elevation of ≥1 mm in ≥2 contiguous leads and positive biomarkers ST-elevation equivalents include new LBBB or posterior MI (tall R waves and ST depressions in V_1-V_3)

Echocardiogram may show regional wall motion abnormalities in ACS. This may be especially useful in patients with LBBB.

STUDY TABLE: ECG Localization of STEMI

Anatomic Location	ST-Segment Change	Indicative ECG Leads
Inferior	Elevation	II, III, aVF
Anteroseptal	Elevation	V_1-V_3
Lateral and apical	Elevation	V_4-V_6, possibly I and aVL
Posterior wall*	Depression	Tall R waves in V_1-V_3
Right ventricle*	Elevation	V_4R-V_6R; tall R waves in V_1-V_3

*Often associated with inferior and/or lateral ST-elevation infarctions.

Unstable Angina/NSTEMI

In patients with **unstable angina**/**NSTEMI**, immediate angiography is indicated if any of the following are present:

- hemodynamic instability
- HF
- recurrent rest angina despite therapy
- new or worsening MR murmur
- sustained VT

Risk stratification: Otherwise, in patients with unstable angina and NSTEMI, risk stratification is used to determine whether the patient should receive early angiography (usually within 24 hours during the index hospitalization) or predischarge stress testing with angiography reserved when significant ischemia is seen on stress testing. Several risk scoring systems are available to estimate risk and guide management. One is the Thrombolysis in Myocardial Infarction (TIMI) risk score, a 7-point score for estimating risk in patients with unstable angina/NSTEMI. The rate of death for MI significantly increases with a higher TIMI risk score.

Do not attempt to memorize the scoring system, but understand the difference in approach for a patient with a low-risk score, such as a TIMI score of 0-2, compared with the approach for a patients with a higher score (3-7).

STUDY TABLE: Unstable Angina or NSTEMI Risk Stratification	
TIMI Risk Score	**Strategy**
0-2	Low risk. Begin aspirin, β-blocker, nitrates, heparin, statin, clopidogrel. Predischarge stress testing and angiography if testing reveals significant myocardial ischemia
3-7	Intermediate to high risk. Begin aspirin, β-blocker, nitrates, heparin, statin, clopidogrel, and early angiography followed by revascularization

Cardiac catheterization is indicated for patients with the following post-MI stress test results:

- exercise-induced ST-segment depression or elevation
- inability to achieve 5 METs during testing
- inability to increase SBP by 10 to 30 mm Hg
- inability to exercise (arthritis)

DON'T BE TRICKED

- **STEMI is not the only cause of ST-segment elevations. Consider acute pericarditis, LV aneurysm, takotsubo (stress) cardiomyopathy, coronary vasospasm (Prinzmetal angina), acute stroke, or normal variant.**

STEMI

Patients with **STEMI** should undergo immediate cardiac angiography.

STUDY TABLE: Drug Therapy for ACS	
Drug	**Indication**
Aspirin	ASAP for all patients with ACS Continue indefinitely as secondary prevention
$P2Y_{12}$ inhibitor (clopidogrel, ticagrelor, prasugrel)	ASAP for all patients with ACS Continue for at least 1 year following MI
β-Blockers (metoprolol, carvedilol)	Administer for ACS within 24 hours Continue indefinitely as secondary prevention
Anticoagulant (UFH, LMWH, bivalirudin)	ASAP for definite or likely ACS
ACE inhibitors	Administer within 24 hours Continue indefinitely in patients with reduced LVEF or clinical HF, diabetes, hypertension, or CKD
ARB	Administer if intolerant of ACE inhibitor
Nitroglycerin	Administer in presence of ongoing chest pain or HF
Statin	Administer high-intensity statin early, even in patients with low LDL levels Continue indefinitely as secondary prevention
Eplerenone or spironolactone	Administer 3 to 14 days after MI if LVEF ≤40% and clinical HF or diabetes
GP IIb/IIIa antagonists (abciximab, eptifibatide, tirofiban)	Generally reserved for short-term infusion after difficult or failed PCI in patients at high risk with a large clot burden Usually not administered to patients with ACS who have received aspirin and a $P2Y_{12}$ inhibitor

For **patients with STEMI**, **percutaneous coronary intervention (PCI)** is the preferred strategy. PCI should be performed as soon as possible, with first medical contact to PCI time ≤90 minutes in a PCI-capable hospital and ≤120 minutes if transferred from a non–PCI-capable hospital to a PCI-capable hospital.

Other indications for PCI are:

- failure of thrombolytic therapy (continued chest pain, persistent ST elevations on ECG)
- thrombolytic therapy is contraindicated
- new HF or cardiogenic shock

Thrombolytic agents: Administer thrombolytic agents when PCI is not available and cannot be achieved within 120 minutes with transfer. The most commonly encountered contraindications include active bleeding or high risk for bleeding (recent major surgery). BP >180/110 mm Hg on presentation is a relative contraindication.

CABG surgery: CABG is indicated acutely for STEMI in the presence of thrombolytic PCI failure or mechanical complications (papillary muscle rupture, VSD, free wall rupture).

Right ventricular infarction: Patients with a right ventricular/posterior infarction may present with hypotension or may develop hypotension following the administration of nitroglycerin or morphine. Look for JVD with clear lungs, hypotension, and tachycardia. The most predictive ECG finding is ST-segment elevation on right-sided ECG lead V_4R. Treat these patients with IV fluids.

Cardiogenic shock: Place an intra-aortic balloon pump for patients with cardiogenic shock, acute MR or VSD, intractable VT, or refractory angina.

DON'T BE TRICKED

- Do not choose thrombolytic therapy for patients with NSTEMI or for asymptomatic patients with onset of pain >24 hours ago.
- Unlike medical therapy for stable CAD, routine use of nitrates, calcium channel blockers, or ranolazine generally has no role in the post-STEMI setting.
- Do not choose ranolazine for treatment of ACS.

Pacing in Acute MI

Recommendations for temporary pacing in the setting of acute MI are:

- asystole
- symptomatic bradycardia (including complete heart block)
- alternating LBBB and RBBB
- new or indeterminate-age bifascicular block with first-degree AV block

Complications of Acute MI

Mechanical complications (VSD, papillary muscle rupture, and LV free wall rupture) may occur 2 to 7 days after an MI. Emergency echocardiography is the initial diagnostic study. Patients with VSD or papillary muscle rupture develop abrupt pulmonary edema or hypotension and a loud holosystolic murmur and thrill. LV free wall rupture causes sudden hypotension or cardiac death associated with pulseless electrical activity.

Patients with papillary muscle rupture and VSD should be stabilized with an intra-aortic balloon pump, afterload reduction with sodium nitroprusside, and diuretics followed by emergency surgical intervention.

Cardiogenic shock: Emergency revascularization supported by intra-aortic balloon pump and LVAD may be necessary.

Postinfarction angina: Cardiac catheterization is indicated.

In patients with recurrent **ventricular arrhythmias**, an underlying cause, such as recurrent ischemia, should be sought. Repetitive and sustained bouts of postinfarction ventricular arrhythmias may warrant ICD therapy.

ICDs are also indicated in post-MI patients meeting all of the following criteria:

- >40 days since MI
- LVEF ≤35% and NYHA functional class II or III or LVEF ≤30% and NYHA functional class I
- >3 months since PCI or CABG

Depression: All post-MI patients should be screened for depression, because it is associated with increased hospitalization and death.

TEST YOURSELF

A 56-year-old woman has a 3-hour history of chest pain. BP is 80/60 mm Hg, respiration rate is 30/min, and pulse rate is 120/min. Physical examination shows JVD, inspiratory crackles, and an S_3 gallop. ECG shows 2-mm ST-segment elevation in leads V_2-V_6.

ANSWER: For diagnosis, choose STEMI and cardiogenic shock. For management, choose cardiac catheterization and PCI.

A 58-year-old man with acute chest pain has ST-segment elevation in leads II, III, and aVF. BP is 82/52 mm Hg, and pulse rate is 54/min. Physical examination shows JVD, clear lungs, and no murmur or S_3.

ANSWER: For diagnosis, choose RV MI. For management, select IV fluids, ECG lead V_4R tracing, and cardiac catheterization.

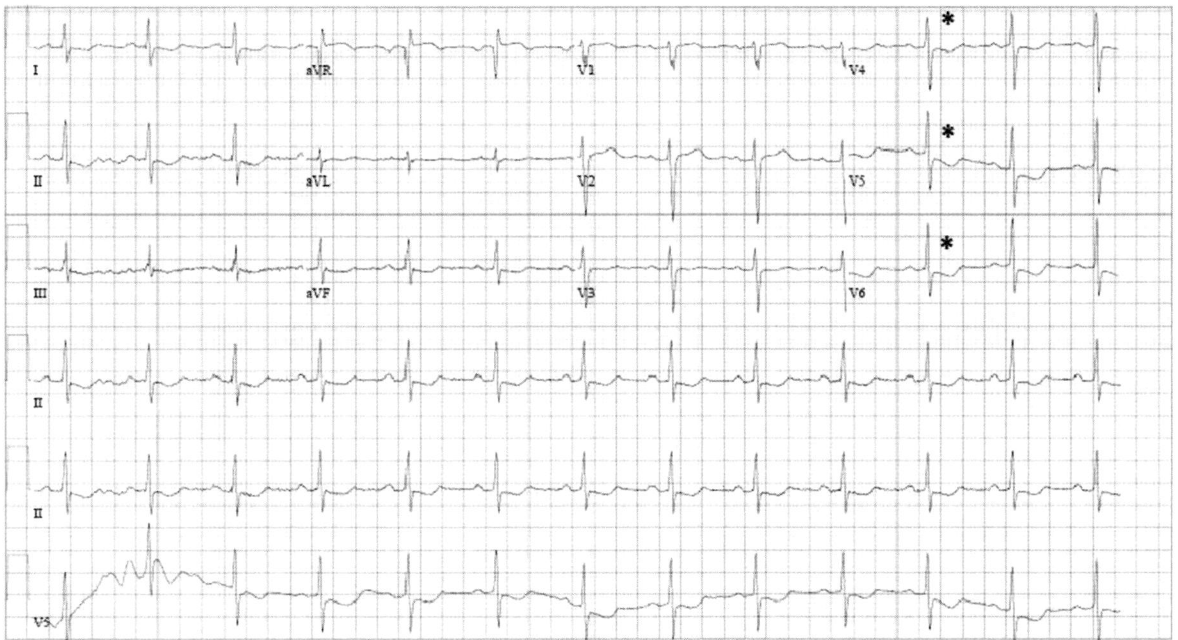

Non–ST-Elevation Myocardial Infarction: The ECG demonstrates a non-ST-elevation myocardial infarction. A 1-mm ST-segment depression is seen in leads V_4-V_6 (asterisks) and nonspecific ST-T wave changes are seen in leads II, III, and aVF.

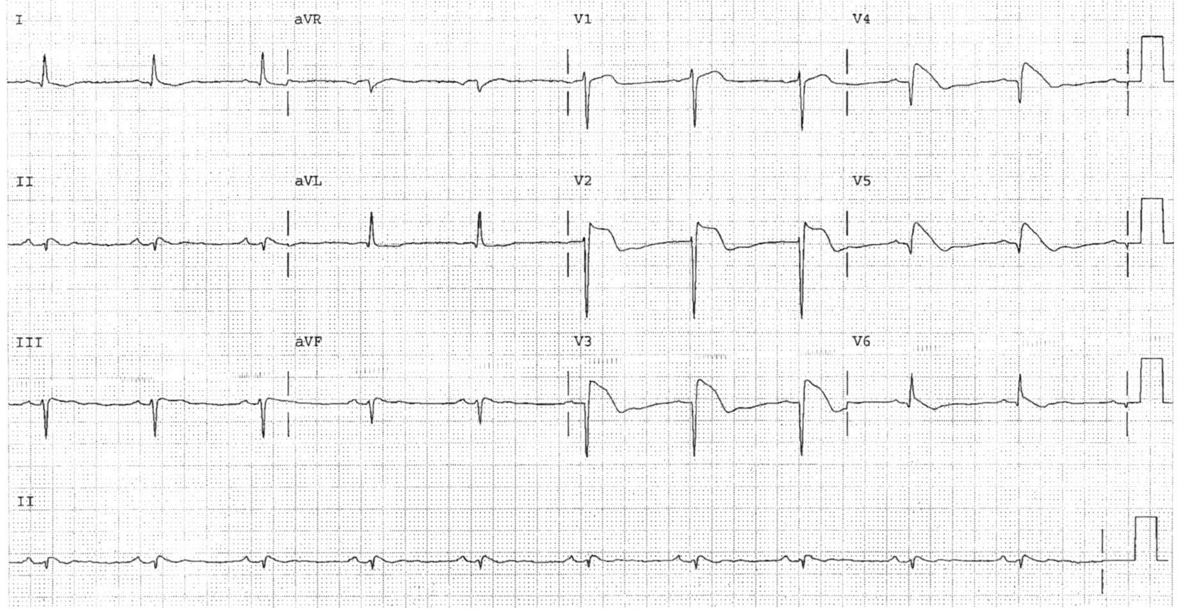

ST-Elevation Myocardial Infarction: The ECG shows abnormal Q waves in leads V_3-V_5 and ST-segment elevation in leads V_2-V_5. The T waves are beginning to invert in leads V_3-V_6. This pattern is most consistent with a recent anterolateral MI.

Follow-Up

Arrange for cardiac rehabilitation. Medications at hospital discharge should include aspirin indefinitely, a $P2Y_{12}$ inhibitor for at least 1 year, a β-blocker, a statin, and an ACE inhibitor or ARB (in patients with LV systolic dysfunction, hypertension, diabetes, or kidney disease).

Chronic Stable Angina

Diagnosis

Stable angina pectoris is defined as reproducible, stable anginal symptoms of at least 2 months' duration precipitated by exertion or stress and relieved by rest.

Testing

Stress testing is most useful in patients with an intermediate pretest probability of CAD (>10% or <90%). Pretest probability is based on a patient's age, sex, and symptoms; risk factors for CAD; and ECG findings.

STUDY TABLE: Selecting the Correct Stress Test[a]

Stress Test	Indications
Exercise ECG without imaging	Patients who can exercise Normal or nonspecific baseline ECG changes (e.g., <0.5 mm ST depression)
Exercise ECG with myocardial perfusion imaging or exercise echocardiography	Patients who can exercise Pre-excitation (WPW) pattern >1 mm ST depression Previous CABG or PCI LBBB LV hypertrophy Digoxin use
Pharmacologic stress myocardial perfusion imaging or dobutamine echocardiography	Unable to exercise Electrically paced ventricular rhythm LBBB

[a]CTA can detect anatomic coronary abnormalities (compared with functional ischemia on stress testing) and has been shown to be effective in the assessment of patients with suspected CAD.

Select coronary angiography for patients with high pretest probability of disease or:

- LV dysfunction
- class III or IV angina despite therapy
- highly positive stress or imaging test
- high pretest probability of left main or three-vessel CAD (a Duke treadmill score ≤−11)
- uncertain diagnosis after noninvasive testing
- history of surviving sudden cardiac death
- suspected coronary spasm

DON'T BE TRICKED

- **Stress testing is of little value in patients with very low (e.g., <10%) or very high (e.g., >90%) pretest probabilities of CAD.**
- **In patients with LBBB, do not perform exercise ECG for evaluation of possible CAD; stress echocardiography or vasodilator stress radionuclide myocardial perfusion imaging should be performed instead.**

Treatment

Intensive lifestyle modification is selected for all patients with chronic stable angina. Treatment is indicated to achieve the following goals: BP <130/80 mm Hg and glucose control in those with diabetes.

The four major classes of antianginal medications for stable angina are β-blockers, nitrates, calcium channel blockers, and ranolazine. Most patients with stable angina will require combination therapy.

Cardioselective β-blockers are first-line therapy in patients with chronic stable angina. Dosage should be adjusted to achieve a resting HR of approximately 60/min. Absolute contraindications to β-blockers include severe bradycardia, advanced AV block, decompensated HF, and severe reactive airways disease.

Calcium channel blockers should be initiated as first-line therapy for patients with absolute contraindications to β-blockers. In the setting of continued angina despite optimal doses of β-blockers and nitrates, calcium channel blockers can be added. Avoid short-acting calcium channel blockers. Bradycardia and heart block can occur in patients with significant conduction system disease.

Nitrates are as effective as β-blockers and calcium channel blockers in reducing angina. Prevent nitrate tachyphylaxis by establishing a nitrate-free period of 8 to 12 hours per day (typically overnight), during which nitrates are not used. For patients using nitrates, sildenafil, vardenafil, and tadalafil are contraindicated.

Ranolazine should be considered in patients who remain symptomatic despite optimal doses of β-blockers, calcium channel blockers, and nitrates.

Cardioprotective drugs reduce the progression of atherosclerosis and subsequent cardiovascular events.

- Aspirin reduces the risk of stroke, MI, and vascular death in patients with CAD.
- ACE inhibitors reduce cardiovascular and all-cause mortality in patients with diabetes, hypertension, CKD, LVEF ≤40%, HF, or a history of MI.
- High-intensity statins reduce cardiovascular events, including MI and death.

Revascularization therapy with PCI or CABG should be considered in patients with persistent symptoms despite maximal medical therapy. Revascularization with CABG for mortality reduction may also be recommended in patients at high risk, particularly those with triple-vessel disease or left-main disease with LV dysfunction.

DON'T BE TRICKED

- **Do not select hormone replacement therapy (in women), antioxidant vitamins (vitamin E), or treatment of elevated serum homocysteine levels with folic acid or vitamin B_{12}.**

TEST YOURSELF

A 69-year-old man has burning retrosternal discomfort related to exertion. His father died of an acute MI at age 61 years. Physical examination is unremarkable, and the resting ECG is normal.

ANSWER: For treatment, choose aspirin, sublingual nitroglycerin, and a β-blocker, and follow up with an exercise stress test.

Heart Failure

Diagnosis

One half of patients with HF have HF with preserved ejection fraction (HFpEF); the remainder have HF with reduced ejection fraction (HFrEF). Patients with HFrEF often have dilated ventricles and patients with HFpEF have normal systolic contraction and normal-sized ventricles or concentric hypertrophy. Symptoms are the same for HFrEF and HFpEF.

Symptoms and signs that increase the likelihood of HF as a diagnosis include:

- paroxysmal nocturnal dyspnea (>2-fold likelihood)
- an S_3 (11-fold likelihood)

The likelihood of HF as a diagnosis is decreased 50% by:

- absence of dyspnea on exertion
- absence of crackles on pulmonary auscultation

Disease classification systems are part of the diagnosis and can help guide treatment decisions.

STUDY TABLE: NYHA Classification of Heart Failure
NYHA Functional Class
I (structural disease but no symptoms)
II (symptomatic; slight limitation of physical activity)
III (symptomatic; marked limitation of physical activity)
IV (inability to perform any physical activity without symptoms)

Testing

A BNP level >400 pg/mL is compatible with HF, and a level <100 pg/mL effectively excludes HF as a cause of acute dyspnea.

The ECG may show a previous MI, ventricular hypertrophy, arrhythmias, or conduction abnormalities. Chest x-rays may show cardiomegaly, pulmonary edema, or pleural effusion. Echocardiography will estimate EF and may detect valvular heart disease, HCM, and regional wall abnormalities suggesting CAD.

Other studies include stress testing to detect myocardial ischemia, coronary angiography in patients with symptoms or risk factors for CAD, and measurement of serum TSH levels.

Endomyocardial biopsy is rarely indicated but can assist in the diagnosis of giant cell myocarditis, amyloidosis, and hemochromatosis.

A sleep study should be performed on symptomatic NYHA class II-IV HFrEF patients with excessive daytime sleepiness.

DON'T BE TRICKED

- **Routine testing for unusual causes of HF, including hemochromatosis, Wilson disease, multiple myeloma, and myocarditis, should not be performed.**
- **Don't order serial BNPs in hospitalized patients to monitor HF.**
- **Kidney failure, older age, and female sex all increase BNP; obesity reduces BNP.**

Treatment of HFrEF

For making treatment decisions, NYHA functional classification can be implemented.

STUDY TABLE: Treatment of HFrEF	
Therapy	**Indication**
ACE inhibitors	For all stages of HF to reduce mortality ARBs are acceptable if ACE inhibitor cannot be tolerated
Hydralazine plus nitrates	Given in addition to standard therapy for NYHA class III-IV and EF <40% in black and select nonblack patients (low output syndrome, hypertension) to reduce mortality, For patients who cannot tolerate ACE inhibitors or ARBs

(Continued on the next page)

STUDY TABLE: Treatment of HFrEF *(Continued)*	
Therapy	**Indication**
β-Blockers (only metoprolol succinate, carvedilol, and bisoprolol)	For NYHA classes I-IV to reduce mortality
Aldosterone antagonist (spironolactone or eplerenone)	For NYHA class III-IV HF to reduce mortality
Digitalis	Used predominantly in patients who continue to experience symptoms despite guideline-directed medical therapy
Diuretics	Given to improve symptoms of volume overload
Ivabradine	EF ≤35% who are in sinus rhythm with a heart rate ≥70/min
Valsartan-sacubitril	Substitute for an ACE inhibitor or ARB in HFrEF (NYHA class II or III) in patients who have tolerated ACE inhibitor or ARB therapy
ICD	For ischemic and nonischemic cardiomyopathy in patients with an EF ≤35% and NYHA functional class II-III or with an EF ≤30% and NYHA functional class I
	For NYHA class II-III symptoms
Cardiac resynchronization therapy	For NYHA class II-IV, LVEF ≤35%, and LBBB with QRS duration >150 ms
Cardiac transplantation	For patients with refractory HF symptoms despite maximal medical therapy
Exercise training	Recommended in all patients with newly diagnosed HF

DON'T BE TRICKED

- Do not begin β-blocker therapy in patients with decompensated HF.
- Continuous IV infusion of furosemide provides no advantage vs. bolus therapy in decompensated HF.
- Do not prescribe or continue NSAIDs or thiazolidinediones because they worsen HF.
- Nondihydropyridine calcium channel blockers (diltiazem or verapamil) may be harmful to patients with HF.

TEST YOURSELF

A 64-year-old woman with previously stable HF now has increasing orthopnea. Medications are lisinopril 10 mg/d and furosemide 20 mg/d. BP is 140/68 mm Hg and HR is 102/min. Pulmonary crackles and increased JVD are present.

ANSWER: For treatment, increase the furosemide and lisinopril dosages and add a β-blocker when the patient is stable.

Follow-Up

In patients with chronic HF who are clinically stable, follow-up echocardiography more frequently than every 1 to 2 years is not recommended.

Heart Failure with Preserved Ejection Fraction

Diagnosis

Diagnose HFpEF (also known as diastolic HF) when signs and symptoms of HF are present but the echocardiogram reveals EF >50% and significant valvular abnormalities are absent.

Treatment of HFpEF

The primary treatment goals in HFpEF are to treat the underlying cause (hypertension, AF), to manage potentially exacerbating factors (e.g., tachycardia), and to optimize diastolic filling (control HR and avoid decreased effective circulating blood volume). Diuretics should be used when volume overload is present.

DON'T BE TRICKED

- Pharmacologic agents (β-blockers, ACE inhibitors, ARBs, aldosterone antagonists) have not been shown to decrease morbidity and mortality in patients with HFpEF.

Nonischemic Dilated Cardiomyopathy

Diagnosis

Dilated cardiomyopathy is characterized by dilation and reduced function of one or both ventricles manifesting as HF, arrhythmias, and sudden death. The most common cause is idiopathic dilated cardiomyopathy (50%), but the differential diagnosis is broad.

STUDY TABLE: Differential Diagnoses of Nonischemic Dilated Cardiomyopathy

Condition	Distinguishing Characteristics
Acute myocarditis	Associated with bacterial, viral, and parasitic infections and autoimmune disorders. Cardiac troponin levels are typically elevated; ventricular dysfunction may be global or regional. Can cause cardiogenic shock and ventricular arrhythmias. Choose supportive care in the acute phase, then standard HF therapy.
Alcoholic cardiomyopathy	Associated with chronic heavy alcohol ingestion, but other manifestations of chronic alcohol abuse may be absent. Typically, the LV (and frequently both ventricles) is dilated and hypokinetic. Choose standard HF therapy and total abstinence from alcohol.
Drug-induced cardiomyopathy	Illicit use of cocaine and amphetamines has been associated with myocarditis and dilated cardiomyopathy, as well as MI, arrhythmia, and sudden death. Choose standard HF treatment. In patients with stimulant-induced acute myocardial ischemia, β-blockers may exacerbate coronary vasoconstriction; labetalol, a β-blocker with α-blocker activity, is preferred.
Giant cell myocarditis	Rare disease characterized by biventricular enlargement, refractory ventricular arrhythmias, and rapid progression to cardiogenic shock in young to middle-aged adults. Histologic examination demonstrates the presence of multinucleated giant cells in the myocardium. Choose immunosuppressant treatment and/or LVAD placement or cardiac transplantation.
Hemochromatosis	Caused by excess iron deposition in the myocardium. Characterized by symptoms of heart failure and by conduction defects.
Peripartum cardiomyopathy	Presence of HF with an LVEF <45% diagnosed between 1 month before and 5 months after delivery. Management includes early delivery (when identified before parturition) and HF treatment. ACE inhibitors, ARBs, and aldosterone antagonists (e.g., eplerenone) should be avoided (teratogenicity) during pregnancy. Anticoagulation with warfarin is recommended for women with peripartum cardiomyopathy with LVEF <35%. Women with persistent LV dysfunction should avoid subsequent pregnancy.
Stress-induced (takotsubo) cardiomyopathy	Characterized by acute LV dysfunction in the setting of intense emotional or physiologic stress. May mimic acute STEMI. Dilation and akinesis of the LV apex occur in the absence of CAD. Resolves in days to weeks with supportive care.
Tachycardia-mediated cardiomyopathy	Occurs when myocardial dysfunction develops as a result of chronic tachycardia. Primary treatment is to slow or eliminate the arrhythmia.

Treatment

In addition to reversal of the underlying cause (alcohol, drug, and tachycardia-mediated cardiomyopathies), if possible, choose standard medical therapy for HF.

TEST YOURSELF

A 35-year-old man develops abdominal discomfort and swelling in both legs. He has an 18-pack-year smoking history and drinks a six-pack of beer daily but has no other significant medical history. Physical examination shows an elevated JVD, a displaced apical impulse, distant heart sounds, a grade 2/6 apical holosystolic murmur, an enlarged and tender liver, and peripheral edema.

ANSWER: For diagnosis, choose alcoholic cardiomyopathy. For management, select echocardiography and alcohol cessation.

Hypertrophic Cardiomyopathy

Diagnosis

HCM is an uncommon primary cardiac disease characterized by diffuse or focal myocardial hypertrophy. The disease is genetically inherited in an autosomal dominant pattern in approximately 60% of patients. Patients may present with syncope (often arrhythmogenic), exertional syncope, or syncope associated with volume depletion, chest pain, and sudden cardiac death.

STUDY TABLE: Distinguishing HCM from AS

Assessment/Finding	HCM	AS
Carotid pulse	Rises briskly, then declines, followed by a second rise (pulsus bisferiens)	Rises slowly and has low volume (pulsus parvus et tardus)
Ejection sound	None	Present
Aortic regurgitation	None	May be present
Valsalva maneuver	Increased murmur intensity	No change or decreased murmur intensity
Squatting to standing position	Increased murmur intensity	Decreased murmur intensity
Carotid radiation	None	Usually present
Apex beat	"Triple ripple"	Sustained single

Testing

The ECG shows LV hypertrophy and left atrial enlargement. Deeply inverted, symmetric T waves in leads V_3-V_6 are present in the apical hypertrophic form of the disease (mimics ischemia). Echocardiography is the diagnostic technique of choice.

Treatment

Patients with HCM should avoid competitive sports and intense isometric exercise. β-Blockers are first-line agents for patients with an EF ≥50%, dyspnea, and/or chest pain. Calcium channel blockers (verapamil or diltiazem) may be substituted for β-blockers. ACE inhibitors are used only if systolic dysfunction is present.

Treat all patients with HCM and AF with warfarin (first line) or one of the NOACs (dabigatran, rivaroxaban, apixaban) (second-line therapy) regardless of CHA_2DS_2-VASc score. Surgery or septal ablation is indicated for patients with an outflow tract gradient of >50 mm Hg and continuing symptoms despite maximal drug therapy. Patients at high risk for sudden death (one or more major risk factors) are candidates for an ICD (see Study Table following). The absence of any risk factors has a high negative predictive value (>90%) for sudden death.

STUDY TABLE: Sudden Death Risk Factors in HCM

Major Risk Factors
Previous cardiac arrest
Spontaneous sustained VT
Family history of sudden death (first-degree relative)
Unexplained syncope
LV wall thickness ≥30 mm
Blunted increase or decrease in SBP with exercise
Nonsustained spontaneous VT ≥3 beats

DON'T BE TRICKED

- Electrophysiologic studies are not useful in predicting sudden cardiac death.
- Do not prescribe digoxin, vasodilators, or diuretics, which increase LV outflow obstruction, for patients with HCM.

Screening

All first-degree relatives of patients with HCM should have genetic counseling and, in the absence of a documented genetic mutation in the proband, echocardiographic screening. Ongoing screening is recommended throughout adulthood starting at age 12 years because of the possibility of disease expression at any age.

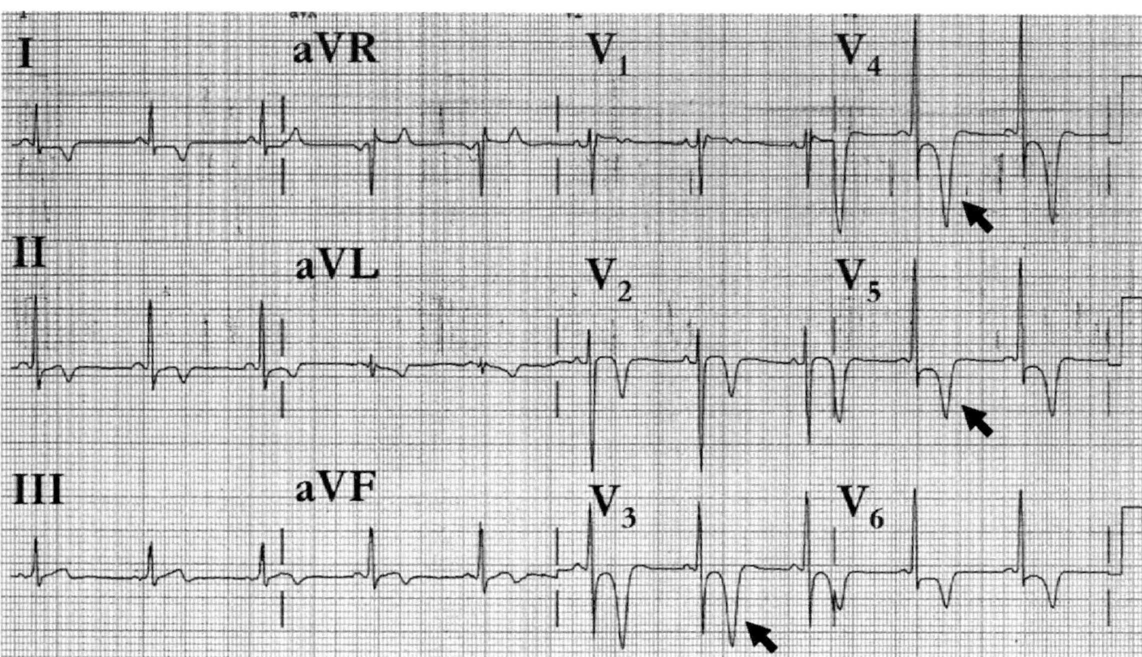

Hypertrophic Cardiomyopathy: The ECG shows ST-segment depression and deeply inverted T waves (*arrows*) in the precordial leads consistent with marked apical hypertrophy.

Restrictive Cardiomyopathy

Diagnosis

In restrictive cardiomyopathy, abnormally rigid ventricular walls cause diastolic dysfunction in the absence of systolic dysfunction, manifesting as impaired ventricular filling and elevated diastolic ventricular pressures. Pulmonary venous congestion, PH, and right-sided HF ensue. Jugular veins may engorge with inspiration (Kussmaul sign).

Testing

Echocardiogram shows normal ejection fraction/systolic function. Cardiac catheterization shows elevated LV and RV end-diastolic pressures and a characteristic early ventricular diastolic dip and plateau.

STUDY TABLE: Clues to Underlying Systemic Diseases Causing Restrictive Cardiomyopathy

Disease	Clues
Amyloidosis	Neuropathy, proteinuria, hepatomegaly, periorbital ecchymosis, bruising, low-voltage ECG. Diagnosis can be confirmed with abdominal fat pad aspiration.
Sarcoidosis	Bilateral hilar lymphadenopathy; possible pulmonary reticular opacities; and skin, joint, or eye lesions. Cardiac involvement is suggested by the presence of arrhythmias, conduction blocks, or HF. Diagnosis is supported by CMR imaging with gadolinium.
Hemochromatosis	Abnormal aminotransferase levels, OA, diabetes, erectile dysfunction, and HF; elevated serum ferritin and transferrin saturation level.

Restrictive cardiomyopathy must be differentiated from constrictive pericarditis (see Cardiac Tamponade and Constrictive Pericarditis).

Treatment

Treat any underlying disease that affects diastolic function (hypertension, diabetes, ischemic heart disease, amyloidosis). Loop diuretics are used to treat dyspnea and peripheral edema. β-Blockers or nondihydropyridine calcium channel antagonists may enhance diastolic function and should be considered if diuretic therapy is not effective or in the presence of atrial tachyarrhythmias. ACE inhibitors and ARBs may improve diastolic filling and may be beneficial in patients with diastolic dysfunction.

TEST YOURSELF

A 63-year-old man develops dyspnea and fatigue. Physical examination shows JVD, a prominent jugular *a* wave, a prominent S_4, and a grade 2/6 holosystolic murmur at the left sternal border. The lungs are clear. Other findings include an enlarged, tender liver; petechiae over the feet; and periorbital ecchymoses.

ANSWER: The diagnosis is amyloid cardiomyopathy, indicated by the noncardiac symptoms and signs.

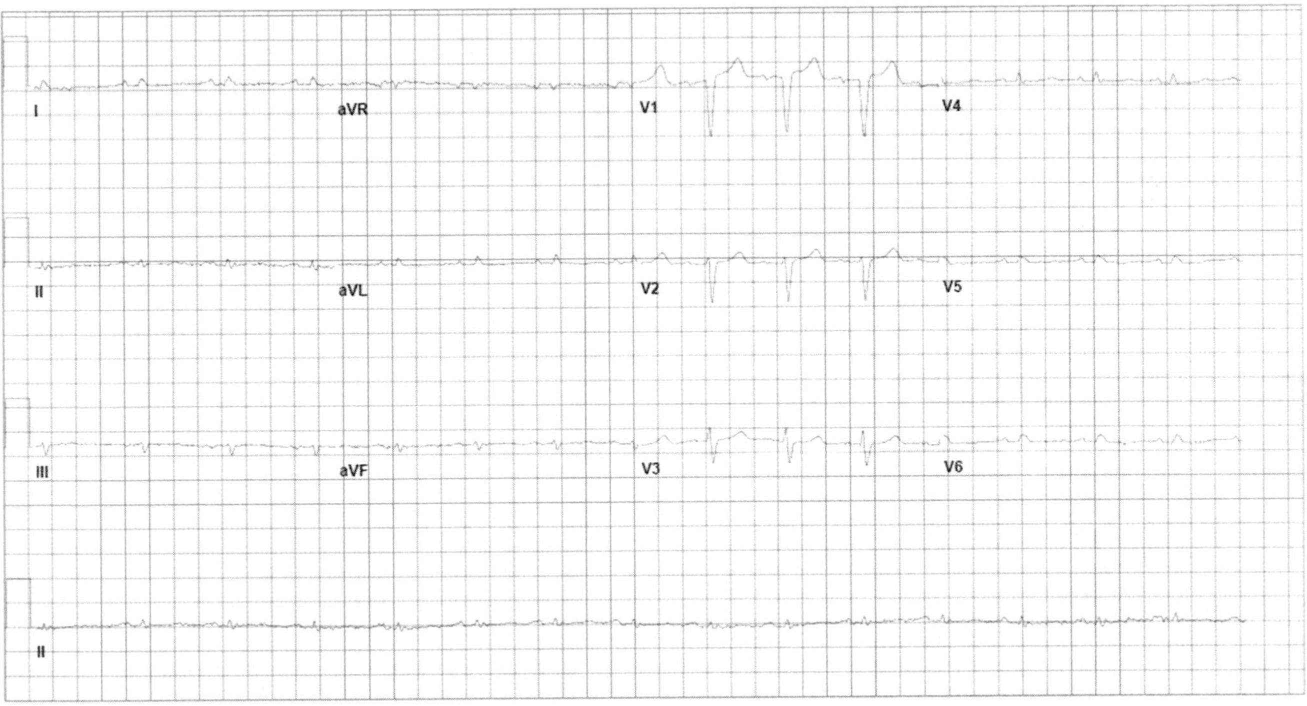

Cardiac Amyloidosis: The ECG shows low voltage, the most common ECG abnormality associated with cardiac amyloidosis.

Palpitations and Syncope

Testing

In a patient with palpitations and syncope, the key diagnostic test is an ECG recorded during the clinical event. Obtain an echocardiogram in patients with suspected structural heart disease. See General Internal Medicine chapter for major causes of syncope.

STUDY TABLE: Diagnostic Studies for Suspected Arrhythmias

Diagnostic Test	Utility	Advantages	Limitations
Resting ECG	Initial diagnostic test in all patients	Diagnostic if recorded during the arrhythmia	Most arrhythmias are intermittent and not recorded on a resting ECG
Ambulatory (24-hour) ECG	Indicated for frequent (at least daily) arrhythmias	Records every heart beat during a 24-hour period	Not helpful if arrhythmia is infrequent

(Continued on the next page)

STUDY TABLE: Diagnostic Studies for Suspected Arrhythmias *(Continued)*			
Diagnostic Test	**Utility**	**Advantages**	**Limitations**
Exercise ECG	Indicated for arrhythmias provoked by exercise	Allows diagnosis of exercise-related arrhythmias	Physician supervision required
Event monitor	Indicated for infrequent arrhythmias >1-2 min in duration	Small recorder is held to the chest when symptoms are present	Limited to symptomatic arrhythmias that persist long enough for patient to activate the device; not a viable choice for patients with syncope
Loop recorder	Indicated for infrequent symptomatic brief arrhythmias	Saves previous 30 s to 2 min ECG signal when patient activates the recorder; can be activated following syncopal event to capture arrhythmia	ECG leads limit patient activities
Implanted recorder	Indicated for very infrequent arrhythmias	Long-term continuous ECG monitoring	Invasive procedure with some risk
Electrophysiology study	Can be used for inducing, identifying, and clarifying mechanism of arrhythmia as well as for treatment (e.g., catheter ablation); EP studies are not used for initial diagnosis	The origin and mechanism of an arrhythmia can be precisely defined	Invasive procedure with some risk

Sinus Bradycardia and Heart Block

Diagnosis

Sinus bradycardia occurs when the AV nodal impulses fire at a rate lower than expected (less than 60/min). Common causes are medications, hypothyroidism, and inferior MI.

AV nodal block results from functional or structural abnormalities at the AV node or in the His-Purkinje system. Potentially reversible causes include acute or chronic myocardial ischemia, Lyme disease, sarcoidosis, and amyloidosis.

STUDY TABLE: Heart Block	
Type	**Diagnostic Criteria**
First-degree block	PR interval >0.2 s without alterations in HR
Second-degree block	Intermittent P waves not followed by a ventricular complex; further classified as Mobitz type 1 or type 2
Third-degree block (complete heart block)	Complete absence of conducted P waves (P-wave and QRS complex rates differ, and the PR interval differs for every QRS complex) and an atrial rate that is faster than the ventricular rate; most common cause of ventricular rates 30-50/min
LBBB	Absent Q waves in leads I, aVL, and V_6; large, wide, and positive R waves in leads I, aVL, and V_6; QRS >0.12 s
RBBB	rsR′ pattern in lead V_1 ("rabbit ears"), wide negative S wave in lead V_6, QRS >0.12 s
Bifascicular block	Right bundle branch and one of the fascicles of the left bundle branch are involved
Trifascicular block	Characterized by bifascicular block and prolongation of the PR interval
Left anterior hemiblock	Left axis usually -60°, upright QRS complex in lead I, negative QRS complex in aVF, and normal QRS duration
Left posterior hemiblock	Right axis usually +120°, negative QRS complex in lead I, positive QRS complex in lead aVF, and normal QRS duration

STUDY TABLE: Second-Degree AV Block: Mobitz Type 1 and Type 2		
Type	**Characteristics**	**Significance**
Mobitz type 1 (Wenckebach block)	Constant P-P interval with progressively increased PR interval until the dropped beat; grouped beating is classic	Rarely progresses to third-degree heart block
Mobitz type 2	Usually associated with RBBB or LBBB; constant PR interval in the conducted beats; R-R interval contains the nonconducted (dropped) beat equal to two P-P intervals	May precede third-degree heart block

Treatment

Sinus bradycardia requires no treatment for asymptomatic patients. For hemodynamically stable patients, treat the underlying condition (e.g., MI, thyroid disease, medications).

Initial therapy of AV block includes correcting reversible causes of impaired conduction such as ischemia, increased vagal tone, and elimination of drugs that alter electrical conduction, (digitalis, calcium channel blockers, β-blockers).

Guidelines for permanent pacemaker implantation include absence of reversible cause and:

- symptomatic bradycardia
- asymptomatic sinus bradycardia with significant pauses (>3 s) or heart rate <40/min
- AF with 5-second pauses
- complete heart block
- Mobitz type 2 second-degree AV block
- alternating bundle branch block

Choose IV atropine and/or transcutaneous or transvenous pacing for symptoms of hemodynamic compromise caused by bradycardia or heart block.

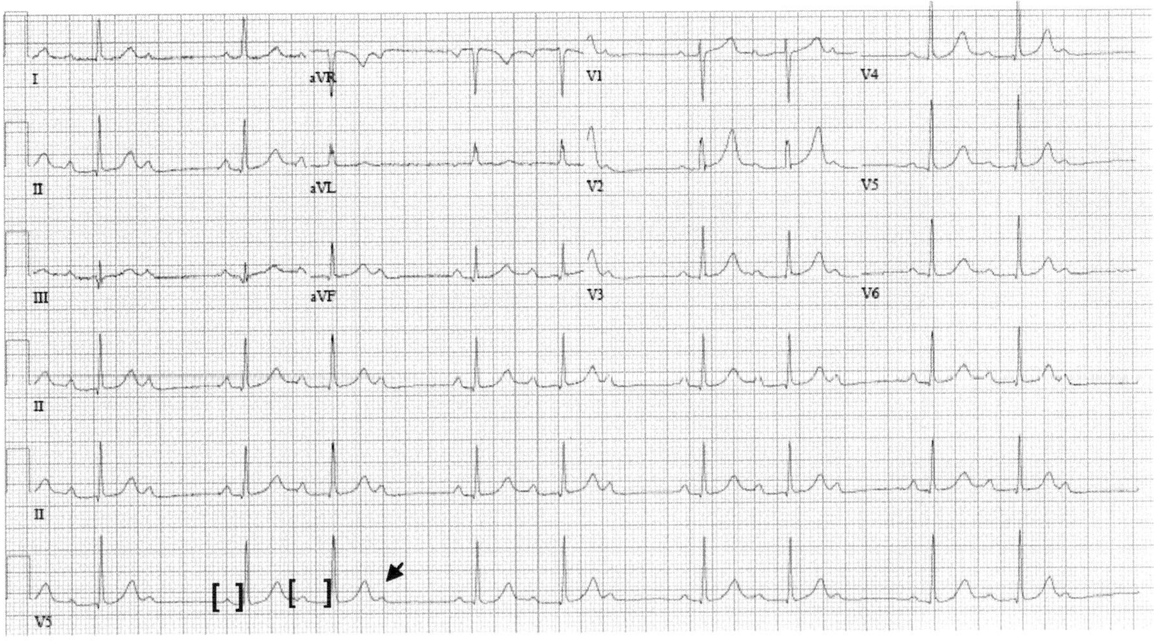

Mobitz Type 1 Heart Block: The rhythm strip shows progressive prolongation of the PR interval until the dropped beat.

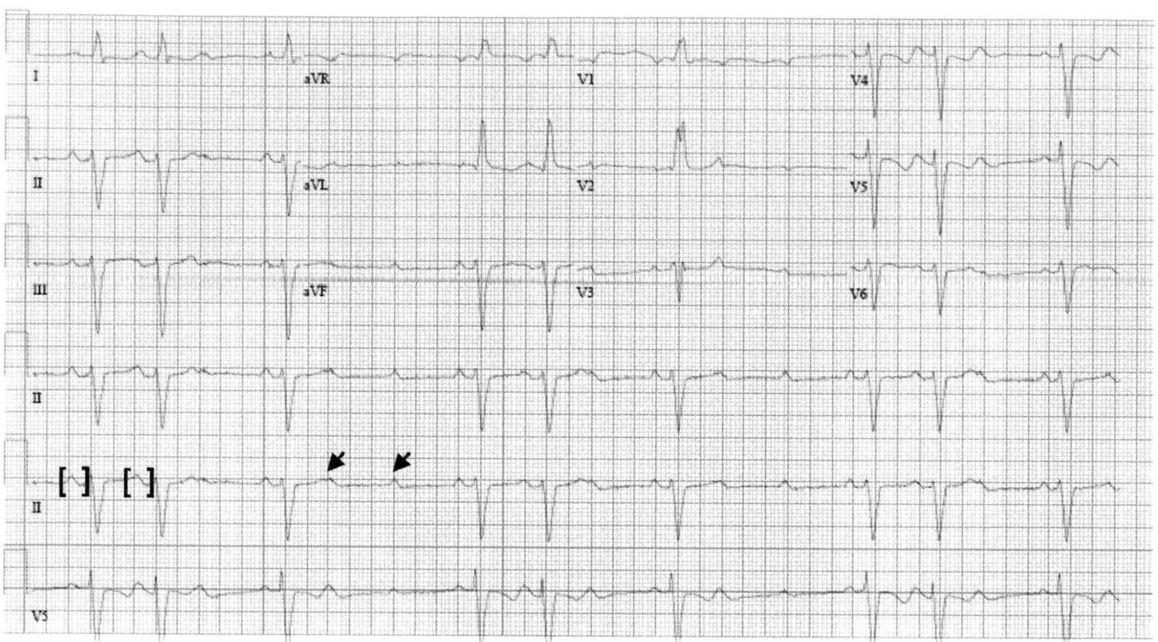

Mobitz Type 2 Heart Block: The rhythm strip shows constant PR interval. The R-R interval containing the nonconducted beat is equal to two P-P intervals.

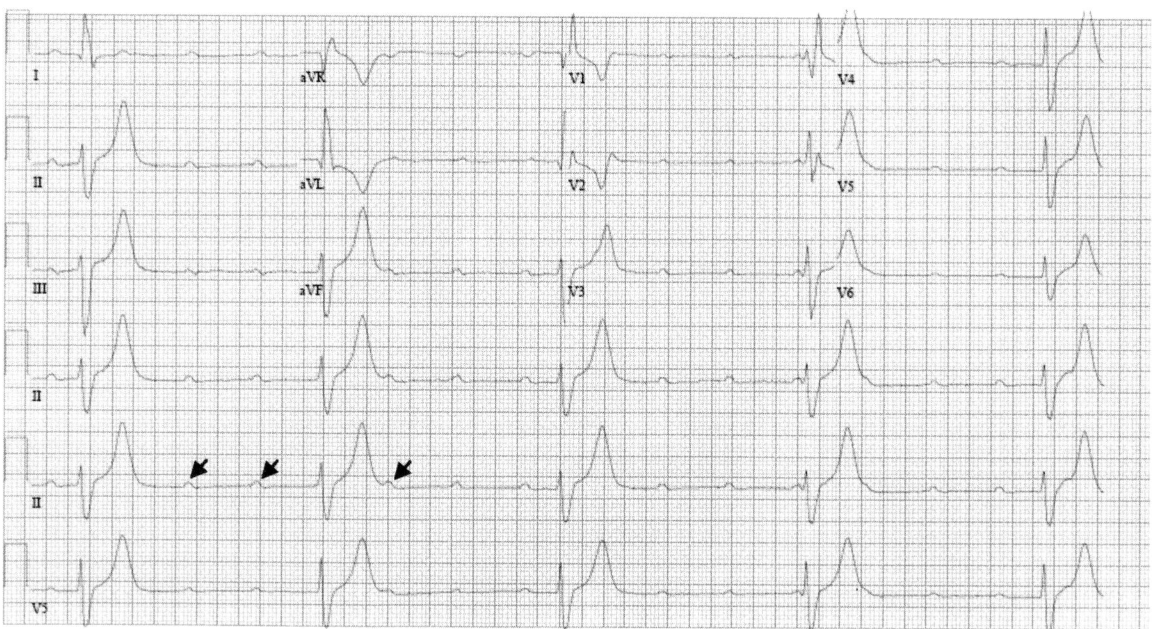

Complete Heart Block: The rhythm strip shows third-degree heart block with three nonconducted atrial impulses and a pause of 3.5 seconds.

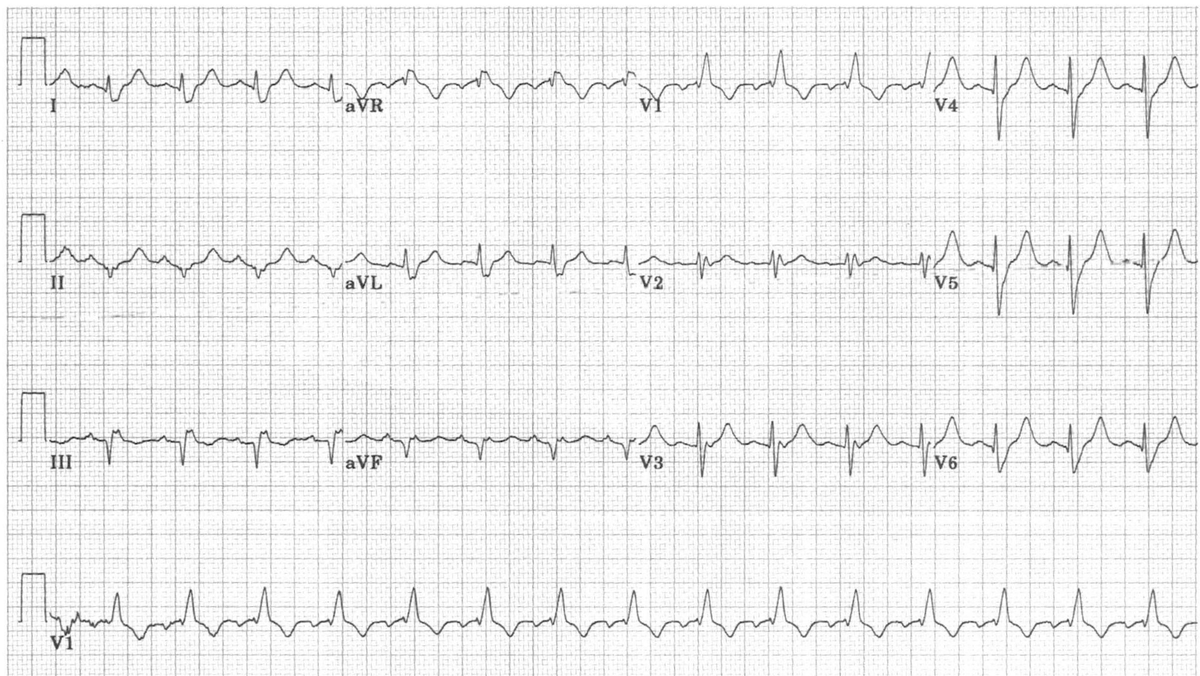

Bifascicular Block: The ECG shows RBBB and left anterior hemiblock characteristic of bifascicular block.

DON'T BE TRICKED

- Don't place a pacemaker for asymptomatic bradycardia in the absence of second- or third-degree heart block.

Atrial Fibrillation

Diagnosis

Findings of AF include an irregularly irregular ventricular rhythm with absence of P waves in all ECG leads.

Do not confuse AF with:

- sinus tachycardia with premature atrial beats
- MAT in patients with COPD
- Mobitz type 1 second-degree AV block (Wenckebach) with characteristic group-beating
- arrhythmia caused by digitalis toxicity (atrial tachycardia with block)
- atrial flutter with variable conduction

AF can appear as irregular, wide-complex tachycardia mimicking VF in the setting of underlying intraventricular conduction delay or in the presence of an accessory pathway.

Diagnostic studies include serum TSH and digoxin level measurement (if appropriate), pulse oximetry, sleep apnea evaluation, and echocardiography.

Treatment

Perform emergency electrical cardioversion for patients with hemodynamically unstable AF.

Rhythm control is an appropriate management for younger patients with persistent symptomatic AF. Rhythm control may be achieved with medications, synchronized cardioversion, or both. If rhythm control is unsuccessful or not tolerated, catheter-based AF ablation is an option.

Patients with infrequent paroxysmal AF will benefit from the "pill-in-the-pocket" approach: flecainide or propafenone with a β-blocker or calcium channel blocker.

No mortality benefit is evident from restoration of sinus rhythm ("rhythm control") compared with **rate control**. Older patients with chronic AF or AF of unknown duration should have rate control (resting HR <110/min) with calcium channel blockers or β-blockers.

Almost all patients with AF require chronic **anticoagulation**. The risk of stroke in patients who have nonvalvular AF plus one other risk factor (other than sex) exceeds the risk of hemorrhage from anticoagulation.

The most common method of assessing stroke risk in patients with nonvalvular AF is by calculating the CHA_2DS_2-VASc score.

1 point each is given for:

- HF
- hypertension
- diabetes
- vascular disease (previous MI, PAD, aortic plaque)
- female sex
- age 65 to 74 years

2 points each are given for:

- previous stroke, TIA, or thromboembolic disease
- age ≥75 years

Provide anticoagulation for a score ≥1 in men and ≥2 in women.

STUDY TABLE: Anticoagulants Approved for Stroke Prevention in Atrial Fibrillation

Medication	Type of AF	Cautions
Warfarin (vitamin K antagonist)	Valvular[a] or nonvalvular	Avoid in pregnancy
Dabigatran (direct thrombin inhibitor)	Nonvalvular	Caution with P-glycoprotein inhibitors Reduce dose with CrCl 15-30 mL/min
Rivaroxaban (factor Xa inhibitor)	Nonvalvular	Avoid with CrCl <30 mL/min, moderate hepatic impairment, strong P-glycoprotein inhibitors, and strong cytochrome P-450 inducers and inhibitors Reduce dose with CrCl 30-49 mL/min
Apixaban (factor Xa inhibitor)	Nonvalvular	Avoid with strong P-glycoprotein inhibitors or strong cytochrome P-450 inducers and inhibitors Reduce dose with creatinine ≥2.5 g/dL, age ≥80 years, or weight ≤60 kg
Edoxaban (factor Xa inhibitor)	Nonvalvular	Avoid with strong cytochrome P-450 inducers and inhibitors Reduce dose with CrCl 30-50 mL/min, weight ≤60 kg, or concomitant use of verapamil or quinidine (potent P-glycoprotein inhibitors)

[a]Valvular AF refers to AF in the presence of a mechanical heart valve or moderate-severe rheumatic mitral valve stenosis.

Bridging anticoagulation is discussed in the General Internal Medicine section.

DON'T BE TRICKED

- NOACs are preferred for most patients with nonvalvular AF; warfarin is indicated for valvular AF.
- Do not begin calcium channel blockers, β-blockers, or digoxin in patients with AF and WPW syndrome; use procainamide instead.
- Adenosine is not effective for cardioversion of AF.

TEST YOURSELF

A 55-year-old woman has dyspnea and chest pain of 12 hours' duration. BP is 75/44 mm Hg, and bibasilar crackles are heard. ECG shows a wide-complex tachycardia of 160/min.

ANSWER: For management, always choose cardioversion in patients with any arrhythmia who are hemodynamically unstable.

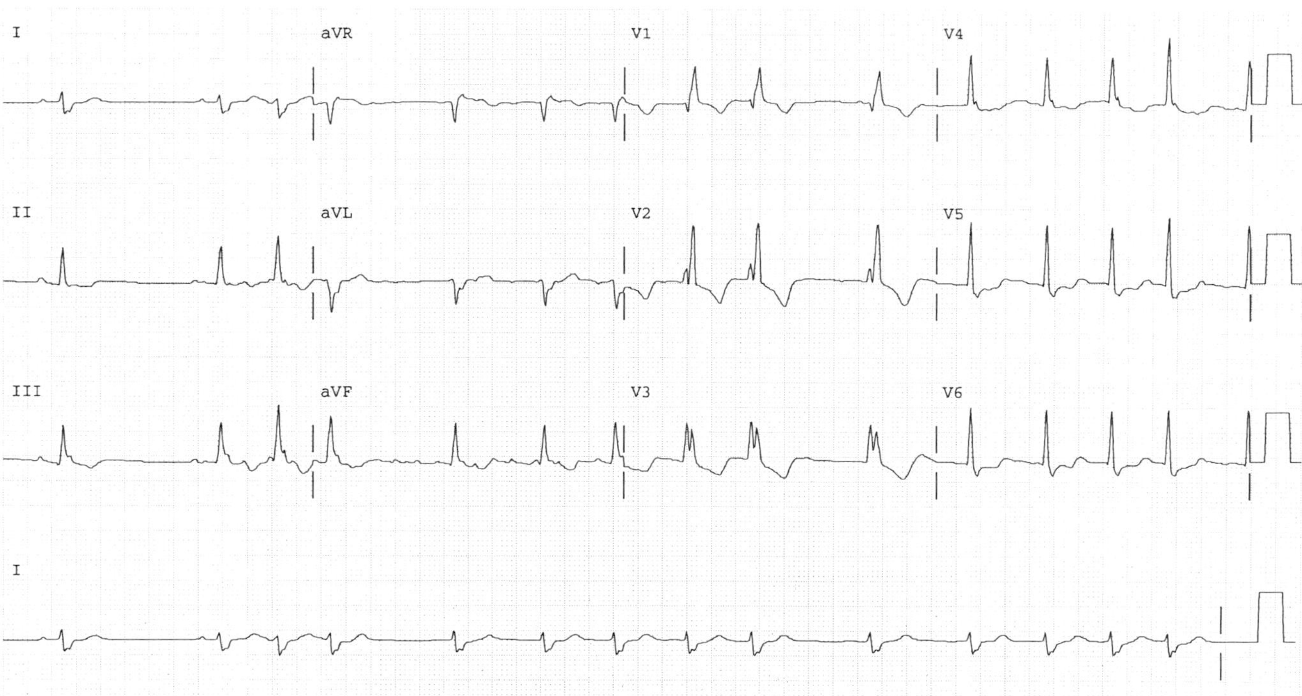

Atrial Fibrillation: The rhythm strip (*bottom*) shows two sinus beats followed by AF. The AF rhythm is irregular, and fibrillatory waves are clearly seen. RBBB is also present.

Atrial Flutter

Diagnosis

Atrial flutter is a reentrant arrhythmia with atrial rates typically between 250 and 300/min. ECG typically shows a saw-tooth pattern on the inferior leads and a positive deflection in lead V_1. The ventricular response is often regular, although it may be irregular and can be confused with AF. Classically, patients have 2:1 conduction resulting in a ventricular response close to 150/min. Atrial flutter may be seen interspersed with AF or may follow treatment of AF.

Treatment

Atrial flutter may be managed with rate or rhythm control and can be successfully eliminated with radiofrequency catheter ablation, which is superior to medical therapy. Guidelines for anticoagulation for atrial flutter are similar to those for AF.

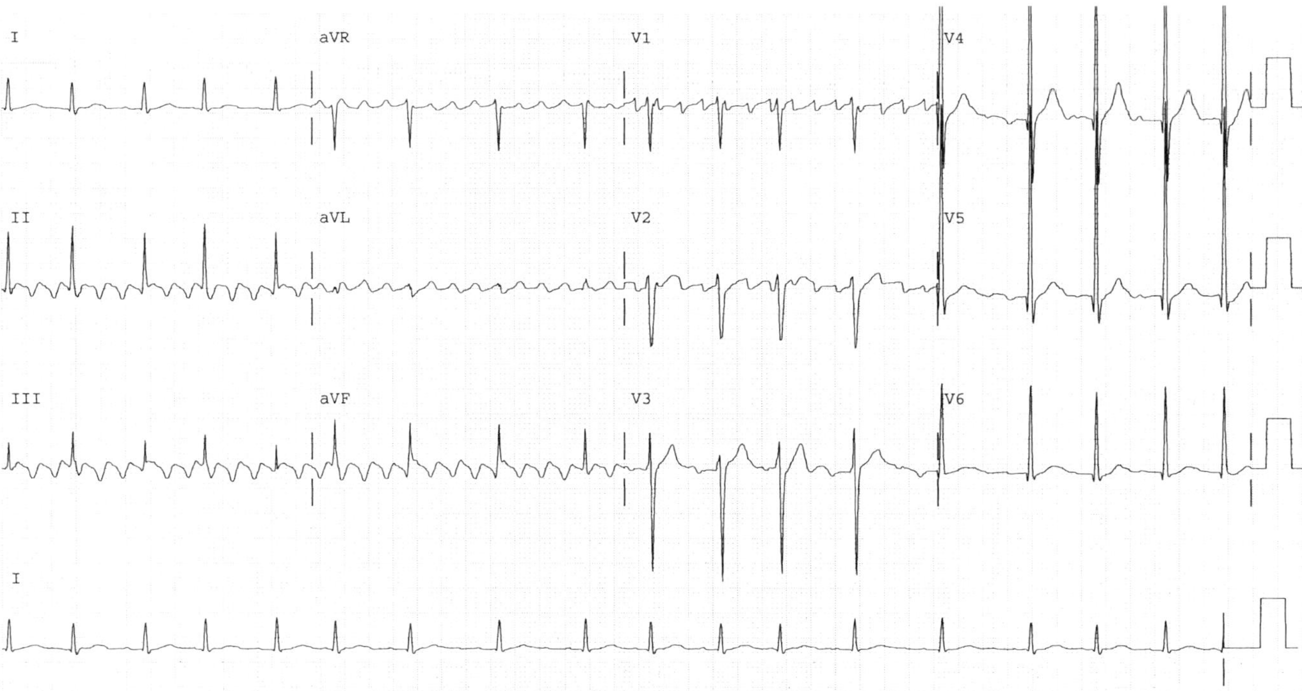

Atrial Flutter: The ECG shows a "saw-tooth" pattern in leads II and III characteristic of atrial flutter.

Supraventricular Tachycardia

Diagnosis

SVTs are a group of arrhythmias that arise in atrial tissue or the AV node. The most common SVTs, exclusive of AF and atrial flutter, are AVNRT, AVRT, and atrial tachycardia. The ECG usually reveals a narrow-complex tachycardia, although the QRS complexes can be wide in the presence of bundle branch block, aberrancy, pacing, or anterograde accessory pathway conduction.

The most common paroxysmal SVT is AVNRT. Typical AVNRT often has an RP interval so short that the P wave is buried within the QRS complex, but it may be seen as a pseudo R in lead V_1 and a pseudo S wave in the inferior leads.

AVRT is a reentrant circuit that includes a bypass pathway and the AV node. If a bypass pathway conducts antegrade, a preexcitation pattern may be seen on the ECG. When this pattern is accompanied by a symptomatic tachycardia, it is termed WPW syndrome (see Wolff-Parkinson-White Syndrome).

MAT is an irregular SVT that demonstrates three or more P waves of different morphologies and is often seen in end-stage COPD.

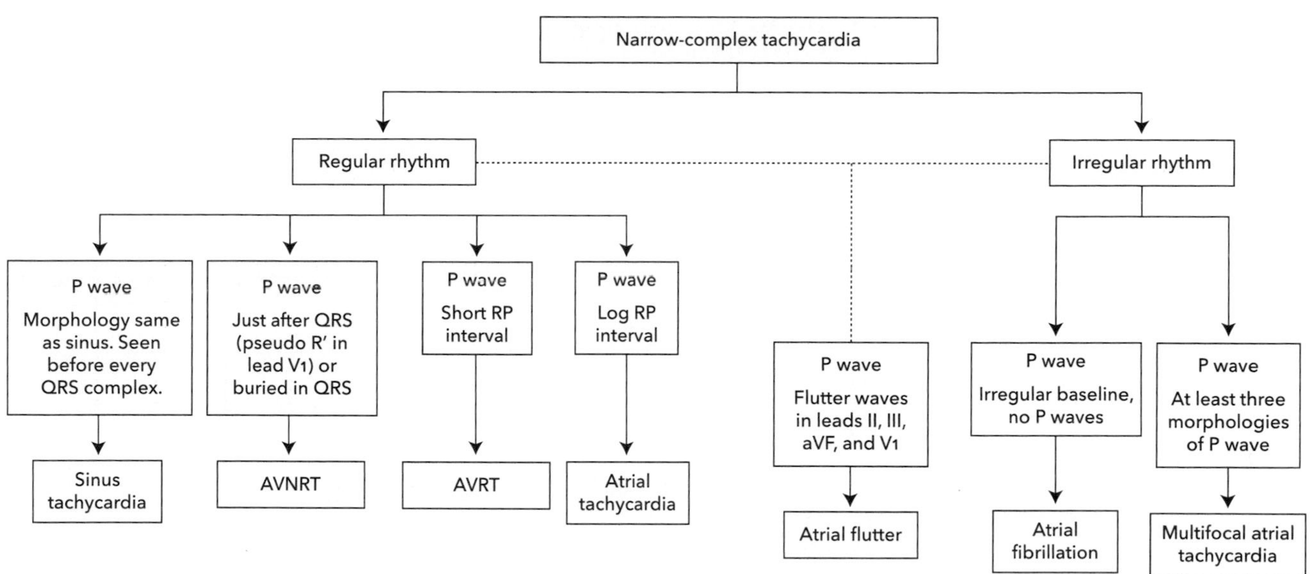

Classification of Narrow-Complex Tachycardia: AVNRT = atrioventricular nodal reentrant tachycardia; AVRT = atrioventricular reciprocating tachycardia.

Treatment

Episodes of SVT can often be terminated with Valsalva maneuvers, carotid sinus massage, or facial immersion in cold water.

Adenosine can be used to terminate SVT and to help diagnose the cause. Termination with adenosine often suggests AV node dependence (AVNRT and AVRT), whereas continued P waves during AV block can help identify atrial flutter and atrial tachycardia. Rate control for atrial tachycardia can be achieved with β-blockers or calcium channel blockers.

Use oral calcium channel blockers and β-blockers to prevent recurrent AVNRT. For recurrent AVNRT despite drug therapy or intolerance of drug therapy, select catheter ablation therapy.

Treatment of MAT is directed at correcting associated pulmonary and cardiac disease, hypokalemia, and hypomagnesemia. Drug therapy is indicated for patients who are symptomatic or experience complications such as HF or chest pain secondary to cardiac ischemia. Metoprolol is the drug of choice followed by verapamil in patients with bronchospastic disease.

DON'T BE TRICKED

- **Do not treat irregular wide-complex tachycardia or polymorphic tachycardia with adenosine.**

TEST YOURSELF

A 32-year-old woman has a 4-hour history of palpitations. BP is 80/50 mm Hg. An ECG shows regular, narrow-complex tachycardia of 180/min and normal QRS complex morphology. No P waves are seen.

ANSWER: The diagnosis is AVNRT. Choose the Valsalva maneuver, carotid sinus massage, verapamil, or IV adenosine.

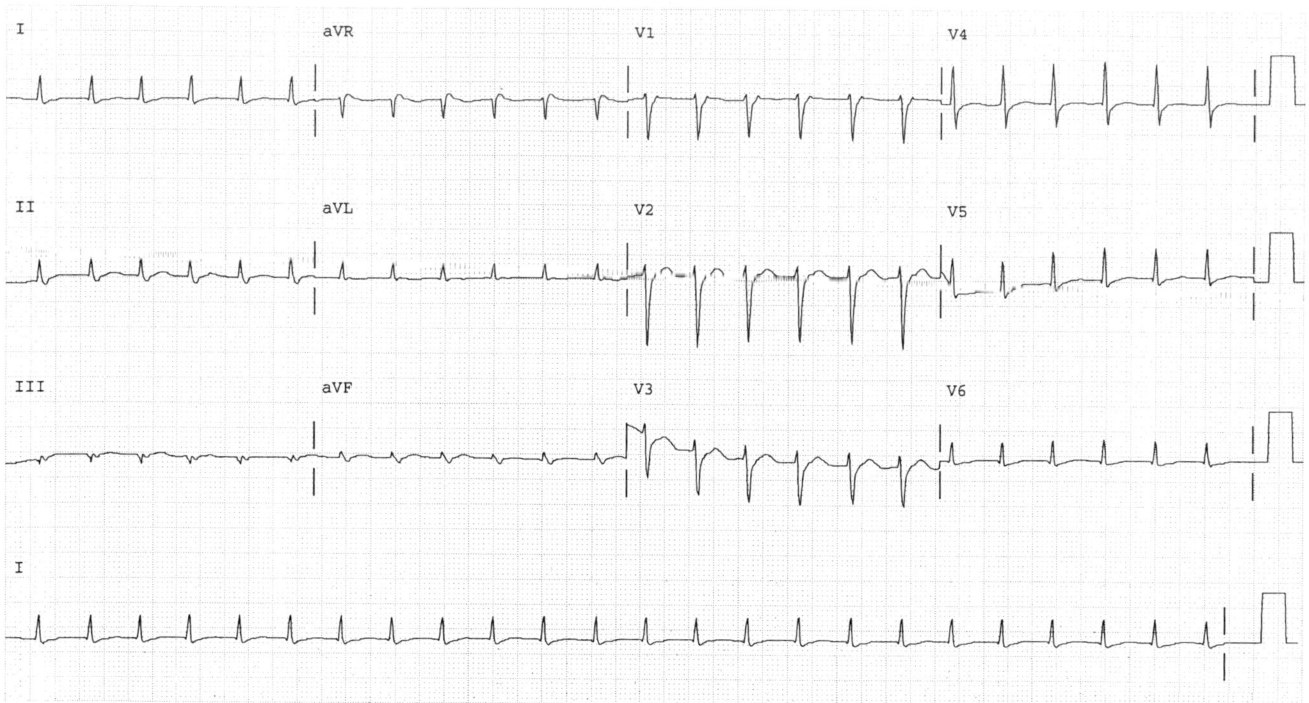

AV-Nodal Reentrant Tachycardia: The ECG shows a narrow-complex tachycardia at 144/min and no visible P waves.

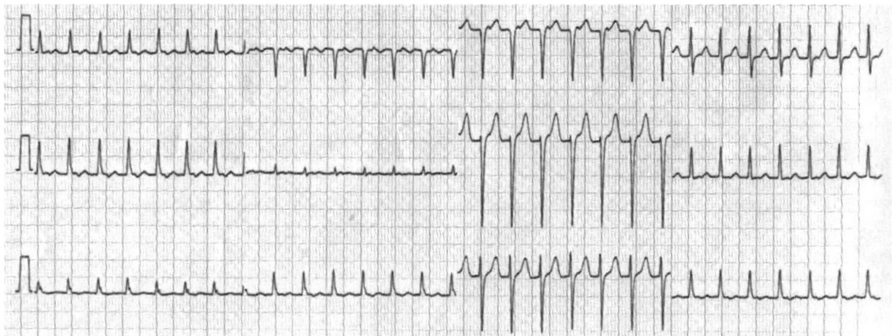

AV Reciprocating Tachycardia: The ECG shows a narrow-complex tachycardia with the P wave buried in the ST segment.

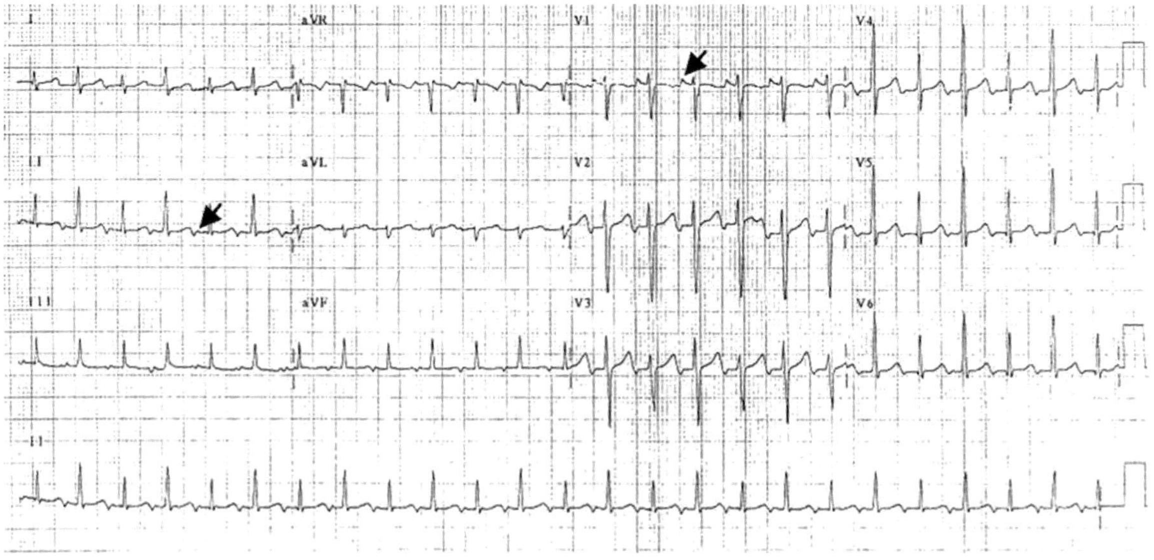

Atrial Tachycardia: The ECG shows a narrow-complex tachycardia with P waves most clearly seen in lead V_1 and at the end of the T wave in other leads.

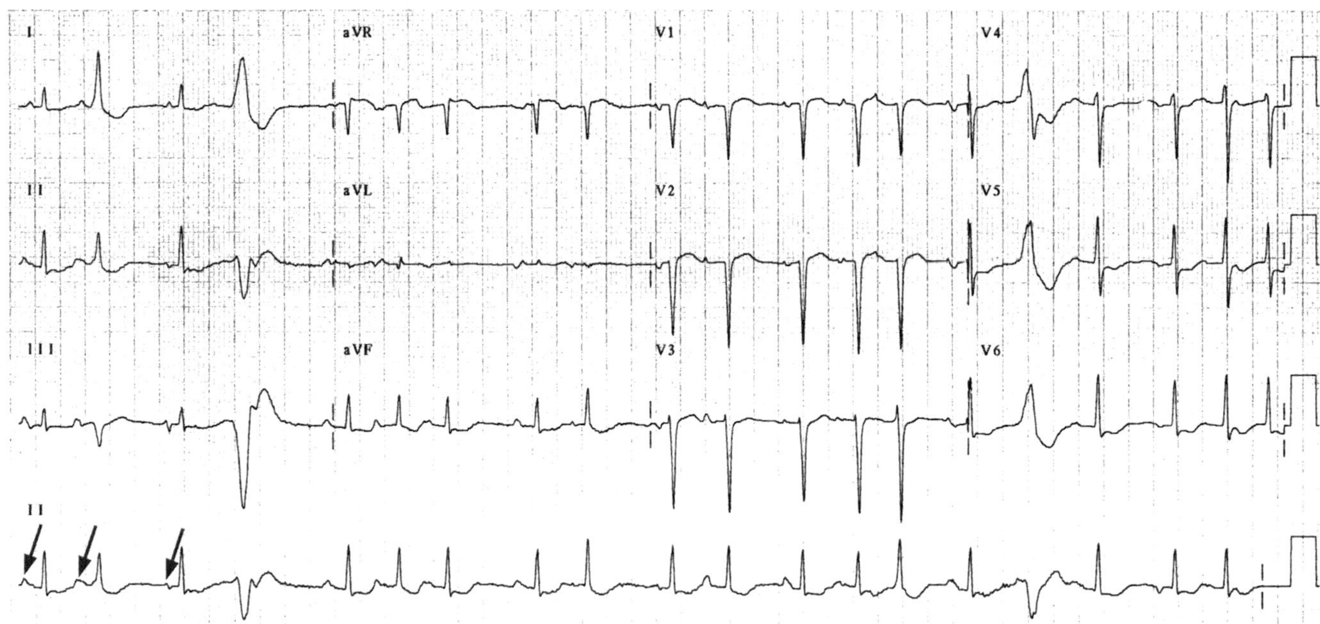

Multifocal Atrial Tachycardia: The ECG shows an irregular tachycardia with three distinct P wave morphologies characteristic of MAT (*arrows*).

Wolff-Parkinson-White Syndrome

Diagnosis

WPW syndrome is a symptomatic AVRT caused by an accessory AV conduction pathway that is:

- usually antegrade to the ventricles, resulting in the delta wave that indicates ventricular preexcitation (in this situation, WPW is described as "manifest")
- occasionally concealed or retrograde; ventricles are depolarized over the normal AV node-His-Purkinje network, resulting in a normal surface ECG (in this situation, WPW is described as "concealed")

ECG findings include a short PR interval, delta wave, and normal or prolonged QRS. AF associated with WPW syndrome is a risk factor for VF. Look for an irregular, wide-complex tachycardia.

Treatment

Begin procainamide or another class I or class III agent for patients with wide-complex tachycardia, especially when AF and preexcitation are present. Cardioversion is the preferred treatment for any unstable patient with WPW syndrome.

Ablation of the accessory bypass tract is first-line therapy for patients with preexcitation and symptoms. Antiarrhythmic agents are second-line therapy.

DON'T BE TRICKED

- Asymptomatic WPW conduction without arrhythmia does not require investigation or treatment.
- Do not select calcium channel blockers, β-blockers, or digoxin for patients who have AF with WPW syndrome; such treatment may convert AF to VT or VF.

TEST YOURSELF

A 28-year-old woman has a 4-hour history of palpitations. Physical examination shows a BP of 132/80 mm Hg, an irregularly irregular HR of 140/min, and no other abnormal findings. The ECG shows AF with a ventricular rate of 180 to 270/min. QRS complexes are broad and bizarre.

ANSWER: The diagnosis is WPW syndrome with AF. Begin IV procainamide.

A 30-year-old woman has an episode of palpitations and syncope. ECG shows WPW pattern.

ANSWER: Refer for ablation of the accessory tract.

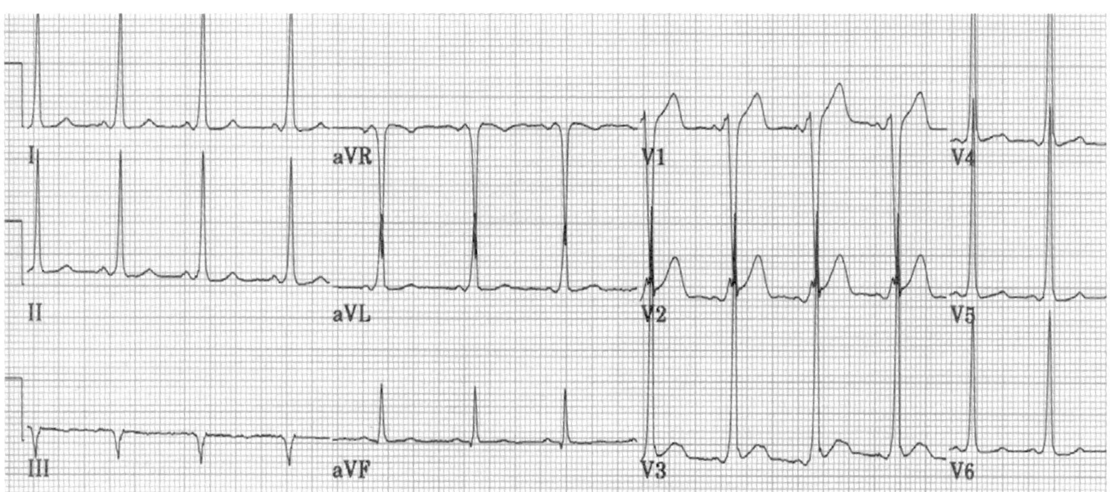

WPW Syndrome: WPW syndrome is diagnosed by a short PR interval, prolonged QRS, and a slurred onset of the QRS (*delta wave*).

Ventricular Tachycardia

Diagnosis

Premature ventricular complexes (PVCs) can be single, in pairs (couplets), or alternating with sinus beats. In healthy adults, PVCs are benign.

Ventricular tachyarrhythmias consist of VT, VF, and torsades de pointes. Ventricular tachyarrhythmias are characterized by:

- QRS >0.12 s
- AV dissociation

The ventricular rate typically ranges from 140 to 250/min in VT, is typically >300/min in VF, and is characteristically 200 to 300/min in torsades de pointes.

VT can be further classified as sustained or nonsustained. Nonsustained VT lasts <30 s.

VT is also categorized by the morphology of the QRS complexes:

- Monomorphic VT: QRS complexes in the same leads do not vary in contour.
- Polymorphic VT: QRS complexes in the same leads do vary in contour.

Differentiating VT from SVT with aberrant conduction is important because the treatment differs markedly. VT is more common than SVT with aberrancy, particularly in persons with structural heart disease. Any wide QRS tachycardia should be considered to be VT until proven otherwise. In the presence of known structural heart disease, especially a previous MI, the diagnosis of VT is almost certain.

Torsades de pointes is a specific form of polymorphic VT associated with long QT syndrome, which may be congenital or acquired (see Sudden Cardiac Death). Torsades de pointes episodes are typically short lived and terminate spontaneously, but multiple successive episodes may result in syncope or VF.

Testing

Evaluation with resting ECG, exercise treadmill testing (to provoke arrhythmias), and cardiac imaging (to identify structural heart disease) is indicated in all patients with VT.

Treatment

Patients without identifiable structural heart disease: In otherwise healthy patients without structural heart disease and non-sustained VT, treatment with β-blockers or calcium channel blockers, especially verapamil, should only be given if disabling symptoms are present.

Patients with structural heart disease: β-Blockers and ACE inhibitors have been shown to reduce the risk of sudden cardiac death in patients with previous MI and cardiomyopathy. In those with recurrent VT despite β-blocker therapy, antiarrhythmic drug therapy with amiodarone may be considered. Catheter ablation should be considered in patients with recurrent VT despite medical therapy. ICD placement is indicated for prevention of sudden cardiac death in patients with structural heart disease or cardiomyopathy who have sustained VT/VF, if reversible causes have been excluded (such as acute coronary ischemia or cocaine ingestion).

Acute treatment of sustained VT:

- For unstable patients, immediate electrical cardioversion is indicated. Pulseless VT is treated in the same way as VF.
- For hemodynamically stable patients with impaired LV function, IV lidocaine or amiodarone is preferred. Procainamide and sotalol are additional therapeutic possibilities.

DON'T BE TRICKED

- In patients with structural heart disease, therapy to suppress PVCs does not affect outcomes.

TEST YOURSELF

A 65-year-old woman with chronic stable angina and a history of an anterior MI is evaluated in the emergency department for palpitations and lightheadedness. Vital signs are stable. ECG shows a wide-complex tachycardia with an RBBB pattern. No previous ECGs are immediately available.

ANSWER: The diagnosis is most likely sustained VT. The acute treatment is IV lidocaine or amiodarone.

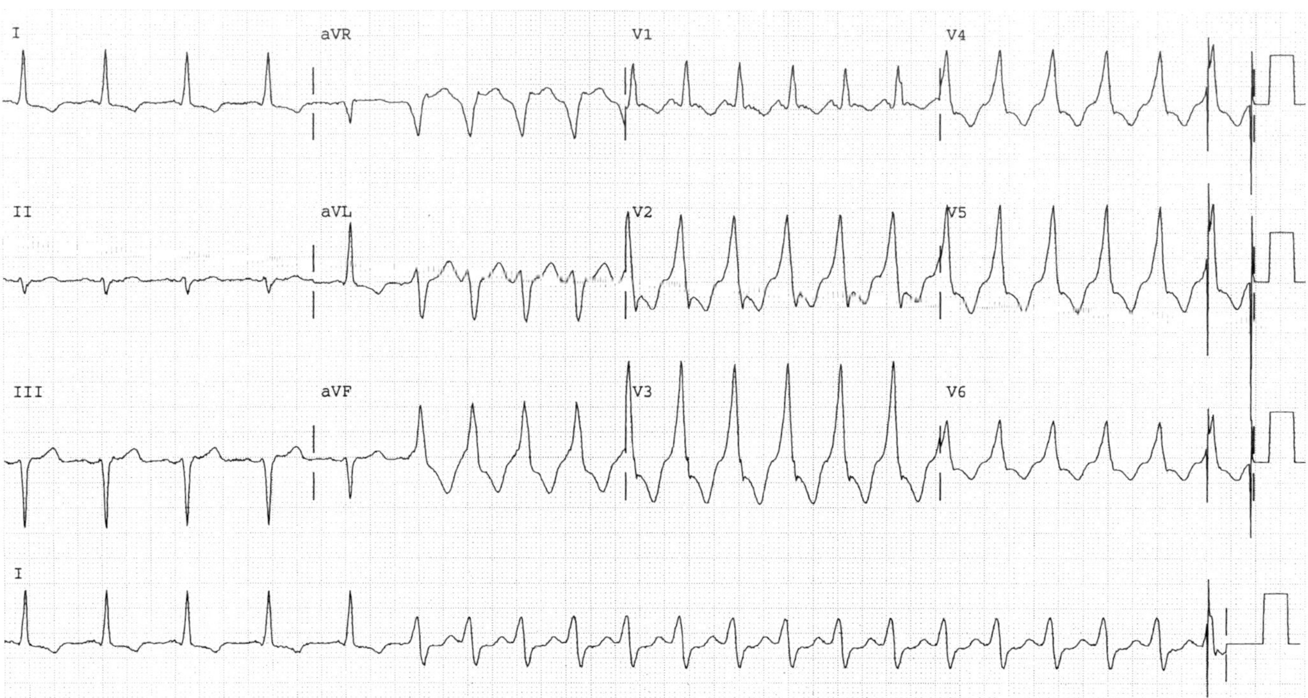

Monomorphic VT: Approximately one quarter of the way into this ECG rhythm strip (*bottom*), monomorphic VT begins; it is associated with an abrupt change in the QRS axis.

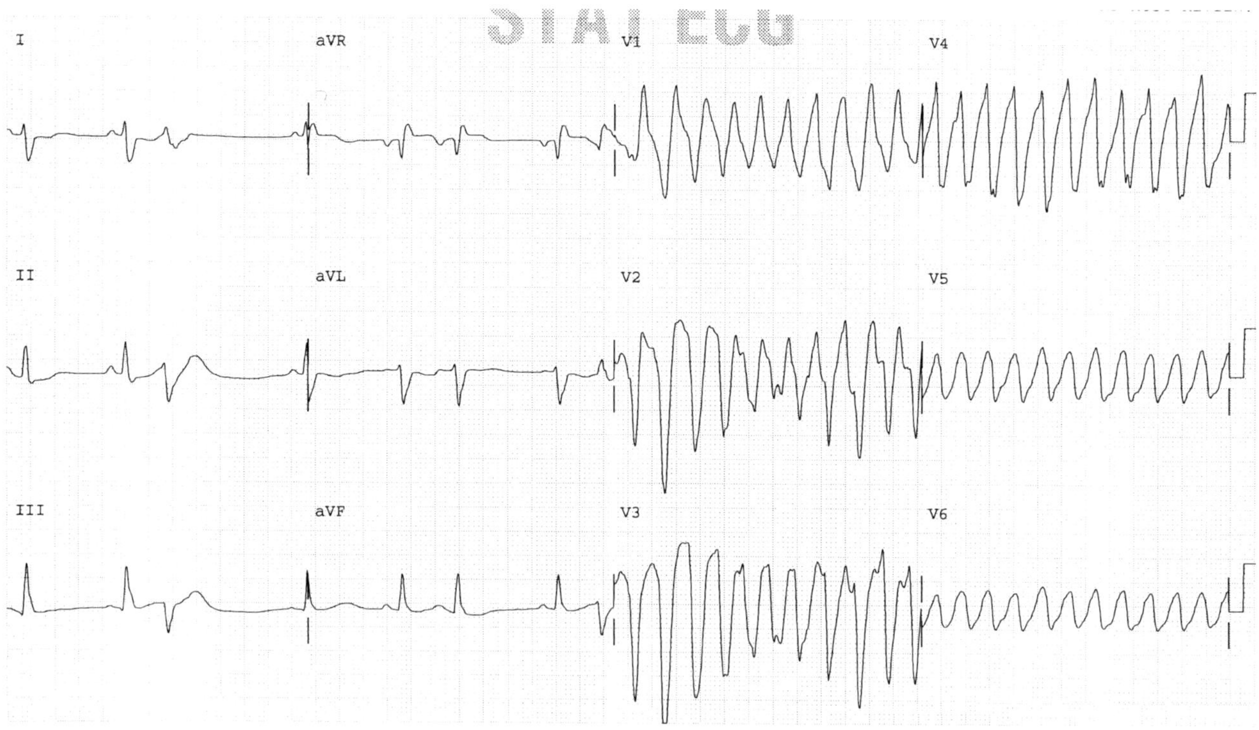

Polymorphic VT: This ECG shows degeneration of the sinus rhythm into polymorphic tachycardia.

Sudden Cardiac Death

Screening

Unexplained premature (age <35 years) death or sudden death in a first-degree family member should raise suspicion for an inherited arrhythmia syndrome.

Diagnosis

Sudden cardiac death is most often associated with structural heart disease or arrhythmogenic substrate, including HCM, abnormal cardiac rhythms or conduction, dilated cardiomyopathy with reduced systolic function, WPW syndrome, Brugada syndrome, and long QT syndrome.

Long QT syndrome may be inherited or acquired. Patients may experience syncope or sudden cardiac death as the result of torsades de pointes. Look for hypokalemia, hypomagnesemia, structural heart disease, medications, and drug interactions. Look specifically for:

- macrolide and fluoroquinolone antibiotics (especially moxifloxacin)
- terfenadine and astemizole antihistamines
- antipsychotic and antidepressant medications
- methadone
- antifungal medications
- class Ia and class III antiarrhythmics

Risk is greatest with a QTc interval >500 ms.

Brugada syndrome is an inherited condition characterized by a structurally normal heart but abnormal electrical conduction associated with sudden cardiac death. Classic Brugada syndrome is recognized as an incomplete RBBB pattern with coved ST-segment elevation in leads V_1 and V_2.

Testing

Select echocardiography for survivors of sudden cardiac death to identify anatomic abnormalities, impaired ventricular function, and/or myopathic processes. Electrophysiologic studies are indicated for patients with suspected ventricular arrhythmias, episodes of impaired consciousness, and structurally abnormal hearts. Patients taking antiarrhythmic agents should have a serum drug level measurement and an ECG to look for long QT syndrome.

Treatment

Therapy includes pharmacologic treatment of underlying CAD and a revascularization procedure if anatomically possible. Inherited long QT syndrome may be treated with β-blockers.

Select an ICD in the following scenarios:

- for survivors of cardiac arrest resulting from VF or VT not explained by a reversible cause
- after sustained VT in the presence of structural heart disease
- after syncope and sustained VT/VF on electrophysiology study
- for ischemic and nonischemic cardiomyopathy with an EF ≤35%, NYHA class II or III symptoms, with guideline-directed medical therapy
- for Brugada syndrome with syncope or ventricular arrhythmia
- for inherited long QT syndrome not responding to β-blockers
- ≥40 days after MI with an EF ≤30%
- for high-risk HCM (familial sudden death; multiple, repetitive nonsustained VT; extreme LVH; a recent, unexplained syncopal episode; and exercise hypotension)

TEST YOURSELF

A 55-year-old man is evaluated 4 months after a large anterior MI. He has no symptoms, and his physical examination is normal. Follow-up echocardiography documents an LVEF of 28%.

ANSWER: For management, choose an ICD, because this patient is at high risk for sudden cardiac death.

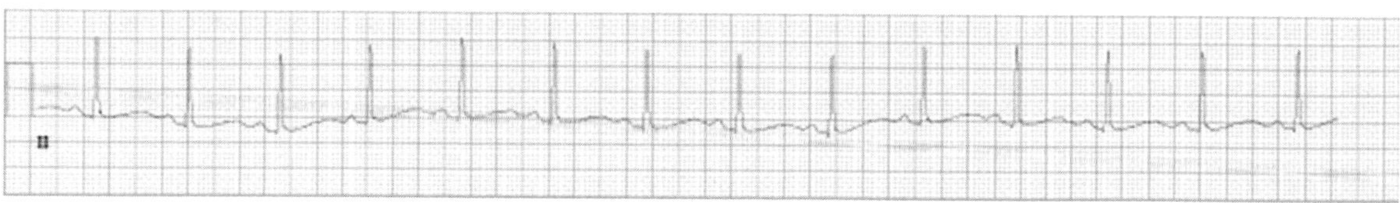

Prolonged QT syndrome: The ECG shows a prolonged QT interval of 590 ms.

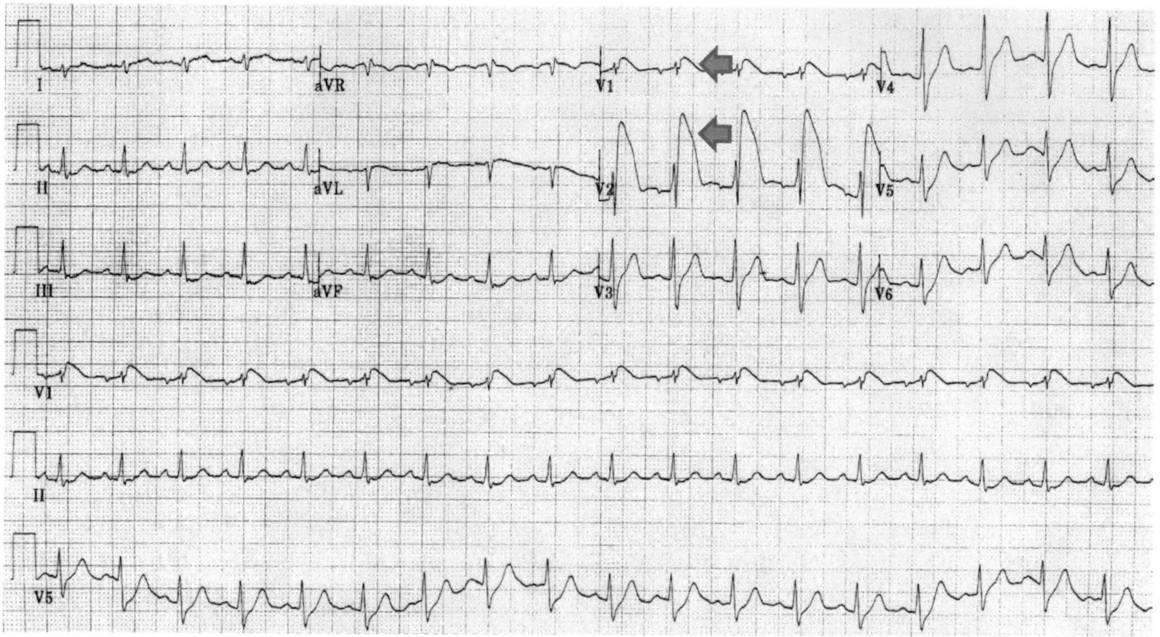

Brugada Pattern on ECG: Incomplete RBBB pattern and elevation of the ST segments that gradually descends to an inverted T wave in leads V_1 and V_2 are characteristic of the classic variety of Brugada syndrome.

Acute Pericarditis

Diagnosis

The most common symptom is acute sharp or stabbing substernal chest pain that worsens with inspiration and when lying flat and is alleviated when sitting and leaning forward. Medical history may include:

- preceding viral symptoms
- cancer (current or in the past)
- recent trauma
- arthralgia, arthritis (suggesting systemic rheumatic disease)
- MI
- recent thoracic surgical procedures
- use of medications, including hydralazine, phenytoin, and minoxidil

A two- or three-component pericardial friction rub is characteristic. Pericardial tamponade (pulsus paradoxus ≥10 mm Hg) may be present. Electrical alternans (alternating high- and low-voltage QRS complexes) may be present in patients with large effusions.

An echocardiogram may show evidence of an effusion or of early tamponade.

STUDY TABLE: ECG Features Differentiating Acute Pericarditis from MI

Feature	Acute Pericarditis	Myocardial Ischemia
ST-segment contour	Concave upwards	Convex upwards
ST-segment lead involvement	Diffuse	Localized
Reciprocal ST-T changes	No	Yes
PR-segment abnormalities	Yes (depression in limb leads, elevation in aVR)	No
Pathologic Q waves	No	Yes

DON'T BE TRICKED

- **Cardiac enzyme values may be slightly elevated in patients with pericarditis (myopericarditis).**
- **Absence of a pericardial effusion on echocardiography does not rule out pericarditis.**

Treatment

First-line treatment is colchicine plus aspirin (preferred after MI) or an NSAID. Choose glucocorticoids for pericarditis that does not respond to colchicine plus aspirin, or an NSAID, or is related to an autoimmune process. Choose emergent pericardiocentesis for tamponade and hemodynamic instability.

TEST YOURSELF

A 57-year-old man has a 2-day history of chest pain that worsens when he lies flat. Cardiac examination shows a three-component friction rub.

ANSWER: For diagnosis, choose pericarditis. Look for diffuse ST-segment elevation and PR-segment depression. Ignore slight elevation of cardiac troponin tempting you to answer "acute MI."

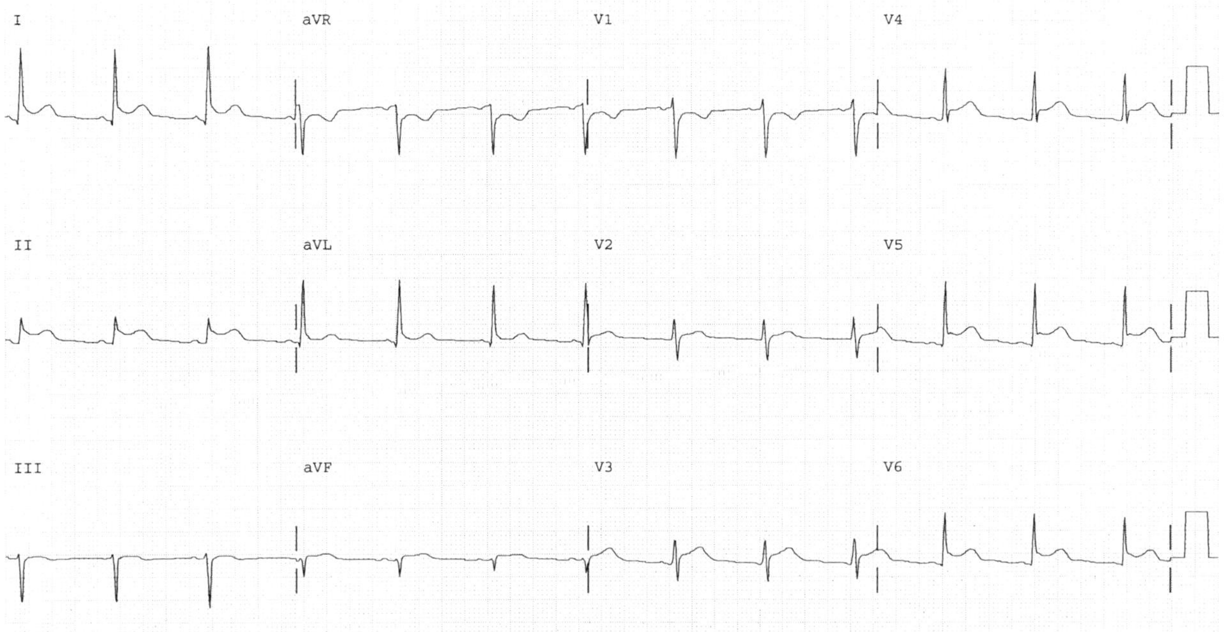

Acute Pericarditis: The ECG shows sinus rhythm with diffuse ST-segment elevation and PR-segment depression in lead II, characteristic of acute pericarditis.

Cardiac Tamponade and Constrictive Pericarditis

Diagnosis

Patients with chronic cardiac tamponade present with dyspnea, fatigue, peripheral edema, hepatomegaly, hepatic dysfunction, and ascites in the absence of pulmonary congestion. The diagnosis may be suggested by risk factors for tamponade, including patients with:

- metastatic lung and breast cancer (most common cause)
- cardiac surgery
- viral or bacterial pericarditis
- systemic rheumatic disease

Physical examination reveals JVD, pulsus paradoxus, tachycardia, reduced heart sounds, and/or hypotension. Chest x-ray shows an enlarged silhouette ("water bottle sign"). Echocardiography can confirm diagnosis.

Absence of a pericardial effusion excludes a diagnosis of cardiac tamponade.

Constrictive pericarditis is characterized by adherent pericardium that restrains ventricular diastolic expansion, leading to impaired filling. Constrictive pericarditis is often a sequela of acute pericarditis. Other causes include chest radiation, previous cardiac surgery, and TB. Physical examination findings in constrictive pericarditis include a pericardial knock (a loud third heart sound that occurs earlier in diastole than a normal S_3), Kussmaul sign (increased JVD on inspiration), and pericardial friction rub. Long-standing constrictive pericarditis may be associated with liver failure and cirrhosis. Imaging findings that support the diagnosis include:

- calcified pericardium on x-ray (specific, but not sensitive)
- pericardial thickening on CT or CMR imaging
- abnormal diastolic motion on echocardiography

Treatment

Acute management of cardiac tamponade includes drainage of pericardial fluid by percutaneous pericardiocentesis or surgery. SBP should be maintained with volume resuscitation and vasopressors.

In patients with chronic constrictive pericarditis, cardiac output depends on a high preload; therefore, diuretics must be used cautiously. Pericardiectomy is the most effective treatment, but it is unnecessary in patients with early disease (NYHA functional class I) and is unwarranted in many patients with advanced disease (NYHA functional class IV).

TEST YOURSELF

A 44-year-old woman with a history of ovarian cancer presents with fatigue, dyspnea, and peripheral edema. Examination shows JVD that increases with inspiration, reduced heart sounds, BP of 94/50 mm Hg, and HR of 132/min. A 20 mm Hg pulsus paradoxus is present.

ANSWER: For diagnosis, choose acute pericardial tamponade, probably secondary to metastatic disease. For management, select pericardiocentesis.

Cardiac Physical Diagnosis

Heart Murmurs

Right-sided heart murmurs increase in intensity during inspiration. Murmurs caused by HCM increase in intensity during the Valsalva maneuver and on standing from a squatting position. The clicks caused by MVP may move closer to S_1, and the murmur lengthens during the Valsalva maneuver and on standing from a squatting position.

Abnormal splitting of S_2 helps differentiate heart murmurs. Normally, a split S_2 is heard only during inspiration. Splitting during inspiration and expiration occurs in conditions that further delay RV ejection, including RBBB, pulmonary valve stenosis, VSD with left-to-right shunt, and ASD with left-to-right shunt. Reversed or expiratory splitting occurs in conditions that prolong LV ejection, including LBBB, AS, HCM, and ACS with LV dysfunction.

Innocent heart murmurs are typically midsystolic, located at the base of the heart, grade 1/6 to 2/6 without radiation, and associated with normal splitting of S_2. Signs of serious cardiac disease include an S_4, murmur grade ≥3/6 intensity, any diastolic murmur, continuous murmurs, and abnormal splitting of S_2. TTE is indicated in symptomatic patients, in those with a systolic murmur grade ≥3/6 intensity, and in those with a diastolic murmur or any continuous murmur (a murmur that begins after S_1 and extends beyond S_2).

DON'T BE TRICKED

- An increased P_2, an S_3, and an early peaking systolic murmur over the upper left sternal border are normal findings during pregnancy.

TEST YOURSELF

A 19-year-old asymptomatic woman has a heart murmur first heard during a college sports physical examination. A nonradiating grade 2/6 midsystolic murmur is heard over the upper left sternal border. Physiologic splitting of S_2 is present, and a soft S_3 is heard at the cardiac apex.

ANSWER: For diagnosis, choose an innocent heart murmur. Do not order echocardiography.

Valvular Lesions

STUDY TABLE: Valvular and Other Cardiac Lesions and Their Associated Examination Findings

Cardiac Condition	Characteristic Murmur	Location	Radiation	Associated Findings	Severity and Pitfalls
Aortic stenosis	Mid-systolic; crescendo-decrescendo	RUSB	Right clavicle, carotid, apex	Enlarged, nondisplaced apical impulse; S_4; bicuspid valve without calcification will have systolic ejection click followed by murmur	Severe aortic stenosis may include decreased A_2; high-pitched, late-peaking murmur; diminished and delayed carotid upstroke Radiation of murmur down the descending thoracic aorta may mimic mitral regurgitation
Aortic regurgitation	Diastolic; decrescendo	LLSB (valvular) or RLSB (dilated aorta) (heard best sitting and leaning forward)	None	Enlarged, displaced apical impulse; S_3 or S_4; increased pulse pressure; bounding carotid and peripheral pulses	Acute, severe regurgitation murmur may be masked by tachycardia and short duration of murmur Severity in chronic regurgitation is difficult to assess by auscultation
Mitral stenosis	Diastolic; low pitched, decrescendo	Apex (heard best in left lateral decubitus position)	None	Loud S_1; tapping apex beat; opening snap after S_2 if leaflets mobile; irregular pulse if AF present	Interval between S_2 and opening snap is short in severe mitral stenosis Intensity of murmur correlates with transvalvular gradient P_2 may be loud if pulmonary hypertension present

(Continued on the next page)

STUDY TABLE: Valvular and Other Cardiac Lesions and Their Associated Examination Findings *(Continued)*					
Cardiac Condition	**Characteristic Murmur**	**Location**	**Radiation**	**Associated Findings**	**Severity and Pitfalls**
Mitral regurgitation	Systolic; holo-, mid-, or late systolic	Apex	To axilla or back; occasionally anteriorly to precordium	Systolic click in mitral valve prolapse; S_3; apical impulse hyperdynamic and may be displaced if dilated left ventricle; in mitral valve prolapse, Valsalva maneuver moves onset of clicks and murmur closer to S_1; handgrip increases murmur intensity	Acute, severe regurgitation may have soft or no holosystolic murmur, mitral inflow rumble, S_3
Tricuspid regurgitation	Holosystolic	LLSB	LUSB	Merged and prominent *c* and *v* waves in jugular venous pulse; murmur increases during inspiration	Right ventricular impulse below sternum Pulsatile, enlarged liver with possible ascites May be high pitched if associated with severe pulmonary hypertension
Tricuspid stenosis	Diastolic; low pitched, decrescendo; increased intensity during inspiration	LLSB	Nonradiating	Elevated CVP with prominent *a* wave, signs of venous congestion (hepatomegaly, ascites, edema)	Low-pitched frequency may be difficult to auscultate, especially at higher heart rate
Pulmonary stenosis	Systolic; crescendo-decrescendo	LUSB	Left clavicle	Pulmonic ejection click after S_1 (diminishes with inspiration)	Increased intensity of murmur with late peaking
Pulmonary regurgitation	Diastolic; decrescendo	LLSB	None	Loud P_2 if pulmonary hypertension present	Murmur may be minimal or absent if severe because of minimal difference in pulmonary artery and right ventricular diastolic pressures
Innocent flow murmur	Midsystolic; grade 1/6 or 2/6 in intensity	RUSB	None	Normal intensity of A_2; normal splitting of S_2; no radiation	May be present in conditions with increased flow (e.g., pregnancy, fever, anemia, hyperthyroidism)
Hypertrophic obstructive cardiomyopathy	Systolic; crescendo-decrescendo	LLSB	None	Enlarged, hyperdynamic apical impulse; bifid carotid impulse with delay; increased intensity during Valsalva maneuver or with squatting to standing	Murmur may not be present in nonobstructive hypertrophic cardiomyopathy
Atrial septal defect	Systolic; crescendo-decrescendo	RUSB	None	Fixed split S_2; right ventricular heave; rarely, tricuspid inflow murmur	May be associated with pulmonary hypertension with increased intensity of P_2, pulmonary valve regurgitation
Ventricular septal defect	Holosystolic	LLSB	None	Palpable thrill; murmur increases with hand-grip, decreases with amyl nitrite	Murmur intensity and duration decrease as pulmonary hypertension develops (Eisenmenger syndrome) Cyanosis if Eisenmenger syndrome develops

A_2 = aortic valve component of S_2; LLSB = left lower sternal border; LUSB = left upper sternal border; P_2 = pulmonary valve component of S_2; RLSB = right lower sternal border; RUSB = right upper sternal border.

Rheumatic Valvular Heart Disease

Prevention

Give penicillin to patients with group A streptococcal infection (or erythromycin to patients with penicillin allergy). Patients with a history of RF require long-term prophylactic penicillin, and patients with rheumatic valvular disease should continue prophylaxis for at least 10 years after the last episode of RF or until at least 40 years of age (whichever is longer).

Diagnosis

Mitral stenosis and regurgitation are common consequences of RF. The aortic valve is the second most likely affected valve.

STUDY TABLE: Jones Criteria for Diagnosis of Rheumatic Fever	
Manifestations*	
Major	Carditis, polyarthritis, chorea, subcutaneous nodules, erythema marginatum
Minor	Arthralgia, fever
Minor	Elevated ESR, elevated CRP, evidence of group A streptococcal infection, prolonged PR interval on ECG

*Note: Two major manifestations or one major and two minor manifestations establish the diagnosis.

Treatment

Antibiotic therapy is required even if the throat culture is negative for group A streptococci. Salicylates are the drug of choice; nonresponse to salicylates makes RF unlikely.

Aortic Stenosis

Diagnosis

The most common cause of AS is progressive degenerative disease of a normal trileaflet valve that is usually diagnosed in patients ≥60 years. Aortic valve sclerosis, or valve thickening without outflow obstruction, is an earlier phase of calcific aortic valve disease present in more than 20% of persons >65 years. Patients with a congenital bicuspid aortic valve usually present at a younger age (40-60 years).

Cardinal symptoms of AS are dyspnea, angina, and syncope. Findings include:

- midsystolic murmur at the upper right second intercostal space
- murmur that radiates to the carotid arteries
- decreased intensity of S_2
- delayed, low-amplitude carotid pulse (pulsus parvus et tardus)
- chest x-ray showing a boot-shaped cardiac silhouette and poststenotic aortic dilatation
- echocardiogram showing left atrial enlargement and LVH, as well as calcified aortic valve leaflets with restricted motion
- severe AS associated with a valve area <1 cm^2 and a mean transvalvular gradient >40 mm Hg

DON'T BE TRICKED

- Echocardiography may significantly underestimate the transvalvular gradient in patients with severe LV dysfunction.
- Do not select exercise stress testing for symptomatic patients with AS.

Treatment

In the absence of symptoms, patients have a low risk of death. Surgical aortic valve replacement (SAVR) is recommended for symptomatic patients at low operative risk.

Transcatheter aortic valve replacement (TAVR) has a survival benefit similar to that of SAVR for intermediate-risk and high-risk patients and is superior to medical therapy in nonsurgical candidates. Contraindications to TAVR include a bicuspid aortic valve, significant AR, and mitral valve disease.

Medical therapy does not stall the progression of disease but is indicated for patients with symptoms and LV dysfunction who are awaiting valve repair or replacement. Treat these patients with diuretics, digoxin, and ACE inhibitors.

DON'T BE TRICKED

- Do not select balloon valvuloplasty as a definitive treatment for AS in adults.
- Medical therapy with statins does not alter the natural history of AS.

Follow-Up

Use serial echocardiography to evaluate the left aortic valve area, degree of ventricular hypertrophy, and LV function every 6-12 months in asymptomatic patients with severe AS, every 1-2 years in patients with moderate AS, and every 3-5 years in those with mild AS.

TEST YOURSELF

A 71-year-old man is evaluated for HF. On physical examination, the apical impulse is enlarged and displaced laterally, and a grade 2/6 midsystolic murmur is heard at the right upper sternal border that radiates to the carotid arteries. Echocardiography shows hypokinesis and an LVEF of 30%. The aortic valve cusp is calcified with diminished mobility, and the transvalvular mean gradient is 26 mm Hg.

ANSWER: For diagnosis, choose severe AS with cardiomyopathy despite the low transvalvular gradient (which is low because of severe LV dysfunction). For management, select cardiac catheterization and probable valve replacement.

Bicuspid Aortic Valve

Diagnosis

Bicuspid aortic valve disease is the most common congenital heart abnormality. Auscultatory findings include a systolic ejection click at the left lower sternal border and murmur of AS or AR in a young patient. A bicuspid aortic valve may occur with other cardiovascular and systemic abnormalities, including aortic coarctation, aneurysm of the sinuses of Valsalva, PDA, and aortic aneurysm and dissection.

Treatment

Surgical aortic valve replacement is first-line therapy for a stenotic bicuspid aortic valve. Recommendations regarding when to intervene are the same as for tricuspid aortic valves.

For a regurgitant bicuspid aortic valve, valve replacement is the treatment of choice when regurgitation is clinically significant, manifesting as symptomatic HF or asymptomatic LVEF <50%.

Surgery to repair the aortic root or replace the ascending aorta is indicated when the aortic root diameter is >5 cm with additional risk factors for dissection (family history, rate of progression ≥0.5 cm/year) or >5.5 cm without risk factors.

Follow-Up

Asymptomatic patients with severe aortic valve stenosis or regurgitation require echocardiography every 6-12 months; those with mild stenosis or regurgitation require it every 3 to 5 years.

The ascending aortic diameter should be assessed annually by echocardiography if the aortic root or ascending aorta dimension is >4.5 cm and every 2 years if the dimension is <4.0 cm.

Aortic Regurgitation

Diagnosis

AR is classified as chronic or acute. Acute severe AR usually is caused by IE or aortic dissection. Chronic severe AR is most commonly associated with dilated ascending aorta from hypertension or primary aortic disease, calcific AS, bicuspid aortic valve, or rheumatic disease. Findings in chronic, severe AR include:

- angina, orthopnea, and exertional dyspnea
- widened pulse pressure
- soft S_1, soft or absent A_2, and loud S_3
- diastolic murmur immediately after A_2 along the left sternal border (primary aortic valvular disease) or right sternal border (secondary to aortic root dilatation)
- enhanced auscultation when leaning forward and exhaling
- left axis deviation and LVH on ECG
- cardiomegaly and aortic root dilatation and calcification on chest x-ray

Acute AR is associated with a short, soft, and sometimes inaudible diastolic murmur and normal heart size and pulse pressure.

Treatment

Schedule immediate aortic valve replacement for patients with acute AR. Bridging medical therapy includes sodium nitroprusside and IV diuretics. Dobutamine or milrinone are also indicated if the BP is unacceptably low.

For chronic symptomatic AR, valve replacement is indicated regardless of LV systolic function. Valve replacement also is indicated for asymptomatic patients with LVEF <50%. Combined aortic root replacement with aortic valve replacement is used when an associated aortic root aneurysm is present.

ACE inhibitors and nifedipine may be used in patients with chronic severe AR and HF pending valve replacement.

DON'T BE TRICKED

- Do not select β-blockers or intra-aortic balloon pumps for patients with acute AR because both may worsen the AR.
- Therapy with ACE Inhibitors or calcium channel blockers does not delay the need for surgery in asymptomatic patients with chronic AR.

Follow-Up

Recommended follow-up involves obtaining history and physical examination, focusing on findings consistent with HF, and serial echocardiography (TTE), with intervals determined by AR severity (mild, moderate, or severe).

TEST YOURSELF

A 36-year-old man with aortic valve endocarditis is transferred to the ICU because of the abrupt onset of hypotension and hypoxemia. Physical examination findings include a BP of 80/30 mm Hg, HR of 120/min, bilateral crackles, and a gallop. No murmurs are heard.

ANSWER: For diagnosis, choose acute AR. For management, select echocardiography, IV sodium nitroprusside, and dobutamine as a bridge to urgent surgery.

Mitral Stenosis

Diagnosis

Mitral stenosis usually presents 20 to 40 years after an episode of RF, although calcific degenerative mitral stenosis is also common and unrelated to RF. The most common symptoms are fatigue, orthopnea and paroxysmal nocturnal dyspnea, and lower extremity swelling. Patients may have a history of AF or systemic thromboembolism. Physical examination findings include:

- a prominent *a* wave in the jugular pulse
- a prominent tapping apical impulse
- signs of right-sided HF (increased JVD, lower extremity edema)
- accentuation of the P_2 and an opening snap
- a low-pitched, rumbling diastolic murmur with presystolic accentuation

Chest x-ray shows an enlarged pulmonary artery, left atrium, right ventricle, and right atrium. The ECG shows RV hypertrophy and a notched P-wave duration >0.12 s in lead II (P mitrale).

TTE is used to assess disease severity of mitral stenosis by measuring valve area and transvalvular gradient. TEE provides better visualization for the presence of left atrial appendage thrombus.

Treatment

Percutaneous balloon mitral commissurotomy is indicated for symptomatic patients (NYHA functional class II, III, or IV) and for asymptomatic patients when the valve area is <1.0 cm^2.

Valvular characteristics that favor a successful percutaneous commissurotomy include the presence of pliable leaflets, minimal commissural fusion, and minimal valvular or subvalvular calcification. Concurrent MR and left atrial thrombus are contraindications to valvulotomy.

Mitral valve surgery (repair if possible) is indicated in patients with symptomatic (NYHA functional class III-IV) mitral stenosis when balloon valvotomy is unavailable or contraindicated or the valve morphology is unfavorable.

Medical therapy for mitral stenosis consists of diuretics or long-acting nitrates, which may help improve symptoms such as dyspnea. In addition, β-blockers or nondihydropyridine calcium channel blockers can lower HR and improve LV diastolic filling time.

TEST YOURSELF

A 28-year-old woman who is 29 weeks pregnant has progressive dyspnea. Physical examination shows tachycardia, JVD, a parasternal impulse, an opening snap, and a grade 2/6 diastolic rumble with presystolic accentuation.

ANSWER: This is the classic presentation for mitral stenosis with associated increased intravascular volume in a pregnant patient. For management, select metoprolol to allow greater time for LV diastolic filling and relief of PH.

DON'T BE TRICKED

- **Treat all patients with mitral stenosis and AF, regardless of CHA_2DS_2-VASc score, with warfarin.**

Mitral Regurgitation

Diagnosis

MR may be either acute or chronic. Acute MR most often occurs in patients with chordae tendineae rupture resulting from myxomatous valve disease or endocarditis. In the setting of an MI, consider papillary muscle dysfunction or rupture. Characteristic findings in acute MR include the abrupt onset of dyspnea, pulmonary edema, or cardiogenic shock. Physical examination shows left-sided HF associated with a holosystolic murmur at the apex that radiates to the axilla and occasionally to the base. The murmur may be short or absent in patients with acute MR. A soft S_3 and P_2 are usually heard.

Causes of chronic MR include:

- MVP
- IE
- HCM
- ischemic heart disease
- ventricular dilatation
- Marfan syndrome

TTE serves as the main imaging modality in the evaluation and management of MR.

Treatment

Surgery is first-line therapy for:

- acute MR
- chronic symptomatic MR
- asymptomatic MR with LVEF <60% or LV end-systolic diameter >40 mm
- PH caused by MR
- new-onset AF
- chronic severe primary MR when another cardiac surgery is planned

Options are mitral valve repair (preferred) or mitral valve replacement. MR resulting from ischemia-induced dysfunction of the papillary muscle should improve after appropriate revascularization.

Medical therapy is used to stabilize decompensated HF in patients with acute or chronic MR. Nitrates (nitroprusside) and diuretics reduce filling pressures in acute severe MR. Inotropic agents, an intra-aortic balloon pump, or other means of circulatory support may be added in the setting of hypotension.

DON'T BE TRICKED

- **ACE inhibitors and ARBs have not been shown to be effective in preventing progression of LV dysfunction in patients with chronic MR.**

TEST YOURSELF

A 63-year-old man who is asymptomatic and active is found to have MR during a physical examination. LV systolic dimension is 51 mm and the EF is 52%.

ANSWER: For treatment, select mitral valve replacement or repair.

Mitral Valve Prolapse

Diagnosis

MVP is the most common cause of significant MR, but most patients with prolapse have either minimal or no MR. MVP syndrome is usually asymptomatic but can cause chest pain, palpitations, syncope, dyspnea, and embolic phenomena. On physical examination, a high-pitched midsystolic click is heard followed by a late systolic murmur that is loudest at the apex. Standing from a sitting position and performing the Valsalva maneuver causes the click and murmur to occur earlier (closer to S_1). Squatting from a standing position delays the click (moves closer to S_2) and murmur and decreases the intensity. The initial diagnostic study is echocardiography. Patients with symptoms of arrhythmia require ambulatory ECG monitoring.

Treatment

Treat patients with palpitations, chest pain, anxiety, or fatigue with β-blockers. Aspirin is appropriate for patients with unexplained TIA who have sinus rhythm and no atrial thrombi. Warfarin is indicated for patients with recurrent ischemic neurologic events despite aspirin. Surgery is required for significant MR, a flail leaflet caused by a ruptured chorda, or marked chordal elongation.

TEST YOURSELF

A 28-year-old woman has palpitations. Cardiac examination is normal except for an isolated click. Echocardiography is also normal except for mild MR, and 24-hour ECG monitoring shows 728 isolated, unifocal PVCs.

ANSWER: For management, choose to provide reassurance and counsel on lifestyle modification (reduction of caffeine and other stimulants).

Tricuspid Regurgitation

Diagnosis

Primary causes of TR include Marfan syndrome and congenital disorders such as Ebstein anomaly (abnormalities of the tricuspid valve and right ventricle) and AV canal malformations. Common secondary causes include IE, carcinoid syndrome, PH, and RF. Physical examination shows prominent *v* waves in the neck, increased JVD during inspiration, and hepatic pulsations. Patients with severe disease may have ascites and pedal edema. A holosystolic murmur is heard at the left lower sternal border, increasing in intensity during inspiration. Echocardiography is diagnostic.

Treatment

Consider tricuspid valve surgery in patients undergoing left-sided valve surgery who have severe tricuspid regurgitation or in patients with symptomatic tricuspid regurgitation unresponsive to medical management.

DON'T BE TRICKED

- Mild or less severe TR is common, can be easily identified by echocardiography, is physiologically normal, and does not require treatment.

Prosthetic Heart Valves

Characteristics

Mechanical valves are more durable than bioprosthetic valves but require lifelong anticoagulation. Prosthetic valves in the aortic position are more durable and less prone to thromboembolism than valves in the mitral position.

Complications

Common complications include structural valve deterioration, valve thrombosis, embolism, bleeding, and endocarditis. In the immediate postoperative period, valve dehiscence or dysfunction should be suspected in patients who develop acute HF. Valve dysfunction is characterized by new cardiac symptoms, embolic phenomena, hemolytic anemia (with schistocytes on peripheral blood smear), or new murmurs. If valve dysfunction is suspected, TEE is the diagnostic procedure of choice.

Anticoagulation

Lifelong oral anticoagulation with warfarin is recommended for all patients with a mechanical prosthesis. Target INRs are:

- 2.5 for an aortic prosthetic valve without thromboembolism risk factors
- 3.0 for aortic prosthetic valve with thromboembolism risk factors

All patients with mechanical prosthetic valves of any type, and most patients with bioprostheses, should receive aspirin therapy.

Keep the following in mind:

- Interrupt anticoagulation in patients with a prosthetic heart valve before they undergo noncardiac or dental surgery (but not cataract surgery).
- For aortic valve prostheses, stop warfarin 4 to 5 days before the procedure and restart as soon as postprocedure control of bleeding allows.
- In patients at high risk for thrombosis (mitral prostheses, multiple prosthetic valves, AF, or previous thromboembolic events), stop warfarin 4 to 5 days before surgery and begin bridging anticoagulation with IV heparin; resume IV heparin within 24 hours after surgery. Warfarin is also reinitiated after surgery, and heparin is discontinued when INR is therapeutic.

DON'T BE TRICKED

- **Begin long-term anticoagulation only for patients with mechanical heart valves.**
- **Select only warfarin for anticoagulation of mechanical heart valves. Do not select a NOAC (e.g., dabigatran, rivaroxaban).**

Atrial Septal Defect

Diagnosis

Findings of ASD include fixed splitting of the S_2, a pulmonary midsystolic murmur, and tricuspid diastolic flow murmur.

The most common form of ASD is the ostium secundum defect, which usually occurs as an isolated abnormality. The ECG shows right axis deviation and partial RBBB. The ostium primum ASD is often associated with a cleft in the mitral or tricuspid valve with associated valve regurgitation. A VSD may also be present.

Treatment

Closure is indicated for right atrial or right ventricular enlargement, large left to right shunt, or symptoms (dyspnea, paradoxical embolism). Select percutaneous device closure for ostium secundum ASD and surgical closure for ostium primum ASD and associated mitral valve defects. Pregnancy in patients with ASD is generally well tolerated in the absence of PH.

DON'T BE TRICKED

- Closure of an ASD is contraindicated if shunt reversal (right to left) is present.
- A small ASD with no associated symptoms or right heart enlargement can be followed clinically.

TEST YOURSELF

An asymptomatic 26-year-old woman who is 30 weeks pregnant has a recently discovered heart murmur. Physical examination shows a right parasternal lift, a normal S_1, fixed splitting of S_2, and a grade 2/6 early systolic murmur at the upper left sternal border.

ANSWER: For diagnosis, choose ASD. The murmur is often first discovered during pregnancy as a result of increased intravascular volume.

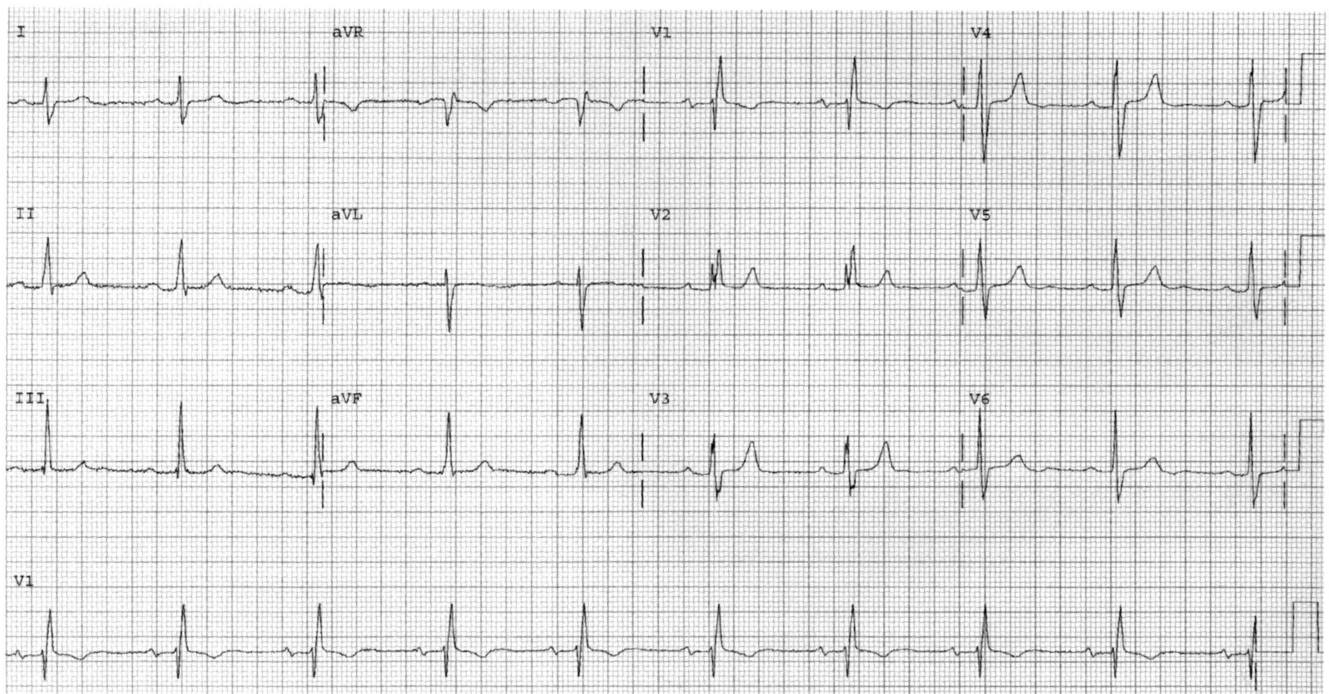

Ostium Secundum Atrial Septal Defect: The ECG shows right axis deviation, partial RBBB, and evidence of RV hypertrophy characteristic of ostium secundum ASD.

Coarctation of the Aorta

Diagnosis

Coarctation of the aorta is a congenital disorder that may not be discovered until young adulthood. Characteristic findings include hypertension, diminished femoral pulses, radial-to-femoral pulse delay, and a continuous murmur audible over the back. In patients with aortic coarctation and a bicuspid aortic valve, an ejection click or a systolic murmur may be heard.

Imaging

A chest x-ray shows the classic "figure 3" sign (an indented aortic wall at the site of the coarctation with dilatation above and below the coarctation) and notching on the undersides of the posterior ribs. TTE is confirmatory. CMR imaging and CT are recommended to identify the anatomy, severity, and location of the coarctation. Cardiac catheterization is used in patients in whom intervention is being considered.

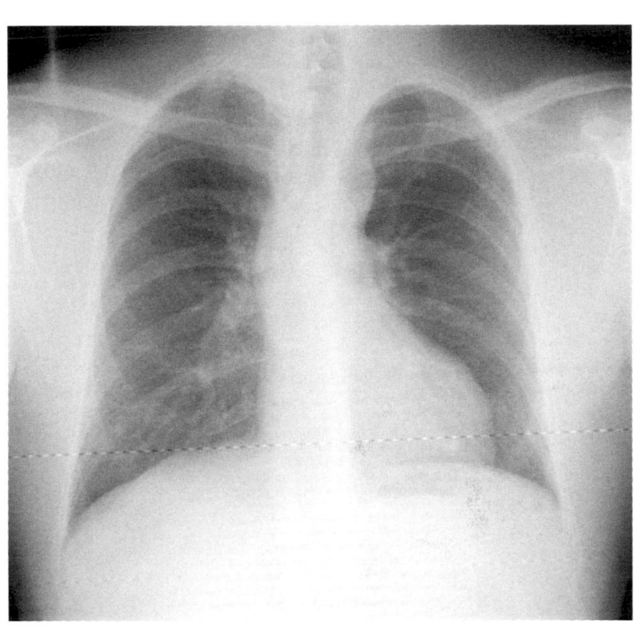

Aortic Coarctation: A chest x-ray shows inferior rib notching and the classic "figure 3" sign (an indented aortic wall at the site of the coarctation with dilatation above and below the coarctation).

DON'T BE TRICKED

- Obtain BP in the legs in young people presenting with unexplained hypertension.

Treatment

Schedule balloon dilation for patients with a discrete area of aortic narrowing, proximal hypertension, and a pressure gradient >20 mm Hg. Hypertension persists or recurs in up to 75% of patients following coarctation repair.

TEST YOURSELF

A 35-year-old female immigrant reports cold feet and leg cramping when walking long distances. BP is 160/90 mm Hg. Cardiac examination shows a sustained apical impulse, an early systolic ejection sound, and an early systolic murmur at the upper right sternal border.

ANSWER: For diagnosis, choose coarctation of the aorta with an associated bicuspid aortic valve. Be alert for congenital heart disease in questions featuring an adult immigrant patient.

Patent Ductus Arteriosus

Diagnosis

Patients with a moderate-sized PDA may present with symptoms of dyspnea and HF. A continuous "machinery" murmur is heard beneath the left clavicle. Bounding pulses and a wide pulse pressure may also be noted. A large PDA causes a large left-to-right shunt and, if unrepaired, may cause PH with eventual shunt reversal from right-to-left (Eisenmenger syndrome).

A characteristic feature of an Eisenmenger PDA is clubbing and oxygen desaturation that affects the feet but not the hands (differential cyanosis).

Treatment

Closure of a PDA is indicated for left-sided cardiac chamber enlargement in the absence of severe PH. A tiny PDA without other findings requires no intervention.

Patent Foramen Ovale

Diagnosis

The foramen ovale usually closes within the first few weeks of life. In 25% to 30% of the population, however, the foramen ovale remains patent. PFO is usually asymptomatic and identified incidentally and, in these cases, no treatment or follow-up is needed. The prevalence of PFO is increased in patients with cryptogenic stroke. PFO is diagnosed by visualizing the interatrial septum by echocardiography, and demonstrating shunting of blood across the defect by color flow Doppler imaging or by using agitated saline.

Treatment

Percutaneous PFO closure plus aspirin therapy is beneficial in the prevention of recurrent stroke in patients with cryptogenic stroke.

Ventricular Septal Defect

Diagnosis

A small VSD causes a loud holosystolic murmur that obliterates the S_2. A displaced apical LV impulse and mitral diastolic flow rumble suggest a hemodynamically important VSD. TTE demonstrates the hemodynamic impact of a VSD.

Treatment

Consider closure in adults with progressive regurgitation of the aortic or tricuspid valve, progressive LV volume overload, and recurrent endocarditis. Device closure is possible in patients with muscular VSD. Without closure, large VSDs cause PH with eventual right-to-left shunt (Eisenmenger syndrome). At this stage, closure is contraindicated. Pulmonary vasodilators may be used for progressive symptoms.

Infective Endocarditis

Prevention

Provide prophylaxis for IE only in patients with the highest risk, including those with:

- prosthetic cardiac valve
- history of IE
- unrepaired cyanotic congenital heart disease
- repaired congenital heart defect with prosthesis or shunt (≤6 months post-procedure) or residual defect
- valvulopathy following cardiac transplantation
- prosthetic material used for cardiac valve repair (annuloplasty rings and chords)

Prophylaxis is only indicated for the highest risk procedures:

- dental procedures that involve mucosal bleeding
- procedures that involve incision or biopsy of the respiratory mucosa
- procedures in patients with ongoing GI or GU tract infection
- procedures on infected skin, skin structures, or musculoskeletal tissue
- surgery to place prosthetic heart valves or prosthetic intravascular or intracardiac materials

Most patients requiring prophylaxis will be undergoing dental procedures, and the indicated antibiotic is oral amoxicillin 30 to 60 minutes before the procedure. If the patient is allergic to penicillin, use cephalexin, azithromycin, clarithromycin, or clindamycin.

Diagnosis

Fever, malaise, and fatigue are sensitive but nonspecific symptoms associated with IE. Suggestive physical examination findings include:

- new cardiac murmur
- new-onset HF
- conduction abnormalities on ECG (suggests perivalvular abscess)
- petechiae, splinter hemorrhages
- Osler nodes (violaceous, circumscribed, painful nodules found in the pulp of the fingers and toes)
- Janeway lesions (painless, erythematous, macular lesions found on the soles and palms)
- Roth spots (hemorrhagic lesions of the retina)
- leukocytosis, anemia, and hematuria
- focal neurologic signs (septic emboli)
- multiple bilateral small nodules on chest x-ray (septic emboli)

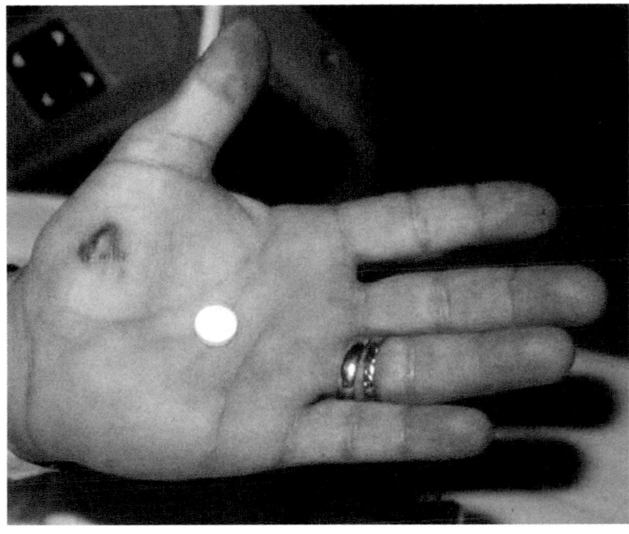

Osler Nodes: Osler nodes are red to purple painful papules, papulopustules, or nodules found in the pulp of fingers or occasionally hands and feet.

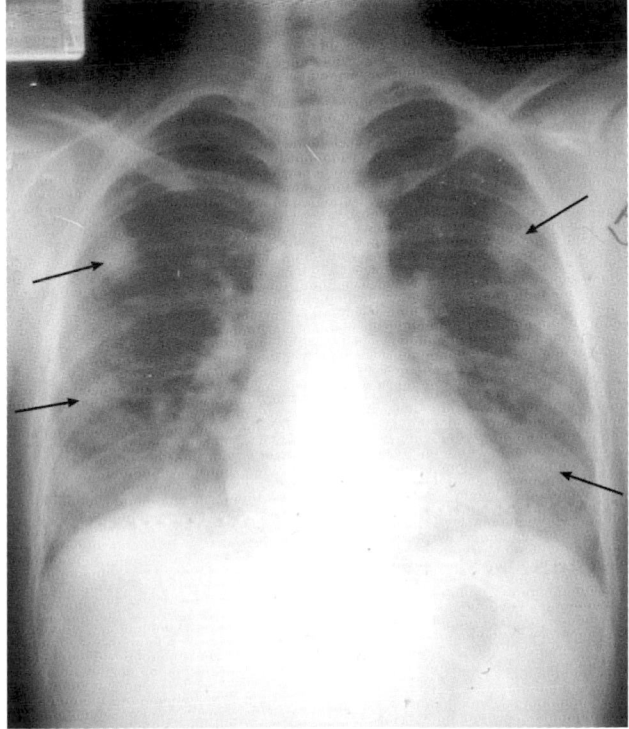

Septic Pulmonary Emboli: Septic pulmonary emboli are characterized by multifocal, patchy, and otherwise ill-defined infiltrates; cavitation may occur.

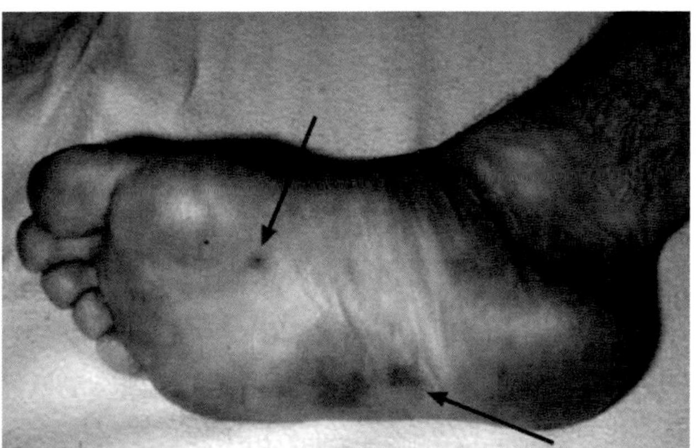

Janeway Lesions: Janeway lesions are macular, erythematous, nontender microabscesses in the dermis of the palms and soles caused by septic emboli that are considered pathognomonic for IE.

TTE is sufficient to rule out IE in low-probability patients, but a TEE is indicated to rule-in IE in patients with high probability of disease. Obtain a TEE particularly in the setting of *Staphylococcus aureus* bacteremia. TEE is the test of choice to identify a paravalvular abscess.

Diagnose endocarditis in patients with two major Duke criteria, one major and three minor criteria, five minor criteria, or pathological confirmation.

STUDY TABLE: Diagnosing Endocarditis with Modified Duke Criteria

Major Duke Criteria	Minor Duke Criteria
Positive blood culture for endocarditis × 2 or single positive blood culture for *Coxiella burnetii* or antiphase I IgG antibody titer >1:800	Predisposing heart condition or injection drug use
Positive echocardiogram	Fever
New valvular regurgitation	Embolic vascular phenomena
	Immunologic phenomena (GN or rheumatoid factor)
	Positive blood culture not meeting major criteria

DON'T BE TRICKED

- Don't give antimicrobial prophylaxis to patients with MVP or other low-risk valvular abnormalities.
- Look for colon cancer in patients with *Streptococcus bovis* or *Clostridium septicum* endocarditis.

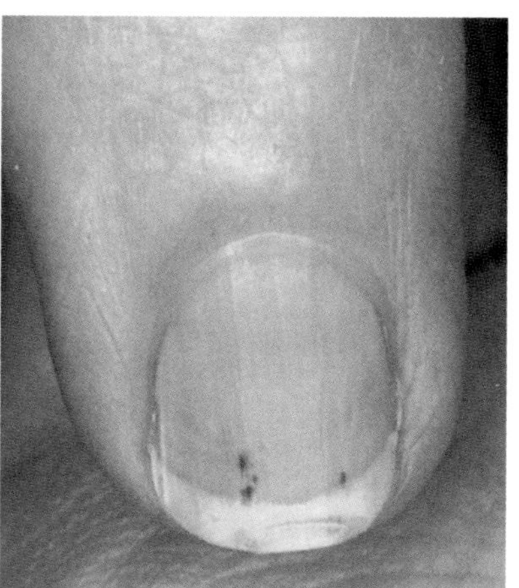

Splinter Hemorrhages: A fingernail with splinter hemorrhages, which are non-blanching, linear, reddish-brown lesions found under the nail bed. Reprinted from Sparkla / Wikimedia Commons / Public Domain.

Treatment

Indications for surgery include:

- valvular dysfunction and acute HF
- left-sided IE caused by *S. aureus*, fungal infection, or highly resistant organisms
- heart block
- annular or aortic abscess
- systemic embolization on antibiotic therapy
- prosthetic valve endocarditis with relapsing infection or dehiscence
- *S. aureus* prosthetic valve endocarditis

Patients with suspected IE and good cardiovascular function do not require empiric treatment before culture results. In decompensated patients, start empiric antibiotics immediately after blood cultures are obtained.

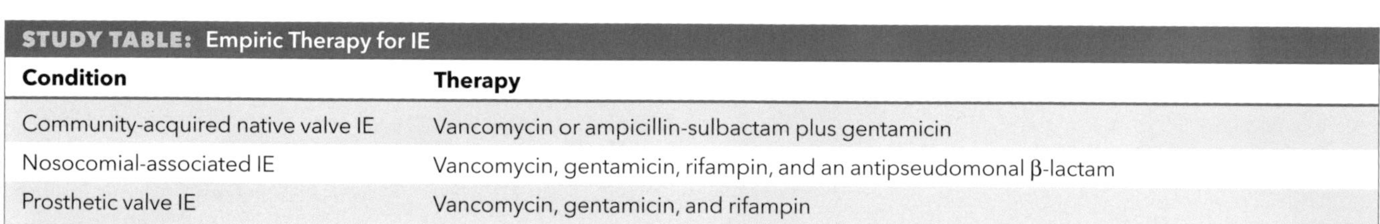

STUDY TABLE: Empiric Therapy for IE

Condition	Therapy
Community-acquired native valve IE	Vancomycin or ampicillin-sulbactam plus gentamicin
Nosocomial-associated IE	Vancomycin, gentamicin, rifampin, and an antipseudomonal β-lactam
Prosthetic valve IE	Vancomycin, gentamicin, and rifampin

Narrow antibiotic selection after susceptibilities are known. Continue treatment for 4 to 6 weeks except in uncomplicated right-sided native valve endocarditis caused by MSSA, which can be treated for 2 weeks with a combination of nafcillin, oxacillin, or flucloxacillin.

DON'T BE TRICKED

- Oral antibiotics are not recommended for treatment of IE.

Thoracic Aortic Aneurysm and Dissection

Screening

Perform screening echocardiography of first-degree relatives of patients with familial thoracic aneurysm syndromes such as familial thoracic aortic aneurysms and aortic dissections (TAAD), bicuspid aortic valve, Marfan syndrome, Turner syndrome, and Loeys-Dietz syndrome.

Diagnosis

Most thoracic aortic aneurysms are asymptomatic and are typically incidental findings on imaging studies. Patients present with symptoms attributable to compression or distortion of adjacent structures, such as hoarseness, dysphagia, recurrent pneumonia, and SVC syndrome. The most common risk factors in younger patients include Marfan syndrome, cocaine abuse, and bicuspid aortic valve. Poorly controlled hypertension is a risk factor in older patients.

Aortic dissection symptoms include chest and tearing back pain. Physical examination findings may include new AR, HF, and a BP differential between the arms. A widened mediastinum is seen on chest x-ray. Patients may also have evidence of thromboembolism, dissection of branch arteries (stroke, MI), or cardiac tamponade. A low D-dimer level (<500 ng/mL) helps rule out an acute aortic syndrome. Dissections involving the ascending aorta are classified as type A, and all other dissections are classified as type B.

The diagnosis is established by TEE, CTA, or MRA. Bedside TEE is used for critically ill patients who cannot be moved.

TEST YOURSELF

A 50-year-old man is evaluated for severe chest pain and left hemiparesis.

ANSWER: For diagnosis, choose aortic dissection with involvement of the right carotid artery.

Treatment

For thoracic aneurysms, β-blockers reduce the rate of thoracic aortic dilation in patients with Marfan syndrome. Prophylactic surgery is recommended for the following clinical situations in patients with ascending thoracic aortic aneurysm:

- aortic diameter >5.0 cm (>4.5-5.0 cm for Marfan syndrome)
- aortic diameter >4.5 cm and undergoing other heart surgery
- rapid growth >0.5 cm/yr

For acute dissection, begin IV β-blocker therapy; add nitroprusside if BP does not respond to IV β-blocker therapy. Emergent surgery is required for type A dissection (involving the ascending aorta) or intramural hematoma. Uncomplicated type B dissection (descending dissection of the thoracic aorta) is treated with continued medical therapy alone with the exception of patients with complications, including end-organ ischemia.

Follow-Up

Annual echocardiography is recommended if the aortic diameter has been stable and <4.5 cm. If the aortic diameter is ≥4.5 cm or the rate of enlargement >0.5 cm/year, imaging should be performed every 6 months.

DON'T BE TRICKED

- **Do not use hydralazine for acute aortic dissection because it increases shear stress.**
- **Schedule surgery for type B dissection if major aortic vessels, such as renal arteries, are involved.**

TEST YOURSELF

A 73-year-old man has a 1-hour history of severe, tearing substernal chest pain. BP is 90/60 mm Hg in the right arm and 130/70 mm Hg in the left arm. A chest x-ray shows a widened mediastinum.

ANSWER: For diagnosis, choose dissection of the aortic arch. For acute management, select β-blockers, sodium nitroprusside, and emergent imaging studies.

Abdominal Aortic Aneurysm

Screening

One-time ultrasonographic screening is indicated to detect an asymptomatic AAA in any man between the ages of 65 and 75 years who has ever smoked and in selected men ages 65 to 75 years who have never smoked (e.g., family history of AAA).

DON'T BE TRICKED

- Do not screen women for AAA.

Diagnosis

Most chronic AAAs are asymptomatic. Signs and symptoms of a ruptured AAA include new abdominal, flank, or back pain; hypotension; syncope; and sudden collapse and shock. The diagnosis is confirmed by MRA or CT.

DON'T BE TRICKED

- Ultrasonography is not accurate for diagnosing a ruptured AAA.

Treatment

Therapy includes treatment of cardiovascular risk factors. Schedule surgical or endovascular repair of AAAs ≥5.5 cm in diameter, those growing ≥0.5 cm per year, or symptomatic AAAs. Ruptured AAA requires emergent surgery or endovascular repair.

Follow-Up

Patients with an unrepaired AAA require ultrasonographic monitoring at 6- to 12-month intervals if the AAA measures 4.0 to 5.4 cm and every 2 to 3 years for smaller AAAs.

Aortic Atheroemboli

Diagnosis

Plaque in the thoracic aorta is associated with an increased risk of clinical thromboembolism, including stroke. Characteristic findings include livedo reticularis, gangrene of the digits (blue toe syndrome), and transient vision loss (a golden or brightly refractile cholesterol body within a retinal artery [Hollenhorst plaque] is pathognomonic). Patients often present with stroke or AKI following recent cardiac or aortic surgery or other intravascular procedures (catheterization).

Testing

Thrombocytopenia, eosinophilia, and urinary eosinophils may be present. Biopsy of muscle, skin, kidney, or other organs confirms the diagnosis.

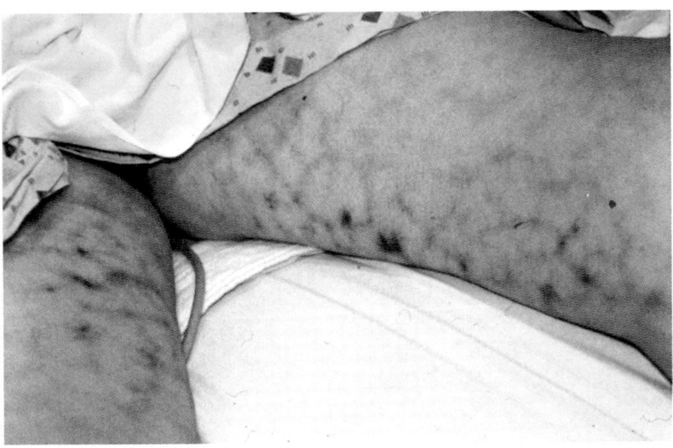

Livedo Reticularis: Livedo reticularis in the lower extremities caused by cholesterol emboli following cardiac catheterization.

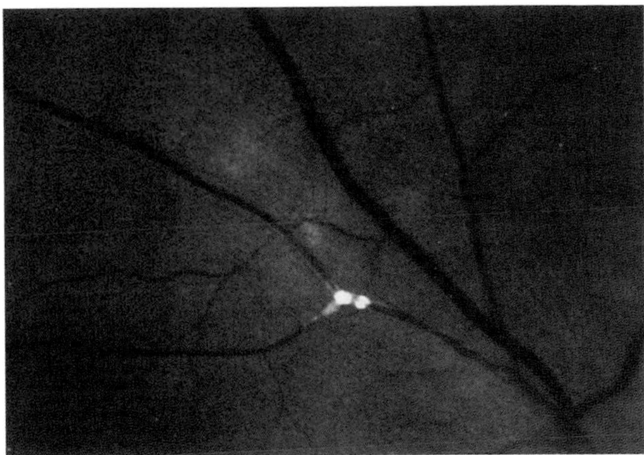

Hollenhorst Plaque: A highly refractile yellow body (cholesterol crystals) within a retinal artery.

Treatment

Treatment is control of cardiovascular risk factors.

DON'T BE TRICKED

- **Asymptomatic aortic atheroma should be aggressively treated with antiplatelet agents and statins to reduce the risk of future cardiovascular events.**

TEST YOURSELF

A 67-year-old man has AKI following coronary angiography 10 days ago. BP is 168/100 mm Hg. Bruits are noted over the abdomen and femoral arteries. His legs have a lacy, purplish discoloration. Urinalysis shows eosinophils.

ANSWER: For diagnosis, choose cholesterol emboli to the skin and renal vasculature. For management, select skin biopsy and control all cardiovascular risk factors.

Peripheral Artery Disease

Screening

The USPSTF has concluded that the current evidence is insufficient to recommend routine screening for PAD. ACC/AHA guidelines suggest that screening is reasonable in high-risk patients, including patients of any age with known atherosclerotic disease in another vascular bed.

Diagnosis

PAD most commonly involves the lower extremities and is the result of atherosclerosis involving the aorta and branch vessels. Clinical risk factors include:

- age
- smoking
- diabetes mellitus
- hyperlipidemia

Intermittent claudication is the classic sign of PAD. Most patients with PAD have coexisting coronary artery and cerebrovascular disease.

Differentiate claudication caused by PAD from claudication caused by spinal stenosis.

STUDY TABLE: Discriminating Claudication from Pseudoclaudication

Characteristic	Claudication	Pseudoclaudication (Spinal Stenosis)
Nature of discomfort	Cramping, tightness, aching, fatigue	Same as claudication plus tingling, burning, numbness, weakness
Location of discomfort	Buttock, hip, thigh, calf, foot	Same as claudication; most often bilateral
Exercise-induced	Yes	Variable
Walking distance at onset of symptoms	Consistent	Variable
Discomfort occurs with standing still	No	Yes
Action for relief	Stand or sit	Sit, flexion at the waist
Time to relief	<5 minutes	≤30 minutes

Testing

Resting ABI should be performed on all patients with a history or physical examination suggesting PAD. Exercise treadmill ABI testing should be performed for patients with normal or borderline resting ABI values and unexplained exertional leg symptoms. Noninvasive angiography with duplex ultrasonography, CTA, or MRA is performed for anatomic delineation of PAD in patients requiring surgical or endovascular intervention.

Interpret the ABI:

- ABI for each side is the ratio of the highest systolic arm BP (regardless of side) compared with the highest systolic ankle BP for that side.
- Normal ABI is >0.9 to ≤1.40.
- ABI ≤0.90 is compatible with PAD.
- ABI ≤0.40 is associated with ischemic rest pain.
- False-normal ABI occurs in patients with diabetes with calcified, noncompressible arteries (ABI >1.40).

Recall the "six Ps" to diagnose acute limb ischemia:

- Pain
- Paresthesias
- Pallor
- Paralysis
- Pulselessness
- Poikilothermia (coolness)

Acute ischemia can be caused by in-situ thrombosis or remote embolization. Diagnostic angiography should be performed immediately in patients with acute limb ischemia to define the anatomic level of occlusion. Angiography is used to locate the embolic source of acute ischemia.

DON'T BE TRICKED

- When the ABI is >1.40, select a toe-brachial index to provide a better assessment of lower extremity perfusion.

Treatment

Exercise training is the most effective treatment for improvement in functional status in patients with PAD.

PAD is a CAD risk equivalent. Therapy includes:

- BP goal <130/80 mm Hg
- aspirin (preferred over clopidogrel)
- high-intensity statin therapy
- cilostazol for patients with intermittent claudication

Select angioplasty or surgery for patients who do not improve with medical therapy or have pain at rest or poorly healing ulcers.

Patients with acute limb ischemia require antiplatelet agents and heparin anticoagulation as well as urgent surgical consultation.

DON'T BE TRICKED

- PAD alone is not an indication for anticoagulation.
- Do not use cilostazol in patients with a low LVEF or history of HF.
- β-Blockers are not contraindicated in patients with PAD.

TEST YOURSELF

A 60-year-old man has a 6-month history of claudication in both thighs and calves. ABI is 0.66 on the right side and 0.55 on the left side. He is symptomatic despite an intensive lifestyle management program.

ANSWER: For treatment, begin cilostazol.

Cardiac Tumors

Diagnosis

The most common cardiac tumors are metastatic. Melanoma, malignant thymoma, and germ cell tumors have the highest metastatic potential.

Primary cardiac tumors are rare. The most common benign primary cardiac tumors in adults are myxomas. Patients with myxomas may have constitutional symptoms such as fever, anorexia, and weight loss. The auscultatory findings resemble mitral stenosis murmur with an accompanying sound of a "tumor plop." Embolization may cause neurologic symptoms.

Testing

Imaging (echocardiography, CT, or CMR imaging) is diagnostic for cardiac tumors. Myxomas characteristically are pedunculated and arise most commonly in the left atrium with the stalk adherent to the fossa ovalis, whereas angiosarcomas typically arise in the right atrium.

DON'T BE TRICKED

- Auscultatory findings of atrial myxoma may mimic those of mitral stenosis.

Treatment

Myxomas should be resected after diagnosis because of the risk of embolization and cardiovascular complications, including the potential for sudden death.

Dermatology

Eczemas

Diagnosis

Eczematous dermatitis is a type of inflammation characterized by inflamed, dry, red, itchy skin. Dry skin, intense pruritus with erythematous papules and vesicles, crusting, and oozing are typical of acute eczema. Lichenification (skin thickening from chronic scratching, with scaling and fissuring) defines chronic eczema.

Common types of eczematous dermatitis include:

- atopic dermatitis
- contact dermatitis
- dyshidrotic eczema
- xerotic (asteatotic) eczema
- venous stasis dermatitis

Atopic dermatitis is the development of eczema in patients with an inherited atopic diathesis. Look for:

- a waxing and waning course
- acute lesions consisting of pruritic, erythematous papules and plaques that may be vesicular and weeping
- chronic lesions that may be lichenified and hyperkeratotic
- involvement of the periocular areas and flexural surfaces, including posterior neck, antecubital and popliteal fossae, wrists, and ankles
- complicating *Staphylococcus aureus* infection evidenced by pustules, crusting, and erosions
- the atopic triad of allergic rhinitis, asthma, and eczema

Contact dermatitis includes allergic contact dermatitis (type IV hypersensitivity reaction) and irritant contact dermatitis.

Allergic contact dermatitis is precipitated by local absorption of an allergen or irritant through the stratum corneum. With repeated exposure, an itchy eczematous dermatitis develops on the area that was exposed. A secondary "id" reaction may develop: a generalized acute eczematous reaction that develops in areas not exposed to the allergen. Causative allergens ("triggers") are identified by epicutaneous patch testing and include:

- nickel
- topical anesthetics
- neomycin and bacitracin
- transdermal medication patches
- strong soaps, fragrances, or personal care products
- rubber
- poison oak, poison ivy

Irritant contact dermatitis occurs as a direct toxic effect from exposure to a chemical such as a cleaning agent or other caustic substance; for example, over-washing.

Dyshidrotic eczema (pompholyx) is an itchy eruption of small vesicles on the sides of the fingers and palms that can occur from wetting and drying, sweating, or allergies.

Xerotic eczema usually occurs on the anterior shins of older persons with dry skin. Affected skin is red, dry, and cracked with multiple fine fissures. The dermatitis is more common in winter or in dry conditions.

DON'T BE TRICKED

- Neomycin and bacitracin, commonly used for wound care, can cause an allergic contact dermatitis that mimics a wound infection.

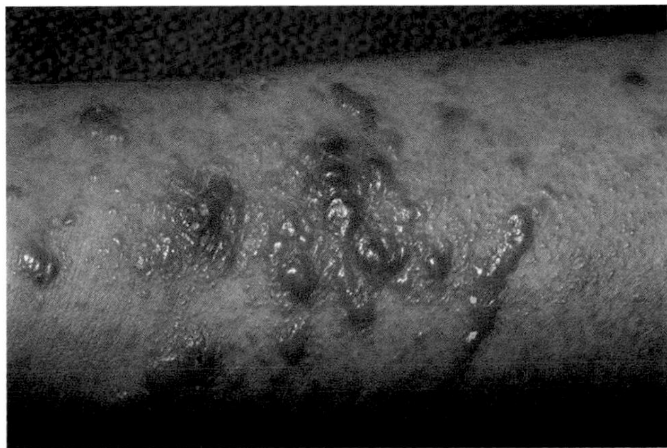

Contact Dermatitis: Discretely grouped red vesicles and bullae in a linear distribution are characteristic of contact dermatitis caused by poison ivy.

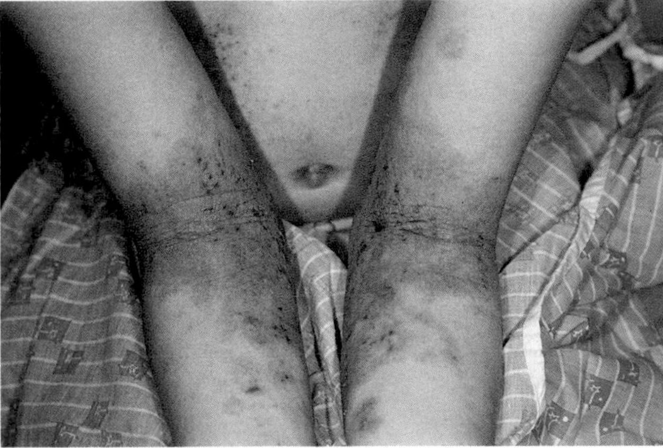

Atopic Dermatitis: Atopic eczema involves the antecubital fossae, with lichenification and surrounding excoriations.

Treatment

For irritant hand dermatitis, treat by washing less and moisturizing with emollients.

Contact dermatitis, atopic dermatitis, and dyshidrotic eczema may benefit from a short course of topical glucocorticoids for symptom relief.

- 1% topical hydrocortisone for the face and intertriginous areas (low-potency glucocorticoid)
- 0.1% triamcinolone for other body sites (medium-potency glucocorticoid)
- potent glucocorticoids for the palms, soles, and extremely thick eruptions

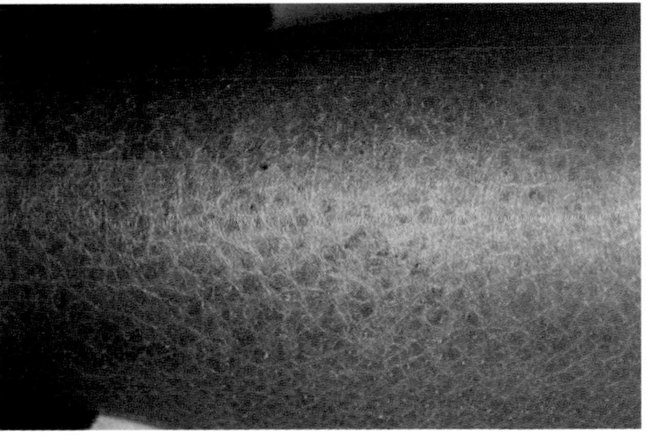

Xerotic (asteatotic) Dermatitis: Xerotic dermatitis is characterized by red, dry, cracked skin with multiple fine fissures, seen here on the anterior thigh.

Other treatments include:

- nighttime sedating antihistamines to reduce scratching
- topical tacrolimus for recalcitrant atopic eczema

Severe allergic contact eruptions may necessitate a 2- to 3-week taper of systemic glucocorticoids, although they have no role in long-term management.

Always select emollients as part of eczema treatment. Emollients work through various mechanisms, including trapping water in the skin (petrolatum), introducing water into the skin (aqueous cream), or increasing the water-holding capacity of the skin (urea).

DON'T BE TRICKED

- Do not select potent glucocorticoids for the face because of the risk of steroid-induced acne and cutaneous atrophy.

TEST YOURSELF

A healthy 40-year-old nurse has a 1-month history of vesicular eruptions on the dorsum and distal areas of her hands.

ANSWER: For diagnosis, choose acute eczema, likely secondary to latex gloves. For treatment, select a topical glucocorticoid and latex product avoidance.

Psoriasis

Diagnosis

Typical findings of chronic plaque psoriasis are erythema, scaling, and induration on the extensor surfaces, scalp, ears, intertriginous folds, and genitalia. The nails may be pitted, thickened, or yellow, with subungual debris and may be the only manifestation of psoriasis. Psoriatic arthritis and spondylitis may coexist in 25% of patients.

Psoriasis is exacerbated by systemic glucocorticoids, lithium, antimalarial drugs, tetracyclines, β-blockers, NSAIDs, and ACE inhibitors.

STUDY TABLE: Clinical Appearance of Common Psoriasis Subtypes

Subtype	Description
Chronic plaque psoriasis	Thick, erythematous lesions with silvery, adherent scale anywhere on the body
Guttate psoriasis	Many small drop-like papules and plaques on the trunk often developing after infection with β-hemolytic *Streptococcus*
Pustular psoriasis	Abrupt onset of generalized erythema and "lakes of pus," typically following abrupt discontinuation of glucocorticoids
Inverse psoriasis	Red, thin plaques with a variable amount of scale in the axillae, under the breasts or pannus, intergluteal cleft, and perineum
Nail psoriasis	Indentations, pits, and oil spots often involving multiple nails

Treatment

Select topical glucocorticoids for limited, localized plaques.

Rotate therapy with topical vitamin D analogues (calcipotriene, tacalcitol), retinoids, anthralin, or tar preparations.

Systemic glucocorticoids are not used to treat psoriasis. Patients receiving systemic glucocorticoids or cyclosporine are at risk for acute erythrodermic or pustular flares with sudden cessation of medication. Erythroderma is a dermatologic emergency because patients are at high risk for infection as well as electrolyte abnormalities secondary to fluid loss.

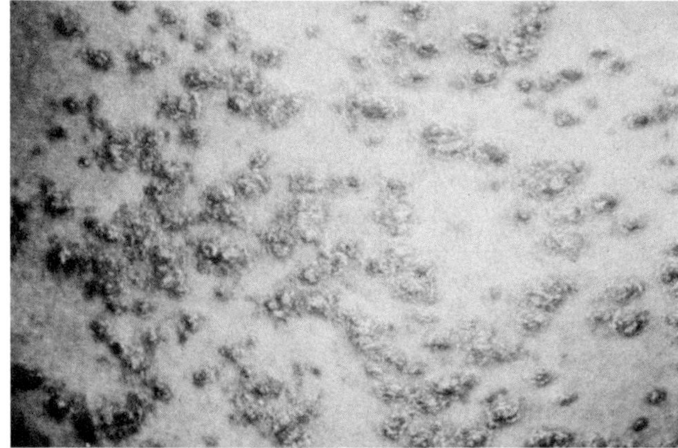

Guttate Psoriasis: Note the characteristic lesions consisting of multiple, discrete, droplike papules with a salmon-pink hue. A fine scale, which is usually absent in early-stage lesions, may be observed on more established lesions. Image reprinted with permission from Hon S. Pak, MD, FAAD, 3M Health Information Systems, published by Medscape Drugs & Diseases (http://emedicine.medscape.com/), Guttate Psoriasis, 2017, available at: https://emedicine.medscape.com/article/1107850-overview.

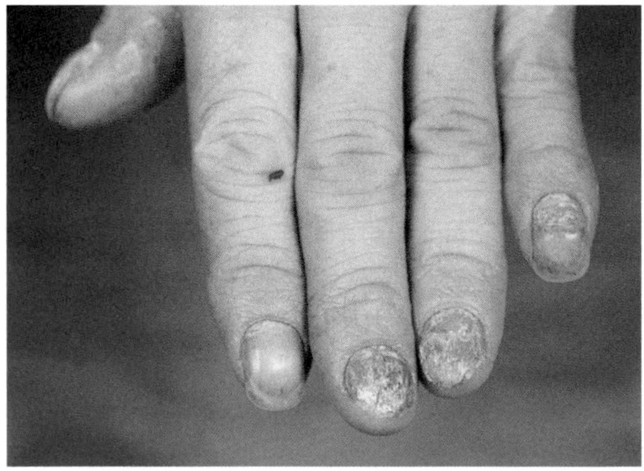

Nail Findings in Psoriasis: Psoriatic nails are shown, with characteristic discoloration, crumbling, subungual debris, and separation of the nail plate from the nail bed (white areas of nail).

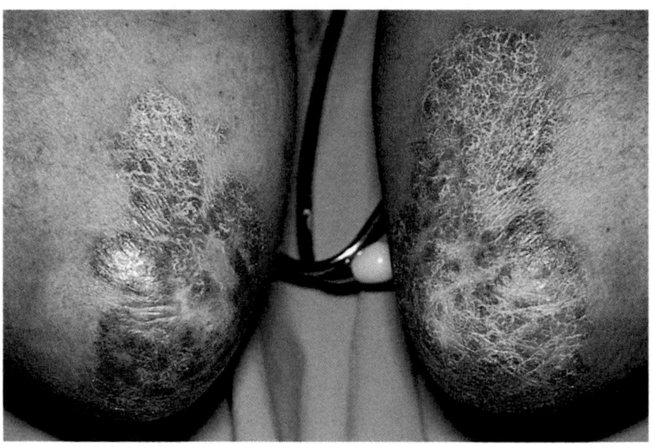

Chronic Plaque Psoriasis: The image depicts classic plaque psoriasis, showing erythematous plaques with a silvery scale on an extensor surface.

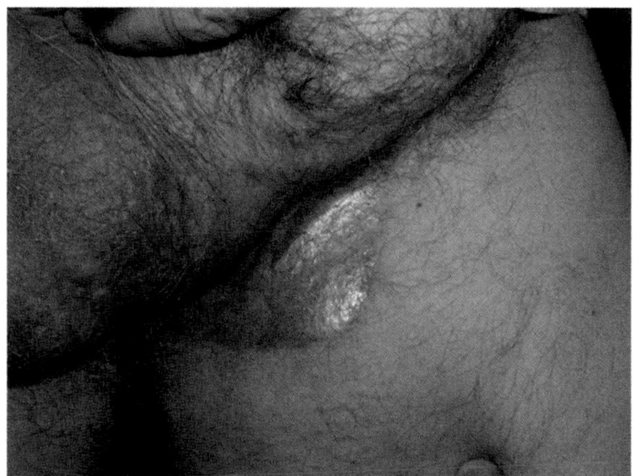

Inverse Psoriasis: Inverse psoriasis presents as a bright red, smooth patch in the folds of the skin, typically occurring under the breasts, in the armpits, near the genitals, under the buttocks, or in abdominal folds.

DON'T BE TRICKED

- Never select systemic glucocorticoids for the treatment of psoriasis.

TEST YOURSELF

A 28-year-old woman has a chronic extensive skin rash consisting of multiple small and large plaques with an adherent, thick, silvery scale.

ANSWER: For diagnosis, select psoriasis.

Other Papulosquamous Disorders

STUDY TABLE: Other Papulosquamous Disorders

Condition	Presentation	Therapy
Lichen planus	Acute eruption of purple, pruritic, polygonal papules that most commonly presents on the wrists and ankles. Lichen planus can also present in the mouth, vaginal vault, penis, and in the nails (leading to thickening and distortion of the nail plate).	Topical glucocorticoids
Pityriasis rosea	Presents with one herald patch that is a few centimeters wide followed by many 0.5- to 2.0-cm red scaling pruritic patches along the skin cleavage lines in a "Christmas tree" distribution on the trunk that last 1-3 months. Can mimic syphilis except for sparing the palms and soles.	Topical glucocorticoids and antihistamines for pruritus
Seborrheic dermatitis	An inflammatory, scaling, itchy dermatosis that most commonly affects the scalp but can also affect the eyebrows, nasolabial folds, chin, central chest, and perineum. Explosive onset with wide distribution may be a sign of HIV infection. Commonly seen in patients with Parkinson disease.	Selenium sulfide or zinc pyrithione shampoos, ketoconazole shampoo

DON'T BE TRICKED

- Extensive seborrheic dermatitis may be a clue to underlying HIV infection.

TEST YOURSELF

A 28-year-old man is evaluated for severe seborrheic dermatitis of acute onset.

ANSWER: For evaluation, order HIV testing.

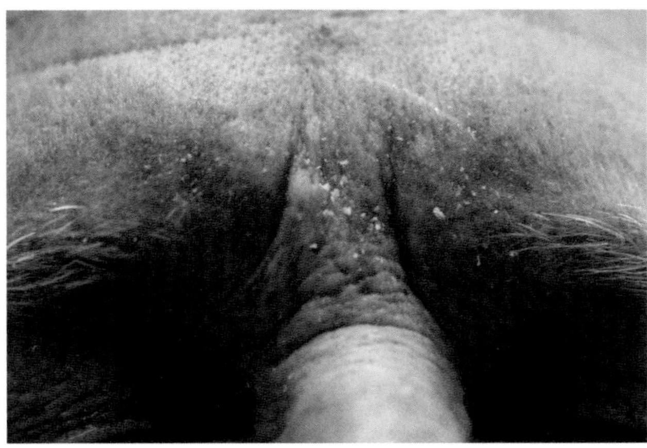

Seborrheic Dermatitis: Seborrheic dermatitis is shown, with fine, oily scale around the medial eyebrows.

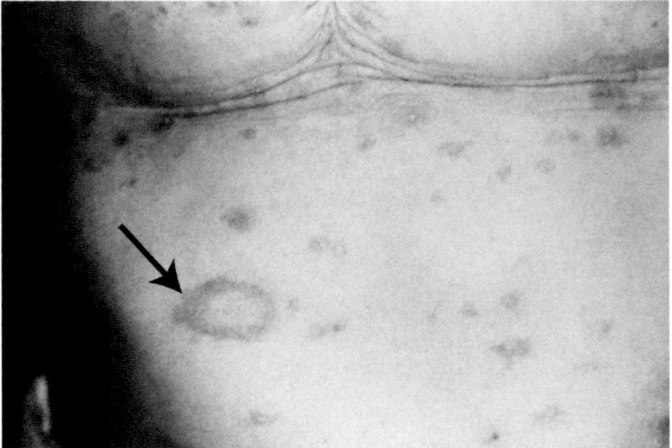

Pityriasis Rosea: Pityriasis rosea, presenting with an oval herald patch on the abdomen, followed by a more generalized rash. Reprinted from the Centers for Disease Control and Prevention Public Health Image Library; https://phil.cdc.gov/default.aspx

DON'T BE TRICKED

- Pityriasis rosea can resemble secondary syphilis but does not involve the palms and soles; obtain RPR in sexually active persons.

Acneiform Lesions

Diagnosis

Acne is a chronic inflammatory skin condition characterized by open and closed comedones (blackheads and whiteheads, respectively) and inflammatory lesions, including papules, pustules, or nodules.

Consider hyperandrogenism in women whose acne is severe, cyclical, or unresponsive to conventional therapy and is associated with hirsutism, menstrual irregularities, virilization, or rapid onset of severe disease.

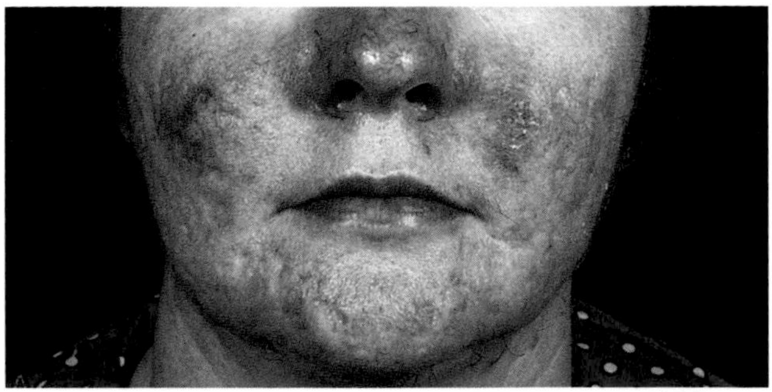

Rosacea: Papules, pustules, and dilated blood vessels involving the central face are typical of rosacea. Rosacea involves the nasolabial folds whereas the malar rash of SLE does not.

Rosacea is a chronic inflammatory skin disorder that affects the cheeks and nose and usually occurs after the age of 30 years. Rosacea is commonly associated with facial flushing in response to certain stimuli such as spicy foods. Erythema with telangiectasias, pustules, and papules without comedones is typically seen.

In early stages, rosacea can resemble the malar rash of SLE. However, the rash of SLE spares the nasolabial folds. The development of papules, pustules, and flushing is inconsistent with SLE and supports the diagnosis of rosacea.

Hidradenitis suppurativa is a chronic inflammatory disease that predominantly affects the axillae, breasts and inframammary creases, inguinal folds, and gluteal cleft. It is characterized by comedones, inflammatory papules, nodules, cysts, and scarring.

STUDY TABLE: Differential Diagnosis of Acne

Disease	Characteristics
Acne (acne vulgaris)	Microcomedones are precursors to acne lesions. They are very common in adolescents but also in preadolescents and adults. Women may have premenstrual flare-ups. Physical examination: coexisting open and closed comedones, papules, pustules, and nodular lesions located primarily on the face, neck, and upper trunk.
Rosacea	Not true acne; primary lesion is not a comedone but an inflammatory papule; rhinophyma (bulbous, red nose) is a variant. Physical examination: central facial erythema, telangiectasias, papules, and pustules.
Bacterial folliculitis	Common in athletes. Physical examination: follicular papules; pustules; occasional furuncles on any hair-bearing area, especially scalp, buttocks, and thighs. Most common cause is *Staphylococcus aureus*.
Gram-negative folliculitis	A) Presents as exacerbation of pre-existing acne, caused by overgrowth of gram-negative bacteria during prolonged systemic antibiotic acne treatment. Physical examination: many inflamed pustules, most often on the face. Positive culture for gram-negative bacteria, often *Escherichia coli*. B) "Hot tub folliculitis" occurring secondary to exposure to inadequately chlorinated pools or hot tub water contaminated with *Pseudomonas aeruginosa*.
Periorificial dermatitis, idiopathic	More common in women. Physical examination: small (<2 mm) papules and pustules around the mouth or eyelids. Similar to acne but without comedones.
Periorificial dermatitis, iatrogenic	Frequent causes are prolonged topical glucocorticoid therapy for atopic dermatitis and inappropriate use of these agents to treat acne. Similar in appearance to idiopathic type. Classically spares the skin around the lips. Differentiation is by history.

DON'T BE TRICKED

- The prominent papules and pustules seen in rosacea are not typical of the maculopapular malar rash seen in SLE.
- The rash of SLE does not involve the nasolabial folds.

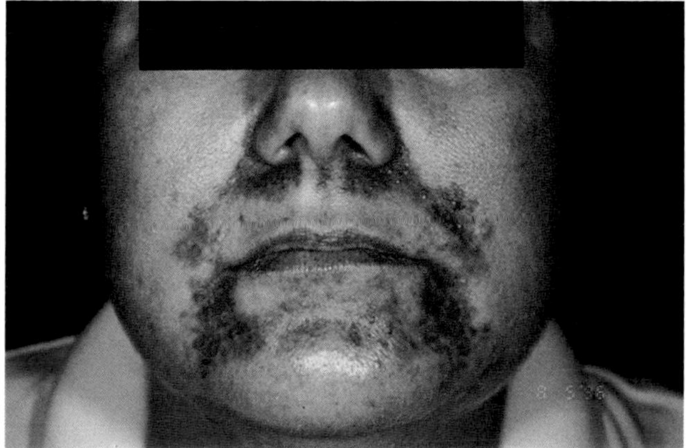

Perioral Dermatitis: Discrete papules and pustules on an erythematous base around the mouth, but typically sparing the skin directly around the lips, are characteristic of perioral dermatitis.

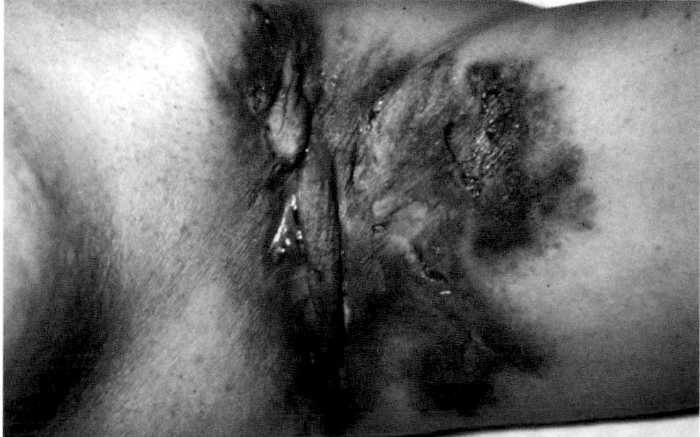

Hidradenitis Suppurativa: Hidradenitis suppurativa is a chronic skin condition characterized by painful, recurrent, chronic, sterile abscesses; sinus tract formation; and scarring.

Treatment

STUDY TABLE: Drug Therapy for Acne	
Indication	**Drug**
Mild noninflammatory acne (comedones)	Comedolytic agent (topical retinoid)
Mild inflammatory acne (papules and pustules)	Topical retinoid and topical antibiotic (erythromycin or clindamycin)
Moderate noninflammatory acne	Topical retinoid and benzoyl peroxide or azelaic acid
Moderate to severe inflammatory acne	Topical retinoid, topical antibiotic, and an oral antibiotic (tetracycline or others)
Acne in women with hyperandrogenism	Oral contraceptive
Severe recalcitrant nodular acne	Oral isotretinoin (women require two forms of birth control when taking this drug because it is teratogenic)
Iatrogenic perioral acne	Discontinue topical glucocorticoid

Rosacea with inflammatory pustules and papules will respond to metronidazole gel and low-dose oral tetracycline.

Hidradenitis suppurativa is best treated with clindamycin-rifampin combination antibiotics, infliximab, and surgical excision.

DON'T BE TRICKED

- Avoid oral or topical antibiotic monotherapy for treatment of moderate to severe acne because of increased antibiotic resistance.
- Do not use tetracycline, any topical retinoids, or oral isotretinoin for acne treatment during pregnancy.

TEST YOURSELF

An 18-year-old man has had nodular and cystic acne. Pustules and nodules with scarring are present on the chin, face, back, and chest.

ANSWER: For diagnosis, choose severe inflammatory acne. For treatment, select isotretinoin.

Dermatophyte and Yeast Infections

Diagnosis

Dermatophytes are types of fungi that invade epidermal stratum corneum, hair, and nails, causing tinea infections.

Yeast infections include *Candida*, the main yeast species infecting humans, and *Malassezia*, causing pityriasis versicolor.

Physical Examination

Dermatophytosis causes the following:

- **Tinea pedis** presents as chronic fissuring and scaling between the toes, but some patients have a chronic "moccasin-type" form of infection with a fine, silvery scale extending from the sole to heel and sides of the feet.
- **Tinea corporis** most typically presents as an annular lesion with an active erythematous border of small vesicles and scales, often with central clearing.
- **Tinea cruris** (jock itch) is a dermatophyte infection of the inguinal folds presenting as erythematous patches with a rim of scale that does not involve the scrotum.
- **Onychomycosis** is usually characterized by a thickened, yellow or white nail with scaling under the elevated, distal free edge of the nail plate. Sometimes, however, the infecting organism invades the surface of the toenail presenting as a white crust.

Cutaneous candidiasis is characterized by red, itchy, inflamed skin. At sites of skin-to-skin contact, lesions have glazed, shiny, and at times eroded surfaces. Satellite pustules (yellow, fluid-filled lesions at the edge of the confluent red eruption) are a key physical finding.

Testing

Diagnosis of dermatophyte infection is made by examination of the scale or subungual debris with KOH demonstrating the presence of branching hyphae.

Pityriasis versicolor is associated with yeast spores characterized by "spaghetti and meatballs" microscopic appearance.

Candida is associated with pseudohyphae and spores (see General Internal Medicine section for figure).

DON'T BE TRICKED

- *Candida* intertrigo can involve the scrotum, whereas tinea cruris does not.
- Two feet–one hand tinea is a common presentation of tinea pedis.
- Nail dystrophy may be caused by psoriasis, aging, or peripheral vascular disease.

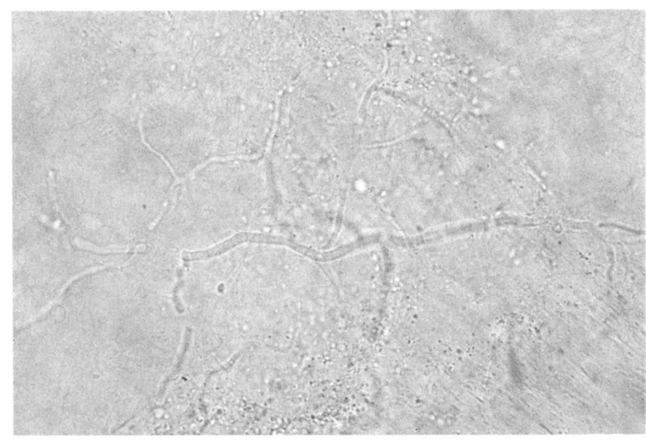

Pityriasis Versicolor KOH: Hyphae and yeast cells are recognized as a "spaghetti and meatballs" pattern.

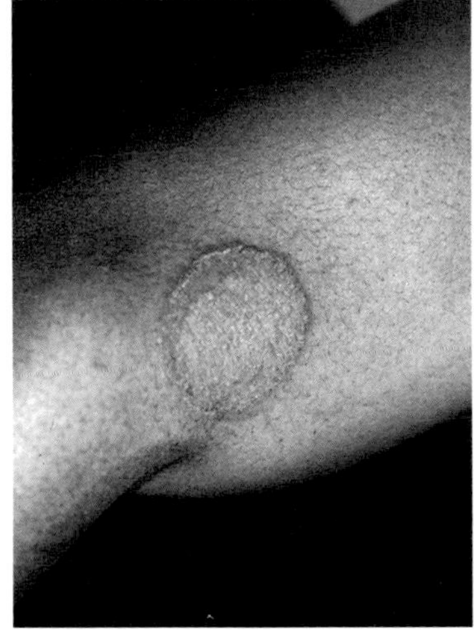

Tinea Infection: Tinea most commonly presents as a round or oval erythematous scaling patch that spreads centrifugally with central clearing. It has an active border that is raised, consisting of tiny papules or vesicles and scale.

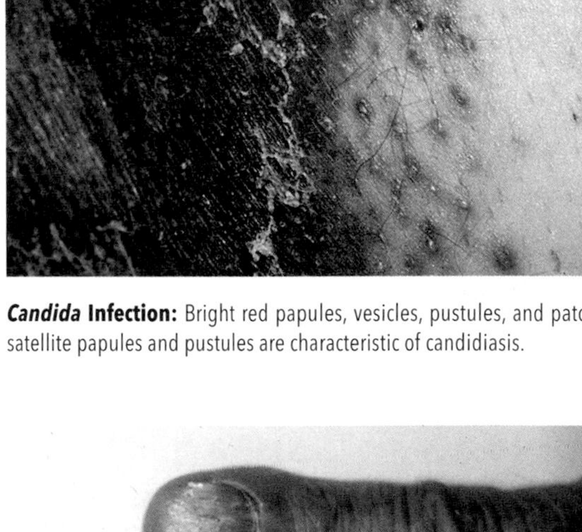

***Candida* Infection:** Bright red papules, vesicles, pustules, and patches with satellite papules and pustules are characteristic of candidiasis.

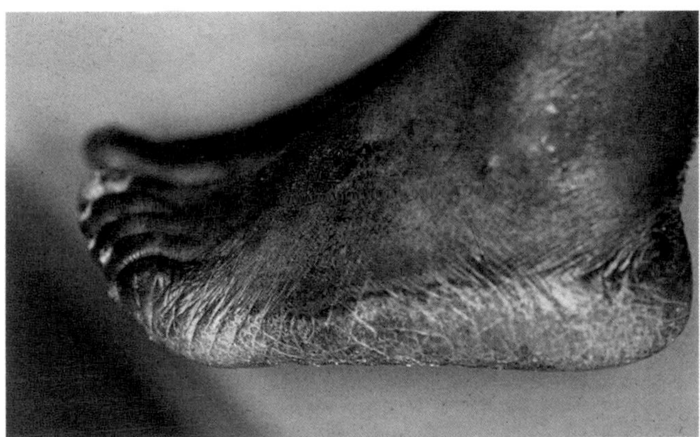

Tinea Pedis: Extension of tinea pedis onto the sole and sides of the foot ("moccasin" appearance) presents as chronic scaling.

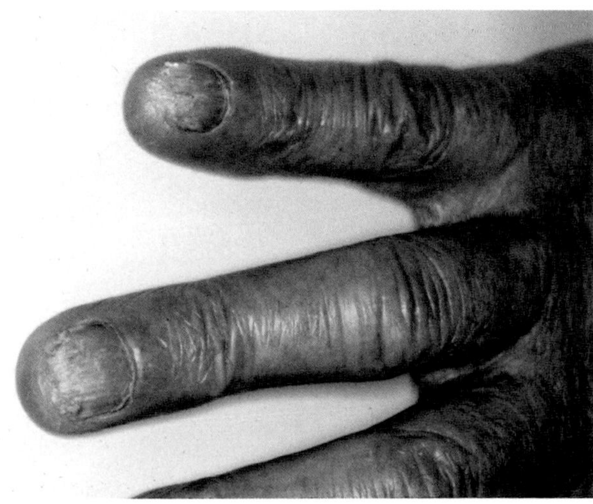

Onychomycosis: Distal subungual thickening and nail separation (white areas of nail) involving most of the nails are associated with onychomycosis.

Treatment

STUDY TABLE: Treatment for Dermatophyte and Yeast Infections	
Treatment	**Indication**
Topical antifungal cream (clotrimazole, terbinafine)	Most dermatophyte infections, except tinea capitis and onychomycosis
Oral terbinafine or itraconazole	Confirmed onychomycosis, tinea capitis, extensive tinea corporis, treatment-resistant dermatophytosis
Topical ketoconazole, selenium sulfide, zinc pyrithione	Initial treatment of pityriasis versicolor
Itraconazole or fluconazole, single dose	Recurrent pityriasis versicolor
Topical nystatin, miconazole, clotrimazole, ketoconazole, econazole	*Candida* infections

Treatment of onychomycosis is typically not necessary but is recommended for patients with peripheral vascular disease or diabetes mellitus to prevent the development of cellulitis.

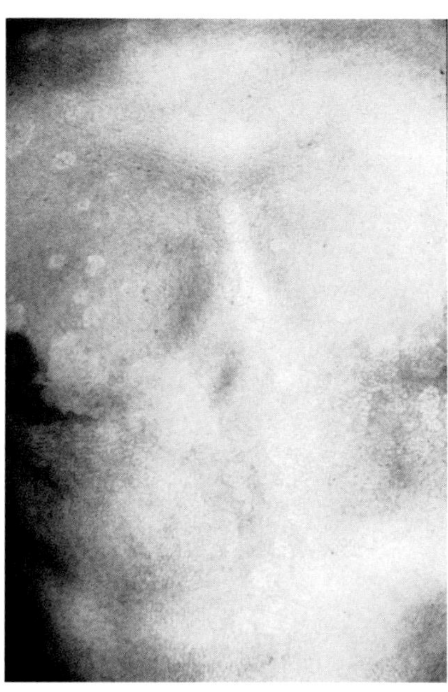

Pityriasis Versicolor: Hypopigmented, scaly macules are present on the chest.

DON'T BE TRICKED

- Do not select antifungal treatment for thick, yellow, and crumbling toenails without KOH scraping or positive culture for dermatophytes.
- Never select a combination of a topical antifungal agent and a glucocorticoid for treatment of an unknown skin rash or dermatophyte infection.
- Do not choose oral ketoconazole as initial antifungal treatment because of the risk of severe hepatotoxicity.

TEST YOURSELF

A 35-year-old man has a nonpruritic rash on his chest. He previously had a similar rash that became hypopigmented when he became suntanned.

ANSWER: For clinical diagnosis, choose pityriasis versicolor. For management, order KOH preparation of the scale with demonstration of a "spaghetti and meatballs" hyphae pattern.

Molluscum Contagiosum

Diagnosis

Molluscum contagiosum is a self-limited viral infection characterized by skin-colored, umbilicated papules that are typically found in children and sexually active adults. Associated HIV infection may cause multiple large, disfiguring lesions.

Treatment

Treatment may involve destructive techniques such as cryosurgery or curettage.

In patients with HIV, the lesions may resolve with initiation of ART.

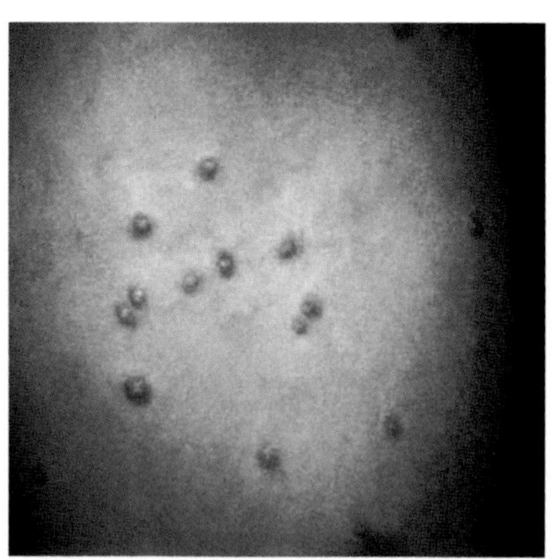

Molluscum Contagiosum: Molluscum contagiosum presents as small, flesh-colored, umbilicated papules in sexually active adults.

Leishmaniasis

Diagnosis

Leishmaniasis is a parasitic infection caused by several species of *Leishmania* and is transmitted by the sandfly. Military personnel returning from Afghanistan and Iraq and travelers to Saudi Arabia, Brazil, and Peru are at risk. The cutaneous form of the disease begins as a small, red, painless papule on the limb or face, usually 2 to 4 weeks after the sandfly bite. The papule enlarges to approximately 2 cm over the next 2 to 4 weeks, becomes dusky red to violaceous in color, and may ulcerate. Diagnosis is based on finding parasites on biopsy of the skin.

TEST YOURSELF

A 30-year-old man who recently returned from active military duty in Afghanistan is seen for an enlarging, ulcerated, purple papule on his arm of 2 weeks' duration.

ANSWER: For diagnosis, select leishmaniasis. For laboratory evaluation, choose skin biopsy.

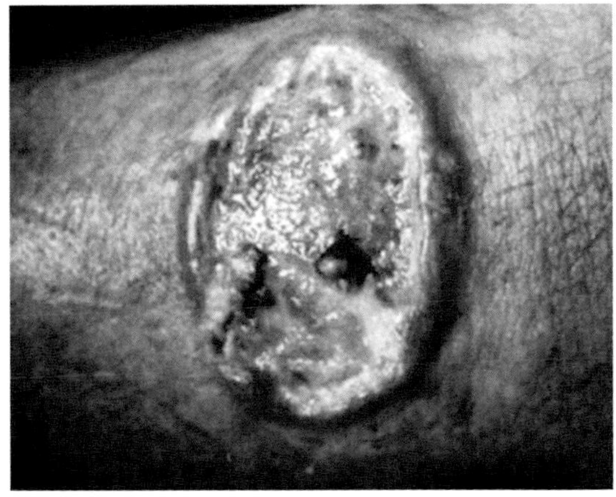

Leishmaniasis: The characteristic shallow ulcer of leishmaniasis is shown on an arm.

Herpes Zoster

Prevention

Administer the recombinant zoster vaccine to adults 50 years and older (rather than the live attenuated zoster vaccine, which is indicated for immunocompetent adults 60 years and older) to prevent or attenuate illness caused by herpes zoster infection and to reduce the risk of postherpetic neuralgia.

Physical Examination

Localized pain and a vesicular rash in a dermatomal distribution are characteristic features. Dermatomal neuropathic pain may develop before skin lesions occur.

Severe, complicated, or recurrent herpes zoster should trigger testing for possible associated HIV infection.

Be alert for two special syndromes:

- Lesions along the first division of the trigeminal nerve (zoster ophthalmicus), including the tip of the nose, may require urgent referral to an ophthalmologist.
- Vesicles in the ears, diminished taste on the anterior two thirds of the tongue, and ipsilateral facial paralysis (Ramsay Hunt syndrome) require referral to an ENT specialist.

Testing

Obtain rapid tests, such as direct-fluorescent antibody and PCR studies on scrapings from active vesicular skin lesions that have not yet crusted, or viral culture from a vesicle when the diagnosis is unclear.

Treatment

Give valacyclovir, famciclovir, or acyclovir if lesion onset is within 72 hours of contemplated treatment.

Disseminated zoster requires intravenous therapy and both contact and airborne precautions.

Antiviral agents are used to treat zoster ophthalmicus, even if more than 72 hours have elapsed.

Treat postherpetic neuralgia with gabapentin, pregabalin, tricyclic antidepressants, or topical lidocaine or capsaicin.

DON'T BE TRICKED

- Administer recombinant varicella-zoster vaccine to patients 50 years and older regardless of previous history of varicella infection or previous immunization with live attenuated vaccine.
- Do not select topical acyclovir or penciclovir for the treatment of herpes zoster.
- Do not select glucocorticoids to treat herpes zoster.

TEST YOURSELF

A 72-year-old man has a 4-day history of a painful vesicular rash in the distribution of the first division of the trigeminal nerve and conjunctival inflammation.

ANSWER: Choose zoster ophthalmicus for diagnosis. Select an antiviral agent (valacyclovir, famciclovir, or acyclovir) and ophthalmologist referral as treatment.

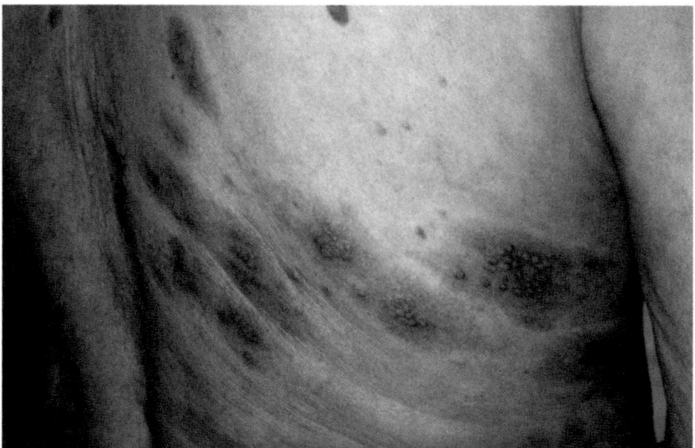
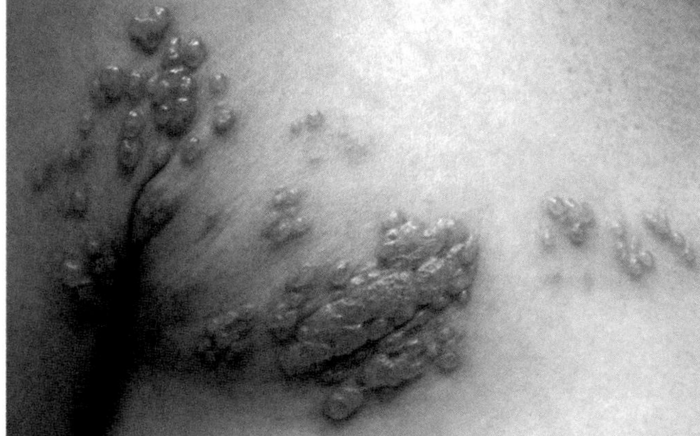

Herpes Zoster: Herpes zoster is characterized by the dermatomal distribution of painful grouped vesicles on an erythematous base.

Scabies

Diagnosis and Physical Examination

Scabies is an "itchy rash" occurring between the fingers and on the penis, scrotum, areolae, and nipples.

Look for burrows appearing as wavy, thread-like, grayish-white skin elevations capped with small vesicles at the terminal ends.

Patients with AIDS and those in institutions such as nursing homes and hospitals may develop widespread scabies with extensive scaling that may not itch.

Testing

Microscopic identification of the mite, feces, or eggs using KOH or simple mineral oil is diagnostic.

A skin biopsy may also establish the diagnosis.

Treatment

Treat all family members and close contacts of the patient simultaneously.

Topical permethrin is the preferred agent.

Oral ivermectin is indicated for relapsed scabies, except when treating children and pregnant or lactating women.

Clothing, linens, and towels must be washed in hot water and dried at high heat.

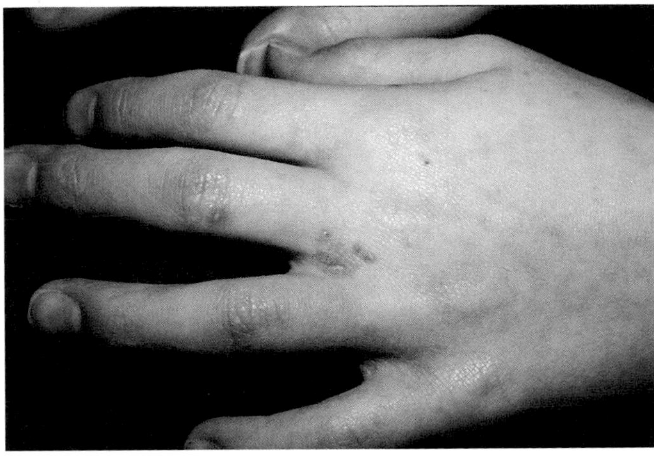

Scabies Rash: Multiple pink to red glistening papules and erosions with diffuse scaling, predominately in the finger webs, characteristic of scabies.

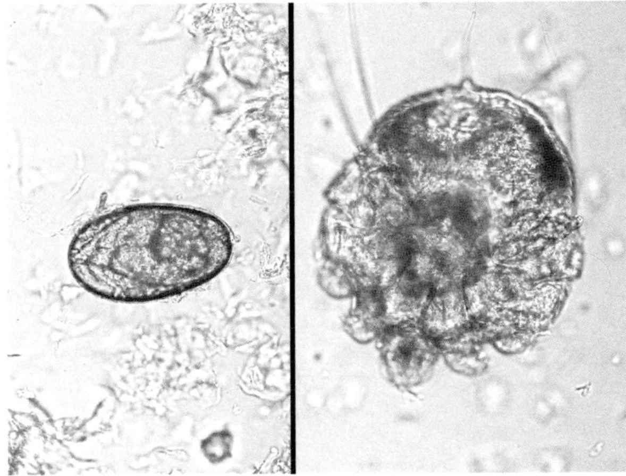

Scabies: *Sarcoptes scabiei*, the organism responsible for scabies, is shown after KOH preparation from skin scraping.

DON'T BE TRICKED

- Do not re-treat scabies because of persistent itching, which can continue for 2 weeks after successful treatment.
- Avoid topical lindane because of its associated neurotoxicity.

TEST YOURSELF

A 67-year-old woman with a recent hospitalization and her 3-year-old granddaughter have a 3-week history of generalized pruritus. Both patients have widespread excoriations and interdigital linear burrows.

ANSWER: For diagnosis, select scabies. For treatment, choose topical permethrin for patients and other close contacts.

Bedbugs

Diagnosis

Classic presentation is grouped, itchy papules in close configuration ("breakfast, lunch, and dinner") on exposed body areas. Bites are typically noticed in the morning, because bedbugs feed at night.

Treatment

Lesions will resolve spontaneously. Symptomatic treatment involves topical glucocorticoids and oral antihistamines.

Eradication of the bedbug is necessary for a "cure."

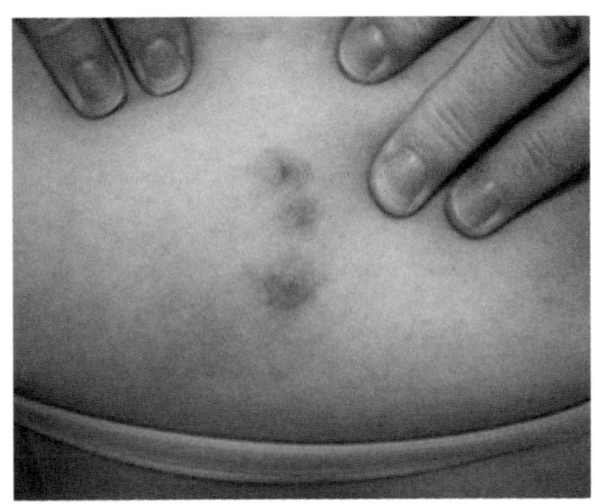

Bedbugs: Classic grouped pruritic papules ("breakfast, lunch, and dinner") presentation of bites from bedbugs.

Seborrheic Keratosis

Diagnosis

Seborrheic keratosis is a painless, nonmalignant growth that appears as a "stuck-on" waxy, brownish patch or plaque.

Treatment

Therapy is not required. A shave excision or liquid nitrogen destruction can be performed for lesions that are irritated (e.g., rubbed by clothing or jewelry).

DON'T BE TRICKED

- **Rapid onset of multiple pruritic seborrheic keratoses can be a sign of GI adenocarcinoma.**

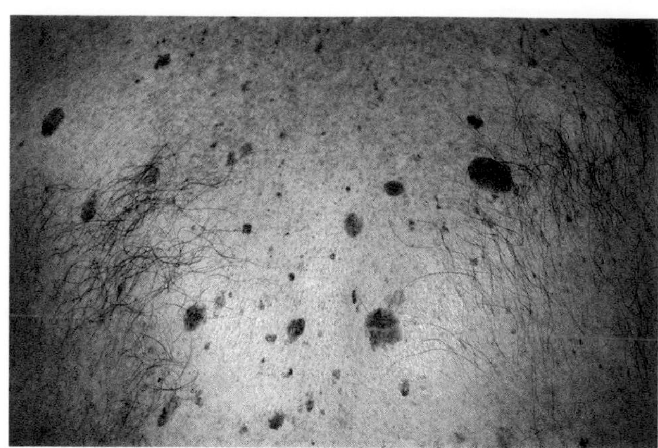

Seborrheic Keratoses: Brown to tan, sharply demarcated, waxy-like papules, plaques, and nodules are characteristic of seborrheic keratoses.

Warts

Diagnosis

Look for flesh-colored, exophytic, hyperkeratotic papules or nodules.

Anogenital warts (condyloma acuminata) present as single or multiple papules on the penis, vulva, or perianal area and may be flat-topped or cauliflower-like papules.

Treatment

Treat common warts with salicylic acid (a keratolytic agent).

Alternatives to drug therapy include cryotherapy.

"No therapy" is an acceptable option because spontaneous resolution is likely.

Podophyllin is often used as the initial therapy for anogenital warts.

Actinic Keratosis

Diagnosis

Lesions are located on sun-exposed sites and appear as 2- to 3-mm, elevated, flesh-colored or red papules with adherent, whitish scale or "rough spots" that may be easier to palpate than visualize.

Actinic keratosis is a precursor to SCC.

Treatment

Destruction by liquid nitrogen or curettage is the preferred treatment for most single lesions.

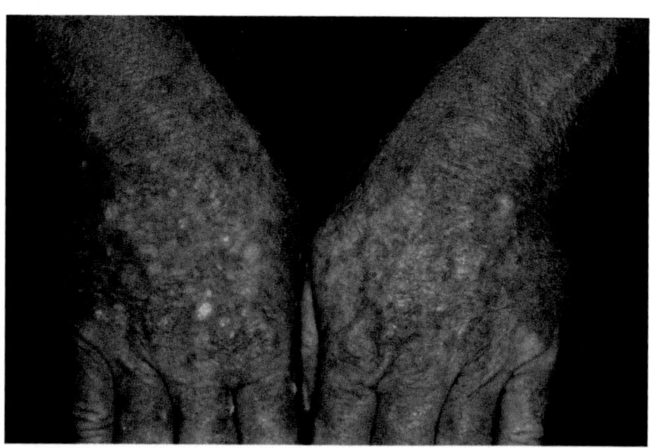

Actinic Keratoses: Multiple white, scaly patches measuring 1-3 mm on the hands are characteristic of actinic keratoses.

Topical 5-FU or imiquimod cream is used for the treatment of numerous lesions.

Excision is indicated for larger lesions (>5 mm); thick, indurated papules; lesions that have grown rapidly; and lesions that bleed, itch, or are painful.

Skin Cancer

Prevention

Sun avoidance and sun-protective clothing are first-line preventions. Use of sun screening agents is adjunctive therapy.

DON'T BE TRICKED

- Do not choose annual screening for the prevention of skin cancer in low-risk adults.

Squamous Cell Carcinoma

Diagnosis

SCC presents as a slowly evolving, isolated, keratotic, or eroded macule, papule, or nodule that commonly appears on the scalp, neck, pinna, or lip. Bowen disease is a form of anaplastic in situ SCC that presents as circumscribed erythematous or pigmented patches that typically have a keratotic surface. Shave or punch biopsy confirms the diagnosis of SCC.

Keratoacanthoma is a form of SCC generally appearing as a rapidly growing red nodule with a prominent central plug of scale and crust; its appearance is "volcaniform," resembling the cinder cone of a volcano.

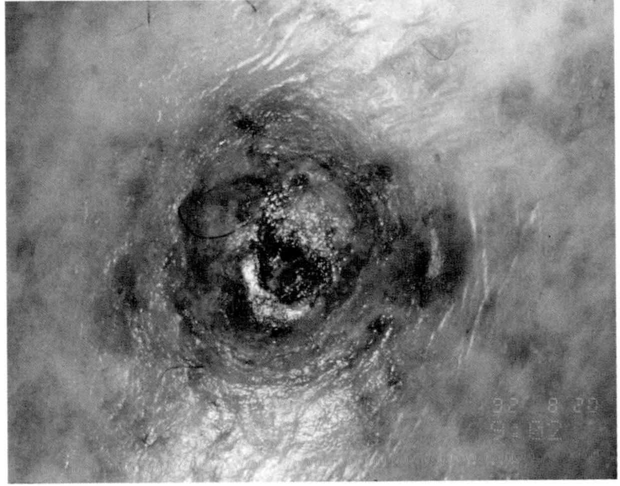

Cutaneous Squamous Cell Carcinoma: Typically presents as a slowly evolving, isolated, keratotic, or eroded macule, papule, or nodule that commonly appears on the scalp, neck, pinna, or lip.

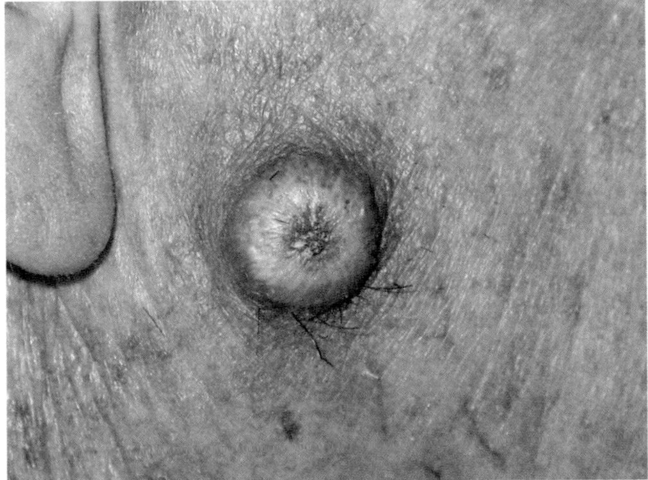

Keratoacanthoma: A form of SCC that appears as a rapidly growing, red, "volcaniform" nodule with a prominent central plug of scale and crust.

Treatment

Small lesions can be treated with electrodesiccation and curettage.

Most lesions require excision.

Basal Cell Carcinoma

Diagnosis

The most characteristic lesion is a pink, pearly, translucent papule or nodule with telangiectasias, rolled borders, and central depression with ulceration. Superficial BCCs are well demarcated, irregularly bordered, red patches; they tend to enlarge radially rather than invading into deeper structures. Biopsy should be performed for clinically suspicious lesions.

Treatment

Most BCCs are treated with simple excision.

Ill-defined lesions, high-risk histologic types, and tumors on the face and hands are often best treated with Mohs micrographic surgery.

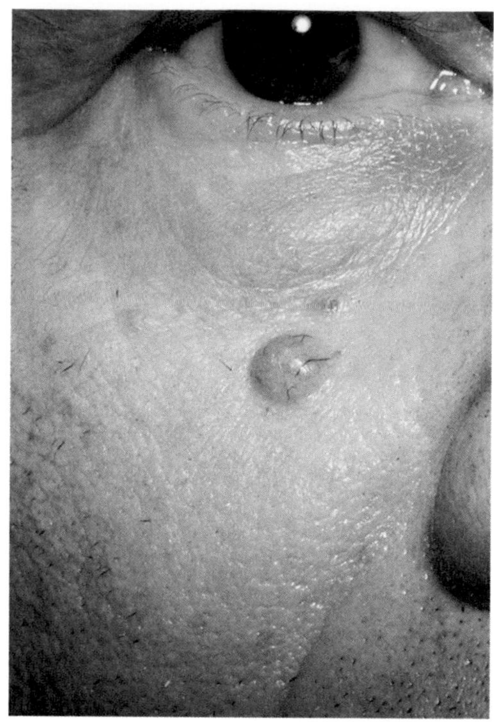

Basal Cell Carcinoma: This pink, pearly, translucent, dome-shaped papule with telangiectasias is characteristic of BCC.

Dysplastic Nevi

Diagnosis

Dysplastic nevi have some features of melanoma, including:

- diameter ≥5 mm
- asymmetric shape with indistinct borders
- a "fried egg" appearance with a darker, elevated, central portion and tan, flat shoulders blending into the surrounding skin
- pigmentation ranging from light tan to dark brown and occasionally black

Dysplastic nevi are markers for an increased risk of melanoma.

Autosomal-dominant familial melanoma/dysplastic nevus syndrome is defined by the presence of melanoma in at least two relatives; more than 50 nevi, with multiple nevi having atypical clinical and histologic features; and dysplastic nevi in other family members.

Treatment

Dysplastic nevi that develop increased characteristics associated with melanoma (fuzzy or ill-defined borders, multiple colors, diameter ≥5 mm), have otherwise changed, or stand out from other nevi must be removed and sent for pathology.

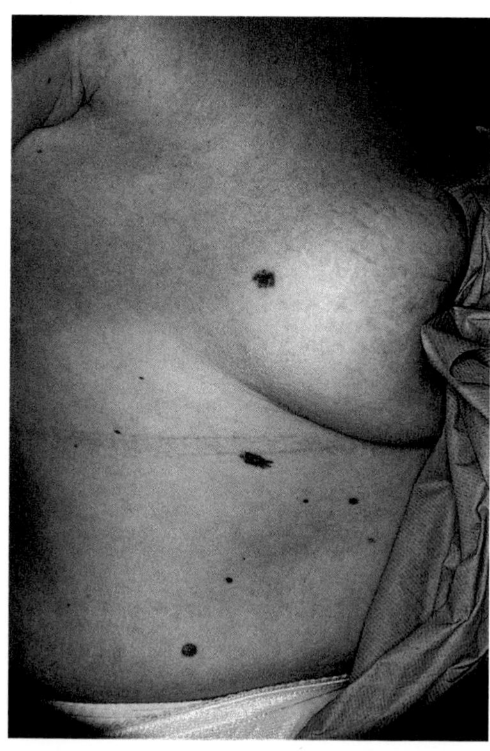

Dysplastic Nevi: Dysplastic nevi share similar characteristics with melanoma including asymmetry, indistinct and irregular borders, and variation in pigmentation.

Melanoma

Diagnosis

STUDY TABLE: "ABCDE" Rule to Diagnose Melanoma	
Characteristic	**Description**
Asymmetry	Not regularly round or oval
Border irregularity	Notching, scalloping, or poorly defined margins
Color variegation	Shades of brown, tan, red, white, blue-black, or combinations
Diameter	Size >6 mm (early melanomas may be diagnosed at a smaller size)
Evolution	Lateral expansion or vertical growth

There are several subtypes of melanoma.

- Lentigo maligna begins as a uniformly pigmented, light brown patch on the face or upper trunk that is confined to the epidermis and resembles a solar lentigo. Over time, the lesion expands and becomes more variegated in color.
- Superficial spreading melanoma presents as a well-defined asymmetric patch or plaque with an irregular border, variation in color, and an expanding diameter. This type tends to occur on the back in men and the legs in women (areas that receive intermittent sun and are prone to sunburn).
- Nodular melanomas are the most aggressive form (invading deeper structures); they are responsible for most deaths from melanoma.
- Acral lentiginous melanomas are the most common type of melanoma seen in patients with dark skin; they usually occur on the hands and feet.

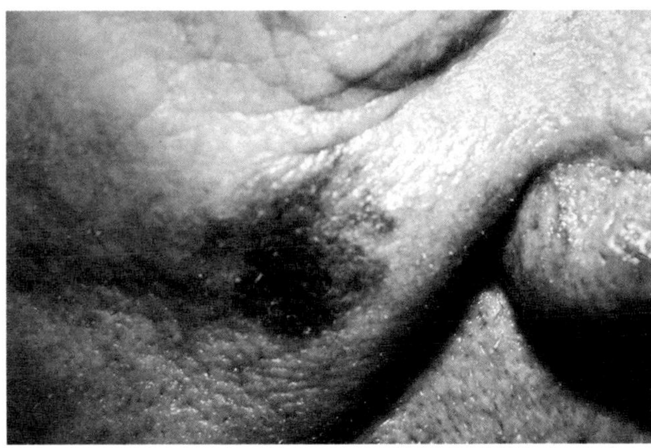

Lentigo Maligna: This melanoma in situ appears as a brown patch on sun-exposed skin.

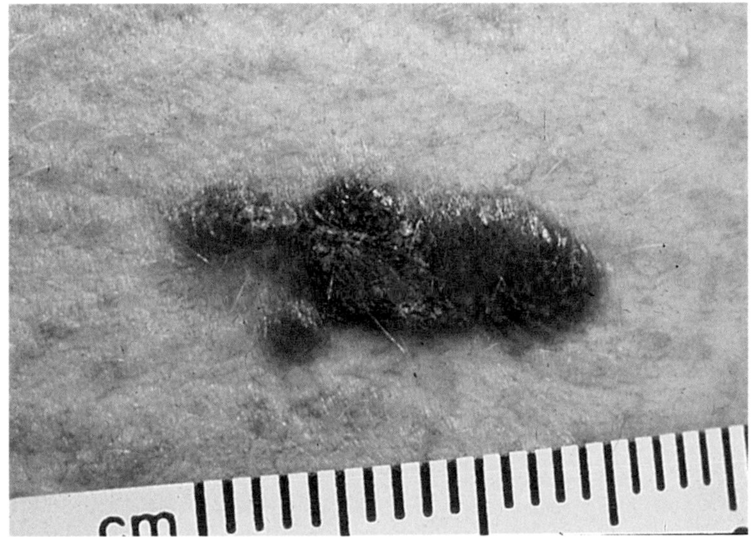

Melanoma: This asymmetric pigmented skin lesion has irregular, scalloped, notched, and indistinct borders with variegated coloration.

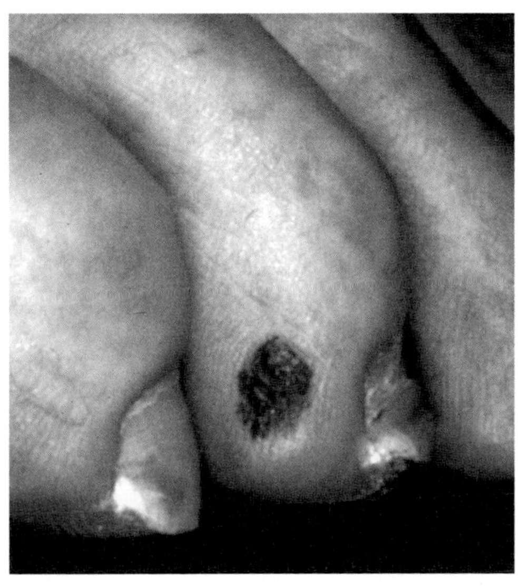

Acral Melanoma: Acral melanoma on the toe.

Treatment

Complete excision is the preferred biopsy technique for most varieties of melanoma, and sentinel lymph node biopsy is indicated for melanomas >1 mm thick. The extent of the surgical excision depends on the thickness of the primary melanoma.

DON'T BE TRICKED

- Routine blood tests are not recommended in patients with nonmetastatic melanoma treated with complete excision, and the value of screening radiography, CT, or PET/CT scanning is questionable.

Urticaria

Diagnosis

The hallmark of urticaria (hives) is the wheal, a superficial, pruritic, erythematous, well-demarcated, intermittently present plaque.

Wheals involving the skin around the mouth are considered an emergency, requiring careful observation and investigation for airway obstruction.

In acute urticaria, intermittent hives are present for 6 weeks or less. In chronic urticaria, intermittent hives are present for greater than 6 weeks.

Individual lesions usually disappear within hours without residual skin discoloration. More than two thirds of cases of new-onset urticaria resolve within 6 weeks. β-Lactams, sulfonamides, NSAIDs, opioids, insect stings, contrast dyes, latex (including condoms), nuts, fish, and eggs are common causes. Urticaria can also be initiated by pressure, cold, heat, vibration, water, or sunlight.

In most patients with chronic urticaria, a definite cause is not identified. Limited targeted laboratory testing is indicated when clinical suspicion suggests a cause, but routine, extensive testing should not be performed.

DON'T BE TRICKED

- Do not select ANA, patch testing, or specific IgE measurements for acute or chronic urticaria.
- Painful lesions persisting >24 hours with purpura/ecchymoses on resolution are likely the result of urticarial vasculitis. Definitive diagnosis is made by skin biopsy.

STUDY TABLE: Differential Diagnosis of Urticaria

If you see this...	Select this...
↑ESR, ↑CRP, lesions persisting >24 hours; purpuric papules	Vasculitic urticaria; perform skin biopsy and obtain serum complement levels, hepatitis B and C serology, cryoglobulins, and SPEP
Fever, adenopathy, arthralgias, and antigen or drug exposure	Serum sickness; measure CRP, ESR, and complement levels
Features of anaphylaxis, obvious allergen exposure	Immediate hypersensitivity reaction; treat emergently with epinephrine
Marked eosinophilia	Parasitic infection, possibly strongyloidiasis, filariasis, or trichinosis (especially with periorbital edema)

Treatment

Avoid aspirin and other NSAIDs. Select nonsedating antihistamines as first-line therapy.

Short-term oral glucocorticoids are indicated in very symptomatic patients with acute urticaria or in refractory disease.

DON'T BE TRICKED

- Measurement of C1 inhibitor levels is not indicated in patients with urticaria, because C1 inhibitor deficiency, seen in hereditary angioedema, is not associated with hives.

TEST YOURSELF

A 31-year-old man has a 2-week history of hives. Individual lesions persist for less than 24 hours and are not worsened by cold, sunlight, or pressure.

ANSWER: For diagnosis, choose acute urticaria. For laboratory evaluation, order no additional diagnostic studies. For treatment, select an H_1-blocker such as cetirizine.

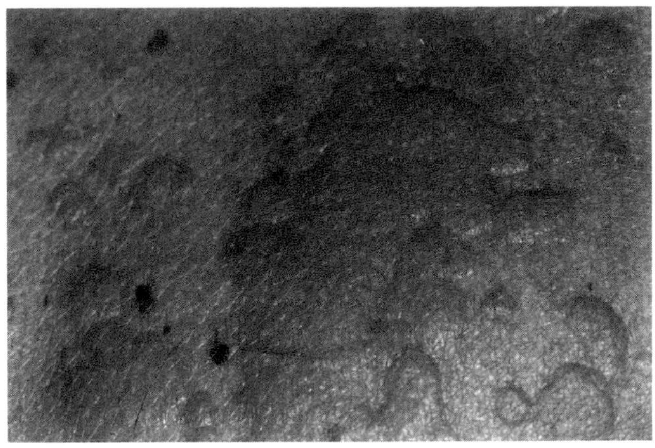

Urticaria: Urticaria is characterized by small white, pink, or flesh-colored pruritic papules.

Drug Allergy

Diagnosis

Immediate drug reactions (type I reactions) are usually IgE-mediated hypersensitivity reactions and cause symptoms of anaphylaxis within minutes to hours. Commonly implicated drugs are β-lactams, neuromuscular blocking agents, and platinum-containing chemotherapies.

Delayed drug reactions (type II-IV) typically present several days to months after treatment. Typical presentations include:

- cytopenias (type II)
- vasculitis or serum sickness (type III)
- prominent rash, fever, and multiorgan involvement (type IV)

Common causes include β-lactams, sulfa drugs, anticonvulsants, allopurinol, and abacavir. Radiocontrast agents, opiates, and NSAIDs cause a non–IgE-mediated degranulation of mast cells.

Penicillin is the most common self-reported medication allergy. Penicillin or one of its analogues should be avoided if the patient has a history of anaphylactic symptoms. If penicillin or one of its analogues must be used (treatment of neurosyphilis) in a patient with a penicillin allergy, choose skin testing, which identifies 95% of patients at risk for immediate reaction; do not select RAST or ELISA.

IgE-mediated cephalosporin reaction occurs in 2% of patients who are allergic to penicillin. Cephalosporins and carbapenems should be avoided in those with a positive skin test for penicillin or a convincing history of anaphylactic penicillin allergy.

Antibiotic therapy for syphilis or Lyme disease may precipitate the Jarisch-Herxheimer reaction, characterized by fever, headache, myalgia, rash, and hypotension. This reaction, related to dying spirochetes releasing endotoxin, begins within 2 hours of treatment and resolves by 48 hours. Management is supportive. Continue antibiotic therapy.

STUDY TABLE: Common Drug-Mediated Skin Eruptions

Type	Description
Acute generalized exanthematous pustulosis	Acute onset of widespread pustules, fever, leukocytosis, and possibly eosinophilia Usually self-limiting and clears without residual skin changes approximately 2 weeks after drug cessation
DRESS (also known as hypersensitivity syndrome)	Acute onset of generalized papular eruption, facial edema, fever, arthralgia, generalized lymphadenopathy, elevated serum aminotransferase levels, eosinophilia, and lymphocytosis

(Continued on the next page)

STUDY TABLE: Common Drug-Mediated Skin Eruptions *(Continued)*	
Type	**Description**
EM, SJS, TEN	Spectrum ranges from classic target lesions (EM), to involvement of mucous membranes with systemic symptoms (SJS), to a life-threatening loss of epidermis (TEN) SJS involves <10%, SJS/TEN overlap involves 10% to 30%, and TEN involves >30% skin detachment
Erythema nodosum	Tender subcutaneous nodules on lower leg; often preceded by a prodrome of fever, malaise, and/or arthralgia Causes fall into three broad categories: infections, drugs, and systemic diseases (usually inflammatory disorders)
Exfoliative and erythrodermic	Widespread generalized redness and scaling reaction
Fixed drug eruption	Discrete, often round or oval lesions that recur in exactly the same spot when rechallenged with the drug
Maculopapular and morbilliform (small discrete papules)	Most common type of drug reaction; symmetric distribution, usually truncal, hardly ever on palms or soles, and associated with fever and pruritus
Photosensitive skin reaction	Phototoxic reaction consists of severe sunburn after drug exposure (tetracycline) Photoallergic reaction presents as a rash after days or months of use (sulfonamides)
Red man syndrome	Body flushing, hypotension, and muscle pain associated with vancomycin and ciprofloxacin
Urticarial	Second most common drug reaction type, with or without angioedema

The appearance of a maculopapular rash is associated with the use of ampicillin in EBV and CMV infections or underlying ALL. This is not a drug allergy. Duration of the rash is independent of whether the drug is continued.

DON'T BE TRICKED

- The absence of eosinophilia does not rule out drug reaction or DRESS.

Treatment

Discontinue the offending medication.

Treat anaphylaxis, if present, with epinephrine.

Treat DRESS with glucocorticoids or IV immune globulin.

SJS/TEN treatment is supportive (fluid and electrolyte management, wound care); the effectiveness of IV immune globulin and glucocorticoids is uncertain.

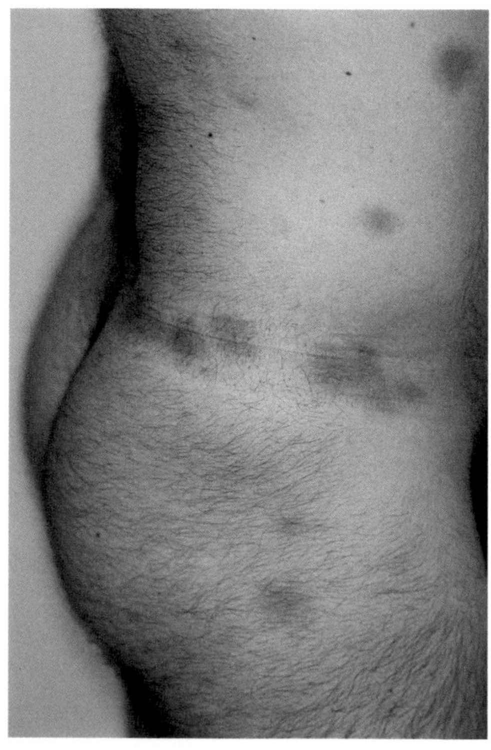

Fixed Drug Eruption: Discrete round to oval lesions are characteristic of a fixed drug eruption.

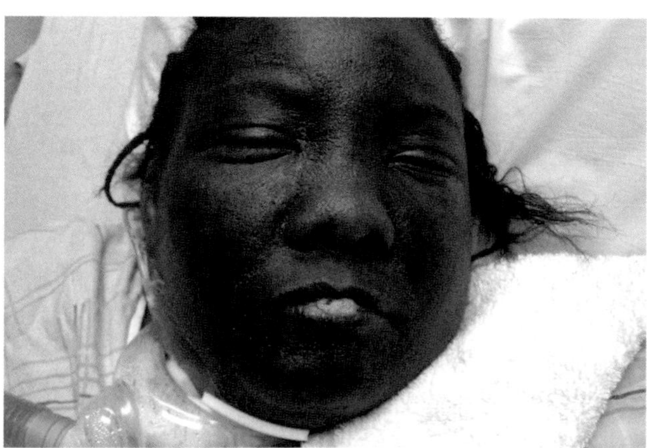

Drug Reaction with Eosinophilia and Systemic Symptoms: Acute facial edema in a patient with anticonvulsant-induced DRESS.

TEST YOURSELF

A 37-year-old man is prescribed ceftriaxone and azithromycin for CAP. Five days later, he is feeling better, coughs less, and produces less sputum, but he continues to have daily temperatures of up to 38.3 °C (101.0 °F.)

ANSWER: Suspect drug fever as the cause of persistent fever despite improvement in all other clinical parameters.

A 15-year-old student is given ampicillin for headache, pharyngitis, cervical lymph node enlargement, fever, and lymphocytosis on CBC. He develops a diffuse maculopapular rash.

ANSWER: Choose EBV infection (infectious mononucleosis) for diagnosis; do not select drug rash.

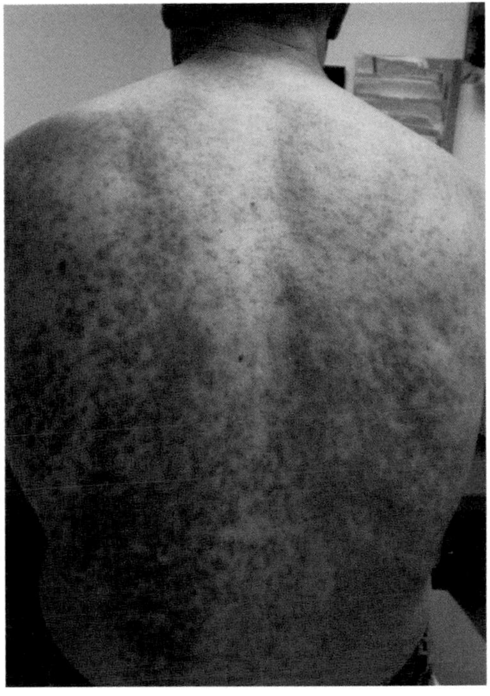

Morbilliform Drug Eruption: Morbilliform drug eruption consisting of symmetrically arranged erythematous macules and papules, some discrete and others confluent.

Pemphigus Vulgaris and Pemphigoid

Diagnosis

Pemphigus vulgaris often presents initially as painful, nonhealing oral erosions. Also look for flaccid, hemorrhagic, or seropurulent bullae and denuded areas that ooze serous fluid, bleed, or are covered with crusts. The esophagus and vulva may also be involved.

Look for a positive Nikolsky sign (erosion of normal-appearing skin by application of sliding pressure) or a positive Asboe-Hansen sign (ability to laterally extend bullae by applying gentle pressure).

STUDY TABLE: Differential Diagnosis of Blisters

Condition	Key Features
Pemphigus vulgaris	Flaccid blisters that rapidly transform to large, weeping, denuded areas and appear most commonly on the oral mucosa, trunk, and proximal extremities. Only erosions may be clinically apparent. Nikolsky sign is positive. Direct immunofluorescence shows intercellular IgG deposition.
Bullous pemphigoid	Tense blisters most commonly seen in older adults on the trunk, limbs, and flexures. Oral lesions are uncommon. Nikolsky sign is negative. Direct immunofluorescence shows linear IgG deposition at the basement membrane.
Dermatitis herpetiformis	Severely pruritic vesicles on elbows, knees, back, and buttocks associated with celiac disease. Lesions occur in crops and are symmetrically distributed. Direct immunofluorescence shows granular IgA deposition.
Porphyria cutanea tarda	Vesicles and bullae form in sun-exposed areas following minor trauma (typically the back of the hands). Urine fluoresces dark orange with Wood lamp illumination. Direct immunofluorescence shows deposition of immunoglobulins and complement around the dermal capillaries and linear at the basement. Look for hepatitis C infection.

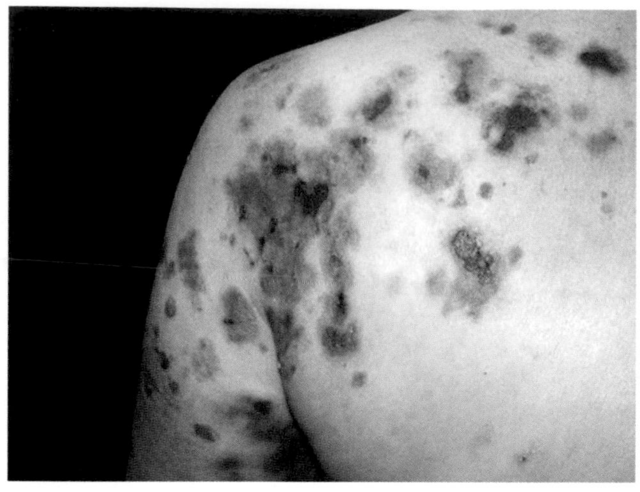

Pemphigus: This patient has multiple erosions and crusting with only an occasional intact blister; mucosal surfaces are typically involved.

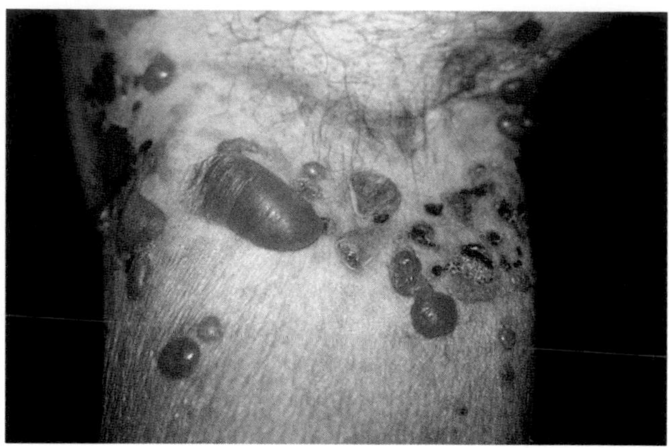

Bullous Pemphigoid: An autoimmune blistering disease characterized by multiple tense bullae and occasional erosions; mucosal surfaces are typically not involved.

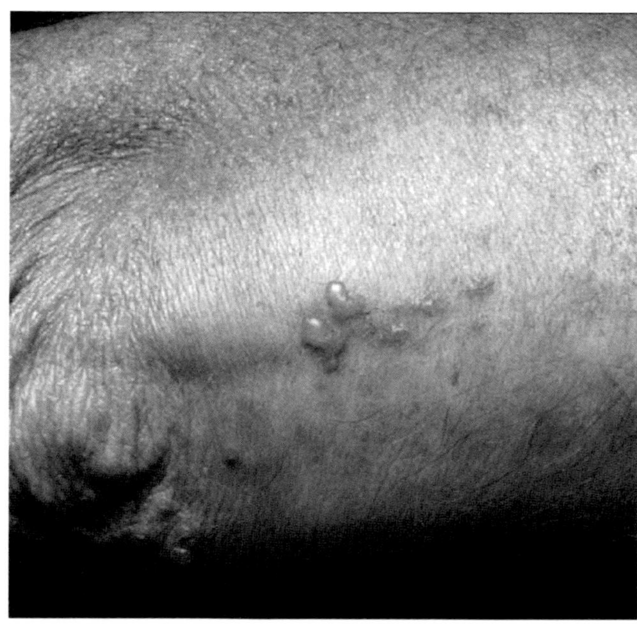

Dermatitis Herpetiformis: Dermatitis herpetiformis is characterized by pruritic papulovesicles over the external surface of the extremities and on the trunk; test for celiac disease.

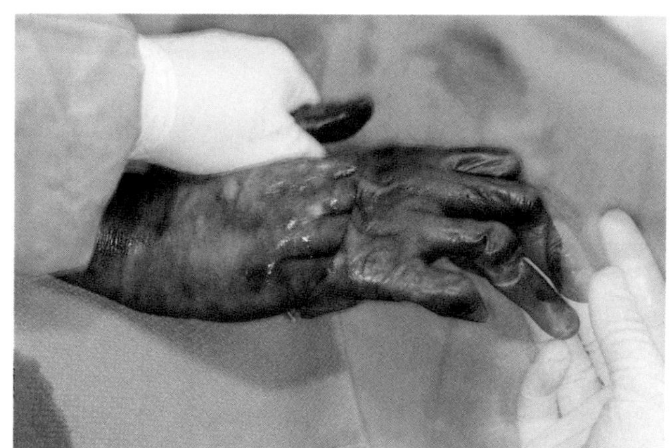

Toxic Epidermal Necrolysis: Shedding of entire sheets of skin is characteristic of TEN.

DON'T BE TRICKED

- The blisters of pemphigus vulgaris are so fragile that they are rarely seen; look instead for erosions, crusting, and sores in the mouth.

Treatment

Oral glucocorticoids are first-line therapy for pemphigus vulgaris and pemphigoid.

Patients who do not respond to conventional drug treatment may require plasmapheresis.

Dermatitis herpetiformis is always treated with a gluten-free diet, even in the absence of GI symptoms.

Dapsone may be added initially to hasten symptom resolution. Before using dapsone, check for G6PD deficiency.

TEST YOURSELF

A 72-year-old man has a 1-week history of a rash on his trunk and upper arms. He has lost 5 kg (11 lbs). Oral erosions and bullae are present on his trunk. Pressure applied to the edge of one of the blisters causes it to extend laterally without eruption.

ANSWER: Choose pemphigus for diagnosis. Biopsy is required for diagnosis.

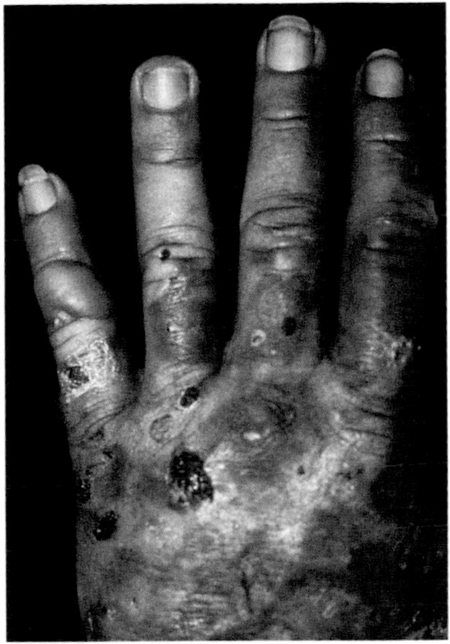

Porphyria Cutanea Tarda: Bullae and erosions on the dorsal hands are typical findings in porphyria cutanea tarda. Approximately 50% of such patients test positive for hepatitis C infection.

Erythema Multiforme

Diagnosis

Look for target-like erythematous macules or papules, each with pale and erythematous outer rings around a violaceous or dark center, blister, or erosion. Mucosal erosions may also be found.

Recurrent HSV infection is the most common inciting factor. Drug allergy (most often to sulfonamides, penicillin, and phenytoin) is another common cause.

Treatment

Treat EM by removing the offending agent and providing supportive care.

Antihistamines and topical or systemic glucocorticoids may be helpful depending on the severity.

If EM is caused by an active mycoplasma infection, antibacterial drugs may be helpful.

Recurrent episodes of EM may be managed with antiviral suppressive therapy for HSV infection.

DON'T BE TRICKED

- Do not confuse EM with erythema migrans, the rash of Lyme disease (red macule with central clearing as the macule expands).
- Do not treat acute EM-associated HSV with antivirals.

TEST YOURSELF

A 24-year-old man is evaluated for target lesions on his hands and arms, which he says he has had twice before in recent years.

ANSWER: For diagnosis, select recurrent EM caused by HSV.

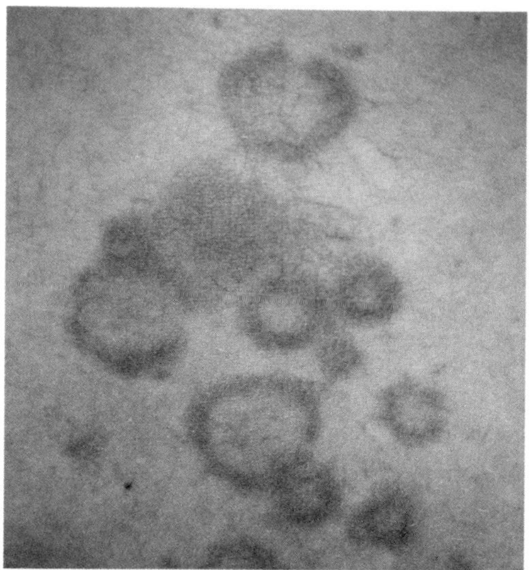
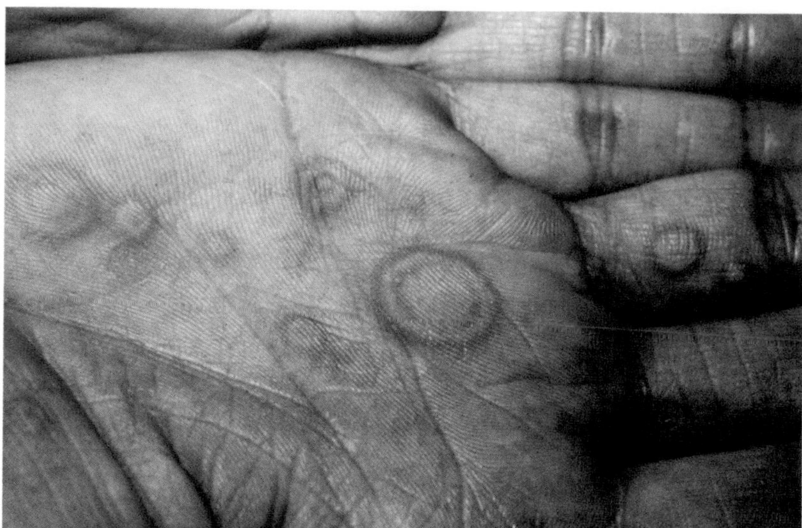

Erythema Multiforme: These images show the targetoid lesions of erythema multiforme.

Stevens-Johnson Syndrome/Toxic Epidermal Necrolysis

Diagnosis

SJS and TEN are severe mucocutaneous reactions, most commonly to a drug. These conditions are differentiated by the amount of epidermal detachment or necrosis.

- SJS: <10%
- TEN: >30%
- SJS-TEN overlap: 10% to 30%

When caused by drugs, SJS and TEN often occur between 1 and 3 weeks after exposure. Flu-like symptoms precede the skin eruption by 1 to 3 days. Initially, red-purple macules or papules develop on the trunk and extremities, which enlarge and coalesce. Skin pain is prominent. Vesicles, bullae, and Nikolsky sign are present. Two or more mucosal surfaces (eyes, nasopharynx, mouth, and genitals) are involved in >80% of patients.

Treatment

Stop the offending drug.

The role of glucocorticoids or IV immune globulin is controversial.

Patients with TEN (>30% skin involvement) represent medical emergencies and may need treatment in an intensive care or burn unit experienced in caring for this condition.

Dermatologic Signs of Systemic Disease

Diagnosis

Pruritus in the absence of primary skin lesions suggests an occult internal disease or medication effect. Causes of generalized pruritus without rash include liver disease (cholestatic and noncholestatic), CKD, Hodgkin disease, lymphoma, leukemia, and PV.

STUDY TABLE: Skin Disorders and Associated Systemic Diseases	
Description	**Diagnosis**
Violaceous papules around the nose, including the ala, or periorbitally and periorificially (lupus pernio)	Sarcoidosis
Painful subcutaneous nodules or plaques with overlying red-brown discoloration, superimposed angulated purpuric patches with central necrosis in patients with end-stage kidney disease	Calciphylaxis
Tightening and thickening of the skin following gadolinium administration in patients with chronic kidney disease (becoming rare now because of increased awareness by radiologists)	Nephrogenic systemic fibrosis
Painful, exudative ulcer with a purulent base and ragged, edematous, violaceous, "overhanging" border	Pyoderma gangrenosum
Pruritic eruption of papules and transient, almost immediately excoriated blisters on the elbows, knees, and buttocks	Dermatitis herpetiformis
Skin fragility and small, transient, easily ruptured vesicles in sun-exposed areas, mainly on the hands, and hypertrichosis	Porphyria cutanea tarda
"Juicy" indurated edematous red-purple plaques and nodules, sharply demarcated from the adjacent skin	Sweet syndrome (acute febrile neutrophilic dermatosis)

STUDY TABLE: Important Associations	
If you see this...	**Consider diagnosis of...**
Porphyria cutanea tarda, palpable purpura	Hepatitis C
Severe or recalcitrant seborrheic dermatitis or abrupt onset of severe psoriasis	Initial manifestation of HIV infection
Erythema nodosum	IBD, TB, sarcoidosis, coccidioidomycosis, streptococcal infection; look particularly for Löfgren syndrome (bilateral hilar lymphadenopathy, erythema nodosum, and lower extremity arthralgia)
Dermatitis herpetiformis	Celiac disease
Livedo reticularis (see Cardiovascular Medicine section for image)	Atheroemboli (previous vascular catheterization), thrombophilia, hyperviscosity syndrome, vasculitis
Pyoderma gangrenosum	IBD, inflammatory arthritis, lymphoproliferative disorders
Acanthosis nigricans (hyperpigmentation and velvety hyperkeratosis on flexural surfaces)	Diabetes
Xanthomas	Familial hypercholesterolemia
Mechanic's hands (hyperkeratotic, fissured skin on the palms)	Dermatomyositis/antisynthetase syndrome (myositis, Raynaud syndrome, interstitial lung disease with anti-Jo-1 antibodies)
Heliotrope rash	Dermatomyositis

STUDY TABLE: Skin Conditions and Associated Malignancies	
Skin Condition	**Malignancy**
Acanthosis nigricans	Gastric cancer, genitourinary cancer
Acute febrile neutrophilic dermatosis (Sweet syndrome): acute onset of erythematous papules or plaques	Leukemia, especially AML
Amyloidosis (primary systemic): pinch purpura, macroglossia, raccoon's eyes, and waxy skin	Multiple myeloma
Dermatomyositis: heliotrope-violaceous periorbital eruption; scaly red papules and plaques over bony prominences (Gottron papules)	Various cell types, but ovarian cancer is overrepresented
Paraneoplastic pemphigus: polymorphous erythematous plaques, blisters, and mucosal erosions	Lymphoma, Castleman disease, and CLL
Paget disease of the breast: nipple "eczema"	Breast cancer
Necrolytic migratory erythema: eczematous or psoriasiform eruption located around orifices and flexural and acral areas	Glucagonoma
Keratoderma of the palms and soles: bilateral thickening of the epidermis	SCC of the esophagus
Explosive onset of multiple pruritic seborrheic keratoses (Leser-Trélat sign)	GI adenocarcinoma, breast cancer, lung cancer
Rugal folds on palms and soles (tripe palms)	GI adenocarcinoma; SCC; head, neck, and lung cancer
Erythematous scaly plaque or patch on the perineal skin, scrotum, or perianal area (extramammary Paget disease)	GI or genitourinary cancer; dermatosis is also a malignancy and requires removal

DON'T BE TRICKED

- Ecthyma gangrenosum is a characteristic skin lesion of *Pseudomonas* and other systemic bacterial, fungal, or viral infections. It begins as a painless, erythematous macule and quickly develops into a large necrotic ulcer. It is usually seen in an immunocompromised patient.

TEST YOURSELF

A 36-year-old woman has a rash around the left nipple that she attributes to irritation from jogging. No discharge, mass, or other abnormality of either breast is noted.

ANSWER: For diagnosis, select Paget disease of the breast. For management, biopsy the rash and order mammography.

A 25-year-old man presents with a painful leg ulcer and persistent, bloody diarrhea.

ANSWER: For diagnosis, choose pyoderma gangrenosum. For management, order colonoscopy to look for IBD.

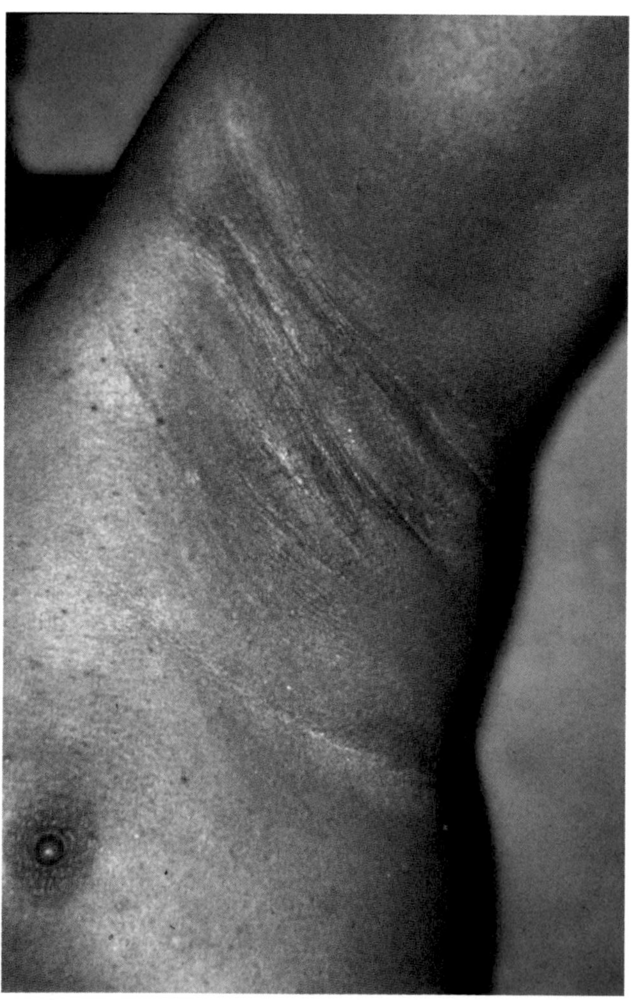

Acanthosis Nigricans: Acanthosis nigricans presents as a hyperpigmented hyperkeratosis on flexural surfaces and is most commonly associated with conditions such as diabetes mellitus and obesity.

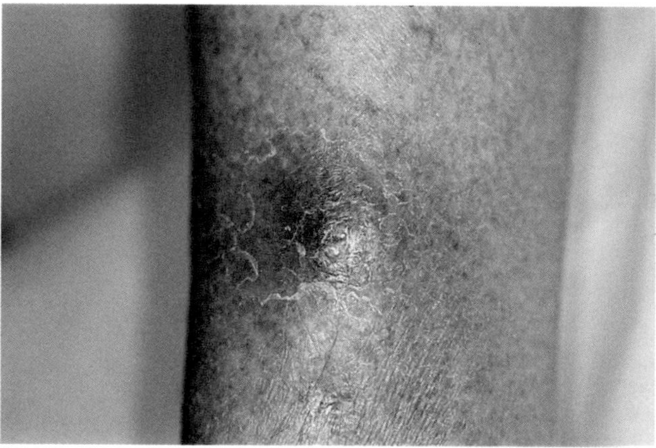

Erythema Nodosum: Tender pink to dusky red, deep, subcutaneous nodules located on the anterior leg are characteristic of erythema nodosum.

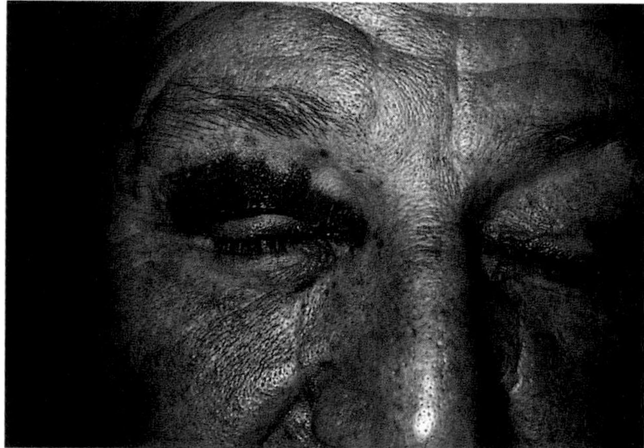

Pinch Purpura: "Raccoon's eyes" are characterized by purpura in the periorbital region, which is associated with amyloidosis.

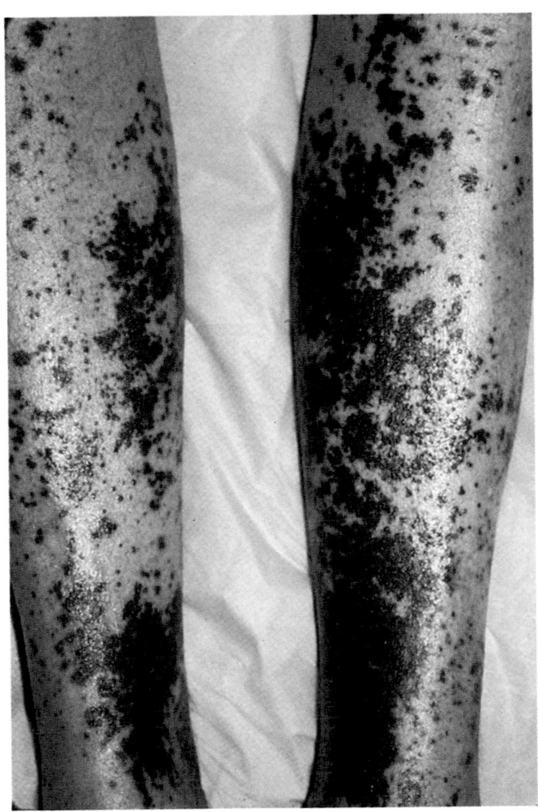

Palpable Purpura: The hallmark of leukocytoclastic vasculitis is palpable purpura consisting of bright red macules and papules and occasionally hemorrhagic bullae confined to the lower leg and foot.

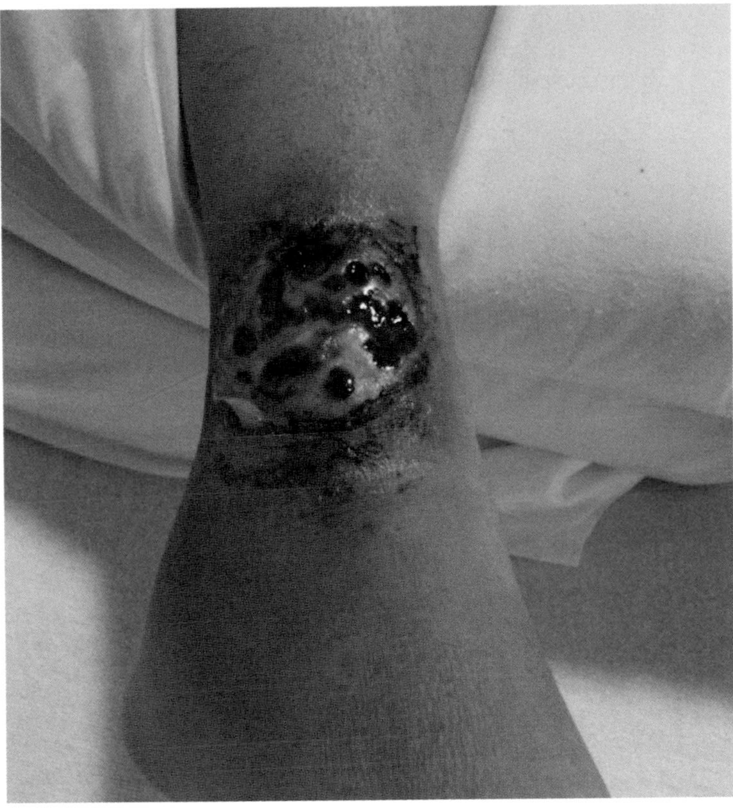

Pyoderma Gangrenosum: Nonhealing ulcer, often occurring on the lower extremities, with a purulent base and ragged, edematous borders; it is often seen in association with inflammatory bowel disease.

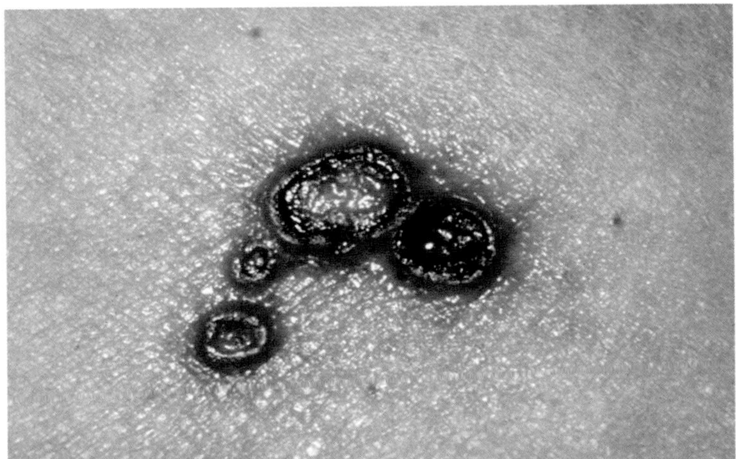

Ecthyma Gangrenosum: A characteristic skin lesion of *Pseudomonas* and other systemic bacterial, fungal, or viral infections, beginning as a painless, erythematous macule and quickly developing into a large necrotic ulcer. It is usually seen in immunocompromised patients.

Endocrinology and Metabolism

Diabetes Mellitus

Type 1 Diabetes Mellitus

Diagnosis

Type 1 diabetes is characterized by a β-cell destructive process that may eventually lead to absolute insulin deficiency. The onset of type 1 diabetes is typically abrupt and severe, with marked hyperglycemia developing over several days to weeks, and may be associated with a precipitating event, such as infection, pregnancy, or MI. Look for fatigue, polyuria, polydipsia, blurring of vision, weight loss, and dehydration.

More than 90% of cases of type 1 diabetes are autoimmune (type 1A). Several autoantibodies are directed against β cells or their products. Measuring antibodies to GAD65 and IA-2 are recommended for initial confirmation. Approximately 20% of patients with type 1 diabetes develop other organ-specific autoimmune diseases, such as celiac disease, Graves disease, hypothyroidism, Addison disease, pernicious anemia, and vitiligo.

Type 1B diabetes is idiopathic, has no autoimmune markers, and occurs more commonly in patients of Asian or African ancestry.

Treatment

Patients with type 1 diabetes are treated with **intensive insulin** therapy, which includes intermediate-acting or long-acting insulin for basal coverage and preprandial analog or regular insulin injections throughout the day. Intensive insulin therapy can also include continuous subcutaneous insulin infusion with an insulin pump and meal-time boluses.

Basal insulin dose accounts for 40% to 50% of the total daily dose of insulin; the remaining insulin is divided to cover the preprandial doses. Examples of **basal insulin** options:

- Insulin glargine, insulin detemir, or insulin degludec: A single 10 PM dose controls nocturnal plasma glucose levels and glucose levels between meals. It also counters the early morning rise in glucose level ("dawn phenomenon") caused by hepatic gluconeogenesis.
- Isophane (NPH) intermediate-acting insulin: This insulin can be used in the morning and evening to provide basal plasma insulin levels and to suppress hepatic gluconeogenesis.

Examples of short-acting **preprandial insulin** options:

- Insulin aspart, insulin glulisine, and insulin lispro: Rapid-acting insulin given 5 to 15 minutes before meals to modulate the postprandial rise in glucose level.
- Regular insulin: Given 30 minutes before meals to prevent postprandial elevations in blood glucose.

Correctional insulin is the use of additional analog or regular insulin beyond the usual dose to treat preprandial glucose that is not at target. For example, a correction for type 1 diabetes is an additional 1 U of insulin for every 50 mg/dL that the glucose level is above the preprandial target.

Insulin pumps: Subcutaneous infusion of rapid-acting insulin is delivered continuously for basal insulin requirements and given in intermittent boluses for prandial needs.

STUDY TABLE: Adjusting Insulin Dose in Diabetes Mellitus	
Condition	**Cause**
Fasting hyperglycemia	Not enough basal insulin
Prelunch hyperglycemia	Not enough rapid-acting insulin at breakfast or not enough morning NPH insulin
Predinner hyperglycemia	Not enough rapid-acting insulin at lunch or not enough morning NPH insulin
Bedtime hyperglycemia	Not enough rapid-acting insulin at dinner
Fasting or nocturnal hypoglycemia	Too much basal insulin
Prelunch hypoglycemia	Too much rapid-acting insulin at breakfast or too much morning NPH insulin
Predinner or bedtime hypoglycemia	Too much rapid-acting insulin at lunch or dinner or too much morning NPH

Hypoglycemia unawareness describes the presence of severely low plasma glucose levels that occur without warning symptoms followed by sudden loss of consciousness. Treat immediately with rapid-acting carbohydrates or a glucagon injection followed by food. Lowering the insulin dose and allowing the average plasma glucose level to increase for several weeks restores sensitivity to hypoglycemia.

Type 2 Diabetes Mellitus

Diagnosis

Type 2 diabetes is characterized by a combination of insulin resistance and a β-cell secretory defect. With time, progressive β-cell dysfunction can develop, leading to absolute insulin deficiency.

In general, type 2 diabetes presents less dramatically than type 1 diabetes. DKA is rare because patients maintain some degree of insulin secretion allowing for suppression of lipolysis. Because symptoms may be subtle, the time to diagnosis may be delayed. Consequently, approximately 20% of patients with type 2 diabetes have microvascular complications of the disease at presentation; an even higher percentage may have CAD or peripheral vascular disease. Most patients with type 2 diabetes are obese or at least have abdominal obesity. Characteristic findings of long-standing diabetes include:

- polyuria, polyphagia, and polydipsia
- retinal microaneurysms, dot-and-blot hemorrhages, macular edema
- symmetric sensory "stocking-glove" peripheral neuropathy
- cardiovascular and kidney disease

Five percent of patients with diabetes in the United States have an autosomal dominant form of the disease known as maturity-onset diabetes of youth (MODY). Presentation is generally before age 25 years.

Screening for Type 2 Diabetes

The USPSTF recommends screening for abnormal blood glucose as part of cardiovascular risk assessment in adults aged 40 to 70 years who are overweight or obese, and clinicians should consider screening earlier in persons with one or more risk factors for diabetes. Risk factors include positive family history, history of gestational diabetes or PCOS, or are members of certain racial or ethnic groups (African American, American Indian or Alaskan Native, Asian American, Hispanic or Latino, or Native Hawaiian or Pacific Islander).

The American Diabetes Association recommends screening overweight adults (BMI ≥25; ≥23 in Asian Americans) with at least one additional risk factor and all patients >45 years.

Screen using the following tests: fasting plasma glucose, 2-hour postprandial glucose during an oral glucose tolerance test (OGTT), or hemoglobin A_{1c}. If two separate tests are done simultaneously and both are abnormal, diagnose diabetes. If only one of the two tests is abnormal, repeat the abnormal test.

DON'T BE TRICKED

- A random plasma glucose level ≥200 mg/dL with hyperglycemic symptoms is diagnostic of diabetes and does not warrant repeat measurement.

STUDY TABLE: Diagnosis and Classification of Type 2 Diabetes Mellitus				
Diagnosis	**Fasting Glucose**	**Random Glucose**	**2-Hour Glucose During OGTT**	**Hemoglobin A_{1c}**
Increased risk for diabetes (prediabetes)	100-125 mg/dL	140-199 mg/dL	140-199 mg/dL	5.7%-6.4%
Diabetes	≥126 mg/dL	≥200 mg/dL with symptoms	≥200 mg/dL	≥6.5%

Treatment

Intensive lifestyle modification (exercise, weight loss) is appropriate for all patients with prediabetes or type 2 diabetes.

Medication, such as metformin, reduces the risk of diabetes in patients with prediabetes, although not as effectively as lifestyle interventions.

Bariatric procedures should be considered in obese patients.

Blood glucose monitoring includes self-monitoring of blood glucose (SMBG), hemoglobin A_{1c}, or continuous glucose monitoring.

- Use SMBG for patients taking multiple daily injection insulin therapy or continuous subcutaneous insulin infusion therapy.
- Obtain postprandial blood glucose levels in patients with at-goal preprandial readings but with hemoglobin A_{1c} not at goal.
- Obtain overnight blood glucose monitoring to detect hypoglycemia or dawn phenomenon.

Although guidelines vary, a reasonable individualized goal for most patients is a hemoglobin A_{1c} of 7% to 8%.

DON'T BE TRICKED

- If a patient is nonadherent with multiple insulin injections, adherence is unlikely to increase because a pump is prescribed.
- Hemoglobin A_{1c} will be falsely low in patients with hemolytic anemia, patients taking erythropoietin, or patients with kidney injury.

STUDY TABLE: Treatment for Type 2 Diabetes Mellitus	
First-Tier Validated Treatment (in suggested order)	**Notes**
1. Lifestyle changes plus metformin	Metformin is contraindicated in patients with an eGFR ≤30 mL/min/1.73 m^2. Some 5%-10% of patients taking metformin develop vitamin B_{12} deficiency. Periodic monitoring may be indicated, especially in patients with anemia or peripheral neuropathy.
2. Add basal insulin (± preprandial insulin) or begin dual therapy with metformin plus a second pharmacologic agent	Insulin and sulfonylureas can cause hypoglycemia.

Empagliflozin, a sodium-glucose cotransportor 2, significantly reduces the rates of death by CVD, all-cause mortality, and hospitalization for HF and is FDA approved for reduction of cardiovascular death in adults with type 2 diabetes and CVD.

Liraglutide, a glucagon-like peptide 1 analogue, significantly reduces cardiovascular death and all-cause mortality and is FDA approved for the reduction of major cardiovascular events and cardiovascular deaths in adults with type 2 diabetes and CVD.

STUDY TABLE: Adverse Effects Associated with Common Noninsulin Diabetes Medications		
Class	**Adverse Effect**	**Caution/Avoid**
Sulfonylureas (glipizide, glimepiride, others)	Weight gain, hypoglycemia, skin rashes	Reduced drug clearance in kidney failure for some sulfonylureas
Biguanides (metformin)	Diarrhea, abdominal discomfort, lactic acidosis	Contraindicated in patients with an eGFR ≤30 mL/min/1.73 m^2
α-Glucosidase inhibitors (acarbose, miglitol, voglibose)	Abdominal discomfort	Avoid in kidney injury
Thiazolidinediones (rosiglitazone, pioglitazone)	Weight gain, edema, HF, macular edema, osteoporosis, bladder cancer risk	Possible increase in cardiovascular events and mortality with rosiglitazone
Meglitinides (repaglinide, nateglinide)	Weight gain, hypoglycemia	Reduced drug clearance in kidney failure
Amylinomimetics (pramlintide)	Nausea, vomiting	Increases hypoglycemia associated with insulin
GLP-1 mimetics (exenatide, liraglutide)	Nausea, vomiting	Possible increased risk of pancreatitis and kidney failure
DPP-4 inhibitors (sitagliptin, saxagliptin, vildagliptin, linagliptin, alogliptin)	Nausea, skin rashes, increased risk of infections	Possible increased risk of pancreatitis, HF exacerbation
SGLT2 inhibitors (dapagliflozin, empagliflozin, canagliflozin)	Increased genital candidal infections and UTIs	Hypoglycemia with insulin secretagogues and insulin; possible increase in DKA; canagliflozin associated with increased risk of lower extremity amputation. Use with caution in patients with a history of peripheral vascular disease, previous amputations, diabetic ulcers, or neuropathy.

DPP-4 = dipeptidyl peptidase-4; GLP-1 = glucagon-like peptide-1; SGLT2 = sodium-glucose transporter-2.

If weight loss is a desired effect, GLP-1 mimetics, pramlintide, and SGLT2 inhibitors are the best choices.

Screening recommendations for chronic complications of diabetes: Patients with type 1 and type 2 diabetes should be screened regularly for diabetic complications, including retinopathy (comprehensive eye examination), nephropathy (albumin-to-creatinine ratio), neuropathy (10 g monofilament, 128-Hz tuning fork, pedal pulses, and ankle reflex), and cardiovascular disease (BP and fasting lipid profile measurements).

Screening for complications in patients with type 1 diabetes should begin at 5 years after diagnosis and should be performed annually thereafter. Screening for complications in patients with type 2 diabetes should begin at the time of diagnosis and be performed annually thereafter.

STUDY TABLE: Treatment of Diabetes Complications		
Condition	**Goal or Indication**	**Treatment**
Hypertension	BP goal <130/80 mm Hg (ACC/AHA hypertension guideline)	All first-line antihypertensive drug classes (ACC/AHA)
	BP goal <140/90 mm Hg (ADA guideline)	ACE inhibitor or ARB should be considered in patients with albuminuria
Diabetes and average cardiovascular risk	Age >40 years, diabetes, and a 10-year ASCVD risk <7.5% (ACC/AHA guideline)	Moderate-intensity statin
Diabetes and increased cardiovascular risk	CAD, peripheral vascular disease, or ASCVD risk ≥7.5% (AHA/ACC guideline)	High-intensity statin
	Age 40-75 years, diabetes, and a calculated 10-year risk of a cardiovascular event ≥10% (USPSTF recommendation)	Moderate- to high-intensity statin
Nephropathy	Urine albumin excretion ≥30 mg/g of creatinine	ACE inhibitor or ARB

(Continued on the next page)

STUDY TABLE: Treatment of Diabetes Complications (Continued)		
Condition	**Goal or Indication**	**Treatment**
Diabetic retinopathy	Proliferative and nonproliferative retinopathy	Excellent blood glucose and BP control and smoking cessation Panretinal laser photocoagulation for PDR and severe NPDR Intraocular injections of bevacizumab or ranibizumab for severe NPDR and PDR or macular edema
Diabetic peripheral neuropathy	Numbness, tingling, burning, heaviness, pain, or sensitivity in stocking-glove distribution	Amitriptyline, venlafaxine, duloxetine, paroxetine, pregabalin, gabapentin, valproate, or capsaicin cream
Sexual dysfunction	Erectile dysfunction	Oral phosphodiesterase inhibitor (sildenafil, vardenafil, tadalafil)
Gastroparesis	Early satiety, nausea and vomiting	Small feedings; metoclopramide or erythromycin
Diabetic foot	Ulcer or osteomyelitis	See Infectious Disease, Diabetic Foot Infections

ACC/AHA = American College of Cardiology/American Heart Association; ADA = American Diabetes Association; NPDR = nonproliferative diabetic retinopathy; PDR = proliferative diabetic retinopathy; USPSTF = U.S. Preventive Services Task Force.

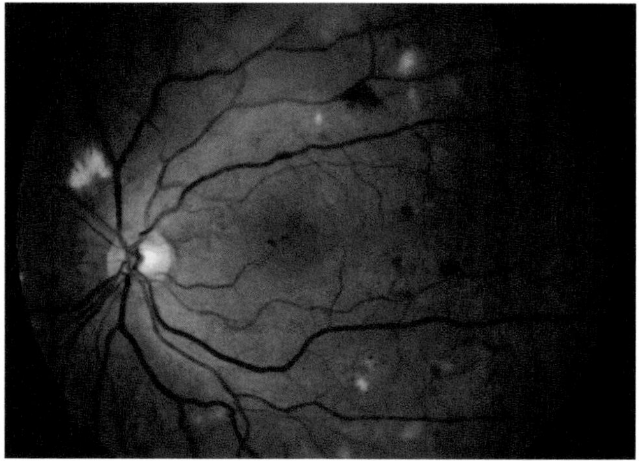

Nonproliferative Diabetic Retinopathy: Dot-and-blot hemorrhages and clusters of hard, yellowish exudates are characteristic of nonproliferative diabetic retinopathy.

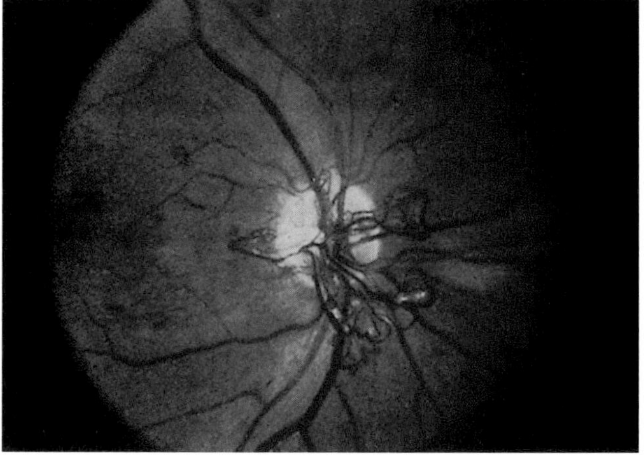

Proliferative Diabetic Retinopathy: A network of new vessels (neovascularization) is shown protruding from the optic nerve.

DON'T BE TRICKED

- Do not treat diabetic mononeuropathy (e.g., third nerve palsy); symptoms resolve spontaneously.

TEST YOURSELF

A 29-year-old woman with a 10-year history of type 1 diabetes has nocturnal hypoglycemia. Her insulin schedule includes 24 units NPH insulin/10 units regular insulin before breakfast and 14 units NPH insulin/10 units regular insulin before dinner. Her hemoglobin A_{1c} is 7.2%. What change should be made to her insulin regimen?

ANSWER: For management, three answers are possible: delay the NPH insulin until bedtime, lower the evening NPH dose, or (an even better choice) stop the NPH insulin and substitute insulin glargine at bedtime.

A 58-year-old man with type 2 diabetes has a hemoglobin A_{1c} value >9%. He takes metformin 1000 mg/d and glyburide 10 mg/d. His fasting and preprandial plasma glucose levels are >130 mg/dL.

ANSWER: For management, choose to add evening basal insulin.

Hyperglycemic Hyperosmolar Syndrome

Diagnosis

Hyperglycemic hyperosmolar syndrome is defined as a plasma osmolality >320 mOsm/kg H_2O, a plasma glucose level >600 mg/dL, either no or low serum levels of ketones, and a relatively normal arterial pH and bicarbonate level. The diagnosis should be considered in any older adult patient with altered mental status and hypovolemia.

Treatment

Manage hyperglycemic hyperosmolar syndrome mainly by identifying the underlying precipitating illness and restoring the contracted plasma volume. Choose normal saline first to replenish the extracellular space. When BP is restored and urine output is established, administer hypotonic solutions. Administer IV insulin only after expansion of the intravascular space has begun. After the plasma glucose level decreases to <200 mg/dL and the patient is eating, begin subcutaneous insulin injections.

Diabetic Ketoacidosis

Diagnosis

The major manifestations of DKA (hyperglycemia, ketosis, and hypovolemia) are directly or indirectly related to insulin deficiency.

Laboratory findings include a plasma glucose level ≥250 mg/dL, arterial blood pH ≤7.30, bicarbonate level ≤15 mEq/L, widened anion gap, and positive serum ketone levels. Evaluate patients for underlying precipitants of DKA, such as medication nonadherence, infection, and MI.

Treatment

Give normal saline solution for immediate volume replacement. Switch to 0.45% sodium chloride after the initial bolus if the serum sodium level is high or normal. Then give:

- insulin infusion (delay if serum potassium level is <3.3 mEq/L)
- potassium replacement when the serum potassium level is <5.5 mEq/L
- glucose infusion (5% dextrose with 0.45% normal saline) when the plasma glucose level is <250 mg/dL
- continued insulin and glucose infusions until the serum anion gap is normal

DON'T BE TRICKED

- DKA can present with abdominal pain.
- Reducing the insulin infusion before complete clearing of ketones will cause a relapse of DKA.
- Treatment of severe acidosis with bicarbonate is controversial, and evidence of benefit is lacking.

Diabetes Care for Hospitalized Patients

Treatment

Insulin is the preferred treatment for achieving inpatient glycemic control. Critically ill patients with type 2 diabetes are treated with IV insulin infusion when plasma glucose levels exceed 180 to 200 mg/dL. Glucose goals are 140 to 180 mg/dL.

For non–critically ill patients, the insulin regimen should incorporate both basal and prandial coverage. Prandial coverage can be supplemented with additional insulin (correction factor insulin) for preprandial hyperglycemia.

DON'T BE TRICKED

- Do not select sliding scale insulin alone to treat in-hospital hyperglycemia.
- Tight inpatient glycemic control (80-110 mg/dL [4.4-6.1 mmol/L]) is not consistently associated with improved outcomes and may increase mortality.

Continuing outpatient oral or noninsulin injectable agents is not recommended when patients are hospitalized because of the potential for hemodynamic or nutritional changes. Begin insulin therapy for management of hyperglycemia. Continuing oral agents should only be considered in a stable inpatient with glycemic control at goal who has no anticipated changes in nutrition or hemodynamic status.

Pregnancy and Diabetes

Screening

Screen women for gestational diabetes at 24 to 28 weeks of gestation with the 75-gram 2-hour OGTT.

DON'T BE TRICKED

- Women with a history of gestational diabetes are at very high risk for developing type 2 diabetes and require annual screening following delivery.

Treatment

Lowering the hemoglobin A_{1c} value to within 1% of normal decreases the risk of congenital malformations and fetal loss. Glycemic targets in pregnancy include premeal plasma glucose <95 mg/dL and 1-hour postprandial values <140 mg/dL and 2-hour postprandial values <120 mg/dL.

Try lifestyle interventions as initial treatment, with the addition of insulin if glycemic targets are not met.

Management strategies in pregnant women are different from those in other patients with diabetes:

- Insulin should replace oral hypoglycemic agents.
- ACE inhibitors, ARBs, and cholesterol-lowering drugs should be stopped before pregnancy.
- A comprehensive eye examination should be completed once per trimester.

Employ aggressive BP control to avoid worsening of diabetic nephropathy and retinopathy. Antihypertensive agents that can be safely used during pregnancy include methyldopa, β-blockers (except atenolol), calcium channel blockers, and hydralazine.

Hypoglycemia in Patients Without Diabetes

Diagnosis

Evaluate for hypoglycemia if the criteria for Whipple triad are met: neuroglycopenic symptoms, hypoglycemia ≤55 mg/dL, and resolution of symptoms with glucose ingestion.

Hypoglycemic disorders are classified as postprandial or fasting.

Postprandial hypoglycemia typically occurs within 5 hours of the last meal and is commonly caused by previous gastrectomy or gastric bypass surgery. Meals consisting of simple carbohydrates (pancakes, syrup, juice) are frequently the cause.

STUDY TABLE: Diagnosis of Nondiabetic Fasting Hypoglycemia	
Condition	**Diagnosis**
Surreptitious use of oral hypoglycemic agents	Patient has access to hypoglycemic agents. Serum C-peptide levels are inappropriately elevated at time of hypoglycemia. Perform urine screen for sulfonylurea and meglitinide metabolites.
Surreptitious use of insulin	Patient has access to insulin. Serum C-peptide levels are low at time of hypoglycemia.
Insulinoma	Perform 72-hour fast and document fasting plasma glucose level <45 mg/dL, serum insulin >5-6 mU/L, and elevated C-peptide levels. If positive, schedule abdominal CT.
Substrate deficiency	Starvation, liver failure, or sepsis; suppressed hepatic glucose production (alcoholism; cortisol or GH deficiencies)

Begin the evaluation of all patients with fasting hypoglycemia with screening for surreptitious use of an oral hypoglycemia agent, such as a sulfonylurea or insulin.

MEN1 can present as hyperparathyroidism, pituitary neoplasms, or pancreatic neuroendocrine tumors (NETs). Pancreatic NETs include gastrinomas that can cause PUD and insulinomas that can cause hypoglycemia.

DON'T BE TRICKED

- **Home glucometers may be inaccurate in the hypoglycemic range.**
- **Asymptomatic hypoglycemia with a plasma glucose level <60 mg/dL is often found after fasting in patients without underlying disease and does not require evaluation.**

Treatment

Treat acute hypoglycemia with oral carbohydrates, IV glucose, or IM glucagon.

For management of postprandial hypoglycemia associated with previous gastrectomy or gastric bypass surgery, choose small mixed meals containing protein, fat, and high-fiber complex carbohydrates.

TEST YOURSELF

A previously healthy 28-year-old female registered nurse is found unconscious on the ward where she works. Her plasma glucose level is 28 mg/dL. She regains consciousness following IV glucose administration. Serum insulin level is 42 mU/L (normal, 2-20 mU/L), and serum C-peptide level is 7.2 ng/mL (normal, 0.9-4.0 ng/mL).

ANSWER: For diagnosis, select factitious hypoglycemia. For management, choose screening for surreptitious ingestion of hypoglycemic agents such as sulfonylureas.

Hypopituitarism

Diagnosis

Hypopituitarism may be partial or complete and acute or chronic. Most commonly, hypopituitarism is the result of a pituitary tumor that causes progressive hypofunction by applying pressure to the normal gland. Pituitary surgery and cranial irradiation are other common causes.

Pituitary apoplexy results from sudden pituitary hemorrhage or infarction, which causes acute hypopituitarism and is often associated with sudden headache, visual change, ophthalmoplegia, and altered mental status.

Postpartum pituitary necrosis (Sheehan syndrome) is caused by silent pituitary infarction and is usually associated with obstetric hemorrhage and hypotension. Acutely, vascular collapse may occur, but more commonly the syndrome presents with amenorrhea, a postpartum inability to lactate, and fatigue.

Lymphocytic hypophysitis causes hypopituitarism and, possibly, symptoms of a mass lesion. Most cases of lymphocytic hypophysitis occur during or after pregnancy.

Symptoms of anterior hypopituitarism are identical to primary target-organ hypofunction. However, the presence of headache and loss of peripheral vision suggest a pituitary mass effect.

Look for:

- amenorrhea, loss of libido, or erectile dysfunction (FSH/LH deficiency)
- fatigue, nausea, vomiting, weight loss, or abdominal pain (ACTH deficiency)
- cold intolerance, weight gain, or constipation (TSH deficiency)
- loss of muscle mass (GH deficiency)
- polydipsia, polyuria, and nocturia (DI secondary to ADH deficiency)
- visual field diagram showing bitemporal loss of vision (mass effect on the optic chiasm)

Testing

Diagnosis is confirmed by documenting target-organ hormone deficiency and a corresponding low or "normal" serum pituitary hormone level. Stimulation testing may be needed to document hypopituitarism.

STUDY TABLE: Key Hormone Tests for Hypopituitarism

Hormone	Findings
GH	Depressed IGF-1
	Diminished response to insulin tolerance test (insulin-induced hypoglycemia)
FSH/LH	Depressed FSH, LH, and estradiol or testosterone levels
TSH	Depressed free T_4 and TSH
ACTH	Low cortisol level and depressed ACTH
	Depressed response of 11-deoxycortisol and cortisol to metyrapone
	Positive cortisol response to ACTH
Prolactin	Level may be elevated from loss of tonic inhibition

After documenting hypopituitarism or hyperprolactinemia, select MRI of the pituitary gland.

DON'T BE TRICKED

- **It is not necessary to measure serum FSH/LH levels in women who have normal menstrual cycles.**
- **Do not measure GH because its release is pulsatile; measure the serum marker of GH instead (IGF-1).**

Treatment

Hydrocortisone is indicated for patients with adrenal insufficiency. Androgen replacement is appropriate for men with hypogonadism, and estrogen replacement is used for premenopausal women with hypogonadism. Consider GH replacement for biochemically confirmed deficiency and consistent symptoms.

Pituitary apoplexy requires acute administration of glucocorticoids until acute adrenal insufficiency has been ruled out and may also require urgent neurosurgical decompression.

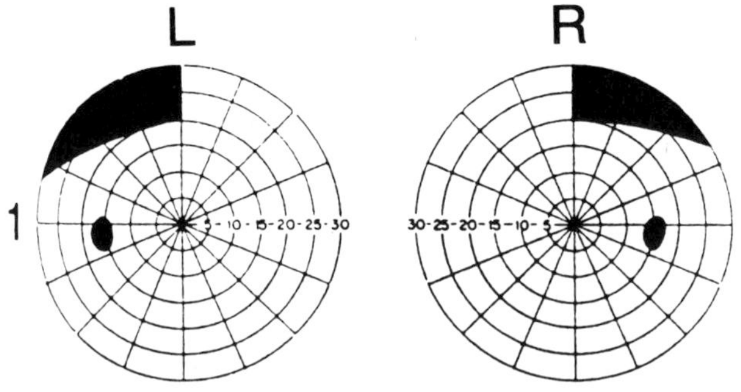

Visual Field Defects: Bitemporal quadrant visual field defects secondary to a pituitary mass.

DON'T BE TRICKED

- **Thyroxine dosing for central hypothyroidism is based on serum free T_4 rather than TSH levels.**
- **T_4 replacement is indicated only after hypoadrenalism has been ruled out or treated.**

TEST YOURSELF

A 65-year-old man was diagnosed with SCLC 20 years ago and received chemotherapy and chest and cranial irradiation. Physical examination shows hypotension, tachycardia, and small testes. Serum sodium is 123 mEq/L.

ANSWER: For diagnosis, choose hypopituitarism. For management, select immediate replacement with stress doses of hydrocortisone followed by confirmatory testing.

Pituitary Adenomas

Diagnosis

Pituitary adenomas are benign tumors that originate from one of the different anterior pituitary cell types. They are classified based on size as microadenomas (<10 mm) or macroadenomas (≥10 mm).

Pituitary adenomas become symptomatic by two different mechanisms:

- mass effect causing hypopituitarism (anterior hormone deficiencies more common than posterior), headaches, visual disturbance/visual field defects, and cranial nerve dysfunction
- endocrine hyperfunction caused by excess secretion by the tumor

DON'T BE TRICKED

- **The pituitary gland is enlarged diffusely in untreated primary hypothyroidism and during normal pregnancies.**

Testing

STUDY TABLE: Diagnosis of Pituitary Adenomas

If you see this...	Think this...	Order this...
Galactorrhea, amenorrhea	Prolactinoma	Serum prolactin level
Enlargement of hands, feet, nose, lips, or tongue; increased spacing of teeth	Acromegaly	Serum IGF-1 OGTT (fails to suppress GH)
Proximal muscle weakness, facial rounding, centripetal obesity, purple striae, diabetes mellitus, and hypertension	Cushing disease	24-hour urine cortisol excretion, dexamethasone suppression test, or late night salivary cortisol level (elevated), serum ACTH level (elevated or inappropriately "normal")
Goiter and hyperthyroidism	TSH-secreting adenoma (rare)	TSH normal or elevated; increased T_4

Test all patients with an incidentally discovered pituitary adenoma for hormone hypersecretion.

Order MRI if testing indicates hormonal hypersecretion from a pituitary source.

If mass effect is the presenting symptom (headache, visual disturbances), obtain MRI first and endocrine testing later.

Evaluate patients with at least one component of MEN1 (usually hyperparathyroidism) and a family history of MEN1 for a pituitary adenoma.

Psychotropic agents, tricyclic antidepressants, antiseizure medications, metoclopramide and domperidone, calcium channel blockers, methyldopa, opiates, and protease inhibitors can cause hyperprolactinemia.

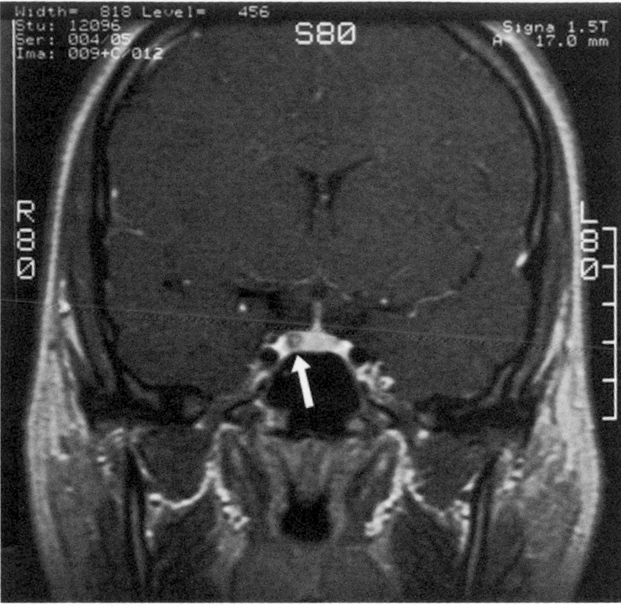

Prolactinoma: A discrete area of hypolucency (*arrow*) is seen in an otherwise normal-sized pituitary gland of homogeneous density.

DON'T BE TRICKED

- **The prolactin level influenced by drugs and other nonprolactinoma conditions is usually <150 ng/mL.**
- **Obtain a pregnancy test in all women with hyperprolactinemia.**
- **Obtain a serum TSH level in all patients with hyperprolactinemia (hypothyroidism can cause hyperprolactinemia).**

Treatment

Choose **observation** for women with microprolactinoma and normal menses or for patients with nonfunctioning pituitary microadenomas.

Choose **medication** such as a dopamine agonist (cabergoline preferred to bromocriptine) for symptomatic prolactinoma. Consider withdrawal of dopamine agonist therapy for prolactinomas no longer visible on neuroimaging if the prolactin level has normalized. Close follow-up is required because of recurrence rates of up to 50%.

Choose **surgery** for adenomas secreting GH, ACTH, or TSH; for adenomas associated with mass effect, visual field defects, or hypopituitarism; and for prolactinomas unresponsive to dopamine agonists.

TEST YOURSELF

A 32-year-old woman has a 4-mm hypointense area in the pituitary gland discovered incidentally on an MRI. Medical history, including menstrual function, and physical examination are normal. The serum prolactin level and thyroid function tests are normal.

ANSWER: For diagnosis, choose an incidental nonfunctioning pituitary adenoma. For management, repeat the MRI in 1 year.

Diabetes Insipidus

Diagnosis

DI is characterized by an inability to concentrate urine because of insufficient arginine vasopressin (AVP, ADH) release (central DI) or activity (nephrogenic DI).

History includes recent head trauma or neurosurgery, pituitary mass lesion, evidence of anterior hypopituitarism (adrenal insufficiency, hypothyroidism), history of an infiltrative disorder (such as sarcoidosis), kidney disease (tubulointerstitial disease), or medications such as lithium.

Symptoms and signs of central DI are cravings for water or cold liquids, urinary frequency, nocturia, and, depending on mass effect of a pituitary tumor, visual field deficits.

Testing

Patients typically have large-volume polyuria. Measure the plasma glucose level to rule out diabetes mellitus and the serum calcium level to rule out hypercalcemia as causes of polyuria.

Urine osmolality <200 mOsm/kg H_2O and the inability to increase the urine concentration during a water deprivation test confirm the diagnosis. When DI has been confirmed, a desmopressin challenge test is done to differentiate between central and nephrogenic forms. If the desmopressin challenge test is positive (urine concentrates, indicating central DI), order an MRI of the pituitary gland. If the test is negative (urine does not concentrate, indicating nephrogenic DI), order kidney ultrasonography.

Treatment

STUDY TABLE: Treating Diabetes Insipidus

If you see...	Choose...
DI after neurosurgery or head trauma	If unable to drink, 5% dextrose in 0.45% sodium chloride IV Add desmopressin if urine output is high or hypernatremia develops
Chronic central DI	Intranasal or oral desmopressin
Lithium-induced nephrogenic DI	Stop lithium or add amiloride
Non-drug-induced nephrogenic DI	Thiazide diuretic and salt restriction

TEST YOURSELF

A previously healthy 27-year-old woman has a 1-month history of polydipsia and polyuria. She has had amenorrhea since giving birth 9 months ago. Her plasma glucose level is 90 mg/dL, urine output is 4 L/d, and urine osmolality is 95 mOsm/kg H_2O.

ANSWER: For diagnosis, choose central DI.

Empty Sella Syndrome

Diagnosis

Empty sella is diagnosed when the normal pituitary gland is not visualized or is excessively small on MRI. Causes include:

- increased CSF entering and enlarging the sella
- tumor
- previous pituitary surgery, radiation, or infarction

Testing

In asymptomatic persons, obtain measures of cortisol, TSH, and free (or total) T_4. A patient with symptoms of hormone deficiency requires testing of all pituitary hormones.

If examination reveals normal hormone functioning, repeated imaging is not necessary.

Hyperthyroidism

Diagnosis

The term **thyrotoxicosis** encompasses any cause of thyroid hormone excess, including primary and secondary hyperthyroidism, excessive thyroid hormone release resulting from thyroid destruction, and excessive exogenous thyroid hormone ingestion.

Thyrotoxicosis occurs in destructive thyroiditis because thyroid damage results in release of preformed thyroid hormone into the circulation. Forms of destructive thyroiditis include subacute (de Quervain), silent (painless), and postpartum thyroiditis. Subacute thyroiditis is a nonautoimmune inflammation that generally presents with a firm and painful thyroid gland. Postpartum thyroiditis is a painless autoimmune thyroiditis occurring within a few months of delivery. Permanent hypothyroidism may follow all forms of destructive thyroiditis.

Look for symptoms of thyrotoxicosis:

- nervousness, emotional lability
- increased sweating, heat intolerance
- palpitations
- increased defecation
- weight loss
- menstrual irregularity

Look for signs of thyrotoxicosis:

- tachycardia
- lid lag
- fine tremor
- muscle wasting, proximal muscle weakness
- hyperreflexia

The term **hyperthyroidism** refers specifically to disorders of increased thyroid hormone production and release, such as destructive thyroiditis, Graves disease, autonomous thyroid nodules, and toxic multinodular goiter.

The most common causes of hyperthyroidism are Graves disease and toxic adenoma(s). Symptoms and signs of thyrotoxicosis are usually present in patients with hyperthyroidism. Physical examination findings specific for Graves disease include goiter, ophthalmopathy (proptosis, chemosis, and extraocular muscle palsy), and pretibial myxedema.

Older adult patients with hyperthyroidism may present with depression, AF, and HF.

Thyroid storm is the development of life-threatening hyperthyroidism associated with cardiac decompensation, fever, delirium, and psychosis. It may occur following surgery, infection, or administration of an acute iodine load (contrast agents) and may also develop in patients with untreated Graves disease. Thyroid storm is a clinical diagnosis; no level of thyroid hormone elevation is diagnostic.

Testing

Order serum TSH and free T_4 levels to make the diagnosis of thyrotoxicosis. If TSH is suppressed but T_4 is normal, order free T_3 to diagnose T_3 toxicosis (rare). Ancillary laboratory testing may reveal mild hypercalcemia, elevated alkaline phosphatase level, and low total and HDL cholesterol levels.

Thyroglobulin levels can be elevated in hyperthyroidism and thyroiditis. Intake of exogenous thyroid hormone suppresses thyroglobulin levels, which makes its measurement useful in patients with thyrotoxicosis caused by surreptitious use of thyroid hormone.

An elevated serum ESR supports thyroiditis, whereas TSH-receptor antibodies are associated with Graves disease. However, antibodies need not be checked routinely in the evaluation of hyperthyroidism unless the diagnosis is unclear.

STUDY TABLE: Interpreting Thyroid Function Tests in Hyperthyroidism

If you see this...	Choose this...
↓TSH, ↑free T_4	Primary hyperthyroidism
↓TSH, ↑T_3, normal free T_4	Primary hyperthyroidism with T_3 toxicosis
↓TSH, normal T_3 and free T_4, without symptoms	Subclinical hyperthyroidism
↑TSH, ↑T_3, ↑free T_4	Secondary hyperthyroidism from a pituitary tumor (central hyperthyroidism)

Imaging

STUDY TABLE: Radioactive Iodine Uptake and Scan Interpretation

Result	Diagnosis
Diffuse homogeneous increased uptake	Graves disease
Patchy areas of increased uptake	Toxic multinodular goiter
Focal increased uptake with decreased uptake in the rest of the gland	Solitary adenoma
Decreased or no uptake	Iodine load (IV contrast or amiodarone)
	Thyroiditis (silent, subacute, postpartum, or amiodarone induced)
	Surreptitious ingestion of excessive thyroid hormone

Treatment

Available strategies for managing hyperthyroidism include antithyroid drugs, radioactive iodine therapy (^{131}I), and thyroid surgery.

Radioactive iodine therapy is associated with few adverse effects but may lead to painful radiation thyroiditis and sialadenitis; it is not used during pregnancy or breastfeeding. Choose ^{131}I therapy or surgery to treat toxic multinodular goiter or toxic adenoma. With ^{131}I ablation, hyperactive nodules take up iodine preferentially while suppressed normal tissue receives minimal radiation exposure. Treatment frequently restores euthyroidism.

Antithyroid drugs may lead to a drug-free remission of Graves disease in 30% to 50% of patients after 1 year of treatment. Antithyroid drugs may also be used short term as a bridge to more definitive therapy (radioactive iodine or thyroidectomy).

STUDY TABLE: Comparison of Antithyroid Drugs

Treatment	Indicated for...	Watch for...
Methimazole	First-line antithyroid medication for most patients	Agranulocytosis, drug rash, hepatotoxicity
Propylthiouracil	Treatment of choice in first trimester of pregnancy; preferred in thyroid storm (inhibits peripheral T_4 to T_3 conversion)	Same as methimazole, except more frequent hepatotoxicity

Thyroidectomy is preferred when definitive therapy for hyperthyroidism is required in a patient with severe Graves ophthalmopathy. Thyroidectomy may also be considered if radioactive iodine or antithyroid drugs cannot be given or are not tolerated or if a large goiter is causing local symptoms.

STUDY TABLE: Management of Thyrotoxicosis

If you see this...	Choose this...
Sympathetic nervous system symptoms	Atenolol or propranolol
Preparation for thyroidectomy	Methimazole
Severe Graves ophthalmopathy	Methimazole or thyroidectomy
	Avoid radioactive iodine (may cause worsening of ophthalmopathy unless pretreated with glucocorticoids)
Pregnancy	Propylthiouracil in first trimester of pregnancy, methimazole thereafter
	Radioactive iodine is contraindicated
Subclinical hyperthyroidism	Methimazole if TSH <0.1 µU/mL
Subacute thyroiditis	NSAIDs or glucocorticoids for pain management; atenolol or propranolol for symptoms of hyperthyroidism; levothyroxine for symptomatic hypothyroidism; repeat thyroid studies in 4-6 months. In 50% of patients, thyroid studies will normalize without intervention.
Suspicious nodule (malignancy)	FNAB followed by thyroidectomy (if malignant)
Thyroid storm	Propylthiouracil (preferred) or methimazole, iodine-potassium solutions, glucocorticoids, and β-blockers

DON'T BE TRICKED

- A fever or sore throat in a patient taking methimazole or propylthiouracil should be presumed to be agranulocytosis until proven otherwise.

TEST YOURSELF

An asymptomatic 78-year-old woman has a serum TSH level of 0.2 µU/mL. Serum T_3 and T_4 levels are normal.

ANSWER: For diagnosis, choose subclinical hyperthyroidism. For management, choose to repeat thyroid tests in 4 to 6 months.

Hypothyroidism

Diagnosis

Symptoms and Signs

Look for symptoms suggesting hypothyroidism:

- weakness, lethargy, fatigue
- depression, impaired concentration
- myalgia
- cold intolerance
- constipation
- weight gain
- menstrual irregularity or menorrhagia
- carpal tunnel syndrome

Examination findings include bradycardia, hypothermia, diastolic hypertension, husky voice, goiter, cool dry skin, brittle hair, edema, and delayed relaxation phase of deep tendon reflexes.

Causes

The most common causes of hypothyroidism include:

- chronic lymphocytic (Hashimoto) thyroiditis
- thyroidectomy
- previous radioactive iodine ablation
- history of external beam radiation to the neck

Hashimoto thyroiditis increases in prevalence with age and is usually associated with a goiter.

Transient mild hypothyroidism typically occurs during the second phase of **destructive thyroiditis** (initial phase is hyperthyroidism). Permanent hypothyroidism may follow either postpartum thyroiditis (more common) or subacute thyroiditis (less common).

Medication-induced hypothyroidism can occur with the use of certain drugs, including lithium carbonate, interferon alfa, interleukin-2, and amiodarone.

Central hypothyroidism results from pituitary disease or from previous surgery or radiation therapy to the sella. TSH and free T_4 are suppressed.

Myxedema coma is defined as severe hypothyroidism leading to decreased mental status, hypothermia, hypotension, bradycardia, hyponatremia, hypoglycemia, hypoxemia, and hypoventilation. It occurs in patients with severe, long-standing, untreated hypothyroidism and may be precipitated by an acute medical or surgical event or the administration of opiates.

Testing

Order TSH and free T_4 to make the diagnosis. Measurement of T_3 levels is generally not necessary. An antithyroid peroxidase antibody assay is associated with Hashimoto thyroiditis but is not needed to make the diagnosis; high levels are associated with an increased risk of permanent hypothyroidism.

Hypothyroidism may be associated with hyperprolactinemia, hyponatremia and increased CK, AST, and cholesterol levels.

Nonthyroidal illness syndrome occurs in patients who are acutely ill with a nonthyroidal illness. Testing reveals low or normal free T_4 and suppressed TSH (initially) followed by elevated TSH (recovery phase). Normalization of thyroid function tests occurs 4 to 8 weeks after recovery.

DON'T BE TRICKED

- **Thyroid scan and radioactive iodine uptake tests are not needed to make the diagnosis of hypothyroidism.**

STUDY TABLE: Interpreting Thyroid Function Tests in Hypothyroidism

If you see this...	Choose this...
↑TSH, ↓free T_4	Primary hypothyroidism
↑TSH, normal T_4	Subclinical hypothyroidism
↓TSH, ↓free T_4	Secondary (central) hypothyroidism; consider hypopituitarism

Treatment

Levothyroxine is the only agent used to treat hypothyroidism. Treatment is indicated for subclinical hypothyroidism when the serum TSH is >10 µU/mL.

Treat women with subclinical hypothyroidism who are pregnant or who want to become pregnant because greater maternal and fetal risk is associated with this disorder.

Recall that celiac disease, calcium and iron supplements, and PPIs can decrease levothyroxine absorption.

DON'T BE TRICKED

- **No treatment is required for nonthyroidal illness syndrome.**
- **Check thyroid function tests frequently during pregnancy in women with a known diagnosis of hypothyroidism taking thyroxine, because maternal thyroxine demand increases by 30% to 50%.**

STUDY TABLE: Levothyroxine Treatment of Hypothyroidism

Condition	Treatment
Age <60 years	Begin full-dose levothyroxine (about 100 µg/d)
Age >60 years	Begin levothyroxine at 25-50 µg/d
	Increase by 25 µg every 6 weeks until TSH level is 1.0-2.5 µU/mL
Heart disease	Begin levothyroxine at 12.5-25 µg/d
	Increase by 12.5-25 µg every 6 weeks until TSH level is 1.0-2.5 µU/mL
Myxedema coma	Begin levothyroxine and hydrocortisone
	Hydrocortisone should be given until concomitant adrenal insufficiency has been ruled out
Pregnancy	The levothyroxine dose should be increased by 30% initially in pregnant patients with existing hypothyroidism; check thyroid function frequently during pregnancy

Thyroid Nodules

Diagnosis

Thyroid nodules are common and are often found incidentally on physical examination or imaging tests.

History: Look for risk factors for thyroid cancer, including family history of thyroid malignancy, personal history of radiation therapy to the head and neck, or other radiation exposure in childhood.

Imaging and Testing

Thyroid ultrasonography allows for accurate detection and sizing of all nodules, and ultrasound characteristics can be used to further delineate cancer risk.

When a nodule is discovered, assess thyroid function with a serum TSH level.

A low TSH level suggests a benign, autonomously functioning thyroid adenoma. If TSH is suppressed, order a radioisotope scan to confirm the diagnosis and to rule out additional nonfunctioning nodules within a multinodular goiter. The serum TSH level is normal (and unhelpful) in most other patients with thyroid nodules.

Evaluate patients with multinodular goiter for compressive symptoms:

- dysphagia
- hoarseness
- dyspnea (tracheal compression from substernal goiter)

Consider evaluation with barium swallow, direct vocal cord visualization, spirometry with flow volume loops, and/or chest CT as needed.

FNAB is indicated for:

- all thyroid nodules >1 cm with suspicious sonographic features and a normal TSH level
- nodules <1 cm in patients with risk factors for thyroid cancer or suspicious ultrasound characteristics

In patients with multinodular goiter, the risk for malignancy is the same for multiple nodules as it is for a solitary nodule; therefore, evaluation and management is identical.

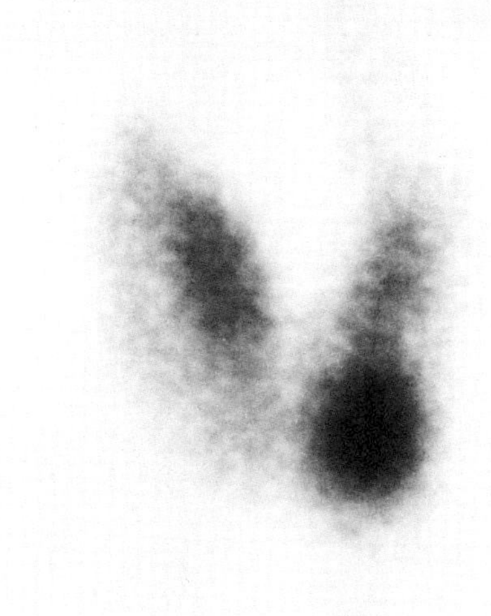

Thyroid Nodule: A hyperfunctioning nodule is shown on the lateral aspect of the left thyroid lobe on thyroid scan.

DON'T BE TRICKED

- **Serum thyroglobulin measurement is not helpful in distinguishing benign from malignant thyroid nodules.**
- **Calcitonin measurement is only considered in patients with hypercalcemia or a family history of thyroid cancer or MEN2.**

Management and Treatment

Observation: Follow benign nodules with periodic ultrasonography. Although one third of benign nodules may increase in size, malignancy must be ruled out when a nodule increases in size or if a nodule develops concerning ultrasound characteristics.

Radioactive iodine or surgery: Treat hyperfunctioning solitary thyroid nodules with radioactive iodine ablation or hemithyroidectomy.

Surgery is indicated for patients with continued nodule growth despite normal initial FNAB results or nondiagnostic results on repeat FNAB and for patients with malignant cytology. Surgery is also indicated for large multinodular goiters associated with compressive symptoms.

DON'T BE TRICKED

- Do not prescribe T_4-suppression therapy for benign thyroid nodules.

TEST YOURSELF

An 18-year-old man has a 2-cm right-sided thyroid nodule. The serum TSH level is 1.4 µU/mL.

ANSWER: For management, choose FNAB.

Hypercortisolism (Cushing Syndrome)

Diagnosis

Cushing syndrome results from ongoing exposure to excess glucocorticoid.

The most common cause of Cushing syndrome is iatrogenic, specifically the use of systemic, topical, intra-articular, or inhaled glucocorticoids. Doses of prednisone (or equivalent) ≤5 mg/d are unlikely to cause clinically significant hypothalamic-pituitary-adrenal axis suppression, whereas those >10-20 mg/d can cause hypothalamic-pituitary-adrenal axis suppression after ≥3 weeks of consecutive use.

Endogenous causes of Cushing syndrome can be ACTH-dependent or ACTH-independent.

ACTH-dependent causes of Cushing syndrome are defined by ACTH levels elevated or inappropriately "normal" in relation to the cortisol level:

- ACTH-secreting pituitary adenomas (Cushing disease)
- ACTH-secreting carcinomas and carcinoid tumors

ACTH-independent causes of Cushing syndrome are defined by low or "normal" ACTH levels in relation to the cortisol level:

- adrenal adenomas
- adrenal carcinomas

Clinical findings highly specific for Cushing syndrome include:

- centripetal obesity
- facial plethora
- supraclavicular or dorsocervical ("buffalo hump") fat pads
- wide (>1 cm) violaceous striae

Testing

First-line diagnostic studies include:

- 1-mg overnight dexamethasone suppression test (failure to suppress serum cortisol to <3 µg/dL)
- 24-hour urine cortisol level (elevated)
- late night salivary cortisol level (elevated)

If the cortisol level is elevated (or not suppressible), order an ACTH level to differentiate ACTH-dependent from ACTH-independent hypercortisolism.

STUDY TABLE: Evaluation of Hypercortisolism

If you see this...	Do this...
Morning ACTH elevated (>20 pg/mL)	Pituitary MRI or CT
Morning ACTH suppressed or normal (<5 pg/mL)	Adrenal CT

If ACTH is elevated but no pituitary tumor is visualized, perform high-dose (8-mg dexamethasone) suppression test to differentiate between pituitary and ectopic tumor ACTH production.

If high-dose dexamethasone does not suppress cortisol production, an ectopic tumor is releasing ACTH. The most common ACTH-secreting malignant tumors are SCLC, bronchial carcinoid, pheochromocytoma, and medullary thyroid carcinoma. Begin investigation with chest and abdomen CT.

If high-dose dexamethasone suppresses pituitary ACTH production and adrenal cortisol secretion, the source is the pituitary. In this case, obtain intrapetrosal sinus sampling for ACTH to confirm pituitary source.

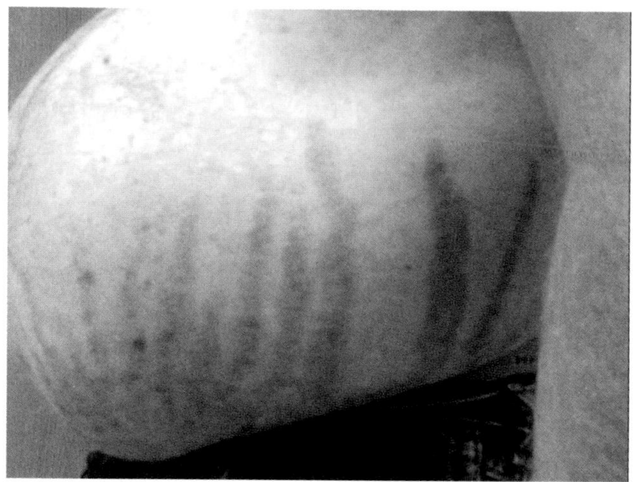

Cushing Syndrome: Wide purple striae characteristic of Cushing syndrome.

DON'T BE TRICKED

- **False-positive results (failure to suppress cortisol) with the 1-mg dexamethasone suppression test are commonly owing to alcohol use, obesity, and psychological disorders.**

Treatment

Surgical resection of the adrenal gland, pituitary gland, or ectopic tumor is the optimal therapy for Cushing syndrome. Bisphosphonates are the treatment of choice for low bone density caused by hypercortisolism.

TEST YOURSELF

A 43-year-old woman has diabetes mellitus, hypertension, hirsutism, and central obesity. The serum cortisol level is 26 µg/dL after administration of 1 mg of dexamethasone and 8.2 µg/dL after 8 mg of dexamethasone. The serum ACTH level is 50 pg/mL.

ANSWER: For diagnosis, choose pituitary tumor. For testing, select pituitary gland MRI.

Adrenal Incidentaloma

Diagnosis

An adrenal incidentaloma is a mass >1 cm that is discovered incidentally.

Testing

The two goals of evaluation are to determine if an adenoma is functioning and if it is malignant. All asymptomatic patients with adrenal incidentaloma should have a 1-mg overnight dexamethasone suppression test and a measurement of 24-hour urine levels of metanephrines and catecholamines. Patients with hypertension or spontaneous hypokalemia also require measurement of the plasma aldosterone–plasma renin activity ratio.

Adrenal metastases are common in patients with a known nonadrenal malignancy. Adenomas >6 cm are more likely to be malignant.

Treatment

Although controversy exists over optimal management, surgery may be recommended for adrenal masses >4 cm in diameter or functioning tumors. Masses <4 cm in size are monitored radiographically.

Follow-Up

For all patients with nonfunctioning tumors not treated surgically, repeat imaging should be performed in 6 to 12 months, and repeat screening for hormonal hypersecretion.

Hypoadrenalism

Diagnosis

Adrenal insufficiency may be caused by disease of the adrenal glands (primary) or disorders of the pituitary gland (secondary). Primary disease (Addison disease) results in loss of cortisol, aldosterone, and adrenal androgens; secondary insufficiency causes only cortisol and adrenal androgen deficiencies (aldosterone synthesis is not ACTH-dependent).

Symptoms and Signs

Characteristic findings include:

- weight loss
- fatigue, anorexia, nausea, vomiting, abdominal pain
- orthostatic hypotension
- hypoglycemia
- eosinophilia
- hyperpigmentation (primary adrenal insufficiency only)
- hyponatremia and hyperkalemia (primary adrenal insufficiency only)
- hypercalcemia

Causes

Autoimmune adrenalitis is the most common cause of primary insufficiency (also look for type 1 diabetes, hypothyroidism, and vitiligo).

Glucocorticoid use is the most common cause of secondary insufficiency (hypothalamic-pituitary suppression). Look for patients who recently discontinued glucocorticoid therapy or did not increase their glucocorticoid dose in times of stress.

Testing

An 8:00 AM serum cortisol <3 µg/dL diagnoses cortisol deficiency and values >18 µg/dL exclude the diagnosis.

For patients with unequivocally low cortisol levels, a morning ACTH level can help distinguish between primary and secondary adrenal insufficiency.

STUDY TABLE: Evaluation of Hypocortisolism

If you see this...	Do this...
Morning ACTH elevated (>20 pg/mL)	Adrenal CT
Morning ACTH suppressed or "normal" (<5 pg/mL)	Pituitary MRI

For nondiagnostic cortisol values, select stimulation testing with synthetic ACTH (cosyntropin). A stimulated serum cortisol >18 µg/dL excludes adrenal insufficiency.

DON'T BE TRICKED

- **Approximately 50% of patients with autoimmune adrenal insufficiency have other autoimmune endocrine disorders (thyroid disease, type 1 diabetes); testing for these disorders is indicated.**

Treatment

If acute adrenal insufficiency is suspected, treat empirically with high-dose (4 mg) dexamethasone and IV saline before obtaining cortisol and ACTH levels and without waiting for the ACTH and cortisol level results to return from the laboratory. Dexamethasone does not interfere with the serum cortisol assay.

After a diagnosis is made, hydrocortisone 10 to 30 mg/d is the standard treatment. Oral fludrocortisone is only appropriate for treatment of primary adrenal insufficiency. Increase the hydrocortisone dose 2 to 10 times the standard replacement dose during periods of physiological stress, including surgery. Fludrocortisone is not required in primary adrenal insufficiency if the hydrocortisone dose >40 mg/d.

DON'T BE TRICKED

- Do not prescribe dexamethasone for chronic replacement therapy.

TEST YOURSELF

A 32-year-old man with hypothyroidism has a 3-month history of fatigue, weakness, nausea, and a 13.9-kg (30-lb) weight loss. He has orthostatic hypotension and increased pigment in the palmar creases. The serum sodium level is 132 mEq/L and the serum potassium level is 5 mEq/L.

ANSWER: For diagnosis, choose autoimmune adrenalitis.

Pheochromocytoma

Diagnosis

Pheochromocytomas are rare tumors arising in the chromaffin cells of the adrenal medulla that secrete biogenic amines (norepinephrine, epinephrine, or dopamine) or their metabolites.

Symptoms and Signs

Characteristic findings may be remembered by the 7 H's:

- Hypertension
- Headache
- Hypermetabolism
- Hyperhidrosis
- Hyperglycemia
- Hypokalemia
- Hypotension (during anesthesia induction)

Orthostatic hypotension (caused by vasoconstriction-related volume depletion) is also a helpful physical examination clue.

Pheochromocytoma is associated with MEN2, von Hippel-Lindau disease, and neurofibromatosis type 1. Suspect a familial form in patients with a family history of pheochromocytoma, those with bilateral disease or an extra-adrenal location, and younger patients with a history of MEN2 or neurofibromatosis.

Testing

24-hour urine measurements of metanephrines and catecholamines are recommended when the pretest probability of disease is relatively low (adrenal mass without typical radiographic appearance or symptoms), whereas measurement of plasma metanephrines is preferred when clinical suspicion is higher (known hereditary syndrome or compatible symptoms).

Positive biochemical tests are followed by MRI or CT of the abdomen and pelvis. A ^{131}I or ^{123}I-MIBG scan may aid in localization when CT or MRI scans are negative.

Treatment

Surgery is the treatment of choice. Use phenoxybenzamine to control BP preoperatively. Give IV normal saline to maintain intravascular volume; nitroprusside or phentolamine is indicated for treating intraoperative hypertensive crisis.

DON'T BE TRICKED

- **For control of hypertension in patients with pheochromocytoma, select α-adrenergic blockers first. β-adrenergic blockade before adequate α-adrenergic blockade can result in severe paroxysmal hypertension.**

Primary Hyperaldosteronism

Diagnosis

Primary hyperaldosteronism is diagnosed in up to 14% of unselected patients with hypertension. Primary hyperaldosteronism is caused by aldosterone-producing adrenal adenomas (40%) or by bilateral adrenal hyperplasia. Characteristic findings are:

- difficult-to-treat or resistant hypertension
- unprovoked or difficult-to-treat hypokalemia
- family history of primary hyperaldosteronism

Testing

Evaluate patients using simultaneous measurements of plasma aldosterone and plasma renin activity.

A plasma aldosterone–plasma renin activity ratio >20, with a plasma aldosterone level >15 ng/dL, strongly suggests primary hyperaldosteronism. The diagnosis is confirmed by demonstrating nonsuppressibility of elevated plasma aldosterone in response to a high salt load given intravenously or orally. In patients without an adenoma, the plasma aldosterone level is suppressed to <5 ng/dL.

Testing can be done in patients receiving treatment with all antihypertensive agents except spironolactone and eplerenone, both of which antagonize the aldosterone receptor.

After autonomous hyperaldosteronism is diagnosed, select either CT or MRI of the adrenal glands. Adrenal vein sampling is needed before surgery to determine the source of aldosterone secretion when imaging is unrevealing and to confirm lateralization when imaging demonstrates an adrenal adenoma.

DON'T BE TRICKED

- **Almost 50% of patients with hyperaldosteronism do NOT have hypokalemia.**

Treatment

Spironolactone or eplerenone is the treatment of choice for adrenal hyperplasia. Laparoscopic adrenalectomy is indicated for an aldosterone-producing adenoma. If additional antihypertensive medications are required to control BP, select a thiazide diuretic agent.

Primary Amenorrhea

Diagnosis

Primary amenorrhea is the failure of menstruation (never occurred). Approximately 50% of primary amenorrhea is caused by chromosomal disorders, commonly Turner syndrome, in which part or all of an X chromosome is lost. Approximately 15% of these patients have an anatomic abnormality of the uterus, cervix, or vagina such as müllerian agenesis, transverse vaginal septum, or imperforate hymen.

STUDY TABLE: Most Common Causes of Primary Amenorrhea	
Diagnosis	**Characteristics**
Turner syndrome	45 XO karyotype Lack of secondary sexual characteristics, growth retardation, webbed neck, and frequent skeletal abnormalities
Hypothalamic/pituitary disorders	Functional (stress, excessive exercise, weight loss), developmental defects of cranial midline structures, tumors, or infiltrative disorders (sarcoidosis)
Androgen-resistance syndromes	XY karyotype Absence of or minimal pubic and axillary hair, a shallow vagina, and often a labial mass (testes)
PCOS	Most commonly associated with secondary amenorrhea but can cause primary amenorrhea. See Polycystic Ovary Syndrome

Testing

Most important studies:

- pregnancy test
- karyotype
- FSH, LH, TSH, prolactin level
- pelvic ultrasound

Secondary Amenorrhea

Diagnosis

Look for absence of menstruation for three cycle intervals or 6 consecutive months in women with previous menstrual flow.

History and physical examination include:

- history of obstetric complications, which could lead to endometrial damage, scarring, or adhesions
- stress, weight loss, significant exercise, anorexia nervosa
- newly initiated oral contraceptives, antipsychotics, or metoclopramide
- symptoms of pituitary adenoma (secondary to mass effect or hyperfunction)
- hirsutism, acne, history of PCOS

Testing

Test all women with secondary amenorrhea for pregnancy, the most common cause.

Look for structural causes, such as Asherman syndrome (see study table following).

If no structural cause is evident, assess hormonal status with estradiol, FSH, LH, TSH, and prolactin levels.

Low estradiol and **low or inappropriately normal FSH and LH** indicate hypogonadotrophic hypogonadism. Causes include:

- hypothyroidism
- hyperprolactinemia
- hypothalamic (stress, weight loss, exercise)
- pituitary (tumor, Sheehan syndrome)

A progesterone challenge test is performed in these patients.

- No bleeding following a progesterone challenge indicates low estrogen because of hypothalamic hypogonadism; measure estradiol level to confirm.
- Bleeding following progesterone challenge indicates a normal estrogen state and suggests possible hyperandrogenism (e.g., PCOS).

Low estradiol and **elevated FSH and LH** levels indicates hypergonadotrophic hypogonadism. Consider:

- premature ovarian insufficiency (autoimmune)
- chemotherapy
- pelvic radiation

STUDY TABLE: Common Causes of Secondary Amenorrhea

Diagnosis	Characteristics	Evaluation
PCOS	Ovulatory dysfunction, evidence of hyperandrogenism, and polycystic ovaries on ultrasonography See Polycystic Ovary Syndrome	Mild elevation in testosterone and DHEAS (not needed for diagnosis)
Hyperprolactinemia	May be associated with galactorrhea Related to medications (tricyclic antidepressants, phenothiazines, and metoclopramide), tumors that secrete prolactin or compress the pituitary stalk, history of cranial radiotherapy	First, rule out hypothyroidism If TSH is normal and serum prolactin level >100 ng/mL, obtain brain MRI to diagnose tumor
Hypothalamic amenorrhea	Most commonly functional (related to stress, weight loss, excessive exercise)	Low or normal LH level, and low estradiol level
Hypothyroidism	Causes secondary increase in serum prolactin levels	High TSH, high prolactin
Adrenal tumor	Signs of hyperandrogenism and virilization, usually acute onset and severe	Decreased LH and FSH, increased or normal estradiol, and increased testosterone and DHEAS levels
Sheehan syndrome (postpartum pituitary necrosis)	History of difficult delivery (blood loss, hypotension) and inability to breastfeed	Varying levels of panhypopituitarism
Asherman syndrome (uterine synechiae)	History of previous dilatation and curettage amenorrhea caused by fibrous uterine scarring	Normal LH and estradiol levels; no response to estrogen and progesterone challenge Abnormal pelvic ultrasound or hysterogram

Treatment

Treat the underlying disorder. Prevent osteoporosis by choosing estrogen and progesterone replacement until menstruation returns to normal or age 50 years. For hypothalamic amenorrhea, choose reduced exercise, improved nutrition, and attention to emotional needs.

Polycystic Ovary Syndrome

Diagnosis

PCOS is the most common cause of hirsutism with oligomenorrhea. Symptoms normally start at puberty or several years later and are slowly progressive. Diagnosis requires two of the following:

- ovulatory dysfunction (amenorrhea, oligomenorrhea, infertility)
- laboratory or clinical evidence of hyperandrogenism (hirsutism, acne)
- ultrasonographic evidence of polycystic ovaries

Testing

Insulin resistance is an important feature of the disorder, as is being overweight or obese. A mild elevation in testosterone and DHEAS levels and an LH/FSH ratio greater than 2:1 are typical.

DON'T BE TRICKED

- **Do not routinely order testosterone or DHEAS testing because PCOS is a clinical diagnosis and laboratory evaluation is only necessary when androgen-producing neoplasms must be ruled out.**
- **An androgen-secreting ovarian or adrenal tumor should be suspected in a woman with acute onset of rapidly progressive hirsutism or virilization.**

Treatment

Instruct patients in intensive lifestyle modification to reduce weight, control abdominal obesity, and restore insulin sensitivity. Treatment follows two models:

- If fertility is not desired, first-line treatment of hirsutism and regulation of menses is an oral contraceptive; spironolactone can be added if hirsutism remains a problem.
- If fertility is desired, ovulation induction can be brought about with clomiphene citrate or letrozole.

TEST YOURSELF

A 27-year-old woman has had oligomenorrhea since age 14 years. She also has acanthosis nigricans and hirsutism but no galactorrhea; she is obese. She does not desire pregnancy.

ANSWER: For diagnosis, choose PCOS. For management, choose intensive lifestyle modification and an oral contraceptive.

Infertility

Diagnosis

Infertility is defined as the inability to conceive after 1 year of intercourse without contraception in women <35 years and after 6 months in women ≥35 years. Regular menses is correlated with regular ovulation. If oligomenorrhea is present, evaluate like secondary amenorrhea. Consider structural abnormalities and evaluate with pelvic ultrasonography or hysterography.

Semen analysis can be performed at any time.

Male Hypogonadism

Diagnosis

Male hypogonadism is present when sperm or testosterone production is decreased. It can be a primary or secondary condition.

Characteristic findings are fatigue, decreased strength, poor libido, hot flushes, erectile dysfunction, and gynecomastia.

Causes and Testing

Testosterone deficiency is diagnosed with two 8:00 AM total testosterone levels below the reference range.

- If the testosterone measurement is equivocal, measure free testosterone level by equilibrium dialysis or mass spectrometry.
- If the testosterone level is low, measure LH, FSH, and prolactin levels.

Elevated LH and FSH values indicate primary testicular failure. Some common causes include:

- Klinefelter syndrome (check karyotype)
- atrophy secondary to mumps orchitis
- autoimmune destruction
- previous chemotherapy or pelvic irradiation
- hemochromatosis

Low or normal LH and FSH levels indicate secondary hypogonadism. Important causes include:

- sleep apnea
- hyperprolactinemia
- hypothalamic or pituitary disorders (hemochromatosis, pituitary/hypothalamic tumor)
- use of opiates, anabolic steroids, or glucocorticoids

If secondary hypogonadism is confirmed, in addition to measuring prolactin, check iron studies to rule out hemochromatosis and obtain an MRI to evaluate for hypothalamic or pituitary lesions.

Men who self-administer anabolic steroids can come to medical attention because of infertility. Physical examination typically reveals acne, muscular hypertrophy, testicular atrophy, and gynecomastia (if the patient is using testosterone). Aromatase inhibitors are frequently used concurrently with testosterone preparations to prevent adipose conversion of androgens to estrogens and development of gynecomastia. Laboratory data show suppressed LH and FSH levels, variable testosterone levels, and otherwise normal pituitary function.

DON'T BE TRICKED

- **Do not measure serum testosterone if a patient is having regular morning erections, has no gynecomastia on examination, and the genital examination is normal.**

Treatment

Testosterone can be administered as a transdermal (preferred by patients but expensive), buccal, implantable, or IM preparation. Before initiation of testosterone replacement and during therapy, routinely monitor hematocrit and PSA to screen for the development of erythrocytosis and prostate cancer, respectively.

DON'T BE TRICKED

- **Don't provide testosterone replacement therapy for nonspecific symptoms such as fatigue and weakness in the absence of unequivocal testosterone deficiency.**
- **Testosterone replacement therapy (and anabolic steroid abuse) results in small testicles and male infertility.**

Hypercalcemia and Hyperparathyroidism

Diagnosis

Primary hyperparathyroidism is the most common cause of hypercalcemia in outpatients. Primary hyperparathyroidism commonly presents as asymptomatic hypercalcemia. Less common presentations are kidney stones, osteoporosis, pancreatitis, and fractures (osteoporosis).

Malignancy is the most common cause of hypercalcemia in hospitalized patients. Hypercalcemia may also occur with the use of lithium (PTH-mediated) or thiazide diuretics (non-PTH-mediated) and in the setting of excessive ingestion of vitamin D and calcium.

Sarcoidosis may be associated with hypercalcemia (10% of patients) and hypercalciuria (50% of patients).

STUDY TABLE: Causes of Hypercalcemia	
Diagnosis	**Key features include hypercalcemia and...**
Primary hyperparathyroidism	PTH elevated (80%) or inappropriately normal (20%); phosphorus low X-rays may show chondrocalcinosis or osteitis fibrosa cystica (rare)
Humoral hypercalcemia of malignancy	PTH suppressed; phosphorus normal or low PTH-related protein may be elevated but is not needed for diagnosis
Local osteolytic lesions	PTH suppressed; phosphorus normal or low Lytic bone metastases result in increased mobilization of calcium from the bone
Multiple myeloma	PTH suppressed; phosphorus elevated Look for patients presenting with new kidney injury and anemia Diagnose with serum and urine protein immunoelectrophoresis
Granulomatous disease (sarcoidosis and TB) and B-cell lymphoma	PTH suppressed; phosphorus elevated; calcitriol elevated (particularly in sarcoidosis)
Milk-alkali syndrome	PTH suppressed; phosphorus, creatinine, carbon dioxide elevated Consider in healthy persons in whom primary hyperparathyroidism has been excluded Excessive ingestion of calcium-containing antacids is a cause (rare)
Hyperthyroidism	Hypercalcemia is a frequent incidental finding in hyperthyroidism caused by direct stimulation of osteoclasts by thyroid hormone

Hypercalcemia requiring acute intervention is most often associated with a rapid rise in serum calcium level and serum calcium >14 mg/dL. Symptoms may include change in mental status and coma. It is most common in the setting of malignancy.

Testing

Measure the ionized calcium level to exclude pseudohypercalcemia caused by an increase in plasma proteins capable of binding calcium; total calcium will be increased and ionized calcium will be normal.

If hypercalcemia is confirmed, check calcium, PTH, phosphate, creatinine, and 25-hydroxyvitamin D levels. If PTH is elevated or inappropriately normal in the setting of elevated serum calcium, the most likely cause is primary hyperparathyroidism.

DON'T BE TRICKED

- **In patients with hypercalcemia and normal PTH levels, measure urinary calcium excretion to exclude familial hypocalciuric hypercalcemia.**

If hyperparathyroidism is confirmed and surgery is indicated, do a sestamibi parathyroid scan to look for an adenoma.

Primary hyperparathyroidism is the most common manifestation of MEN1.

Treatment

For hypercalcemia, select:

- volume resuscitation with normal saline
- IV bisphosphonates and serum calcitonin
- oral glucocorticoid therapy (if caused by multiple myeloma or sarcoidosis)

DON'T BE TRICKED

- **Loop diuretics are not recommended in the treatment of hypercalcemia unless kidney failure or heart failure is present, in which case volume expansion should precede the administration of loop diuretics to avoid hypotension and further kidney injury.**

Multiple Endocrine Neoplasia

Diagnosis

STUDY TABLE: Multiple Endocrine Neoplasia Types 1 and 2	
MEN1	**MEN2**
Multigland hyperparathyroidism is the most common manifestation	Multigland hyperparathyroidism is the least common manifestation
Pituitary neoplasms associated with prolactinoma (amenorrhea and erectile dysfunction), acromegaly (enlargement of hands, feet, tongue, frontal bossing), Cushing disease (bruising, hypertension, central obesity, hirsutism)	Medullary thyroid cancer is the most common manifestation and may be associated with a palpable neck mass
Pancreatic NETs associated with gastrinoma (diarrhea, ulcers), insulinoma (fasting hypoglycemia), vasoactive intestinal polypeptide-secreting tumor (watery diarrhea, hypokalemia), carcinoid syndrome (diarrhea, flushing, right heart valvular lesion)	Pheochromocytoma (hypertension and palpitations)

DON'T BE TRICKED

- **About 50% of patients with primary hyperparathyroidism have coexisting vitamin D deficiency, and serum and urine calcium levels may be decreased. Select measurement of serum vitamin D levels in all patients with hyperparathyroidism.**

Treatment

Parathyroidectomy is indicated for patients with primary hyperparathyroidism and hypercalcemic complications, such as kidney stones, bone disease, or previous episodes of hypercalcemic crisis. Asymptomatic patients are surgical candidates if they have any of the following:

- serum calcium level >1 mg/dL above the upper limit of normal
- estimated GFR <60 mL/min/1.73 m^2
- reduction in bone mineral density (T-score <−2.5)
- age <50 years

Watch for a precipitous fall in the serum calcium level caused by relative hypoparathyroidism after parathyroidectomy ("hungry bone" syndrome). Monitor serum calcium after surgery, and give oral calcium if mild hypocalcemia develops.

Treat patients who are not candidates for parathyroidectomy with cinacalcet or bisphosphonates.

TEST YOURSELF

A 44-year-old man has a 1-year history of fatigue and poor concentration. His serum calcium level is 10.9 mg/dL, serum phosphorus level is 2.8 mg/dL, and PTH level is 75 pg/mL.

ANSWER: For diagnosis, choose primary hyperparathyroidism and measure serum vitamin D levels. For management, select parathyroidectomy.

Hypocalcemia

Diagnosis

Most cases of hypocalcemia are caused by low serum albumin levels; the ionized calcium concentration is normal. Total calcium declines by 0.8 mg/dL for each 1 g/dL decrement in serum albumin concentration.

Symptoms and Signs

Look for:

- circumoral and acral paresthesias
- carpal-pedal spasm
- positive Trousseau sign
- positive Chvostek sign

Causes

The most common cause of acquired hypocalcemia is surgical excision of or vascular injury to the parathyroid glands. Other causes include:

- neck irradiation
- congenital hypoparathyroidism (DiGeorge syndrome)
- autoimmune destruction
- infiltrative diseases
- complication of plasmapheresis

Autoimmune hypoparathyroidism occurs as an isolated defect or as part of polyglandular autoimmune syndrome type 1 in association with mucocutaneous candidiasis, adrenal insufficiency, hypogonadism, and malabsorption.

In addition to hypoparathyroidism, hypocalcemia may result from pseudohypoparathyroidism, vitamin D deficiency, hypomagnesemia, or pancreatitis, or may occur in the setting of rhabdomyolysis, kidney injury, and tumor lysis syndrome.

Order calcium, phosphate, magnesium, creatinine, PTH, 25-hydroxyvitamin D, albumin, and/or ionized calcium tests. Order an ECG to evaluate for QTc interval prolongation.

STUDY TABLE: Differential Diagnosis of Hypocalcemia

Diagnosis	Key features include hypocalcemia and...
Hypoparathyroidism	Hyperphosphatemia; low PTH and variable vitamin D levels
Pseudohypoparathyroidism (resistance to PTH)	Hyperphosphatemia; elevated PTH and normal vitamin D levels
CKD	Hyperphosphatemia; elevated PTH and low 1,25-dihydroxyvitamin D levels
Vitamin D deficiency	Hypophosphatemia; bone tenderness or fibromyalgia-like syndrome, weakness, gait difficulty, osteomalacia
Impaired PTH secretion and PTH resistance	Magnesium deficiency (small bowel bypass, diarrhea, alcoholism, diuretic therapy)
"Hungry bone" syndrome	Recent parathyroidectomy

Treatment

Treat acute symptomatic hypocalcemia with IV calcium gluconate and vitamin D. Chronic hypocalcemia is treated with oral calcium supplements and vitamin D. Choose the type of vitamin D based on the presence of underlying disease:

- kidney disease: calcitriol (1,25-dihydroxyvitamin D)
- liver disease: 25-hydroxycholecalciferol
- any other cause of hypocalcemia: cholecalciferol (D_3) or ergocalciferol (D_2)

The main side effect of therapy is hypercalciuria and nephrolithiasis. Remember to correct hypomagnesemia with magnesium supplements.

TEST YOURSELF

A 46-year-old woman has cramps in her hands and feet. She has pernicious anemia and Hashimoto thyroiditis. Her serum calcium level is 7.9 mg/dL and her serum phosphorus level is 4.1 mg/dL.

ANSWER: For diagnosis, choose autoimmune hypoparathyroidism and select a serum PTH level.

Osteoporosis

Screening

The USPSTF recommends screening BMD with DEXA in women ≥65 years and in postmenopausal women <65 years who are at increased risk as determined by a formal clinical risk assessment tool (e.g., FRAX). Increased risk is defined using the FRAX tool as a predicted 10-year fracture risk >8.4%.

Screen men and women with risk factors for secondary osteoporosis (glucocorticoid use, hyperparathyroidism, ADT [men], malabsorption).

DON'T BE TRICKED

- **Do not repeat annual DEXA in women with normal DEXA results without risk factors. Although the optimal screening interval is unknown, most experts recommend 10 to 15 years for women with normal or slightly low bone mineral density and no risk factors.**
- **In the absence of fractures, primary osteoporosis is associated with no abnormalities on laboratory testing.**

Diagnosis

Osteoporosis is a silent skeletal disorder characterized by compromised bone strength and an increased predisposition to fractures.

- DEXA T-score of −1.0 to −2.4 defines osteopenia.
- DEXA T-score of ≤−2.5 defines osteoporosis.
- Osteoporosis is also diagnosed by a history of fragility fracture (fracture from a fall at standing height or lower).

Causes

The most common cause of osteoporosis in women is estrogen deficiency and in men is testosterone deficiency.

Secondary causes include:

- hyperthyroidism, hyperparathyroidism, Cushing syndrome
- malabsorption (Crohn disease, intestinal resection, celiac disease)
- rheumatoid arthritis
- medications (excessive thyroid hormone, glucocorticoids, phenobarbital, phenytoin, thiazolidinediones)
- multiple myeloma
- CKD, chronic liver disease
- vitamin D deficiency

Testing

Reasonable tests include: CBC; TSH; calcium, phosphorus, and creatinine levels; liver chemistry tests; ESR; serum 25-hydroxy-vitamin D level (if vitamin D deficiency is suspected); and tTG antibodies (if celiac disease is suspected).

Treatment

Encourage all patients to stop smoking, reduce alcohol intake, and begin resistance exercises. Exposure to sunlight is especially important for home-bound persons or nursing-home residents. Supplement calcium and vitamin D intake.

Indications for antiresorptive therapy:

- osteoporosis
- osteopenia (if additional high-risk factors are present)

- previous fragility fracture
- vertebral or hip fracture

The Fracture Risk Assessment Tool (FRAX) estimates the 10-year probability of hip fracture and major osteoporotic fracture. Antiresorptive treatment is cost effective when the risk of major osteoporotic fracture is ≥20% or the risk of hip fracture is ≥3%.

Treatment options:

- alendronate or risedronate is first-line therapy
- denosumab (monoclonal antibody that inhibits osteoclast activation) may be preferred in patients with stage 4 CKD and in those intolerant of or incompletely responding to bisphosphonates
- teriparatide (synthetic recombinant human PTH 1-34) is approved for use in postmenopausal women, men or women with glucocorticoid-induced osteoporosis who are at high risk of osteoporotic fracture, and men with primary or hypogonadism-related osteoporosis at high risk of fracture
- calcitonin for pain from osteoporotic fractures

Oral bisphosphonates are taken on an empty stomach, and patients must remain upright for at least 30 minutes. These agents are contraindicated in patients with CKD or esophageal disease. IV zoledronate (once yearly) is an alternative therapeutic option.

DON'T BE TRICKED

- The effects of denosumab are not sustained when treatment is stopped.

No recommended duration of therapy is specified. Stopping therapy after 5 years is reasonable in women who have a stable BMI, no history of fracture, and are at low risk for fracture. The duration of the drug holiday is unknown but may be determined by changes in DEXA measurements.

Drugs for osteoporosis have various adverse effects:

- oral bisphosphonate therapy may lead to erosive esophagitis and atypical hip fracture
- IV bisphosphonate therapy and denosumab can lead to osteonecrosis of the jaw; this rarely occurs with oral bisphosphonates
- teriparatide is associated with osteosarcoma

Treatment with teriparatide should be limited to 2 years.

DON'T BE TRICKED

- **Do not use estrogen replacement therapy for osteoporosis in postmenopausal women.**
- **Do not combine teriparatide with a bisphosphonate.**
- **IV bisphosphonates are contraindicated in patients with severe hypocalcemia and CKD.**

Follow-Up

Although no consensus exists, follow-up DEXA 24 months after beginning therapy for osteoporosis is reasonable.

TEST YOURSELF

An 82-year-old woman has been taking thyroid hormone since age 31 years. She has lost about 7.6 cm (3.0 in) in height. Serum TSH level is <0.01 µU/mL (normal 0.5 to 5.0 µU/mL).

ANSWER: For diagnosis, choose thyroid hormone–induced osteoporosis. For management, reduce the thyroid hormone dose and schedule DEXA.

Osteomalacia

Diagnosis

Osteomalacia is a metabolic bone disease resulting from failure of the organic matrix of bone to mineralize because of lack of available calcium or phosphorus. Many cases of osteomalacia are related to abnormalities in vitamin D but may also result from deficiencies of calcium or phosphate.

Symptoms and signs include:

- fatigability, malaise, and bone pain
- generalized bone tenderness
- proximal muscle weakness
- Looser zones (bands perpendicular to the bone surface visible on x-rays)
- hypocalcemia and hypophosphatemia
- elevated serum alkaline phosphatase level

Testing

Evaluate for underlying conditions that may lead to intestinal malabsorption of vitamin D, such as celiac disease, or abnormalities in vitamin D metabolism, such as liver and kidney disease. Diagnosis is confirmed with bone biopsy when necessary.

Treatment

If osteomalacia is secondary to vitamin D deficiency, treat with oral ergocalciferol 1000 to 2000 U/d and elemental calcium 1 g/d.

DON'T BE TRICKED

- **Not all fractures in older adult patients are caused by osteoporosis. Look for osteomalacia, particularly in nursing-home residents.**

Vitamin D Deficiency

Screening

The USPSTF concludes that evidence is insufficient to assess the balance of benefits and harms of screening for vitamin D deficiency in asymptomatic adults.

Diagnosis

Prolonged and severe vitamin D deficiency will cause secondary hyperparathyroidism; osteomalacia in adults; and symptoms of bone pain, muscle weakness (including difficulty walking), and fracture.

Testing

In assessing serum levels of vitamin D, concentrations of 25-hydroxyvitamin D are the best indicator of vitamin D status.

The desired level of vitamin D is disagreed on. Most expert panels define a sufficient level ≥30 ng/mL. The National Academy of Medicine has determined that ≥20 ng/mL is sufficient.

Special populations will have lower levels of vitamin D owing to medical conditions or medication side effects:

- obesity
- glucocorticoids
- orlistat
- malabsorption disorders (including bariatric surgery)

Treatment

The USPSTF concludes that evidence is insufficient to recommend vitamin D and calcium supplementation, alone or combined, for the prevention of fractures in men and premenopausal women.

Supplemental vitamin D ≤400 U and calcium ≤1000 mg alone is inadequate to prevent bone fractures in postmenopausal women, and evidence is insufficient to recommend greater supplemental amounts in fracture prevention.

In treating the deficient patient, 50,000 U of either ergocalciferol or cholecalciferol is recommended, followed by maintenance therapy of 1500 to 2000 U/d.

Paget Disease

Diagnosis

Paget disease is a focal disorder of bone remodeling that leads to greatly accelerated rates of bone turnover, disruption of the normal architecture of bone, and sometimes gross deformities of bone (enlargement of the skull, bowing of the femur or tibia). Most patients are asymptomatic, and the disease is suspected when an isolated elevation of alkaline phosphatase is detected in the absence of liver disease.

Symptoms and signs include:

- bone pain, fractures
- cranial nerve compression syndromes, spinal stenosis, nerve root syndromes
- high-output cardiac failure
- angioid retinal streaks

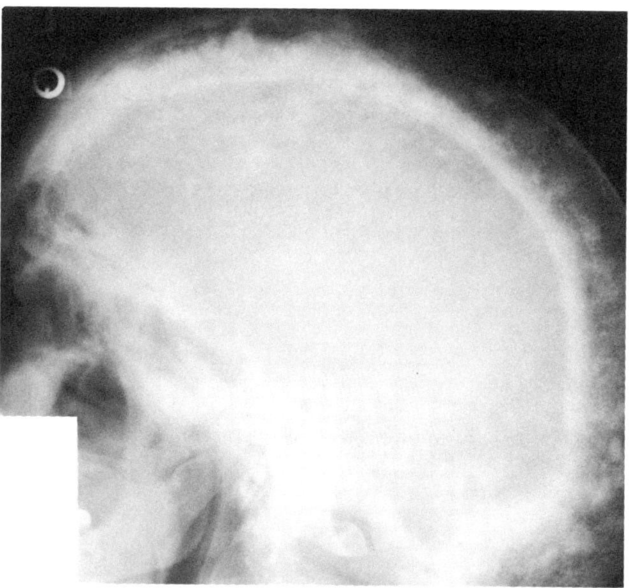

Paget Disease: X-ray showing "cotton wool" appearance of the skull typical of Paget disease.

Testing

If the serum alkaline phosphatase (bone) level is elevated in an asymptomatic patient, order a bone scan and follow-up x-rays of areas that localize radionuclide. In symptomatic patients, obtain x-rays of the painful area. X-rays will reveal these pathognomonic pagetic lesions: focal osteolysis with coarsening of the trabecular pattern, cotton wool skull, and cortical thickening.

Treatment

Indications to treat Paget disease include bone pain, radiculopathy, or involvement of a weight-bearing bone or joint, regardless of symptoms. Bisphosphonates are the first-line agents.

Gastroenterology and Hepatology

Dysphagia

Diagnosis

Dysphagia is defined as difficulty swallowing and is classified as oropharyngeal or esophageal.

Oropharyngeal Dysphagia

- causes patients to have difficulty initiating swallowing.
- presents with coughing, choking, and nasal regurgitation of fluids.
- frequently results from muscular or neurologic disorders, most commonly stroke, Parkinson disease, ALS, MG, and muscular dystrophy.
- frequently causes aspiration pneumonia.

Patients with pharyngoesophageal (Zenker) diverticulum often present with regurgitation of undigested food, gurgling sound in the chest, and severe halitosis.

Videofluoroscopy with liquid and solid phases is used to evaluate suspected oropharyngeal dysphagia.

Esophageal Dysphagia

- is reported as food "sticking" or discomfort in the retrosternal region.
- results from mechanical obstruction or a motility disorder.

Solid-food dysphagia is most often caused by a structural esophageal abnormality.

Dysphagia for solids and liquids or for liquids alone suggests an esophageal motility abnormality such as achalasia.

Solid-food dysphagia that occurs episodically for months to years suggests an esophageal web or a distal esophageal ring (Schatzki ring).

Progressively increasing solid-food dysphagia suggests a peptic stricture or carcinoma.

Treatment

Oropharyngeal dysphagia is managed with dietary adjustment and incorporation of swallowing exercises with the assistance of a speech pathologist.

Therapy for esophageal dysphagia is dictated by the underlying cause.

TEST YOURSELF

A 75-year-old man with Parkinson disease has difficulty initiating a swallow.

ANSWER: For diagnosis, choose pharyngeal dysphagia; for management, order oropharyngeal videofluoroscopy.

Achalasia

Diagnosis

Achalasia is caused by degeneration of the myenteric plexus with failure of the lower esophageal sphincter (LES) to relax in response to swallowing and absent peristalsis. This leads to the retention of food and liquids in the body of the esophagus and the characteristic findings of dysphagia with solids and liquids.

Achalasia often presents with nonacidic regurgitation of undigested food.

Testing

Diagnostic evaluation should be performed in the following order:

- barium swallow: the preferred screening test when diagnosis is suspected clinically; shows "bird's beak" narrowing of the GE junction
- esophageal manometry: documents the absence of peristalsis and incomplete relaxation of the LES with swallows
- upper endoscopy: to rule out adenocarcinoma (pseudoachalasia) at the GE junction

DON'T BE TRICKED

- **Do not select upper endoscopy as the first diagnostic test if achalasia is suspected.**
- **If the patient has a history of travel to South America, suspect Chagas disease as the cause of achalasia.**

Treatment

Laparoscopic surgical myotomy of the LES and endoscopic pneumatic dilation of the esophagus are first-line therapies for achalasia.

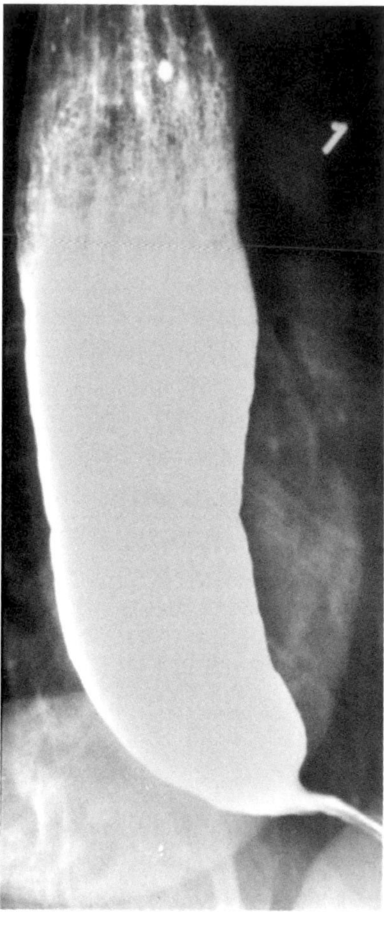

Barium Esophagogram: The "bird's beak" finding reflects narrowing of the distal esophagus and is characteristic of achalasia.

Gastroesophageal Reflux Disease

Diagnosis

Characteristic findings of GERD are heartburn and/or regurgitation.

Extraesophageal symptoms may include chest pain, cough, hoarseness, and wheezing.

In a patient without alarm features (anemia, dysphagia, vomiting, weight loss), symptom relief with PPI therapy confirms the diagnosis.

Testing

STUDY TABLE: GERD Diagnostic Studies

Indication	Test
GERD symptoms refractory to empiric therapy with PPIs	Upper endoscopy; if normal, then choose ambulatory esophageal pH monitoring or impedance pH testing while taking a PPI for symptom-reflux correlation
Dysphagia, odynophagia, and weight loss	Upper endoscopy to rule out cancer

Treatment

PPIs are first-line therapy for GERD and GERD with extraesophageal manifestations (asthma, laryngitis, cough). Lifestyle measures, such as weight loss and not eating before bed, may also be implemented.

Select antireflux surgery for patients with GERD refractory to medical management or patients who have an excellent response to a PPI but do not want long-term medical therapy.

Patients should undergo pH monitoring to demonstrate true reflux with symptom correlation and manometry to rule out a motility disorder before surgery.

DON'T BE TRICKED

- **Chest pain is common in patients with GERD, but a cardiac cause of chest pain must be ruled out first in patients presenting with acute chest pain.**
- **Before ordering upper endoscopy for diagnosis, administer once daily PPI, followed by twice daily PPI for 4 to 8 weeks if no symptomatic response.**
- **Do not order barium x-rays to diagnose GERD.**

TEST YOURSELF

A 34-year-old woman has frequent heartburn. She has tried a PPI, once before breakfast and once before dinner, without improvement.

ANSWER: For management, order upper endoscopy and, if normal, 24-hour esophageal pH monitoring while the patient is taking a PPI.

Barrett Esophagus

BE is a premalignant condition caused by longstanding GERD.

Screening

Screen men aged >50 years with GERD symptoms for more than 5 years and additional risk factors (nocturnal reflux symptoms, hiatal hernia, elevated BMI, tobacco use, and intra-abdominal distribution of fat) to detect esophageal adenocarcinoma and BE.

Diagnosis

The diagnosis of BE is based on the endoscopic finding of columnar epithelium above the normally located GE junction. Low-grade or high-grade dysplasia in biopsy specimens should be confirmed by an expert pathologist.

Treatment

Treat patients with BE without dysplasia with a PPI.

Treatment to remove BE is recommended for patients with confirmed low- or high-grade dysplasia (endoscopic ablation).

Dysplasia can be treated with endoscopic therapies that include radiofrequency ablation, photodynamic therapy, endoscopic mucosal resection, or esophagectomy.

Follow-Up

In patients with BE and no dysplasia, surveillance examinations should occur at intervals no more frequent than 3 to 5 years.

More frequent intervals of every 6 to 12 months are indicated in patients with BE and low-grade dysplasia who do not choose endoscopic ablation.

DON'T BE TRICKED

- **Women with GERD do not require routine screening for BE.**
- **Do not select antireflux surgery to prevent the progression of BE to adenocarcinoma.**

Esophagitis

Diagnosis

Odynophagia is the most common presenting symptom of esophagitis.

Candida albicans is the most common infectious cause, followed by CMV and HSV.

- Two thirds of patients with candidal esophagitis have oral thrush.
- In patients with AIDS and odynophagia, the presence of oral candidiasis is 100% predictive of esophageal candidiasis.
- In patients with odynophagia who are immunosuppressed, begin empiric therapy for esophageal candidiasis.

Patients with viral esophagitis rarely have associated ulcerative oropharyngeal lesions.

Pill-induced esophagitis may be caused by tetracyclines, NSAIDs, potassium chloride, iron, and alendronate. Symptoms of severe substernal chest pain with swallowing occur several hours to days after taking the medication.

Young adults with eosinophilic esophagitis (EE) present with extreme dysphagia and food impaction.

Testing

Perform upper endoscopy with biopsy/brushing if empiric therapy for presumed esophagitis is unsuccessful.

Upper endoscopy in patients with EE may show mucosal furrowing, stacked circular rings, white specks, and mucosal friability. Endoscopic biopsies show marked infiltration with eosinophils.

GERD has been associated with esophageal eosinophilia and can mimic EE.

Evaluation of EE includes an 8-week trial of a PPI; clinical response to the PPI trial indicates GERD-associated eosinophilia rather than EE.

Persistent esophageal eosinophilia following PPI therapy confirms a diagnosis of EE.

TEST YOURSELF

A 30-year-old man has frequent heartburn and recurrent episodes of food impaction.

ANSWER: For diagnosis, choose eosinophilic esophagitis.

DON'T BE TRICKED

- Do not select barium esophagography to evaluate suspected esophagitis.
- The absence of oral *Candida* lesions does not rule out esophageal candidiasis.

Treatment

Address the underlying cause of esophagitis:

- fluconazole or itraconazole for esophageal candidiasis
- acyclovir, famciclovir, or valacyclovir for HSV esophagitis
- ganciclovir and/or foscarnet for CMV esophagitis
- swallowed fluticasone or budesonide for EE
- supportive care for pill esophagitis (spontaneously resolves)

TEST YOURSELF

A 28-year-old man with HIV infection has a 2-month history of odynophagia. On physical examination, oral thrush is present.

ANSWER: For diagnosis, choose *Candida* esophagitis. For treatment, select empiric treatment with fluconazole.

Peptic Ulcer Disease

Diagnosis

Patients with PUD present with dyspepsia or epigastric burning, early satiety, nausea, and postprandial belching or bloating.

Most PUD is caused by *Helicobacter pylori* infection or NSAID use.

All patients with PUD should be tested for *H. pylori* infection regardless of NSAID use.

Complications of PUD:

- **Penetration** is characterized by a gradual increase in the severity and frequency of abdominal pain, with pancreatitis as a common presentation.
- **Perforation** is characterized by severe, sudden abdominal pain that is often associated with shock and peritoneal signs.
- **Outlet obstruction** is characterized by nausea, vomiting, and/or early satiety and a succussion splash.
- **Bleeding** is characterized by hematemesis, melena, or hematochezia (see Upper GI Bleeding).

Testing

In patients aged <60 years with dyspepsia without alarm symptoms, including anemia, dysphagia, persistent vomiting, or weight loss, use the "test-and-treat" approach for *H. pylori* without initially performing upper endoscopy.

Noninvasive strategies for diagnosing *H. pylori* include urea breath tests and stool test for *H. pylori* antigens.

For older patients and those with persistent symptoms or alarm features at any age, obtain upper endoscopy and *H. pylori* testing.

DON'T BE TRICKED

- In patients undergoing upper endoscopy for suspected PUD, biopsy and histologic assessment for *H. pylori* or rapid urease testing for *H. pylori* should be performed.
- False-negative rapid urease tests, urea breath tests, and stool antigen results for *H. pylori* may occur in patients who recently took antibiotics, bismuth-containing compounds, or PPIs; these drugs should be stopped before testing (28 days for antibiotics, 2 weeks for PPIs) or histologic assessment for *H. pylori* should be performed.
- Do not order serum antibody testing for *H. pylori*; it will not differentiate between past and current infection.
- Duodenal ulcers carry little risk of malignancy and do not require biopsy unless they are refractory to therapy.

Treatment

STUDY TABLE: Treating NSAID-Induced Peptic Ulcer Disease

If you see this...	Do this...
Aspirin, NSAID-induced PUD	Stop NSAIDs, treat with H_2 blocker or PPI
Aspirin, NSAID-induced PUD, unable to stop aspirin or NSAID	Treat with long-term PPI
High risk for developing NSAID-induced PUD but needs NSAID treatment*	Initiate prophylaxis with PPI

*High risk = history of PUD or UGI bleeding; dual antiplatelet therapy, anticoagulation, or glucocorticoid therapy; or age ≥60 years.

Initial *H. pylori* therapy should be based on assessment of the probability of high resistance rates to clarithromycin (previous treatment with a macrolide, local resistance rates ≥15%, or eradication rates with clarithromycin-based triple therapy <85%).

- If resistance to clarithromycin is unlikely, use clarithromycin-based triple therapy.
- If resistance to clarithromycin is probable, use bismuth quadruple therapy.

When first-line therapy fails, a salvage regimen should avoid previously used antibiotics.

Surgery for treatment of PUD is reserved for patients with complications.

Follow-Up

Follow-up noninvasive testing to document *H. pylori* eradication should be performed at least 4 weeks after completion of therapy in any patient with a positive *H. pylori* test result.

Follow-up upper endoscopy for gastric ulcers is indicated only if the patient remains symptomatic after treatment, the cause is uncertain, or biopsies were not performed during initial upper endoscopy.

DON'T BE TRICKED

- **A selective COX-2 inhibitor provides no better gastric protection than a nonselective NSAID plus a PPI.**
- **Duodenal PUD without complications does not require follow-up upper endoscopy.**
- **Serologic testing (ELISA test for IgG antibodies) should not be used to confirm *H. pylori* eradication because it can remain positive in the absence of active infection.**
- **Bismuth quadruple therapy should be used as initial treatment for *H. pylori* infection in patients with penicillin allergy.**

TEST YOURSELF

A 42-year-old man was treated with a PPI, amoxicillin, and clarithromycin for an *H. pylori*–positive duodenal ulcer. He returns 9 weeks after treatment because of recurrent symptoms.

ANSWER: For management, select urea breath test. If positive, re-treat with different antibiotics than those prescribed initially.

Nonulcer Dyspepsia

Diagnosis

Nonulcer dyspepsia is defined as nonspecific upper abdominal discomfort or nausea not attributable to PUD or GERD. Diagnosis is based on the presence of one or more of the following symptoms:

- bothersome postprandial fullness
- early satiety
- epigastric burning

Various drugs may cause dyspepsia, including NSAIDs, antibiotics, bisphosphonates, and potassium supplements.

Testing

Patients aged >60 years or patients with alarm features require investigation with upper endoscopy. Alarm features include unexplained iron deficiency anemia, heme-positive stools, progressive dysphagia, weight loss, vomiting, and family history of GI malignancy.

Treatment

If possible, discontinue all medications that cause dyspepsia.

For patients aged ≤60 years without alarm features, a test-and-treat approach for *H. pylori* is reasonable.

For those who test negative for *H. pylori*, an empiric trial of acid suppression using a PPI for 4 to 6 weeks is recommended.

DON'T BE TRICKED

- **Patients with refractory symptoms despite empiric therapy should undergo upper endoscopy.**

Gastroparesis

Diagnosis

Gastroparesis is characterized by delayed gastric emptying and should be considered in patients with recurrent nausea, early satiety, bloating, and weight loss.

Causes include systemic sclerosis, diabetes mellitus, hypothyroidism, administration of anticholinergic agents, and narcotics. A viral cause is suggested by rapid onset of gastroparesis after a presumed viral infection.

Testing

In patients with acute symptoms, upper endoscopy is the initial study to rule out pyloric channel obstruction caused by PUD.

Patients with chronic symptoms or negative findings on upper endoscopy should undergo a nuclear medicine solid-phase gastric emptying study.

DON'T BE TRICKED

- **Patients with diabetes mellitus should have a blood glucose level <275 mg/dL during testing because marked hyperglycemia can acutely impair gastric emptying.**

Treatment

Specific dietary recommendations include small low-fat meals consumed four to five times per day.

Use IV erythromycin for acute gastroparesis and metoclopramide for chronic gastroparesis.

Dystonia and parkinsonian-like tardive dyskinesia are serious complications of metoclopramide; the drug must be stopped at the first sign of these disorders, which may be irreversible.

TEST YOURSELF

A 64-year-old woman with a 20-year history of type 2 diabetes mellitus has a 3-year history of postprandial nausea.

ANSWER: For diagnosis, choose diabetic gastroparesis. For management, order a gastric emptying study.

Complications of Bariatric and Gastric Surgery

Diagnosis

Major complications following Roux-en-Y gastric bypass include cholelithiasis, nephrolithiasis (resulting from increased urinary oxalate excretion), dumping syndrome, anastomotic stricture or ulceration, small-bowel obstruction, and gastrogastric fistula. Small intestinal bacterial overgrowth (SIBO) occurs most often with Roux-en-Y gastric bypass.

Micronutrient deficiencies can develop following bariatric surgery, including deficiencies in calcium, cobalamin (vitamin B_{12}), folate, iron, magnesium, thiamine (vitamin B_1), and vitamins A and D.

Complications following gastrectomy include:

- anastomotic leaks and strictures
- marginal/anastomotic ulcers
- delayed gastric emptying
- dumping syndrome
- fat malabsorption

STUDY TABLE: Complications of Gastric Surgery	
If you see this...	**Do this...**
Abdominal cramps, nausea, and loose stools 15 minutes after eating followed within 90 minutes by lightheadedness, diaphoresis, and tachycardia following gastric resection or bypass surgery	Choose dumping syndrome (a clinical diagnosis) Treat with small frequent feedings and low-carbohydrate meals
Loose stools and malabsorption following bypass surgery	Choose blind loop syndrome (SIBO) Treat with antibiotics and nutritional supplements
Abdominal pain, bloating, difficulty belching following fundoplication	Choose gas-bloat syndrome Treat with diet modification; most treatments are untested

Acute Pancreatitis

Diagnosis

Patients with acute pancreatitis usually have the sudden onset of epigastric pain, often radiating to the back, accompanied by nausea, vomiting, fever, and tachycardia. The major causes of acute pancreatitis in the United States include:

- gallstone biliary obstruction and alcohol (most common)
- sulfonamides, estrogens, didanosine, valproic acid, thiazide diuretics, azathioprine/6-MP, pentamidine, and furosemide
- hypertriglyceridemia (>1000 mg/dL)
- endoscopic retrograde cholangiopancreatography (ERCP)
- CF (young people with pancreatitis)
- hypercalcemia
- infection

Diagnosis of acute pancreatitis requires at least two of the following criteria:

- acute onset of upper abdominal pain
- serum amylase or lipase increased ≥3 × ULN (lipase is more specific and sensitive than amylase)
- findings suggesting pancreatitis on cross-sectional imaging (ultrasonography, CT, MRI)

Risk factors for severe disease include age >55 years, medical comorbidities, BMI >30, SIRS, signs of hypovolemia (serum BUN level >20 mg/dL and rising, hematocrit >44%, or elevated serum creatinine).

Pancreatic pseudocysts are the most common complication of acute pancreatitis.

Repeated episodes of acute pancreatitis may result in chronic pancreatitis.

Testing

All patients with acute pancreatitis require abdominal ultrasonography to evaluate the biliary tract for obstruction.

CT of the abdomen is indicated if the pancreatitis is severe, lasts longer than 48 hours, or complications are suspected.

DON'T BE TRICKED

- Do not routinely obtain abdominal CT for acute pancreatitis.
- Uncomplicated pancreatitis is not typically associated with rebound abdominal tenderness, absent bowel sounds, high fever, or melena. When these findings are present, consider abscess, pseudocyst, or necrotizing pancreatitis.
- Mildly increased amylase values can also be caused by kidney disease, intestinal ischemia, appendicitis, and parotitis.

Treatment

In addition to supportive therapy with vigorous IV hydration and pain relief:

- oral feeding when nausea, vomiting, and abdominal pain resolve
- enteral jejunal feedings (preferred) or total parenteral nutrition for moderate to severe pancreatitis
- antibiotics for cholangitis, infected pancreatic necrosis, and infected pseudocysts
- cholecystectomy before discharge for uncomplicated gallstone pancreatitis
- ERCP within 24 hours of presentation for ascending cholangitis or biliary obstruction
- surgical consultation for pancreatic necrosis (may resolve spontaneously)

Fluid collections that arise from disruption of the pancreatic ductal system are known as acute peripancreatic fluid collections for the first 4 weeks after presentation and pancreatic pseudocysts after becoming encapsulated.

- Most resolve spontaneously.
- Symptomatic fluid collections are treated with transgastric or transduodenal drainage.

DON'T BE TRICKED

- **Fluid resuscitation (250-500 mL/h) is most beneficial in the first 12-24 hours and may be detrimental after this therapeutic window.**
- **Do not withhold oral feeding on the basis of persistent elevations in pancreatic enzyme levels.**
- **Do not select antibiotics for interstitial (nonnecrotizing) pancreatitis without evidence of infection.**

TEST YOURSELF

A 71-year-old woman is admitted to the hospital with gallstone pancreatitis. On the sixth day, she has increased pain, fever, and leukocytosis. A CT scan of the abdomen with contrast shows hypodense, nonenhancing areas involving 50% of the pancreas.

ANSWER: For diagnosis, choose pancreatic necrosis. For management, arrange surgical consultation.

Chronic Pancreatitis

Diagnosis

Common diagnostic criteria:

- history of pain, recurrent attacks of pancreatitis, weight loss
- pancreatic calcifications on imaging
- ductal dilation or inflammatory masses
- exocrine pancreatic insufficiency (steatorrhea)
- diabetes

Chronic alcohol abuse is the most common cause in industrialized countries.

Testing

Pancreas-protocol abdominal CT is the most sensitive imaging test to document pancreatic calcifications.

If calcifications are absent, an MRI, MRCP, or endoscopic ultrasonography should be performed to detect abnormalities of the main and branch pancreatic ducts.

Young adults with chronic pancreatitis require sweat chloride testing for CF.

Disease onset in older patients without risk factors requires exclusion of autoimmune pancreatitis (AIP) and pancreatic cancer.

DON'T BE TRICKED

- **Normal amylase and lipase levels do not rule out chronic pancreatitis.**

Treatment

Treatment of chronic pancreatitis is directed at controlling pain (in the stepwise approach used for chronic pain) and treating diabetes mellitus, malabsorption, and steatorrhea. Administer pancreatic enzymes as initial therapy for malabsorption. If enzyme supplements do not control diarrhea, begin antidiarrheal agents.

Avoid opiates if possible; they may lead to a number of adverse effects, including nausea, vomiting, and constipation.

DON'T BE TRICKED

- In persistent or refractory pain, look for a dilated pancreatic duct and intraductal calcifications; if present,consider endoscopic stenting, lithotripsy, or surgical drainage (pancreaticojejunostomy).

Autoimmune Pancreatitis

Diagnosis

Patients with AIP typically present with painless obstructive jaundice or acute pancreatitis (rare). Cross-sectional imaging reveals "sausage-shaped" pancreatic enlargement with an indistinct border. It is important to exclude pancreatic cancer; biopsy may be necessary.

Type I AIP is seen in older men and is associated with pancreatitis, Sjögren syndrome, PSC, bile duct strictures, autoimmune thyroiditis, and interstitial nephritis. Serum IgG4 level is increased.

Type II AIP is associated with chronic pancreatitis and IBD and less likely to include elevated IgG4 levels.

Treatment

Most patients with type I or II AIP respond to glucocorticoids. Patients with relapsed disease typically respond to glucocorticoid retreatment.

Acute Diarrhea

Diagnosis

Most acute diarrhea in developed countries results from viral gastroenteritis or food poisoning and is self-limited. A careful review of medication history (including nonprescription medications and supplements) is indicated to look for drugs that cause diarrhea.

If diarrhea does not resolve in 1 week, evaluation is recommended with stool testing for common bacterial pathogens and toxins, including *Clostridium difficile.*

Yersinia enterocolitica colitis can mimic appendicitis or Crohn disease. Cryptosporidiosis develops most often in patients with AIDS, but outbreaks also occur in immunocompetent patients and cause a self-limited secretory diarrhea.

Treatment

Supportive care with oral hydration and antidiarrheal medications is sufficient for most patients with acute diarrhea.

Antibiotic treatment is reserved for patients with diarrhea lasting >7 days or with symptoms of fever, abdominal pain, or hematochezia.

Diarrhea caused by parasites (*Giardia lamblia* or *Entamoeba histolytica*) requires therapy with metronidazole.

DON'T BE TRICKED

- Do not order stool cultures for acute diarrhea of <1 week's duration.
- Do not choose antibiotics for EHEC colitis.
- Do not choose loperamide or diphenoxylate for acute diarrhea with fever or blood in the stool. Both agents are associated with HUS in EHEC colitis and toxic megacolon in *C. difficile* infection.

Chronic Diarrhea

Diagnosis

Chronic diarrhea is defined as lasting longer than 4 weeks. Except for *Giardia lamblia*, infectious causes of chronic diarrhea are uncommon in immunocompetent adults in developed countries.

Testing

Select colonoscopy for most patients with chronic diarrhea. The terminal ileum should be viewed to assess for Crohn disease; random biopsies of the colonic mucosa should be performed to assess for microscopic colitis.

If colonoscopy is nondiagnostic, order a 48- to 72-hour stool collection with analysis of fat content. Fat excretion >14 g/d is diagnostic of steatorrhea. Patients with steatorrhea should undergo evaluation for small-bowel malabsorption disorders (e.g., celiac disease), bacterial overgrowth, and pancreatic insufficiency.

Stool electrolytes (sodium and potassium) can be measured in liquid stool to calculate the fecal osmotic gap, which helps to diagnose osmotic diarrhea. The osmotic gap is calculated as 290 − (2 × [Na + K]).

- An osmotic gap >100 mOsm/kg H_2O indicates an osmotic diarrhea.
- A gap <50 mOsm/kg H_2O indicates a secretory diarrhea.
- Measured stool osmolarity <250 mOsm/kg H_2O suggests factitious diarrhea associated with chronic laxative abuse or adding water to the stool.

Osmotic diarrhea is most commonly caused by lactase deficiency. Osmotic diarrhea is associated with eating, improves with fasting, and typically is not nocturnal.

Secretory diarrhea is characterized by large-volume, watery, nocturnal bowel movements and is unchanged by fasting (see also Celiac Disease).

STUDY TABLE: Differential Diagnosis of Chronic Diarrhea

If you see this...	Diagnose or do this...
Bloating, abdominal discomfort relieved by a bowel movement, no weight loss or alarm features	IBS; test for celiac disease
Diarrhea mainly in women aged 45-60 years, unrelated to food intake (nocturnal diarrhea), normal colonoscopy	Microscopic colitis; stop NSAIDs/PPIs, biopsy
Diarrhea with dairy products	Lactose intolerance; dietary exclusion or hydrogen breath test
Use of artificial sweeteners or fructose	Carbohydrate intolerance; dietary exclusion or hydrogen breath test
Nocturnal diarrhea and diabetes mellitus or SSc	Small bowel bacterial overgrowth; hydrogen breath test or empiric antibiotic trial
Coexistent pulmonary diseases and/or recurrent *Giardia* infection	CVI and selective IgA deficiency; measure immunoglobulins
Somatization or other psychiatric syndromes, history of laxative use	Self-induced diarrhea; obtain tests for stool osmolality, electrolytes, magnesium, and laxative screen
Severe secretory diarrhea and flushing	Carcinoid syndrome; obtain test for 24-hour urinary excretion of 5-HIAA

DON'T BE TRICKED

- Don't forget other causes of diarrhea such as sorbitol (added as a sweetener to gum, candy) and medications, including PPIs, magnesium-containing antacids, metformin, colchicine, and antibiotics.
- Infection with *Giardia lamblia* should be considered in patients with exposure to young children or potentially contaminated water (lakes and streams).

TEST YOURSELF

A 36-year-old woman has watery diarrhea that is not nocturnal. She has six to seven high-volume bowel movements daily, and her symptoms improve with fasting. Stool cultures are negative. Stool sodium is 70 mEq/L and stool potassium is 10 mEq/L.

ANSWER: For diagnosis, choose osmotic diarrhea.

A 55-year-old woman who takes NSAIDs daily has watery diarrhea without weight loss. Colonoscopy is grossly normal.

ANSWER: For diagnosis, select microscopic colitis.

Malabsorption

Diagnosis

Patients with chronic diarrhea, especially those who report an oily residue in their stool, should be evaluated for possible fat malabsorption. The four most common disorders causing malabsorption with steatorrhea are celiac disease, SIBO, short-bowel syndrome, and pancreatic insufficiency.

STUDY TABLE: Chronic Diarrhea and Malabsorption Syndromes

If you see this...	Do this...
History of IBS and iron deficiency anemia	Diagnose celiac disease. Obtain IgA anti-tTG antibody assay and small bowel biopsy if positive. Order a gluten-free diet.
Chronic pancreatitis, hyperglycemia, history of pancreatic resection, CF	Diagnose pancreatic insufficiency. Obtain test for excess fecal fat and x-rays for pancreatic calcifications. Treat with pancreatic enzyme replacement therapy.
Previous surgery, small bowel diverticulosis, dysmotility (SSc or diabetes mellitus), combination of vitamin B_{12} deficiency and elevated folate level	Diagnose bacterial overgrowth. Order empiric trial of antibiotics or hydrogen breath test.
Resection of >200 cm of distal small bowel (or viable small bowel <180 cm)	Diagnose short-bowel syndrome. Replace nutrient and electrolyte deficiencies.
History of resection of <100 cm of distal ileum, with voluminous diarrhea, weight loss, and malnutrition	Diagnose short-bowel syndrome with bile acid enteropathy. Order empiric trial of cholestyramine.
Arthralgia; fever; neurologic, ocular, or cardiac disease	Diagnose Whipple disease. Select small bowel biopsy and PCR for *Tropheryma whippelii.* Order antibiotics for 12 months.
Travel to India or Puerto Rico, malabsorption, weight loss, malaise, folate or vitamin B_{12} deficiency, steatorrhea	Diagnose tropical sprue. Order a small bowel biopsy. Treat with a sulfonamide or tetracycline and folic acid.
Prolonged traveler's diarrhea, diarrhea after a camping trip, outbreak in a day-care center	Diagnose giardiasis. Identify *Giardia* parasites or *Giardia* antigen in the stool. Treat with metronidazole.

DON'T BE TRICKED

- Do not use cholestyramine if ileal resection is >100 cm (will worsen bile salt deficiency and steatorrhea).
- Use cholestyramine if diarrhea begins after cholecystectomy.

Celiac Disease

Diagnosis

Celiac disease occurs secondary to ingestion of wheat gluten or related rye and barley proteins in genetically predisposed persons. Characteristic findings are:

- chronic diarrhea or steatorrhea
- bloating, weight loss, and abdominal pain
- pruritic papulovesicular rash on the extensor surfaces (dermatitis herpetiformis; see Dermatology, Pemphigus Vulgaris and Pemphigoid)
- isolated abnormalities of liver chemistry tests
- iron deficiency anemia
- fat-soluble vitamin deficiencies
- osteoporosis

Celiac disease is often misdiagnosed as IBS.

Type 1 diabetes mellitus and autoimmune thyroid disease occur more commonly in patients with celiac disease.

Patients with celiac disease can have problems absorbing thyroid hormone; the first sign of celiac disease may be malabsorption of thyroid hormone (total T_4 does not increase with increasing doses of thyroxine).

Small bowel lymphoma is more common in patients with celiac disease.

Testing

Diagnostic tests include an IgA anti-tTG antibody assay with small bowel biopsy for those with a positive antibody assay.

Measure bone mineral density in all patients with newly diagnosed celiac disease.

Treatment

After diagnosis, select a gluten-free diet for treatment of celiac disease or dermatitis. The effectiveness of diet therapy is determined by remeasuring IgA anti-tTG antibody titers or repeating small bowel biopsies.

Patients with osteomalacia should also receive supplemental vitamin D and calcium.

Nonadherence is the most common reason for failure of a gluten-free diet. Adherent patients with recurrent malabsorption should be evaluated for intestinal lymphoma.

Other causes of continued symptoms include inadvertent exposure to gluten and microscopic colitis.

DON'T BE TRICKED

- Empiric treatment with a gluten-free diet before serologic testing may result in false-negative serologic test results.
- An association between celiac disease and IgA deficiency can lead to false-negative IgA-based tests. In patients with IgA deficiency, assays for IgG anti-tTG or IgG-deamidated gliadin peptides are necessary.
- Definitive diagnosis of celiac disease requires small bowel biopsy.
- All patients, regardless of symptoms, should be treated with a gluten-free diet to prevent intestinal lymphoma, including patients with isolated dermatitis herpetiformis.

TEST YOURSELF

A 54-year-old woman has a 4-month history of diarrhea and weight loss. Laboratory studies show hypocalcemia, microcytic anemia, and an increased PT.

ANSWER: For diagnosis, choose celiac disease. For management, order an IgA anti-tTG antibody assay and, if positive, follow with a small bowel biopsy.

Inflammatory Bowel Disease

Diagnosis

IBD comprises a group of related conditions characterized by idiopathic inflammation of the GI tract. The two most common IBDs are Crohn disease and ulcerative colitis, both of which cause macroscopic inflammation. Microscopic colitis is the least common IBD and does not cause significant macroscopic abnormalities. Although several features may differentiate Crohn disease from ulcerative colitis, overlap is significant.

STUDY TABLE: Differentiating Ulcerative Colitis from Crohn Disease

Ulcerative Colitis	Crohn Disease
Mucosal edema, erythema, and loss of the vascular pattern, granularity, friability, ulceration, and bleeding	Linear, stellate, or serpiginous ulcerations with "skip" areas of inflammation involving entire GI tract
Altered crypt architecture with shortened, branched crypts and crypt abscesses	Granulomas are characteristic but are often not found. Transmural involvement.
Diarrhea (prominent), tenesmus, urgency hematochezia, weight loss, and fever	Abdominal pain (prominent), diarrhea, inflammatory masses, fever, weight loss, intestinal strictures and fistula (to skin, bladder, vagina, or enteric-enteric)
Smoking alleviates symptoms	Smoking is a risk factor for disease

The most common extraintestinal manifestations are oral aphthous ulcers, arthralgia, and back pain (indicating ankylosing spondylitis or sacroiliitis). Eye redness, pain, and swelling may result from uveitis or scleritis. Skin manifestations include pyoderma gangrenosum and erythema nodosum. Liver involvement most commonly includes PSC.

Testing

Colonoscopy and biopsy confirm the diagnosis. Stool studies are indicated for *Shigella*, *Salmonella*, *Campylobacter*, *Escherichia coli* O157:H7, ova and parasites, and *Clostridium difficile* toxin.

DON'T BE TRICKED

- **Do not perform a barium enema examination in patients with moderate to severe ulcerative colitis, because this procedure may precipitate toxic megacolon.**
- **In patients with Crohn disease and cystitis, consider the possibility of enterovesical fistula.**

Treatment

Treatment of Crohn disease and ulcerative colitis is divided into active and maintenance strategies. Specific treatment choices depend on the type, extent, and severity of the disease.

The 5-ASA drugs are first-line therapy for inducing and maintaining remission in ulcerative colitis. They deliver 5-ASA topically to the bowel lumen, primarily to the colon, with the exception of the time-release formulation of mesalamine, which is able to deliver the drug throughout the small bowel as well as the colon.

Patients with IBD should receive seasonal influenza, 13-valent pneumococcal conjugate, and 23-valent pneumococcal polysaccharide vaccines. Ideally, pneumococcal vaccination should occur before beginning immunosuppressive therapy.

STUDY TABLE: Treatment of Ulcerative Colitis

Indications	Principal Therapy
Mild disease: <4 bowel movements daily; occasional blood in stool; normal vital signs, hemoglobin, and ESR	5-ASA agents: mesalamine for pancolitis and topical sulfasalazine for proctitis or left-sided colitis
Moderate disease	Prednisone or budesonide for remission induction Maintenance therapy with a 5-ASA agent (topical and oral), 6-MP, or azathioprine
Severe disease: >6 bowel movements daily, bleeding, fever, pulse rate >90/min, ESR >30 mm/h, anemia	IV glucocorticoids followed by anti-TNF antibody Surgery for refractory disease

Anti-TNF antibodies are approved for inducing and maintaining remission in ulcerative colitis (e.g., infliximab, adalimumab, and golimumab). Patients whose symptoms do not respond to glucocorticoids are treated with an anti-TNF biologic agent or colectomy.

STUDY TABLE: Treatment of Crohn Disease

Indications	Principal Therapy
Mild to moderate disease: No fever or abdominal tenderness, <10% weight loss	Budesonide or mesalamine (for limited, mild ileocolonic disease) for remission 6-MP, azathioprine, or methotrexate for maintenance
Moderate to severe disease: Fever, >10% weight loss, anemia, abdominal pain, and nausea or vomiting	Prednisone for remission induction 6-MP, azathioprine, or methotrexate for maintenance Anti-TNF antibodies (infliximab, adalimumab, and certolizumab) for refractory disease; ustekinumab and vedolizumab for disease refractory to anti-TNF antibodies
Severe to fulminant disease: Despite oral glucocorticoids, high fever, cachexia, vomiting, rebound tenderness, obstruction, or abscess	IV glucocorticoid for remission Anti-TNF antibodies in glucocorticoid-refractory disease; ustekinumab and vedolizumab for disease refractory to anti-TNF antibodies Surgical intervention if patient has extremely toxic disease or does not benefit from medications
Fistula	Azathioprine, 6-MP, anti-TNF antibodies

The level of thiopurine methyltransferase should be checked before starting azathioprine or 6-MP; 1 in 300 patients lacks enzyme activity and is at high risk of drug toxicity; azathioprine and 6-MP should not be used in these patients.

Follow-Up Surveillance

Beginning 8 years after diagnosis, surveillance colonoscopy for colon cancer should be performed every 1 to 2 years for patients with ulcerative pancolitis or Crohn disease involving most of the colon. If dysplasia is found, proctocolectomy is required.

DON'T BE TRICKED

- **Before initiating an anti-TNF agent, all patients should be evaluated for TB and HBV.**

TEST YOURSELF

An 18-year-old man has a 3-month history of five or more bowel movements daily, fever, and abdominal pain. Vital signs are stable. Colonoscopy shows ulcerative colitis.

ANSWER: For treatment, select prednisone for remission and oral sulfasalazine for maintenance.

Microscopic Colitis

Diagnosis

Microscopic colitis is characterized by chronic diarrhea without abdominal pain or weight loss, most commonly in women aged 45 to 60 years.

In certain cases, NSAIDs, PPIs, and SSRIs have been implicated as causative agents.

Testing

Colonoscopy with biopsies is required for diagnosis. The colonic mucosa appears normal on gross examination. Microscopic colitis is further classified into collagenous colitis or lymphocytic colitis based on histology.

Treatment

Microscopic colitis is best treated with antidiarrheal agents such as loperamide or bismuth subsalicylate; diphenoxylate may be effective for mild cases. Otherwise, budesonide has the best documented efficacy. Stop NSAIDs, which may contribute to symptoms.

DON'T BE TRICKED

- **Symptoms of microscopic colitis and celiac disease are similar; in patients with celiac disease or microscopic colitis whose symptoms do not respond to appropriate therapy, the other condition must be considered and ruled out with appropriate testing.**
- **Unlike IBD, patients with microscopic colitis are not at increased risk for colon cancer.**

Chronic Constipation

Diagnosis

Diagnosis of chronic constipation requires ≥3 months of symptoms.

Medications, particularly opioids, are the most common cause of secondary constipation.

Treatment

Chronic constipation can be approached in a stepped fashion:

- eliminate implicated medications, if possible
- increase physical activity and dietary fiber
- soluble fibers such as psyllium and methylcellulose
- surfactants such as docusate sodium or docusate calcium (most appropriate for very mild, intermittent constipation)
- osmotic laxatives include magnesium hydroxide, lactulose, sorbitol, and PEG 3350 (PEG is superior)
- stimulant laxatives such as anthraquinone, senna, and the diphenylmethanes (fastest-acting agents)

If chronic constipation does not respond to initial stepped approach, prosecretory agents, including lubiprostone and linaclotide, are available by prescription.

DON'T BE TRICKED

- **Chronic senna use can lead to benign pigmentation of the colon, known as melanosis coli.**

Irritable Bowel Syndrome

Diagnosis

IBS is defined as abdominal pain associated with altered bowel habits (change in stool form or frequency) over a period of at least 3 months.

Other symptoms include urgency, straining, a feeling of incomplete evacuation, passing mucus, and bloating.

A clinical diagnosis of IBS can be made in the absence of alarm symptoms (anemia; weight loss; and family history of colorectal cancer, IBD, or celiac disease).

IBS is further subtyped based on the predominant stool pattern as IBS with constipation (IBS-C), IBS with diarrhea (IBS-D), or mixed IBS (IBS-M).

DON'T BE TRICKED

- **In the absence of alarm symptoms, CBC, serum chemistry studies, TSH, stool studies, and abdominal imaging are unnecessary.**
- **Patients older than 50 years or with severe or refractory symptoms require diagnostic colonoscopy.**
- **Screen for celiac disease with serum tTG in patients with IBS-D or IBS-M symptoms.**
- **Screening colonoscopy should be pursued only in patients who otherwise meet criteria for colon cancer screening.**

Treatment

Management of IBS focuses on controlling symptoms rather than on cure.

- diet modification
- hyoscyamine and dicyclomine for the short-term treatment of abdominal pain in IBS-D or IBS-C
- tricyclic antidepressants (preferred in IBS-D) and SSRIs (preferred in IBS-C) for abdominal pain
- lubiprostone (FDA approved for women with IBS-C) and linaclotide (guideline preferred; FDA approved for treatment of IBS-C in adults) for IBS-C unresponsive to PEG
- loperamide for IBS-D
- eluxadoline for abdominal pain and stool consistency in IBS-D
- rifaximin for global symptoms associated with IBS-D

DON'T BE TRICKED

- **Alosetron should not be used as first-line therapy for IBS-D because of the risk of ischemic colitis; prescribing is limited to providers in an FDA-mandated Risk Evaluation and Mitigation Strategy program.**

Diverticular Disease

Diagnosis

Diverticular disorders of the colon include diverticulosis, diverticular bleeding, and diverticulitis.

Diverticulosis refers to an asymptomatic herniation (diverticulum) of the intestinal wall.

Diverticulitis is an inflammatory response following microperforation of a diverticulum and is characterized by LLQ abdominal pain and fever.

Diverticular bleeding occurs following rupture of an artery that has penetrated a diverticulum, is typically painless, and usually stops without therapy.

Dysuria, urinary frequency, and urgency may reflect bladder irritation. Pneumaturia, fecaluria, or recurrent/polymicrobial UTI suggest a colovesical fistula.

Testing

If clinical features highly suggest diverticulitis, imaging studies are unnecessary.

If the diagnosis is unclear or if an abscess is suspected (severe pain, high fever, palpable mass), CT is indicated.

Treatment

For stable patients with diverticulitis, select a clear-liquid diet and a 7- to 10-day course of antibiotics, such as ciprofloxacin and metronidazole.

Hospitalize patients if they are unable to maintain oral intake for IV fluids and antibiotics.

A small abscess may resolve with antimicrobial therapy alone. CT-guided drainage can facilitate nonsurgical management of larger abscesses.

Emergent surgery is required when conservative treatment fails or for peritonitis, sepsis, or perforation.

After recovering from acute diverticulitis, 30% of patients will have recurrent episodes. After a second episode, the risk of subsequent attacks increases to 50%, and surgical resection of the affected colon is indicated.

DON'T BE TRICKED

- Avoid colonoscopy in the setting of acute diverticulitis; air insufflation may increase the risk of perforation.
- A colonoscopy should be performed following recovery to rule out colon cancer.

Mesenteric Ischemia and Ischemic Colitis

Diagnosis

The two most common GI ischemic disorders are acute mesenteric ischemia (AMI) and ischemic colitis.

Embolism to the mesenteric arteries from AF or left ventricle thrombus causes 50% of AMI. Mesenteric arterial thrombosis is usually caused by atherosclerotic disease.

Nonocclusive mesenteric ischemia is caused by low-flow states such as HF, sepsis, hypotension, or hypovolemia or the use of vasoactive medications (vasopressors, ergots, triptans, cocaine, digitalis). Leukocytosis, hemoconcentration, increased anion gap metabolic acidosis, and elevations in LDH and/or amylase levels are seen.

STUDY TABLE: Differential Diagnosis of GI Ischemic Syndromes

Problem	Symptoms	Diagnosis
AMI	Poorly localized severe abdominal pain, often out of proportion to physical findings; peritoneal signs signify infarction	CTA or selective mesenteric angiography
Chronic mesenteric ischemia	Postprandial abdominal pain, fear of eating, and weight loss; often, signs and symptoms of atherosclerosis in other vascular beds	CTA, selective angiography, or MRA
Ischemic colitis	LLQ abdominal pain and self-limited bloody diarrhea	Colonoscopy: patchy segmental ulcerations

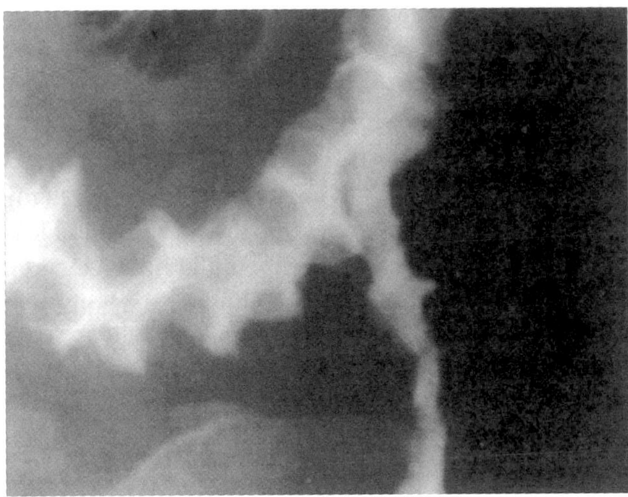

Ischemic Colitis: Thumbprinting (submucosal hemorrhage and edema) is shown in the transverse colon on this barium x-ray.

Treatment

STUDY TABLE: Treatment for Mesenteric Ischemia and Ischemic Colitis	
Condition	**Treatment**
AMI with peritoneal signs	Urgent laparotomy Resection of necrotic bowel Embolectomy or thrombectomy and surgical revascularization
AMI without peritoneal signs	Angiography Surgical embolectomy or intra-arterial thrombolysis Intra-arterial papaverine for nonocclusive mesenteric ischemia
Chronic mesenteric ischemia	Surgical reconstruction or angioplasty with stenting
Ischemic colitis	Supportive care with IV fluids and bowel rest

DON'T BE TRICKED

- The diagnosis of colonic ischemia can be made by clinical history and/or colonoscopy; angiography plays no role.

Differentiating Cholestatic and Hepatocellular Diseases

Key Considerations

Hepatocellular injury primarily results in elevated AST and ALT values, usually >500 U/L.

Virus- or drug-induced acute hepatitis usually causes serum aminotransferase elevations >1000 U/L (ALT > AST) and serum total bilirubin levels >15 mg/dL.

- ALT values >5000 U/L usually result from acetaminophen hepatotoxicity or hepatic ischemia.
- An AST/ALT ratio >2.0 is highly suggestive of AH.
- Prolonged PT/INR and low serum albumin values imply severe hepatocellular dysfunction.
- Minimal ALT and AST elevations in a patient with obesity, hyperlipidemia, and hypertension suggest nonalcoholic liver disease.

Cholestatic liver diseases primarily cause elevated serum bilirubin and alkaline phosphatase values with proportionally lesser elevations of aminotransferase levels. Cholestatic diseases affect microscopic ducts, large bile ducts, or both.

Alkaline phosphatase is also produced in bone and placenta, and high levels are seen in pregnancy. Fractionation of alkaline phosphatase can determine the source.

Overproduction (hemolysis) or impaired uptake (e.g., Gilbert disease) of bilirubin is characterized by >80% indirect (unconjugated) bilirubin, whereas hepatocyte dysfunction or impaired bile flow (obstruction) is characterized by >20% direct (conjugated) bilirubin.

DON'T BE TRICKED

- Extensive testing is not required to establish the diagnosis of Gilbert disease; verify normal aminotransferase levels and the absence of hemolysis.
- Patients with Gilbert disease usually have mild (<3 mg/dL) unconjugated bilirubin levels that increase with stress or fasting.

Hepatitis A

Prevention

Hepatitis A vaccine is indicated for travelers to endemic areas, injection drug users, men who have sex with men, and patients with chronic liver disease and clotting factor disorders.

Immunization or immune globulin should be given within 2 weeks to household, sexual, and day-care contacts of patients with hepatitis A or persons who ate foods contaminated with HAV. Vaccination is preferred in healthy persons aged ≤40 years, immunoglobulin for older and immunocompromised patients.

One dose of hepatitis A vaccine administered to travelers any time before departure provides protection for healthy persons aged ≤40 years. A second dose 6 to 12 months later is recommended. Older adults and those who are immunocompromised or have chronic liver disease and are departing in ≤2 weeks should receive one dose of the vaccine and immune globulin.

Diagnosis

HAV is associated with abrupt onset of fatigue, anorexia, malaise, nausea, vomiting, and jaundice.

Laboratory findings include marked elevations of serum aminotransferases (usually >1000 U/L).

The clinical course of relapsing HAV infection is characterized by clinical recovery with near normalization of serum aminotransferases followed several weeks later by biochemical and sometimes clinical relapse.

Patients with unexplained acute hepatitis or acute liver failure should be tested for IgM anti-HAV.

Hepatitis B

Prevention

HBV vaccination decreases the incidence and prevalence of HBV and results in fewer cases of HCC in endemic areas.

Hepatitis B vaccine plus HBIG is indicated for postexposure prophylaxis after needle-stick injury and for sexual and household contacts of patients with HBV.

Diagnosis

HBV is transmitted by exposure to the blood or body fluids of an infected person, including through injection drug use, sexual contact with an infected person, or transmission by an infected mother to her infant during delivery.

Persons with hepatitis B may have anicteric or subclinical acute infection. Symptoms of acute hepatitis B are similar to those of acute hepatitis A. Characteristic findings are increases in serum aminotransferase (AST/ALT) levels; acute liver failure may occur.

HBV infection includes several stages, but not all patients go through each stage.

- Patients who acquire HBV infection at birth often go through the **immune tolerant phase** characterized by a normal ALT level despite a positive HBeAg and very high HBV DNA level.
- The **inactive carrier stage** is characterized by a normal ALT level and an HBV DNA level <20,000 U/mL.
- Patients in the HBeAg-positive (**immune active**) or HBeAg-negative (**immune escape**) chronic HBV phases have an elevated ALT level and an HBV DNA level >10,000 U/mL.

DON'T BE TRICKED

- **Hepatitis A is not a cause of chronic hepatitis.**
- **Chronic hepatitis B may present with membranous GN, polyarteritis nodosa, or cryoglobulinemia.**

STUDY TABLE: Interpretation of Hepatitis B Test Results

Clinical scenario	HBsAg	Anti-HBs	IgM anti-HBc	IgG anti-HBc	HBeAg	Anti-HBe	HBV DNA, U/mL
Acute hepatitis B; occasionally reactivation of chronic hepatitis B	+	−	+	−	+	−	>20,000
Resolved previous infection	−	+	−	+	−	+/−	Undetected
Immunity from previous vaccination	−	+	−	−	−	−	Undetected
False-positive or resolved previous infection	−	−	−	+	−	−	Undetected
Chronic hepatitis B inactive carrier state	+	−	−	+	−	+	<20,000
HBeAg-positive chronic hepatitis B	+	−	−	+	+	−	>20,000
HBeAg-negative chronic hepatitis B	+	−	−	+	−	+	>10,000

Treatment

Treatment is recommended for those with:

- acute liver failure or cirrhosis
- infection in the immune-active phase (HBeAg positive, ALT ≥2 × ULN, HBV DNA ≥20,000 U/L)
- infection in the reactivation phase (HBeAg-negative, ALT ≥2 × ULN, HBV DNA ≥2,000 U/L)
- immunosuppression or planned immunosuppression

Treatment usually consists of entecavir or tenofovir (preferred). Pegylated interferon may be used for patients without cirrhosis who have high ALT levels and relatively low HBV DNA levels or who are pregnant.

In patients coinfected with HIV and who have not yet been treated for either disease, emtricitabine-tenofovir is typically used as part of ART.

DON'T BE TRICKED

- **Do not treat HBV infection in patients in the immune tolerant or inactive carrier phases.**
- **Interferon alfa should not be used in patients with active autoimmune disorders, severe cytopenias, decompensated cirrhosis, or major depression.**

Follow-Up Surveillance

The following characteristics are associated with an increased risk for HCC in patients with HBV and are indications for surveillance with ultrasonography every 6 months:

- cirrhosis
- Asian men >40 years and Asian women >50 years
- black patients >20 years
- elevated ALT level and HBV DNA levels >10,000 U/mL
- family history of HCC

TEST YOURSELF

A 55-year-old woman has a 6-month history of fatigue and malaise. She is taking paroxetine for depression. The serum ALT is 109 U/L. HBsAg, HBeAg, and HBV DNA are positive, and anti-HBV is negative.

ANSWER: For diagnosis, choose chronic hepatitis B. For treatment, select entecavir or tenofovir; do not select interferon alfa.

Hepatitis C

Screening

Universal screening is recommended for persons born between 1945 and 1965.

Diagnosis

HCV is the most prevalent bloodborne infection in the United States. HCV manifests as chronic liver disease because the acute infection is asymptomatic. Chronic HCV infection can cause cirrhosis and is a risk factor for HCC.

Test for HCV in patients with chronic liver disease, as well as patients with vasculitis, cryoglobulinemia, GN, and porphyria cutanea tarda.

Other high-risk groups include injection drug users, recipients of blood transfusions before 1992, and those with HIV or an STI.

Testing

Measurement of anti-HCV antibody is the initial diagnostic study.

If positive, test for HCV RNA to determine the presence of active infection.

Patients with spontaneous resolution of acute HCV or who have been treated successfully for HCV will have clearance of HCV RNA but usually remain positive for antibody to HCV.

HCV genotyping should be performed at the time of diagnosis to help in choosing a treatment regimen.

DON'T BE TRICKED

- **Because normal aminotransferase levels occur in up to 40% of patients with chronic HCV, normal levels cannot exclude a diagnosis of HCV.**
- **Reactivation of hepatitis B can occur during antiviral therapy for HCV. Test for hepatitis B before initiating direct antiviral therapy for HCV.**

Treatment

Treatment regimens are based on genotype. Genotype 1 is the most prominent in the United States (70%), and its regimen includes:

- sofosbuvir and ledipasvir (available as a combination tablet)
- ombitasvir, paritaprevir, and ritonavir (available as a combination tablet) plus dasabuvir with or without ribavirin
- sofosbuvir and simeprevir with or without ribavirin
- glecaprevir-pibrentasvir or elbasvir-grasoprevir for patients with end-stage kidney disease

Treatment of patients with HIV coinfection is similar to that for patients with HCV alone. Patients with HCV who have decompensated disease or localized HCC are candidates for liver transplantation.

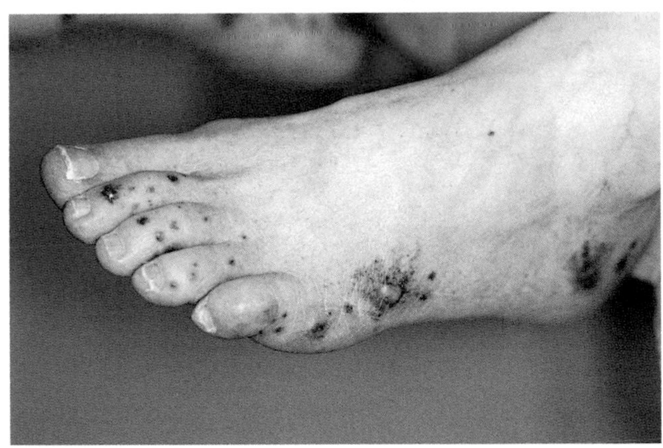

Leukocytoclastic Vasculitis: Palpable purpura consistent with HCV-associated leukocytoclastic vasculitis.

Follow-Up Surveillance

HCV rarely causes HCC in the absence of cirrhosis. Patients with cirrhosis should undergo sonography surveillance for HCC every 6 months.

TEST YOURSELF

A 45-year-old male injection drug user has a 3-month history of recurrent purpuric lesions on his legs. Skin biopsy shows leukocytoclastic vasculitis. HBsAg is negative.

ANSWER: For diagnosis, choose HCV. For management, select anti-HCV testing; if positive, test for HCV RNA and for cryoglobulins.

Alcoholic Hepatitis

Diagnosis

Acute alcoholic binges can cause fatty liver. Hepatic steatosis with inflammation is called alcoholic steatohepatitis. Mild forms of alcoholic steatohepatitis are common, are usually asymptomatic, and are associated with mild elevations in aminotransferase levels. The most severe form of alcoholic steatohepatitis is called AH and is distinguished from alcohol-induced steatosis and steatohepatitis by the presence of symptoms.

- AH usually occurs in patients with daily, heavy alcohol use (>100 g/d) for more than 20 years, although AH can develop in patients who drink moderately.
- The clinical presentation includes jaundice, anorexia, and tender hepatomegaly with or without fever; findings consistent with portal hypertension may be present.
- Patients have AST and ALT measurements <300 to 500 U/L, with an AST/ALT ratio ≥2.0.

Treatment

Abstinence from alcohol is indicated for all patients. Prednisolone is indicated for patients with a Maddrey Discriminant Function (MDF) score ≥32, Model for End-Stage Liver Disease (MELD) score ≥18, or encephalopathy and ascites.

If the bilirubin level does not improve by day 7, prednisolone should be discontinued.

DON'T BE TRICKED

- Do not use glucocorticoids in patients with AH and GI bleeding, infection, pancreatitis, or kidney disease.

TEST YOURSELF

A 46-year-old man has fever and RUQ abdominal pain. He drinks six cans of beer daily. Physical examination discloses ascites. Serum AST is 260 U/L and ALT is 80 U/L. The ascitic fluid leukocyte count is <100/µL.

ANSWER: For diagnosis, choose alcoholic hepatitis.

Autoimmune Hepatitis

Diagnosis

Autoimmune hepatitis primarily develops in women aged 20 to 40 years. The clinical presentation ranges from asymptomatic elevation of aminotransferase levels to acute liver failure. Aminotransferase levels range from mild elevations to >1000 U/L. IgG levels are also elevated. Other findings include positive ANA and anti–smooth muscle antibody titers, positive p-ANCA, or anti-LKM I antibody. Liver biopsy establishes the diagnosis.

Fifty percent of patients with autoimmune hepatitis have other autoimmune diseases such as thyroiditis, ulcerative colitis, or synovitis.

Autoimmune hepatitis has been called "lupoid hepatitis;" although ANA are the most common autoantibodies in autoimmune hepatitis, these patients do not have clinical features consistent with SLE.

DON'T BE TRICKED

- High serum total protein and low serum albumin levels suggest an elevated serum gamma globulin level, which may be the only clue to hypergammaglobulinemia.

Treatment

Patients who have active inflammation on liver biopsy specimens or are symptomatic should be considered for treatment with glucocorticoids and azathioprine. Relapse occurs after stopping treatment in most patients.

Hemochromatosis

Diagnosis

Hereditary hemochromatosis is an autosomal-recessive disorder characterized by increased intestinal absorption of iron and iron deposition in multiple organs.

- The most common symptoms are erectile dysfunction, fatigue, destructive arthropathy of the second and third MCP joints characterized by distinctive hook-like osteophytes, and OA involving unusual joints, such as the shoulders, ankles, and elbows.
- Less commonly, patients may have diabetes, HF, hyperpigmentation (skin bronzing), and panhypopituitarism.

Testing

The most appropriate screening test for hemochromatosis is fasting serum transferrin saturation. Some guidelines suggest diagnosis when the value is >60% in men or >50% in women, and others suggest >55% for all patients. *C282Y* homozygous or *C282Y/H63D* compound heterozygous *HFE* genotypes are diagnostic of hemochromatosis.

DON'T BE TRICKED

- Advanced liver disease commonly causes an elevated ferritin level, but the iron saturation is usually normal.
- A nondiagnostic *HFE* genotype does not rule out a diagnosis of hemochromatosis.

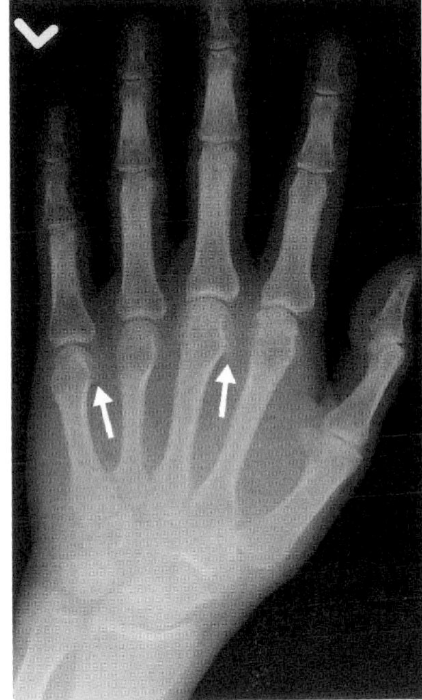

Hemochromatosis: These hook-like osteophytes are characteristic of hemochromatosis.

Treatment

Patients who are *C282Y* homozygous but have normal serum ferritin levels can be monitored without treatment.

Patients with an elevated ferritin level should be treated with phlebotomy.

Family Screening

First-degree relatives of patients with hemochromatosis should undergo screening.

Follow-Up Surveillance

Patients with cirrhosis caused by hereditary hemochromatosis are at increased risk for HCC. Screen for HCC with ultrasonography in patients with cirrhosis every 6 months.

TEST YOURSELF

A 68-year-old man has increasing pain in the second and third MCP joints of both hands. Medical history is significant for type 2 diabetes mellitus and HF.

ANSWER: For diagnosis, select hemochromatosis. For management, order transferrin saturation and serum ferritin measurement.

Nonalcoholic Fatty Liver Disease

Diagnosis

NAFLD is the most common cause of abnormal liver test results. Most patients have insulin resistance, obesity, hypertriglyceridemia, and type 2 diabetes mellitus.

Approximately 20% of patients with NAFLD have nonalcoholic steatohepatitis (NASH), characterized by hepatic steatosis, inflammation, and often fibrosis.

A presumptive diagnosis of NASH can be made in a patient with:

- mild elevations of aminotransferase levels
- risk factors for NAFLD (diabetes, obesity, and hyperlipidemia)
- hyperechoic pattern on ultrasonography or low-density parenchyma on CT

Liver biopsy is indicated when the diagnosis is in doubt.

Treatment

Treatment for NAFLD consists of controlling diabetes, obesity, and hyperlipidemia.

DON'T BE TRICKED

- Patients with fatty liver disease and elevated aminotransferase levels can be treated with statin therapy.

TEST YOURSELF

A 38-year-old woman with type 2 diabetes mellitus develops elevated aminotransferase levels. She is obese. She does not use alcohol excessively. Serum AST is 134 U/L and ALT is 147 U/L. Abdominal ultrasonography shows increased echogenicity of the liver.

ANSWER: For diagnosis, choose NASH.

Primary Biliary Cholangitis

Diagnosis

Primary biliary cholangitis (previously primary biliary cirrhosis) is a chronic progressive autoimmune cholestatic liver disease that occurs predominantly in women aged 40 to 60 years.

Characteristic findings are pruritus, fatigue, weight loss, hyperpigmentation, and/or complications of portal hypertension.

Approximately 50% of patients are asymptomatic.

The diagnostic triad associated with primary biliary cholangitis includes:

- a cholestatic liver profile
- positive antimitochondrial antibody titer
- granulomatous inflammation centered on the septal bile duct

Patients with primary biliary cholangitis may have fat-soluble vitamin deficiencies and osteoporosis or osteomalacia.

Testing

Biliary ultrasonography is required to exclude extrahepatic bile duct obstruction.

Treatment

Ursodeoxycholic acid is the primary therapeutic agent.

Primary Sclerosing Cholangitis

Diagnosis

PSC is a chronic cholestatic liver disease of unknown cause characterized by progressive bile duct destruction and biliary cirrhosis. Eighty percent of patients have an IBD (most often ulcerative colitis). Characteristic findings are:

- pruritus or jaundice
- elevated serum alkaline phosphatase level
- elevated total bilirubin level
- modestly elevated AST and ALT levels

Testing

Abdominal ultrasonography is often the initial diagnostic study.

If intrahepatic biliary dilation is seen, MRCP or ERCP establishes the diagnosis (look for the "string of beads" pattern).

Follow-Up Surveillance

Patients with PSC are at risk for developing cholangiocarcinoma as well as gallbladder carcinoma and colon cancer (when associated with IBD). Screen for colon cancer with colonoscopy every 1-2 years beginning at diagnosis of PSC, regardless of patient age or duration or extent of the IBD.

Annual MRCP and carbohydrate 19-9 level measurement are recommended for cholangiocarcinoma surveillance.

Patients with cirrhosis require screening for HCC with ultrasonography every 6 months.

DON'T BE TRICKED

- **Do not confuse PSC with AIDS cholangiopathy (CD4 cell count <100/µL) caused by CMV or *Cryptosporidium* infection.**

STUDY TABLE: Differentiating Primary Biliary Cholangitis and Primary Sclerosing Cholangitis

	Primary Biliary Cholangitis	Primary Sclerosing Cholangitis
Demographic	Women aged 40-60 years	Men aged 20-30 years
Pathology	Cholestatic liver disease of small bile ducts	Cholestatic liver disease of medium and large bile ducts
Associated conditions	Other autoimmune disease	IBD
Look for...	Positive antimitochondrial antibody titer	"String of beads" on MRCP or ERCP
Treatment	Ursodeoxycholic acid	Endoscopic therapy for extrahepatic dominant strictures Liver transplantation

TEST YOURSELF

A 45-year-old man with a 15-year history of ulcerative colitis develops fatigue and pruritus. Serum alkaline phosphatase level is 750 U/L, AST is 48 U/L, ALT is 60 U/L, and total bilirubin is 2.0 mg/dL.

ANSWER: For diagnosis, choose PSC. For management, select ultrasonography followed by MRCP or ERCP.

Cirrhosis

Diagnosis

Patients with compensated cirrhosis without complications may be asymptomatic or have nonspecific symptoms such as fatigue, poor sleep, or itching.

Patients with **complications of cirrhosis** (hepatic encephalopathy, variceal hemorrhage, ascites, spontaneous bacterial peritonitis, hepatorenal syndrome, jaundice, or HCC) have decompensated cirrhosis.

Portal hypertension is responsible for most of these complications. Portal hypertension also causes splenomegaly and hypersplenism (thrombocytopenia) and loss of hepatic synthetic function (coagulopathy and hypoalbuminemia). Portal hypertension can be divided into prehepatic, intrahepatic, and posthepatic causes. The most common cause of portal hypertension is cirrhosis, an intrahepatic form. Examples of pre- and posthepatic portal hypertension are portal vein thrombosis and Budd-Chiari syndrome, respectively.

STUDY TABLE: Syndromes Associated with Cirrhosis

Syndrome	Comments
Hepatic encephalopathy	Neuropsychiatric syndrome with symptoms ranging from mild cognitive changes to coma
	Measuring plasma ammonia level can be helpful
	Sometimes precipitated by infection, volume depletion, GI bleeding, or sedating medications
Hepatopulmonary syndrome	Dyspnea, hypoxemia increased A-a gradient; may exhibit platypnea (increased dyspnea sitting up and decreased dyspnea lying flat)
	Confirm using transthoracic contrast echocardiography
Portopulmonary hypertension	Pulmonary hypertension with portal hypertension
	Patients should undergo echocardiography
	RV systolic pressure >50 mm Hg requires investigation for causes of pulmonary hypertension.
	Some patients may benefit from liver transplantation.
Hepatorenal syndrome	Diagnostic criteria include: gradual increase in creatinine level to >1.5 mg/dL over days to weeks; lack of response to an albumin challenge of 1 g/kg/d for 2 days; exclusion of other causes of AKI.
	Patients with hepatorenal syndrome not requiring intensive care are treated with midodrine, octreotide, and albumin.
Type 1	More severe, with an increase in serum creatinine of at least 0.3 mg/dL and/or ≥50% from baseline within 48 hours, bland urinalysis, and normal findings on renal ultrasonography
	Lack of improvement in kidney function after withdrawal of diuretics and 2 days of volume expansion with intravenous albumin
	Low urine sodium, low fractional excretion of sodium, and oliguria
	Patients treated in the ICU should receive norepinephrine and albumin.
	Patients who do not respond to medical therapy should undergo liver transplantation.
Type 2	Less severe, with a more gradual decline in kidney function and association with diuretic-refractory ascites.
Hepatic osteodystrophy	Encompasses osteoporosis, osteopenia, and rarely osteomalacia in the context of liver disease.
	Standard evaluation includes calcium, phosphate, and vitamin D levels; DEXA scanning is recommended for patients with cirrhosis or primary biliary cholangitis and before liver transplantation.
	Osteoporosis should be managed with a bisphosphonate (after vitamin D repletion).

Management

To care for patients with cirrhosis, select:

- upper endoscopy for all new patients to evaluate for varices
- ultrasonography to diagnose ascites
- paracentesis for newly discovered ascites and calculation of the serum-ascites albumin gradient (SAAG) to diagnose the cause of ascites
- paracentesis with ascitic fluid granulocyte count and culture for any change in mental status or clinical condition to diagnose spontaneous bacterial peritonitis
- vaccination of nonimmune patients against HAV and HBV as well as other routine vaccinations

STUDY TABLE: Evaluation of Ascites

Ascitic Fluid Protein	SAAG >1.1	SAAG <1.1
<2.5 g/dL	Cirrhosis	Nephrotic syndrome
>2.5 g/dL	Right-sided HF, Budd-Chiari syndrome	Malignancy, TB

Ascitic fluid granulocyte count >250/µL confirms spontaneous bacterial peritonitis.

Follow-Up Surveillance

Patients with cirrhosis should undergo ultrasonography screening for HCC every 6 months.

DON'T BE TRICKED

- Although a plasma ammonia level may be helpful in diagnosing suspected cases of hepatic encephalopathy, monitoring serial ammonia values is not useful.
- Head CT in patients with hepatic encephalopathy and otherwise normal neurologic examination is only warranted with unwitnessed falls or head trauma.
- Use IV, not oral, bisphosphonate therapy in patients with esophageal varices.

Treatment

STUDY TABLE: Treatment of Cirrhosis Complications

Indications	Treatment
Primary prophylaxis of variceal bleeding	First choice: nonselective β-blockers (propranolol, nadolol) or carvedilol (nonselective β-blocker with mild α-1 adrenergic activity) Second choice: endoscopic band ligation if β-blocker not tolerated or contraindicated
Active variceal bleeding	First choice: octreotide with endoscopic band ligation and prophylactic antibiotics such as oral norfloxacin, IV ciprofloxacin, or ceftriaxone Second choice: TIPS or shunt surgery if endoscopic therapy is unsuccessful (portosystemic encephalopathy is primary complication of TIPS)
Transfusion for active bleeding	Hemoglobin transfusion goal of 7 g/dL
Ascites not responding to low-sodium diet	Spironolactone with or without furosemide
Diuretic-refractory ascites	Serial large-volume paracentesis (with albumin if >5 L), TIPS, or liver transplantation
Prevention of spontaneous bacterial peritonitis	Fluoroquinolones chronically if history of spontaneous bacterial peritonitis or otherwise high risk* Fluoroquinolones while hospitalized if ascitic fluid protein <1 g/dL Fluoroquinolones for 7 days if active bleeding
Spontaneous bacterial peritonitis	Cefotaxime and albumin infusion
Acute hepatic encephalopathy	Correct precipitating factors, lactulose; add rifaximin if unresponsive
Prevention of hepatic encephalopathy	Lactulose, titrated to 3 stools per day
Hepatic osteodystrophy	Calcium, vitamin D, and IV bisphosphonate

*High risk = ascitic total protein <1.5 g/dL and any of the following: serum sodium ≤130 mEq/L, creatinine ≥1.2 mg/dL, BUN ≥25 mg/dL, bilirubin ≥3 mg/dL.

Liver transplantation is the definitive treatment for patients with end stage or decompensated liver disease.

DON'T BE TRICKED

- Stop ACE inhibitors, ARBs, and NSAIDs in patients with ascites.
- Blood transfusion to hemoglobin >7.0 g/dL leads to increased portal pressures and risk of further bleeding.
- Antimicrobial prophylaxis should be administered during variceal bleeding even if ascites is absent.
- Do not select prophylactic protein restriction to prevent hepatic encephalopathy.
- Do not select neomycin to treat hepatic encephalopathy because of the significant adverse effects of this drug.

TEST YOURSELF

A 55-year-old man with alcoholic cirrhosis is admitted to the hospital with fever and abdominal pain. Paracentesis is performed. The ascitic fluid granulocyte count is 650/μL and the albumin is <1.0 g/dL.

ANSWER: For diagnosis, choose spontaneous bacterial peritonitis. For management, begin empiric IV cefotaxime and albumin. Do not wait for results of Gram stain or cultures before beginning therapy.

Acute Liver Injury and Acute Liver Failure

Diagnosis

In acute liver *injury*, a sudden increase in serum AST and ALT levels occurs.

Acute liver *failure* refers to acute liver injury complicated by encephalopathy and coagulopathy in patients without previous cirrhosis.

The most common identifiable causes of acute liver injury are acetaminophen hepatotoxicity, idiosyncratic drug reactions, and HBV infection. Other causes include acute HAV infection, hepatic ischemia, herpes infection, mushroom poisoning, Wilson disease. See also Liver Disease Associated with Pregnancy.

Drug-induced liver injury is most commonly caused by acetaminophen, antibiotics (particularly amoxicillin-clavulanate) and antiepileptic medications (phenytoin and valproate).

STUDY TABLE: Differential Diagnosis of Acute Liver Failure

If you see this...	Look for this...	And choose this...
Sudden elevation of serum AST and ALT levels up to 20×	Acetaminophen overdose, which is the most common cause of acute liver failure Acute liver failure is usually caused by acetaminophen ingestion >4 g but can occur with lower doses in patients with alcoholism.	Measure serum acetaminophen level and use nomogram to determine if *N*-acetylcysteine is indicated.
Outbreaks of acute liver failure associated with foods such as raspberries and scallions	Acute HAV infection	Order serologic studies for HAV.
Acute elevation of AST to >1000 U/L while hospitalized	Episode of acute hypotension with associated liver hypoperfusion	Review hospital course.
Acute elevation of liver enzymes and hemolysis in a young patient, Kayser-Fleischer rings, history of psychiatric disorders, and/or athetoid movements	Wilson disease	Measure serum copper and ceruloplasmin levels and urine copper excretion.
Mushroom ingestion	*Amanita* poisoning	Treat with penicillin G or silymarin.
Herpes (simplex or zoster) infection	AST and ALT >5000 U/L in immunocompromised patient or during pregnancy. Often associated with encephalitis. Rash is not always present.	Treat with acyclovir.

Treatment

For patients with acute liver failure, choose:

- immediate contact with liver transplantation center
- chelation with trientine or penicillamine for Wilson disease
- *N*-acetylcysteine for confirmed or suspected acetaminophen poisoning
- penicillin G or silymarin for *Amanita* mushroom poisoning
- arteriovenous hemofiltration to support kidney function
- lactulose for any degree of encephalopathy

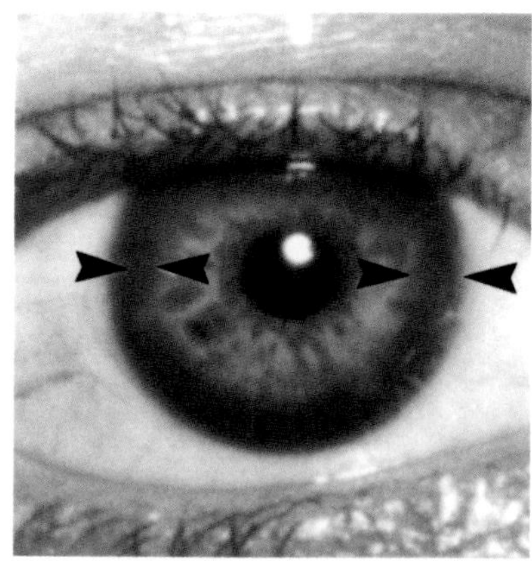

Kayser-Fleischer Ring: A Kayser-Fleischer ring in the cornea is bracketed with arrows.

DON'T BE TRICKED

- **Head CT should be performed in patients with acute liver failure and altered mental status to rule out intracranial hemorrhage.**

TEST YOURSELF

A 24-year-old man has a 1-week history of nausea, jaundice, fatigue, and recent confusion. He is lethargic and confused. The INR is 2.3, serum AST is 940 U/L, and total bilirubin is 12.6 mg/dL. HBsAg and IgM anti-HBc are both positive.

ANSWER: For diagnosis, choose acute liver failure secondary to acute hepatitis B infection. For management, contact liver transplantation center.

Liver Disease Associated with Pregnancy

Several liver diseases are uniquely seen in pregnancy; they are outlined in the table below.

STUDY TABLE: Liver Diseases Unique to Pregnancy

Disease	Trimester	Clinical Features	Laboratory Studies	Bilirubin Level	Management
Hyperemesis gravidarum	1st	Severe vomiting	ALT elevated in 50% of patients, may be 20× upper limit of normal	Normal	Hydration
Intrahepatic cholestasis of pregnancy	2nd or 3rd	Pruritus, often intense	ALT normal to 10-fold increase, elevated serum bile acids, alkaline phosphatase	Normal to mildly elevated	Ursodiol
Preeclampsia	3rd	Hypertension, edema, and proteinuria	Mild increase in ALT	Normal	Delivery
HELLP syndrome	3rd	Features of preeclampsia	Hemolysis, elevated ALT, thrombocytopenia	Usually normal	Delivery
AFLP	3rd	Features of preeclampsia, abdominal pain, nausea	ALT 200-1000 U/L, hemolysis, low platelets, encephalopathy, prolonged INR	Normal unless severe	Delivery

DON'T BE TRICKED

- **HELLP syndrome differs from AFLP in that HELLP syndrome is more closely associated with microangiopathic hemolytic anemia and AFLP is more associated with encephalopathy and coagulation abnormalities.**

Gallstones, Acute Cholecystitis, and Cholangitis

Diagnosis

Biliary pain is the most common cause of upper abdominal pain among patients aged >50 years. Biliary colic is characterized by the episodic onset of acute, severe, epigastric or RUQ pain. Episodes generally last 15 minutes to several hours and are often accompanied by nausea and vomiting. Fever, leukocytosis, and elevated liver enzymes indicate acute cholecystitis or obstruction of the common bile duct.

STUDY TABLE: Biliary Disease Syndromes and Mimics

If you see this...	Diagnose this...
Epigastric or RUQ pain, fever, bilirubin <4 mg/dL, normal or minimally elevated AST or ALT, leukocytosis Sonography shows thickened gallbladder wall and the presence of pericholecystic fluid.	Acute cholecystitis
Biliary colic or pancreatitis and no gallstones or bile duct dilation on imaging studies	Biliary crystals (sludge)
RUQ pain, fever, jaundice, or these findings plus shock and mental status changes; bilirubin >4 mg/dL; AST and ALT >1000 U/L	Acute cholangitis
Critically ill, febrile, or septic patient No gallstones on sonogram, but findings otherwise compatible with acute cholecystitis	Acute acalculous cholecystitis

(Continued on the next page)

STUDY TABLE: Biliary Disease Syndromes and Mimics *(Continued)*	
If you see this...	**Diagnose this...**
Transient elevation of AST or ALT up to 1000 U/L, and cholangitis, or pancreatitis	Passage of common bile duct stone
Midepigastric pain radiating to the back, nausea, vomiting, elevated amylase and lipase	Acute pancreatitis
Recent significant alcohol intake, RUQ pain, fever, jaundice, AST 2-3 × greater than ALT, bilirubin >4 mg/dL	Acute alcoholic hepatitis
RUQ pain, pelvic adnexal tenderness, leukocytosis, cervical smear showing gonococci	Fitz-Hugh-Curtis syndrome (gonococcal or chlamydial perihepatitis)
Impacted gallstone in cystic duct, jaundice, and dilated common hepatic duct caused by extrinsic compression	Mirizzi syndrome
Biliary colic or cholecystitis with small-bowel obstruction and air in biliary tree	Cholecystenteric fistula (gallstone ileus)
RUQ pain, diarrhea, and obstructive jaundice in advanced HIV	AIDS cholangiopathy (*Cryptosporidium* infection)

Testing

Ultrasonography is the initial imaging modality. Dilation of the cystic or biliary duct indicates an obstructing stone. In patients with cholecystitis, ultrasonography will show pericholecystic fluid and a thickened gallbladder wall.

If ultrasonography is nondiagnostic, perform cholescintigraphy (e.g., HIDA scan). Nonvisualization of the gallbladder suggests cystic duct obstruction and cholecystitis.

Cholangitis is potentially life threatening; common bile duct stones should be urgently removed with ERCP.

DON'T BE TRICKED

- HIDA scans can be falsely positive in patients with intrinsic liver disease and elevated serum bilirubin levels.

Treatment

STUDY TABLE: Treatment for Biliary Colic, Cholecystitis, and Acute Cholangitis	
Diagnosis	**Treatment**
Biliary colic	NSAIDs to decrease risk of progression to acute cholecystitis Elective cholecystectomy if gallstones are demonstrated on imaging
Acute cholecystitis	β-lactam/β-lactamase inhibitor or a third-generation cephalosporin plus metronidazole Surgery before hospital discharge
Acute cholangitis	Antibiotic therapy same as for acute cholecystitis ERCP removal of common bile duct stones

DON'T BE TRICKED

- Surgery is not indicated for asymptomatic gallstones.
- Immediate cholecystectomy for acute cholangitis is associated with increased mortality; elective cholecystectomy should be performed within 6 weeks to reduce the risk of complications.

TEST YOURSELF

A 27-year-old woman is evaluated because of cholecystitis. The serum direct bilirubin level is 5.8 mg/dL. Abdominal ultrasonography shows gallbladder stones. The intrahepatic ducts are dilated. The distal common bile duct is not dilated and no stones are present.

ANSWER: For diagnosis, choose Mirizzi syndrome.

Upper GI Bleeding

Diagnosis

Four causes account for 80% of UGI bleeding: PUD, esophagogastric varices, esophagitis, and Mallory-Weiss tear.

PUD caused by *Helicobacter pylori* infection or NSAID use is the most common cause of nonvariceal UGI bleeding. Characteristic findings are hematemesis, melena, or (infrequently) bright red blood per rectum or a high serum BUN/creatinine ratio.

Slow and/or chronic bleeding is suggested by iron deficiency and is typical of erosive disease, tumor, esophageal ulcer, portal hypertensive gastropathy, Cameron lesion (erosions found within large hiatal hernias), and angiodysplasia.

STUDY TABLE: Differential Diagnosis of Upper GI Bleeding

If you see this...	Diagnose this...
Dyspepsia, *H. pylori* infection, NSAID use, anticoagulation, severe medical illness	Peptic ulcer disease
Stigmata of chronic liver disease, evidence of portal hypertension or risk factors for cirrhosis (alcohol use, viral hepatitis)	Variceal bleeding
History of heavy alcohol use and retching before hematemesis, hematemesis following weight lifting, young woman with bulimia	Mallory-Weiss tear
Heartburn, regurgitation, and dysphagia; usually small-volume or occult bleeding	Esophagitis
Progressive dysphagia, weight loss, early satiety, or abdominal pain; usually small-volume or occult bleeding	Esophageal or gastric cancer
NSAID use, heavy alcohol intake, severe medical illness; usually small-volume or occult bleeding	Gastroduodenal erosions

DON'T BE TRICKED

- Do not order a barium x-ray because this will interfere with subsequent upper endoscopy or other studies.

Treatment

Risk-stratification tools guide decisions regarding urgent upper endoscopy (within 12 hours), hospital admission and nonurgent upper endoscopy (within 24 hours), and discharge home from the emergency department. The Glasgow-Blatchford score (range 0-23) is particularly useful when the score is 0, which has a nearly 100% negative predictive value for severe GI bleeding and the need for hospital-based intervention.

Pre-endoscopic management:

- insertion of large-caliber intravenous or central venous catheter
- IV crystalloids targeting HR <100/min, SBP >100 mm Hg, and no orthostasis
- blood transfusion for hemodynamic instability to a target hemoglobin level of 7 g/dL
- PPI therapy (stop if no ulcer found on upper endoscopy)
- Vitamin K or 4f-PCC for supratherapeutic INR
- octreotide and antibiotics before upper endoscopy for suspected variceal bleeding
- aspirin discontinuation if being used for primary prevention, continue if used for secondary prevention

Upper endoscopy evaluation and treatment:

- upper endoscopy within 24 hours; within 12 hours for suspected variceal bleed
- low-risk ulcers are clean-based or have a nonprotuberant pigmented spot; treat low-risk ulcers with oral PPI, begin food, early hospital discharge (12-24 hours)
- high-risk ulcers have active arterial spurting or a nonbleeding visible vessel; treat high-risk ulcers endoscopically (hemoclips, thermal therapy, or injection therapy) and continuous IV PPI infusion for 72 hours
- repeat endoscopic therapy for continued bleeding
- surgery or interventional radiology if endoscopic therapy is unsuccessful

Postendoscopic care:

- test for *H. pylori* and treat if positive; retest if initial test was negative
- provide long-term, daily PPI therapy for patients who must use aspirin and other antiplatelet drugs, NSAIDs, anticoagulants, or glucocorticoids
- see General Internal Medicine section for information on reinitiation of anticoagulation

DON'T BE TRICKED

- **H_2-receptor antagonists are not beneficial in managing UGI bleeding.**
- **Do not select nasogastric tube placement for diagnosis, prognosis, visualization, or therapeutic effect.**
- **Second-look upper endoscopy is not recommended except for rebleeding.**

Lower GI Bleeding

Diagnosis

Acute, painless LGI bleeding in older adult patients is usually caused by colonic diverticula or angiodysplasia.

STUDY TABLE: Differential Diagnosis of Lower GI Bleeding

If you see this...	Diagnose this...
Painless, self-limited, massive hematochezia	Diverticular bleeding (most common overall cause)
Chronic blood loss or acute painless hematochezia in an older adult patient	Colonic tumor, polyp or angiodysplasia
Recent colonic polypectomy	Postpolypectomy bleeding
Evidence of vascular disease in an older adult patient; typically with LLQ abdominal pain	Ischemic colitis
Aortic stenosis	Angiodysplasia (Heyde syndrome)
History of bloody diarrhea, tenesmus, abdominal pain, fever	IBD
Aortic aneurysm repair	Aortoenteric fistula (UGI bleeding most common)
Painless hematochezia in a young patient and normal upper endoscopy and colonoscopy	Meckel diverticulum
Mucocutaneous telangiectasias	Hereditary hemorrhagic telangiectasia

Treatment

Consider outpatient follow-up or early discharge with:

- patient age <60 years
- no hemodynamic instability
- no evidence of gross rectal bleeding
- identification of an obvious anorectal source of bleeding

If the patient is hemodynamically unstable, provide resuscitation before diagnostic studies are performed.

According to expert opinion, the blood transfusion threshold for patients with colonic bleeding is a hemoglobin value <9 g/dL (note this is different than the evidence-based threshold for UGI bleeding).

Most episodes of LGI bleeding resolve spontaneously. Colonoscopy is recommended early, usually within the first 48 hours of admission, and endoscopic therapy is used to control continued bleeding.

If colonoscopy does not identify a discrete lesion or endoscopic therapy does not control the bleeding, interventional angiography or surgery may be indicated.

Patients with angiodysplasia in the setting of AS (Heyde syndrome) may benefit from valve replacement surgery.

DON'T BE TRICKED

- Ten percent of rapid rectal bleeding has a UGI source.

Bleeding of Obscure Origin

Diagnosis

Obscure GI bleeding is recurrent blood loss without an identified source of bleeding despite upper endoscopy and colonoscopy.

Patients aged ≤50 years are more likely to have tumors (adenocarcinoma, carcinoid, leiomyomas, or lymphoma), Dieulafoy lesion, or Crohn disease.

Older patients are more likely to have vascular lesions, such as angiodysplasia. Angiodysplasia is the most common cause of obscure GI bleeding overall (40% of all cases). Patients may present with either melena or hematochezia or positive FOBT.

The first step is to repeat upper endoscopy and/or colonoscopy, which is diagnostic in approximately 25% of patients.

Testing

For patients with obscure **active** GI bleeding:

- perform nuclear studies (technetium 99m-labeled erythrocyte or sulfur colloid nuclear scan) first, followed by angiography
- if unrevealing, consider push enteroscopy or balloon-assisted enteroscopy (deep enteroscopy)
- surgery and intraoperative enteroscopy is a last diagnostic option

For patients with occult GI bleeding:

- perform capsule endoscopy (first choice) or deep enteroscopy
- if unrevealing, repeat endoscopic examinations (upper endoscopy, colonoscopy, capsule endoscopy), or deep enteroscopy

DON'T BE TRICKED

- Do not order small bowel follow-through x-ray as a first-line study in the evaluation of obscure GI bleeding.
- Do not use capsule endoscopy in the setting of obstruction or strictures (severe Crohn disease).

General Internal Medicine

Biostatistics

Sensitivity, Specificity, Predictive Values, Likelihood Ratios and ROC Curves

Sensitivity is the ability of a test to detect a disease when it is truly present. **Specificity** is the ability of a test to exclude disease when it is truly absent.

An ROC curve is a graph of the sensitivity vs. (1 − specificity). In medicine, an ROC analysis helps select tests with optimal performance characteristics. The cut-point with the best combined sensitivity and specificity will be closest to the upper left corner of the graph. When comparing two or more tests, the test with the greatest overall accuracy will have the largest area under the ROC graph.

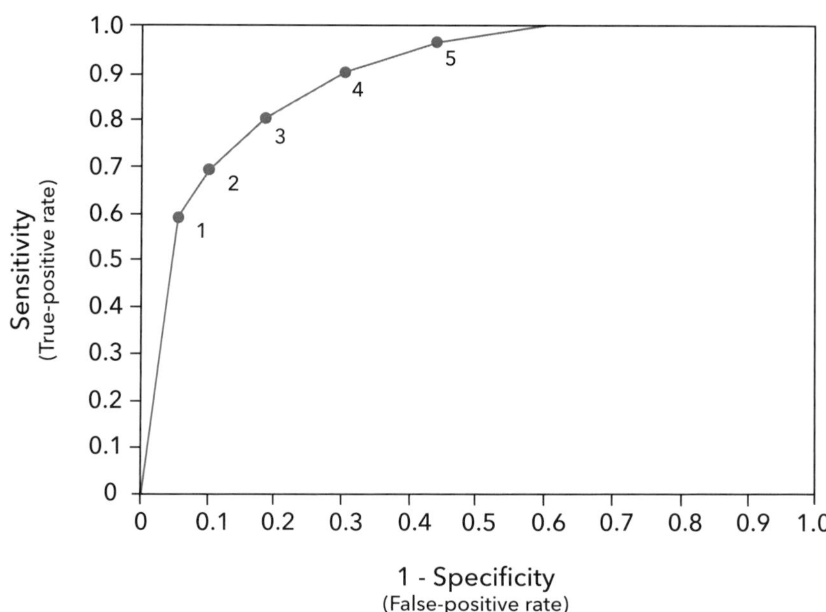

Receiver Operating Characteristic Curve: ROC curve showing sensitivity (true-positive rate) vs. (1 − specificity) (false-positive rate).

DON'T BE TRICKED

- As the prevalence of a condition increases, the positive predictive value increases and the negative predictive value decreases.
- Changes in prevalence do not alter the sensitivity or specificity but do alter the predictive values.

A **likelihood ratio (LR)** is a measurement of the odds of having a disease independent of the disease prevalence. Separate LRs are calculated for use when a test result is positive (LR+) or negative (LR−):

- LR+ = Sensitivity/(1 − Specificity)
- LR− = (1 − Sensitivity)/Specificity
- LR+ of 2, 5, and 10 increase the probability of disease by approximately 15%, 30%, and 45%, respectively.
- LR− of 0.5, 0.2, and 0.1 decrease the probability of disease by approximately 15%, 30%, and 45%, respectively.

Study Designs

STUDY TABLE: Characteristics of Study Designs

Type	Characteristics
Cross-section	The presence of the presumed risk factor and presence of the outcome are measured at one point in time in a population.
Retrospective (case control)	Subjects are divided into groups based on the presence or absence of the outcome of interest, and then the frequency of risk factors in each group is compared.
Prospective (cohort)	Subjects are divided into groups based on the presence or absence of the presumed risk factor and followed for a period of time. At the end of the study, the frequency of the outcome is compared.
Randomized controlled trial	Subjects are randomly divided into groups; one group receives the intervention (patients and researchers may be blinded to treatment, termed *double-blind*) and followed forward in time. At the end of the study, the frequency of the outcome is compared. This study design reduces the effect of unmeasured (confounding) variables that may influence outcomes of a study.
Systematic review with meta-analysis	Usually, multiple clinical trials using similar randomization techniques and interventions can be combined into one large analysis to address very precise clinical questions. The results may be analyzed using the technique of meta-analysis, in which all trial results are combined to create a single point estimate.

STUDY TABLE: Strength of Research Designs in Descending Order (Strongest to Weakest)

Description
RCT including systematic reviews of RCTs
RCT without randomization
Case-control or cohort study
Evidence using many points in time, with or without intervention
Evidence based on experience, descriptive studies, or expert opinion

Risk Estimates

STUDY TABLE: Common Calculations Used in Clinical Research

Term	Definition	Calculation	Notes
Absolute risk (AR)	The probability of an event occurring in a group during a specified time period	AR = patients with event in group / total patients in group	Also known as *event rate*. Often, an experimental event rate (EER) is compared with a control even rate (CER)
Relative risk (RR)	The ratio of the probability of developing a disease with a risk factor present to the probability of developing the disease without the risk factor present	RR = EER / CER	Used in cohort studies and RCTs

(Continued on the next page)

STUDY TABLE: Common Calculations Used in Clinical Research *(Continued)*			
Term	**Definition**	**Calculation**	**Notes**
Absolute risk reduction (ARR)	The *absolute difference* in rates of events between experimental group and control group	ARR = | EER − CER |	Critical to understanding number needed to treat (below)
Relative risk reduction (RRR)	The *ratio* of ARR to the event rate among controls	RRR = | EER − CER | / CER	For very infrequent events, RR can be large while AR is small
Number needed to treat (NNT)	Number of patients needed to receive a treatment for one additional patient to benefit	NNT = 1 / ARR	A good estimate of the effect size in easy-to-understand terms for patients
Number needed to harm (NNH)	Number of patients needed to receive a treatment for one additional patient to be harmed	NNH = 1 / ARR	

An **odds ratio (OR)** estimates the odds of having or not having a particular outcome. When comparing therapeutic outcomes, in most cases OR can be substituted for RR as an equivalent measurement.

AR, RR, and OR are estimates of the cumulative risk over time, usually defined at the end of the study period.

DON'T BE TRICKED

- **A disadvantage of RR is the potential for exaggeration. For example, interventions that reduce the rate of a disease from 40% to 20% and 4% to 2% each have a RR reduction of 50%, but the ARR for the first case is 20% and the ARR for the second case is only 2%. Based on the ARR, the NNT can be calculated. In the first case the NNT is 5 (1/0.2), whereas the NNT for the second case is 50 (1/0.02).**

Confidence Interval

CI provides boundaries within which exists a high probability (95% by convention) of finding the "true" value. For example, if the measured mean difference between two groups is 2.4, and the 95% CI is 1.9 to 3.0, the probability that the true value lies between 1.9 and 3.0 is 95%.

When used in association with RR, if the CI includes the number 1, no risk or benefit exists; the outcomes for the control and experimental groups are the same.

P Values, Type I and Type II Errors in Clinical Research

The *P* value indicates the likelihood of the study result being caused by chance alone. A *P* value of less than 0.05 represents a 1 in 20 chance of obtaining the observed results by chance.

A type I error is incorrectly concluding that a statistically significant difference exists between the experimental and control groups. If the study's *P* value is <0.05, then a <5% chance exists that a type I error has occurred. **A type II error** is incorrectly concluding no difference exists between the experimental and control groups. Studies with small numbers of subjects may not have the statistical "power" to detect true differences between groups and may be subject to type II errors.

DON'T BE TRICKED

- **Do not confuse statistical significance with clinical importance; a study that reports statistically significant *P* values may not be clinically relevant if the effect size is small (absolute difference between outcomes is small).**

TEST YOURSELF

A 19-year-old woman with RLQ abdominal pain and fever has an estimated pretest probability of acute appendicitis of 50%. An appendiceal CT scan shows inflammation and a thickened appendiceal wall. This finding is associated with an LR+ of 13.3 for acute appendicitis. What is the posttest likelihood of acute appendicitis?

ANSWER: >95% (50% plus 45% = 95%). The key to this question is remembering that an LR+ of 10 increases the posttest likelihood of the diagnosis by 45%.

The mortality rate after cardiogenic shock managed with standard care is 72%, but the rate for patients receiving a new medication is 67%. How many patients with cardiogenic shock must be treated with the new medication to save one life?

ANSWER: The NNT is [1/(0.72 − 0.67)] = 1/0.05 = 20.

Screening and Prevention

STUDY TABLE: Summary of Vaccination Recommendations for Adults 19 Years or Older

Disease	Vaccine Type	ACIP Recommendation
Influenza	Live attenuated, inactivated, recombinant	One dose annually (for all persons ≥18 y), including pregnant women and those with HIV infection
Tetanus, diphtheria, and pertussis	Inactivated	One dose Tdap, then Td booster every 10 y for all adults; one dose Tdap each pregnancy between 27 to 36 weeks' gestation
Varicella	Live attenuated	For all immunocompetent persons lacking immunity
Herpes zoster	Recombinant	All nonimmunocompromised persons age ≥50 y, including those previously vaccinated with the inactivated vaccine
Pneumococcal	Inactivated	See Pneumococcal Immunization table, below
HPV	Inactivated	Women aged 19-26 y; men aged 11-21 y; men aged 22-26 y who are immunocompromised or who have sex with other men
MMR	Live attenuated	Adults born in 1957 or later without evidence of vaccination or immunity
Meningococcal (MenACWY)	Inactivated	First-year college students residing in dormitories, travelers to endemic areas, military recruits, and exposed persons; asplenia or complement deficiencies; boost every 5 y if risk remains
Hepatitis A	Inactivated	Any adult requesting immunization and those at high risk
Hepatitis B	Inactivated	Any adult requesting immunization and those at high risk

ACIP = Advisory Committee on Immunization Practices.

DON'T BE TRICKED

- **For pregnant women, do not select live vaccines, including MMR, intranasal influenza, yellow fever, varicella, and zoster vaccines.**
- **All available influenza vaccines are safe in egg-allergic patients.**

STUDY TABLE: Pneumococcal Immunization

Risk Group	PCV13	PPSV23	
	Recommended	**Recommended**	**Revaccination with PPSV23 at 5 years after first dose**
Immunocompetent adults age ≥65 y	Yes	Yes, 1 year after PCV13	Only if originally immunized before age 65 y
Immunocompetent persons with chronic heart, lung, or liver disease, diabetes mellitus, alcoholism, cigarette smoking	No	Yes	Only if originally immunized before age 65 y
Persons with functional (sickle cell disease, hemoglobinopathies) or anatomic asplenia	Yes	Yes	Yes
Immunocompromised persons with HIV, chronic kidney disease, nephrotic syndrome, leukemia, lymphoma, Hodgkin disease, multiple myeloma, generalized malignancy, taking immunosuppressant drugs, congenital immunodeficiencies, solid organ transplant	Yes	Yes	Yes
CSF leaks or cochlear implants	Yes	Yes	No

Aspirin and Prevention

Aspirin is recommended for primary prevention of ASCVD and colon cancer if all the following apply:

- adults aged 50-59 years
- 10-year CVD risk ≥10%
- life expectancy ≥10 years
- no increased risk for bleeding
- willing to take low-dose aspirin daily ≥10 years

STUDY TABLE: USPSTF-Recommended Screening

Condition	Screening Recommendation
Chronic Diseases	
Abdominal aortic aneurysm	One-time abdominal ultrasonography in all men ages 65-75 y who have ever smoked; selectively screen men ages 65-75 y who have never smoked
Depression	All adults, when staff-assisted depression care support is available
Diabetes mellitus	Ages 40-70 y who are overweight or obese as part of risk assessment for cardiovascular disease
Hypertension	All adults; obtain measurements outside of the clinical setting for diagnostic confirmation before starting treatment
Lipid disorders	Universal lipid screening in adults aged 40-75 y as part of risk assessment for cardiovascular disease
Obesity	All adults
Osteoporosis	Women age ≥65 y; postmenopausal women <65 y of age when 10-year fracture risk is ≥9.3%
Infectious Diseases	
Chlamydia and gonorrhea	All sexually active women age ≤24 y; all sexually active older women at increased risk of infection
HCV	One-time screening for adults born from 1945-1965; all adults at high risk
HIV infection	One-time screening for all adults ages 15-65 y; at least annually for adults at high risk
Substance Abuse	
Alcohol misuse	All adults
Tobacco use	All adults
Cancer	
Breast cancer	Biennial screening mammography for women ages 50-74 y; initiation of screening before age 50 y should be individualized
Cervical cancer	Women aged 21-65 y with cytology (Pap smear) every 3 y; in women aged 30-65 y who want to lengthen screening, screen with high-risk HPV testing (preferred) or cytology and high-risk HPV testing every 5 y Do not screen women following hysterectomy and cervix removal for benign disease.
Colon cancer	All adults aged 50-75 y[a]. USPSTF recommendations do not support one form of screening test over another for detecting early stage colorectal cancer in average-risk patients. Available tests include stool-based, direct visualization, and serology tests (see Study Table on screening intervals for average-risk patients).
Lung cancer	Annual low-dose CT scan in high-risk patients (adults ages 55-80 y with a 30-pack-year smoking history, including former smokers who have quit in the last 15 y)
Prostate cancer	Men aged 55-69 y should make an informed decision about prostate cancer screening with their clinician. Routine screening for men ≥70 y is recommended against.

[a]In contrast, the American Cancer Society makes a qualified recommendation to initiate screening for colorectal cancer at age 45 years.

STUDY TABLE: USPSTF Colon Cancer Screening Intervals for Average-Risk Patients	
Method	**Interval**
Guaiac fecal occult blood test (FOBT)	Annually
Fecal immunochemical test (FIT)	Annually
Flexible sigmoidoscopy	Every 5 years
Flexible sigmoidoscopy	Every 10 years when combined with annual FIT (not FOBT)
Colonoscopy	Every 10 years
CT colonography	Every 5 years

Smoking Cessation

Smoking cessation reduces all-cause mortality by up to 50%; when it appears as a potential answer to a test question, it is almost always correct.

Treatment

The Five A's and the Five R's are two motivational interviewing techniques to use when counseling for behavior change, including smoking cessation, at-risk drinking, and other substance abuse.

STUDY TABLE: Behavioral Interventions	
Five A's	**Five R's**
Ask about tobacco use.	Encourage patient to think of **R**elevance of quitting smoking to their lives.
Advise to quit.	Assist patient in identifying the **R**isks of smoking.
Assess willingness to quit.	Assist the patient in identifying the **R**ewards of smoking cessation.
Assist in attempt to quit.	Discuss with the patient **R**oadblocks or barriers to attempting cessation.
Arrange follow-up.	**R**epeat the motivational intervention at all visits.

STUDY TABLE: Pharmacologic Treatments for Smoking Cessation	
Agent	**Notes**
Nicotine gum, patch, spray, inhaler, lozenges	Increases smoking cessation 1.5 times more than control. Avoid with recent MI, arrhythmia, and unstable angina.
Bupropion	Increases smoking cessation rates about 2 times more than control. Avoid with seizure disorder and eating disorder. May be associated with suicidal ideation. Safety in pregnancy is unclear.
Varenicline	Increases smoking cessation rates about 3.5 times more than control and almost 2 times more than bupropion.

Combination therapy is more effective than monotherapy.

- Behavioral intervention and pharmacotherapy are more effective than either therapy used alone.
- Bupropion and varenicline can be used with long-acting (nicotine patches) or short-acting (nicotine gum, lozenges, inhalers, nasal spray) nicotine replacement.
- Combination nicotine replacement therapy (long- and short-acting nicotine replacement) is more effective than nicotine monotherapy.

DON'T BE TRICKED

- **SSRIs show no significant benefit for smoking cessation.**
- **E-cigarettes are not approved by the FDA for smoking cessation.**

Alcohol Use Disorder

Screening

Ask all patients about their level of alcohol consumption and follow up with screening tests for patients with "at-risk drinking." Patients with AUDIT-C scores >6 or a CAGE questionnaire score >1 are candidates for further evaluation and intervention.

Diagnosis

Look for alcoholism in patients with selected conditions, including repeated trauma, hypertension, AF, HF, pancreatitis, alcoholic hepatitis, and cirrhosis. Laboratory clues such as an elevated MCV, γ-glutamyltransferase level, and AST-ALT ratio >2 are suggestive but not diagnostic.

STUDY TABLE: Categories and Patterns of Alcohol Use

Categories	Patterns
At-risk drinking	Men: >14 drinks per week or >4 drinks per occasion Women and adults age ≥65 y: >7 drinks per week or >3 drinks per occasion
Alcohol use disorder	Alcohol use leading to significant impairment or distress, as manifested by multiple psychosocial, behavioral, or physiologic features

In patients undergoing alcohol withdrawal, look for:

- tremor, anxiety, diaphoresis, and palpitations 6 to 36 hours after the last drink
- visual, auditory, and tactile hallucinations 12 to 48 hours after the last drink
- generalized tonic-clonic seizure within 6 to 24 hours after the last drink
- delirium tremens (hallucinations, delirium, agitation, fever, palpitations, and hypertension) 48 to 96 hours after the last drink

DON'T BE TRICKED

- **Alcohol misuse screening begins with quantifying the amount of alcohol consumed, not CAGE or AUDIT-C questions.**
- **Multiple seizures (>1) are not consistent with alcohol withdrawal syndrome and should prompt an evaluation for another disorder.**

Treatment

For management of alcohol use disorder, the USPSTF recommends referral for specialty treatment.

For at-risk drinking, brief behavioral counseling (such as the five A's and the five R's, listed previously) may be useful.

Use naltrexone to prevent relapse of alcohol abuse and dependence and in patients who are actively drinking. Naltrexone is contraindicated in patients receiving or withdrawing from any opioid and in those with liver failure or hepatitis. Acamprosate enhances abstinence but is contraindicated in kidney disease. Disulfiram, second-line treatment, leads to the accumulation of acetaldehyde if alcohol is consumed, resulting in flushing, headache, emesis, and the need to avoid all additional alcohol-containing items.

Hospitalize patients with moderate to severe alcohol withdrawal or another compelling need for hospitalization.

Long-acting benzodiazepines are indicated for hospitalized patients:

- with previous alcohol-related seizures or delirium tremens
- with significant withdrawal symptoms
- who are pregnant
- with acute medical or surgical illnesses

Use a symptom-triggered regimen to treat alcohol withdrawal. Adjunctive therapy with β-blockers and clonidine may help control tachycardia and hypertension but are not used as monotherapy.

DON'T BE TRICKED

- Give thiamine replacement before administering glucose.
- Do not prescribe antipsychotic medications because these agents lower the seizure threshold.
- No evidence supports that continuous infusion therapy with short-acting benzodiazepines provides better outcomes than oral therapy for acute alcohol withdrawal.
- Not all heavy drinkers who stop abruptly experience withdrawal, and treatment with benzodiazepines is not always needed.

TEST YOURSELF

A 36-year-old man with a history of heavy alcohol use is evaluated within 24 hours of his last drink. BP is 172/98 mm Hg, and pulse rate is 120/min. He is tremulous and having visual hallucinations.

ANSWER: For diagnosis, choose alcohol withdrawal syndrome. For management, select hospitalization and treatment with symptom-triggered benzodiazepines.

Opioid Use Disorder

Prescription opioids are a major cause of morbidity and mortality. The risk for overdose is increased with higher doses (>50 morphine mg equivalents/d) and concurrent benzodiazepine prescription. Nonmedical use of prescription opioids is a strong risk factor for heroin use.

Treatment

Most patients with opioid use disorder will require psychosocial support and medication-assisted treatment (buprenorphine-naloxone, buprenorphine, IM naltrexone). Intranasal naloxone is an important adjunct therapy in opioid use disorder. Friends and family members may also receive prescriptions and training in naloxone use.

Intimate Partner Violence

Screening

USPSTF recommends screening for intimate partner violence (IPV) in women of childbearing age (14-46 years). Screening tool examples:

- HITS = Hurt, Insult, Threaten, Scream
- STaT = Slapped, Threatened, and Thrown
- HARK = Humiliation, Afraid, Rape, Kick

Diagnosis

Characteristic findings:

- exacerbations or poor control of chronic medical conditions
- seeming nonadherence to medications
- chronic abdominal pain
- sleep or appetite disturbances, fatigue, reduced concentration
- depression, anxiety, acute or posttraumatic stress, somatization, and eating disorders
- suicide attempts and substance abuse
- frequent appointment changes

- STIs, HIV, unplanned pregnancies
- visible bruises or injuries
- partner unwilling to leave during examination

Assess the risk of homicide, suicide, or serious injury. Inquire about:

- escalating threats or abuse and escalating level of fear
- stalking
- weapons, especially firearms, in the home
- sexual assault and abuse during pregnancy
- recent separation or abuser's awareness of impending separation

Treatment

Initiate safety planning. Determine if the patient wants to leave home, return home, or have the abuser removed from his or her household. Refer the patient to a domestic violence advocate.

Patient Safety

Diagnostic Errors

Reasoning errors can lead to diagnostic errors.

STUDY TABLE: Reasoning Errors

Heuristic	Definition
Availability	Clinician has encountered a similar presentation and jumps to the conclusion that the current diagnosis must be the same as the previous
Anchoring	Clinician accepts at face value a previous diagnosis made by another clinician
Blind obedience	Acceptance of a diagnosis or plan made by another of higher authority
Premature closure	Full differential diagnosis is not considered

Error Analysis

Root-cause analysis is an exercise used to determine the contributors to an adverse event. Often, a cause-effect "fishbone" diagram is used to illustrate causation, beginning with a problem or error at the fish's head. Working back down the spine, the team is asked repetitively, "And what contributed to this?" This continues until as many prime factors as possible are identified.

Quality Improvement

A common methodology to improve quality is the Plan-Do-Study-Act (PDSA) cycle. The clinician might *plan* a test of quality improvement, *do* the test by trying the new protocol on a limited number of patients, *study* the results, and *act* by refining the protocol based on what was learned and planning the next test.

Patient Handoffs

The best practice for handoff includes person-to-person communication, providing an opportunity to ask and respond to questions, and providing information that is accurate and concise (including name, location, history, diagnoses, severity of illness, medication and problem lists, status, recent procedures, a "to-do" list that has "if/then" statements, and contingency plans).

Medical Ethics and Professionalism

Patient Privacy

With the advent of the HIPAA regulations, patients must have control over who has access to their personal health information. The preservation of confidentiality is not absolute. Safeguarding the individual or public from harm or honoring the law prevails over protecting confidentiality. It is important to understand state-specific confidentiality laws regarding adolescents. Some states specifically protect adolescent confidentiality for reproductive health.

TEST YOURSELF

A 78-year-old man is admitted with GI bleeding. Colonoscopy reveals metastatic colon cancer. His daughter wishes to know the results of the colonoscopy.

ANSWER: The information cannot be released unless approved by the patient.

Advance Planning

In advance care planning, the patient articulates and documents his or her values, goals, and preferences for future health care. Advance care planning includes an advance directive, which contains written instructions for health care used in the event that the patient loses decision-making capacity.

Advance directives include:

- the living will, in which the patient lists preferences regarding specific treatments and pain control preferences during terminal illness
- the health care power of attorney, in which the patient designates a surrogate decision-maker
- the combined advance directive, which has features of both a living will and a health care power of attorney

DON'T BE TRICKED

- **The surrogate named by the patient in his or her advance directive is the legal decision-maker regardless of the surrogate's relationship with the patient.**
- **If a surrogate is not specifically named and the patient is incapacitated, then the order of decision making is spouse, adult child, parent, adult sibling.**

Decision-Making Capacity

The physician must assess the patient's decision-making abilities to decide whether a surrogate decision-maker should be enlisted. To make their own decisions, patients need a set of values and goals, the ability to communicate and understand information, and the ability to reason and deliberate about options. The core components of decisional capacity are:

1. understanding the situation at hand,
2. understanding the risks and benefits of the decision being made, and
3. being able to communicate the decision.

DON'T BE TRICKED

- **Minors who are not living independently of their parents, not married, or not in the armed forces cannot legally make their own decisions.**
- **Any physician can determine if a patient has decision-making capacity.**

"Competence" is a legal term; only the courts can determine competence. If a patient is incapable of medical decision making, a surrogate decision-maker is identified. Surrogates can use one of two standards for decision making:

- Substituted judgment standard: The surrogate makes the decision that he or she believes the patient would have made.
- Best interests standard: The surrogate selects the medical treatment that he or she personally feels is best for the patient.

TEST YOURSELF

An 82-year-old woman is hospitalized for the fourth time in 12 months. She lives alone and is unable to take her medications properly. She cannot articulate a plan to manage her disease.

ANSWER: Seek guardianship, because the patient cannot describe realistic plans for living at home alone.

Withholding or Withdrawing Treatment

Withdrawing treatment is reasonable if, from the patient's perspective, the expected benefits of treatment no longer outweigh its burdens. Patients who have do-not-resuscitate orders are still eligible to receive other therapeutic life-prolonging or palliative measures.

Physicians are not obligated to administer interventions that are physiologically futile. Physicians may also disagree with a patient's legitimate choice of care if it violates their ethical principles. If consensus about treatment cannot be reached, options include transfer of the patient to another physician and review by a hospital ethics committee. Administration of nutrients and fluids by artificial means is a life-prolonging measure, guided by the same principles for decision making that are applied to other treatments.

Physician-Assisted Death

In physician-assisted suicide, death occurs when the physician provides a means for the patient to terminate his or her life (lethal prescription is legal in some states). In euthanasia, the physician directly terminates the patient's life (for example, by lethal injection). Euthanasia is illegal in all states.

In caring for patients at the end of life, circumstances may occur in which an intervention may unintentionally hasten death (for example, IV narcotic analgesics).

Disclosing Medical Errors

When patients are injured as a consequence of medical care, whether or not error is involved, they should be informed promptly about what has occurred. An apology should be given if it was a result of error or system failure. Data do not support concerns that disclosure of an error promotes litigation.

The Impaired Physician

Physicians are ethically—and in some states, legally—bound to protect patients from impaired colleagues by reporting such physicians to appropriate authorities, including chiefs of service, chiefs of staff, institutional committees, or state medical boards.

Conflict of Interest

A conflict of interest exists when physicians' primary duty to their patients conflicts or appears to conflict with a secondary interest, which may consist of another important professional responsibility, a contractual obligation, or personal gain. Physicians are obligated to avoid significant conflicts of interest whenever possible. For less serious or unavoidable conflicts of interest, disclosure is appropriate.

Palliative Care

Palliative care may be provided concurrently with life-prolonging therapies or with therapies with curative intent. Hospice, on the other hand, is a specialized type of palliative care that is reserved for patients in the terminal phase of their disease, arbitrarily defined as the last 6 months of life.

Acute and Chronic Pain at the End of Life

Pharmacologic management of pain progresses in a stepwise fashion.

- Use acetaminophen, aspirin, or NSAIDs for mild to moderate pain.
- If pain persists or increases, add a low-dose or low-potency opioid (e.g., oxycodone). Avoid "weak" opioids such as codeine and tramadol.
- Increase opioid potency (e.g., morphine) or add higher doses for persistent or moderate to severe pain at onset.
- Add adjuvant agents at any step (tricyclic antidepressants, anticonvulsants).
- Prescribe around-the-clock analgesics for persistent, chronic pain rather than as needed.

STUDY TABLE: Opioids Commonly Used in Palliative Care

Opioid	Comments
Hydrocodone	Variable efficacy Increased time to analgesic onset in liver failure
Hydromorphone	Better choice if kidney disease is present Reduce dose and frequency in liver failure/cirrhosis
Methadone	Low cost, long acting, available as liquid Long but variable half-life, which contributes to the risk of accumulation and toxicity during initiation
Oxycodone	Increased half-life and variable onset in liver failure; if used, reduce dose and frequency
Morphine	Avoid in liver failure/cirrhosis, kidney injury
Fentanyl	Safest long-acting drug in kidney and liver failure Start lower dose patch in liver failure and opioid-naïve patients

Opioids do not have an analgesic efficacy ceiling and can be titrated upward as needed, until limiting side effects appear. Common side effects of opioids include constipation, sedation, nausea, and itching (not from an allergy).

Warnings about opioid use:

- Fentanyl should only be used in opioid-tolerant patients.
- Meperidine is not recommended for pain because of an increased risk of seizure.
- Tramadol has significant drug interactions, especially with other serotonergic medications.
- Methadone should only be initiated and titrated by experts.

In the administration of opioids, oral routes are preferred (do not use IM).

- Sublingual or subcutaneous routes may be used for patients unable to use an oral route.
- Long-acting formulations are no more effective than short-acting formulations.

Neuropathic pain is characterized by burning, tingling, or lancinating pain. Add tricyclic antidepressants, SNRIs (venlafaxine, duloxetine), and antiepileptic medications (gabapentin, pregabalin, carbamazepine) to the pain regimen.

Treat bone pain with anti-inflammatory medications (NSAIDs or glucocorticoids) or bisphosphonates (pamidronate, zoledronate).

All patients receiving scheduled opioids should be taking a scheduled bowel regimen to prevent constipation, in this order:

- stimulant laxative with or without docusate
- osmotic agent (PEG, sorbitol, or lactulose)
- methylnaltrexone

STUDY TABLE: Treatment of Nausea in Palliative Care	
Cause	**Treatment**
Constipation, bowel obstruction, ileus	Metoclopramide, prochlorperazine, haloperidol
Chemotherapy, radiation, infection, inflammation, direct tumor invasion	Ondansetron, granisetron
Anticipatory nausea	Benzodiazepines
Increased intracranial pressure	Glucocorticoids

Dyspnea

Treat reversible causes of dyspnea, such as pleural effusions, infection, and anemia. Systemic opioids are the standard of care for refractory dyspnea in advanced disease.

DON'T BE TRICKED

- **Oxygen supplementation is helpful if the patient is hypoxic but is otherwise ineffective.**
- **Fans are effective in reducing dyspnea in nonhypoxic patients.**

Depression and Anxiety

It is difficult to distinguish grief from depression. Helplessness, hopelessness, worthlessness, guilt, and anhedonia are signs of depression rather than normal grief.

Depression will respond to typical pharmacologic and nonpharmacologic therapy. If prognosis is less than 6 weeks, use a psychostimulant with a faster onset, such as methylphenidate. Benzodiazepines can help reduce anxiety in a palliative care setting.

Anorexia

Artificial nutrition in cachexia of advanced disease does not improve morbidity or mortality, nor does it reduce aspiration pneumonia risk. Medications used to stimulate appetite (progesterones, dronabinol, glucocorticoids) do not improve morbidity or mortality.

Chronic Noncancer Pain

Diagnosis

Psychological screening for depression, anxiety, and somatization are important adjuncts to a thorough history and physical examination.

Treatment

Evidence-based nondrug treatment includes:

- exercise
- massage
- CBT

Drug treatment for neuropathic pain includes:

- capsaicin cream or a lidocaine patch or cream
- gabapentin and pregabalin
- tricyclic antidepressants (increased drug interactions, poor side effect profile, and potential cardiac toxicities)
- SNRIs (duloxetine and venlafaxine)

Drug therapy for nociceptive pain is primarily NSAIDs (if an inflammatory component is present).

No evidence supports the efficacy of long-term opioids in managing chronic noncancer pain.

Despite the lack of evidence for their efficacy, if opioids are used, an assessment is performed to evaluate for risk of abuse and diversion, and written treatment agreements, adherence monitoring (urine drug screens), and surveillance using prescription monitoring programs are recommended by most guidelines.

DON'T BE TRICKED

- Do not concurrently prescribe opioids and sedative-hypnotics.

Chronic Cough

Diagnosis

Chronic cough lasts ≥8 weeks. Upper airways cough syndrome (UACS) caused by postnasal drip, asthma, and GERD are responsible for approximately 90% of cases of chronic cough but are responsible for 99% in patients who are nonsmokers, have a normal chest x-ray, and are not taking an ACE inhibitor.

All patients should undergo chest x-ray. Smoking cessation and discontinuation of ACE inhibitors is indicated for 4 weeks before additional evaluation.

STUDY TABLE: Causes and Therapy of Chronic Cough

If you see this...	Diagnose this...	Choose this...
Postnasal drainage, frequent throat clearing, nasal discharge, cobblestone appearance of the oropharyngeal mucosa, or mucus dripping down the oropharynx	UACS	First-generation antihistamine-decongestant combination or intranasal glucocorticoid (for allergic rhinitis)
Asthma, cough with exercise or exposure to cold	Cough-variant asthma	Methacholine or exercise challenge if diagnosis is uncertain Standard asthma therapy; may take 6 weeks to respond
GERD symptoms (GERD may be silent)	GERD-related cough	Empiric PPI therapy without testing; may take 3 months to respond
Taking ACE inhibitor	ACE-inhibitor cough	Stop ACE inhibitor, substitute ARB; takes approximately 1 month to respond
Normal chest x-ray findings, normal spirometry, and negative methacholine challenge test	Possible nonasthmatic eosinophilic bronchitis	Sputum induction or bronchial wash for eosinophils Treat with inhaled glucocorticoids; avoid sensitizer

Systemic Exertion Intolerance Disease

Diagnosis

Systemic exertion intolerance disease (SEID; previously chronic fatigue syndrome) is defined as unexplained fatigue lasting more than 6 consecutive months that impairs the ability to perform desired activities, postexertional malaise, unrefreshing sleep, and either cognitive impairment or orthostatic intolerance (symptoms worse in upright position).

Extensive diagnostic evaluation is not needed in patients with typical symptoms and with normal physical examination and basic laboratory study results.

Treatment

Establishing goals of therapy and managing patient expectations are key treatment components of SEID. Focus treatment on minimizing the impact of fatigue through nonpharmacologic interventions (CBT and graded exercise), which are beneficial in improving, but not curing, symptoms. No specific class of medication has been shown to be effective in SEID.

DON'T BE TRICKED

- Do not obtain multiple viral titers to evaluate SEID.

Vertigo

Diagnosis

The first important step is to distinguish central from peripheral causes with the Dix-Hallpike maneuver.

STUDY TABLE: Interpretation of Dix-Halpike Maneuver

Characteristic	Peripheral Disease (benign positional vertigo, vestibular neuronitis, labyrinthitis)	Central Disease (brainstem or cerebellar stroke or tumor, MS)
Latency of nystagmus (lag time between maneuver and onset of nystagmus)	2-40 s	None
Duration of nystagmus	<1 min	>1 min
Severity of symptoms	Severe	Less severe
Fatigability (findings diminish with repetition)	Yes	No
Direction of nystagmus	Horizontal with rotational component; never vertical	Can be vertical, horizontal, or torsional

STUDY TABLE: Diagnosing Common Causes of Peripheral Vertigo

Cause	Findings
Benign paroxysmal positional vertigo	Brief vertigo (10-30 s) and nausea associated with abrupt head movement (turning over in bed). Treat with Epley maneuver (canalith repositioning procedure)
Vestibular neuronitis	Severe and longer lasting vertigo (days), nausea and often vomiting
Labyrinthitis	Similar to vestibular neuronitis but with hearing loss

Less common causes of **peripheral vertigo** are Meniere disease (vertigo, hearing loss, tinnitus), acoustic neuroma (hearing loss, tinnitus, unsteadiness, facial nerve involvement), aminoglycoside toxicity, herpes zoster (Ramsay Hunt syndrome), and migraine.

Diseases associated with **central vertigo** may be life threatening. Vertebrobasilar stroke is usually, but not always, accompanied by dysarthria, dysphagia, diplopia, weakness, ataxia or gait instability, or numbness. It should be considered in older persons with ASCVD risk factors. MS is suggested by relapsing and remitting neurologic abnormalities. Obtain an MRI for suspected central vertigo.

Treatment

Pharmacologic therapies of peripheral vertigo are not curative but may provide symptom relief: glucocorticoids, centrally acting antihistamines (meclizine), vestibular suppressants (benzodiazepines), and antiemetic drugs.

DON'T BE TRICKED

- The Epley maneuver, not drugs, is the primary treatment of benign paroxysmal positional vertigo.

Insomnia

Diagnosis

Insomnia includes problems of sleep initiation, sleep maintenance, early morning waking, or nonrestorative and poor-quality sleep. Insomnia may be associated with shift work and an irregular sleep schedule, obesity, sleep apnea, and restless legs syndrome. Obtain polysomnography for suspected sleep apnea or periodic limb movement disorder.

STUDY TABLE: Differential Diagnosis of Insomnia and Daytime Sleepiness

Condition	Characteristics
Restless legs syndrome	An uncomfortable or restless feeling in the legs most prominent at night and at rest, associated with an urge to move and alleviated by movement Look for iron deficiency Associated with periodic limb movement disorder in most patients
Periodic limb movement disorder	Repetitive stereotypic leg movement during sleep and during quiet wakefulness
Central sleep apnea syndrome	Repetitive pauses in breathing during sleep without upper airway occlusion Associated history of HF or CNS disease
Obstructive sleep apnea syndrome	Upper airway obstruction during inspiration in sleep History of snoring, witnessed pauses in respiration, large shirt collar size, and daytime sleepiness
Shift-work sleep disorder	History of insomnia associated with shift work (permanent night shifts)
Sleep deprivation	Six hours or less of sleep is associated with daytime sleepiness and performance deficits
Narcolepsy	Daytime sleepiness with cataplexy, hypnagogic hallucinations, and sleep paralysis frequently coexisting with other sleep disorders

Treatment

Nondrug treatment of insomnia includes:

- CBT (first-line therapy)
- sleep hygiene practices (regular bedtimes and waking times; spending no more than 8 hours in bed; using bed only for sleep)
- avoiding caffeine, nicotine, alcohol, and electronic devices before sleep
- melatonin for short-term insomnia resulting from travel or shift work

The ACP recommends that physicians engage in a thorough shared decision-making process to decide whether to add pharmacologic therapies in patients with insomnia refractory to CBT. Benzodiazepines (flurazepam, triazolam, temazepam, oxazepam, lorazepam, diazepam) are associated with tolerance, daytime somnolence, falls, rebound insomnia, cognitive impairment, anterograde amnesia, and potential for dependence.

Nonbenzodiazepines (zolpidem, zaleplon, eszopiclone) have fewer side effects, but sedation, disorientation, and agitation may occur as well as (rarely) sleep driving, sleep walking, and sleep eating.

Restless legs syndrome is treated with dopaminergic agents (pramipexole or ropinirole) or with levodopa-carbidopa. Prescribe supplemental iron for patients with restless legs syndrome when the serum ferritin level is <75 ng/mL.

DON'T BE TRICKED

- Do not select antidepressants for insomnia unless the patient is depressed.
- Do not select an antihistamine for insomnia.
- Do not prescribe benzodiazepines for the treatment of insomnia in the elderly (risk of delirium, falls, fractures, cognitive impairment, and motor vehicle accidents).

Syncope

Diagnosis

An uncomplicated faint (vasovagal) is common and can be diagnosed by the history and absence of any suggestion of heart disease from the physical examination and ECG. Look for the 4 P's:

- previous history
- posture (prolonged standing)
- provoking factors (blood draw, pain, emotion)
- prodromal symptoms (sweating, nausea, feeling warm)

A history of heart disease, chest pain before syncope, significant cardiac risk factors, or exertional syncope suggests structural cardiac disease or arrhythmias as the cause of syncope.

STUDY TABLE: Causes of Syncope

If you see this...	Diagnose this...
A prodrome of nausea, diaphoresis, pallor, and brief loss of consciousness (<1 min) with rapid recovery and absence of postsyncopal confusion	Uncomplicated faint (vasovagal syncope)
Preceding pressure on the carotid sinus (tight collar, sudden turning of head)	Carotid sinus hypersensitivity
Association with specific activities (urination, cough, swallowing, defecation)	Situational syncope
On assuming an upright position	Orthostatic hypotension caused by hypovolemia, pharmacologic agents, or autonomic nervous system disorders (e.g., parkinsonism, diabetes)
Brainstem neurologic signs and symptoms	Posterior circulation vascular disease; consider subclavian steal syndrome if preceded by upper extremity exercise
Witnessed "seizure"	Syncope can cause tonic-clonic jerking of extremities; primary seizure is unlikely if findings of diaphoresis or nausea before the event, a brief episode of unconsciousness, and immediate postsyncopal orientation are present
Related to exercise or associated with angina	Obstruction to LV outflow: AS, HCM; also PE and PH
Syncope with sudden loss of consciousness without prodrome	Arrhythmia, sinoatrial and AV node dysfunction (ischemic heart disease and associated with use of β-blockers, calcium channel blockers, and antiarrhythmic drugs)
Syncope following a meal	Postprandial syncope, often in older adult patients

Patients with uncomplicated faint can be discharged home without additional evaluation. Patients with suspected cardiac causes of syncope should be admitted to the hospital.

Testing

Consider the appropriate indications for the following diagnostic tests:

- ECG: Done in all cases. The finding of an arrhythmia and conduction block may establish the diagnosis, but a normal ECG does not rule out a cardiac cause.
- Echocardiography: Obtain if structural heart disease is suspected.
- Ambulatory ECG recording: Indicated if cardiac arrhythmia is suspected or the cause is unclear. The choice of the recording device is determined by the frequency of the patient's symptoms (see Cardiovascular Medicine, Palpitations and Syncope).
- Stress testing: Indicated for patients with exercise-associated syncope or those with significant risks for ischemic heart disease.
- Carotid sinus massage: For suspected carotid sinus syncope or for unexplained syncope in those aged >60 years.
- Tilt-table testing: Most commonly used in patients with suspected recurrent vasovagal syncope or when the initial evaluation of delayed orthostatic hypotension is not diagnostic.
- Electrophysiologic testing: Rarely helpful and almost always the incorrect answer.

DON'T BE TRICKED

- Do not order carotid vascular studies to diagnose cause of syncope.
- Do not order brain imaging, cardiac enzymes, or EEG to evaluate syncope.

Treatment

Treatment of structural cardiac disease and arrhythmias is covered in the Cardiovascular Medicine section. For hypovolemia or orthostatic syncope, eliminate α- and β-blockers and anticholinergic agents, if possible. Increase fluid and sodium intake, and consider compression stockings.

As a last resort, add mineralocorticoids and α-adrenergic receptor agonists. For recurrent neurocardiogenic syncope, choose β-blockers.

TEST YOURSELF

An 18-year-old woman fainted while standing in line to purchase concert tickets. She felt "woozy" and became pale and sweaty before fainting. Friends observed jerking motions of her face and fingers.

ANSWER: For diagnosis, choose vasovagal syncope (uncomplicated faint).

Musculoskeletal Pain

Elbow

Olecranon bursitis is inflammation of a bursa that lies in the posterior aspect of the elbow and presents as a fluid-filled mass. This condition can result from repetitive trauma, infection, or systemic inflammatory conditions. Olecranon bursitis does not cause restriction or pain with range of motion of the elbow whereas joint pathology will cause pain and restricted movement.

Aspirate a bursa if tender or warm to analyze fluid for crystals and infection. NSAIDs and rest (if noninfectious) are first-line treatments.

Epicondylitis involves pain and tenderness at either the insertion of the extensor radii tendons (lateral epicondylitis) or the flexor carpi radialis tendons (medial epicondylitis). Lateral epicondylitis ("tennis elbow") is caused by overuse that involves pronation and supination with the wrist flexed. First-line treatment is stretching and strengthening exercises and avoidance of activities that cause pain. Braces may be useful when exacerbating activities cannot be avoided. Oral and topical NSAIDs provide short-term relief. Do not inject glucocorticoids.

DON'T BE TRICKED

- Do not obtain imaging studies in patients with findings compatible with epicondylitis.

Back

Patients with low back pain can be grouped into one of three broad categories:

- nonspecific pain (85%)
- radiculopathy or spinal stenosis (7%)
- specific spine disorder such as cancer, fracture, infection, or ankylosing spondylitis (8%)

Look for the "red flags" related to malignancy, spinal infection, fracture, and cauda equina syndrome, which suggest the need for early imaging.

The "red flags" of **cauda equina syndrome** include:

- urinary retention or incontinence
- diminished perineal sensation
- bilateral motor deficits

Also perform diagnostic imaging and testing for patients with low back pain when severe or progressive neurologic deficits are present and the patient is a candidate for surgery.

Look for a **herniated disk** when acute back pain radiates down the leg and is associated with:

- positive straight leg raising
- weakness of the ankle and great toe dorsiflexion (L5)
- loss of ankle reflexes (S1)
- less commonly, loss of knee reflex (L4)

Spinal stenosis usually occurs in older adults and is characterized by neurogenic claudication—radiating back pain and lower extremity numbness—that is exacerbated by walking and spinal extension but improved by sitting and leaning forward. A wide-based gait and/or abnormal Romberg test are highly specific (>90%) for spinal stenosis. MRI establishes the diagnosis.

Recovery is generally quick for **acute, nonspecific low back pain** regardless of the intervention used. The first step is self-care (remain active, application of superficial heat). Other interventions include:

- massage
- spinal manipulation
- pharmacologic NSAIDs (first-line treatment)

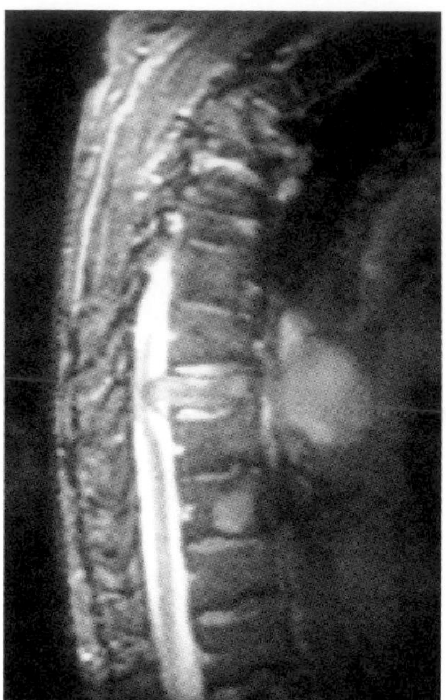

Collapsed Vertebral Body: Unenhanced T2-weighted MRI of the thoracic spine shows collapse of the vertebral body and compression of the spinal cord from posteriorly displaced bony fragments in a patient with metastatic breast cancer.

Muscle relaxants and benzodiazepines may be modestly beneficial for pain relief but dizziness and sedation limit their usefulness. Systemic glucocorticoids or epidural injections have not been shown to be effective in the treatment of low back pain.

Sciatica can be treated conservatively, and most patients are substantially improved within 1 to 3 months. Patients with sciatica assigned to early surgery and those assigned to conservative treatment have similar 1-year outcomes. Patients with spinal stenosis treated surgically have greater improvement in pain and function at 2 years compared with patients treated nonsurgically.

Neoplastic epidural spinal cord compression, including the cauda equina syndrome, is a surgical emergency. Begin management by administering dexamethasone and obtaining immediate MRI of the entire spine.

DON'T BE TRICKED

- **Do not obtain imaging for patients with nonspecific low back pain.**
- **Opioids have not been shown to be more effective than NSAIDs in chronic low back pain, and their use is limited by many potential side effects, including abuse potential. Several guidelines recommend against their use in the treatment of chronic low back pain.**

Knee

The most common cause of knee pain in patients aged <45 years, especially women, is the **patellofemoral pain syndrome**. The pain is peripatellar and exacerbated by overuse (running), descending stairs, or after prolonged sitting. Diagnosis is confirmed by firmly compressing the patella against the femur and moving it up and down along the groove of the femur, reproducing pain. The condition is self-limited. Minimizing high-impact activity, performing quadriceps strengthening exercises, and treatment with NSAIDs improve symptoms.

Prepatellar bursitis is associated with anterior knee pain and swelling anterior to the patella and is often caused by trauma or repetitive kneeling. Perform a joint aspiration to rule out infection if warmth and erythema are present.

Anserine bursitis can cause knee pain that is worse with activity and at night. The anserine bursa is located medially about 6 cm below the joint line. Anserine bursitis is common in patients with OA.

In general, bursitis treatment includes:

- rest
- ice
- NSAIDs
- local glucocorticoid injection for persistent symptoms

Iliotibial band syndrome is a common cause of knife-like lateral knee pain that occurs with vigorous flexion-extension activities of the knee (running). Treat with rest and stretching exercises.

Trauma may result in a **ligament tear**, which produces a noticeable "popping" sensation in 50% of patients. Typically, a large effusion collects rapidly. Check for stability of major ligaments by stressing the ligament; normal knees will have minimal give.

Meniscal tears present with pain, locking, and clicking. Tenderness usually localizes to the joint line on the affected side and with tibial rotation as the leg is extended. No physical examination maneuver reliably establishes or excludes the diagnosis. Initial therapy for acute meniscal tears includes rest, ice, and physical therapy. Surgery for acute meniscal tears is reserved for mechanical symptoms that persist beyond 4 weeks. MRI is reserved for patients in whom surgery is being considered and in patients with persistent locking and catching despite appropriate initial management.

Hip

Most patients with chronic hip pain have degenerative arthritis associated with other large-joint arthritis symptoms.

Look for **greater trochanter pain syndrome**, characterized by lateral point tenderness and full range of motion except for painful resisted abduction. Manage with acetaminophen or NSAIDs. Glucocorticoid injection can be considered for persistent symptoms.

Risk factors for **osteonecrosis** include alcoholism, sickle cell disease, SLE, and prolonged glucocorticoid use. Diagnose early osteonecrosis with hip MRI. Advanced disease will show flattening of the femoral head on x-ray. Treatment of osteonecrosis is often hip replacement for recalcitrant pain and disability.

Consider **bone metastases** to the hip in patients with a history of cancer.

DON'T BE TRICKED

- **True hip joint pain usually presents as groin pain.**

Ankle

For a **ligament tear**, look for ecchymoses around the joint, suggesting bleeding in the region of the torn ligament, and any swelling or obvious deformity. Ability to bear weight rules out fracture or severe sprain.

Look for **Achilles tendon rupture** (a snapping sound followed by posterior ankle pain and inability to plantarflex). Rarely this can occur in older men who are taking a fluoroquinolone antibiotic.

DON'T BE TRICKED

- **Select ankle x-ray following ankle trauma only if the patient cannot bear weight or if bone pain is localized to the lateral or medial malleolus, base of the fifth metatarsal, or the navicular bone.**

Foot

Plantar fasciitis, the most common cause of inferior heel pain, is characterized by pain that worsens with walking, especially with the first steps in the morning or after resting, in addition to localized tenderness along the plantar fascia or the calcaneal insertion site. Manage with weight loss, rest, and calf/heel stretching.

Symptoms of a **Morton neuroma** include pain, numbness, and tingling in the forefoot, usually between the third and fourth toes, aggravated by walking on hard surfaces and wearing tight or high-heeled shoes. Compressing the forefoot or space between the third and fourth toes reproduces the symptoms. Initial therapy includes wearing wider shoes and arch support.

DON'T BE TRICKED

- Do not order heel radiography for plantar fasciitis.

Hand

De Quervain tenosynovitis is typically seen in young women with pain on the radial side of the wrist during pinch grasping or thumb and wrist movement. The diagnosis is established with a positive Finkelstein test. Initial management includes rest, NSAIDs, and splinting; glucocorticoid injections provide symptomatic relief if conservative therapy is ineffective.

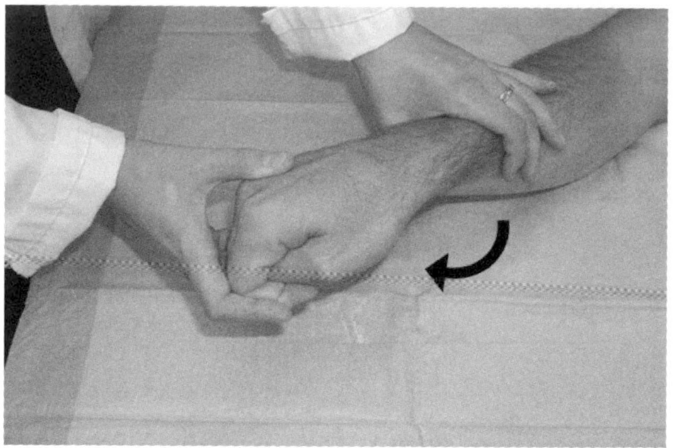

Finkelstein Test: Finkelstein test for de Quervain's stenosing tenosynovitis. Pain elicited by flexing the thumb into the palm, closing the fingers over the thumb, and then bending the wrist in the ulnar direction is confirmatory.

Consider **carpal tunnel syndrome** for pain and paresthesias, particularly at night, localized to the thumb, first two fingers, and the radial half of the ring finger. Keep in mind secondary causes of carpal tunnel syndrome, especially in patients with bilateral symptoms, such as hypothyroidism, diabetes mellitus, pregnancy, paraproteinemias, and RA of the wrist. Splinting at night plus NSAIDs is first-line therapy for carpal tunnel syndrome. Carpal tunnel release surgery is indicated for severe carpal tunnel syndrome (muscle weakness or EMG evidence of nerve injury).

Shoulder

Patients with **rotator cuff tendinitis and subacromial bursitis** typically have gradually worsening pain, especially with overhead activity that limits range of motion. The pain is worse at night and may extend down the arm but rarely below the elbow. Consider the following:

- Pain without weakness is consistent with tendinitis.
- Pain with weakness is consistent with a tendon tear.
- Severe pain and frank weakness (inability to maintain the arm at 90 degrees of abduction) suggest complete rupture of the rotator cuff tendon.

Consider other causes of shoulder pain:

- Impingement syndrome involves lateral deltoid pain that is aggravated by reaching.
- Frozen shoulder presents with an impingement pain pattern accompanied by stiffness and loss of active and passive external rotation or abduction.
- Causes of anterior shoulder pain (acromioclavicular joint, glenohumeral joint, or long head of the biceps)

Acromioclavicular joint pain is localized to the distal end of the clavicle and is most pronounced when the patient reaches across the body to the opposite shoulder.

Glenohumeral joint pain is aggravated by any shoulder movement. Pain owing to **biceps tendinitis** is aggravated by lifting and wrist supination.

Biceps tendon rupture is often associated with a traumatic event but may be spontaneous and presents with a visible or palpable mass near the elbow or mid arm ("Popeye sign") and ecchymosis.

Testing

MRI is the best imaging modality for complete or partial rotator cuff tears, although ultrasonography is more cost effective.

Treatment

Conservative therapy is indicated for patients with suspected rotator cuff tendinitis, incomplete tears, and subacromial bursitis. NSAIDs and exercises that strengthen the rotator cuff muscles and improve flexibility are effective in improving pain.

Immediate surgery is indicated for an acute full-thickness tear in younger patients. Such tears are frequently managed conservatively in older patients.

DON'T BE TRICKED

- **Constant shoulder pain with normal shoulder examination suggests referred pain (e.g., Pancoast tumor) or neuropathic pain (e.g., cervical spine radiculopathy).**

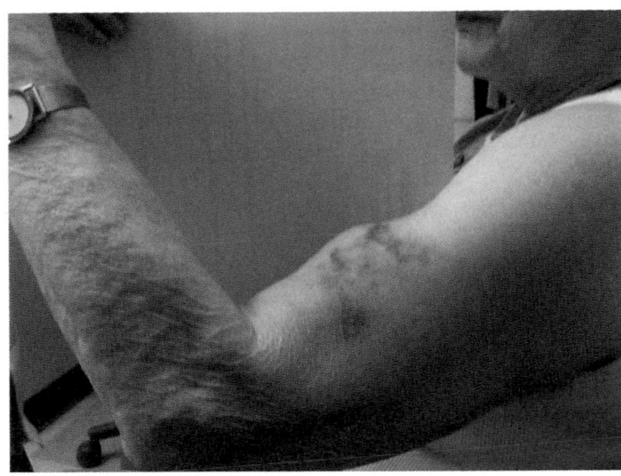

Biceps Tendon Rupture: Biceps tendon rupture showing a visible mass ("Popeye sign") at the mid arm with associated ecchymoses.

Dyslipidemia

Diagnosis

The 2013 ACC/AHA and 2016 USPSTF guidelines do not focus on LDL cholesterol treatment targets, but rather on a person's overall risk of developing ASCVD. The 2017 American Association of Clinical Endocrinologists and American College of Endocrinology (AACE/ACE) guideline recommends treating to specific targets depending on risk factors and calculated cardiovascular risk.

DON'T BE TRICKED

- **Do not obtain lipoprotein(a), apolipoprotein B, or LDL particles in the evaluation of dyslipidemia.**

Prevention and Treatment

The ACC/AHA recommend initiating statin therapy to reduce risk of ASCVD in:

1. patients with clinical ASCVD,
2. patients with an LDL cholesterol level of 190 mg/dL or higher,
3. patients with diabetes mellitus who are aged 40 to 75 years with an LDL cholesterol level of 70 to 189 mg/dL and no clinical ASCVD, and
4. patients without clinical ASCVD or diabetes and an LDL cholesterol level of 70 to 189 mg/dL and estimated 10-year ASCVD risk of 7.5% or higher.

The USPSTF recommends that adults use a low- to moderate-dose statin for the primary prevention of CVD events and mortality when all of the following criteria are met:

- age 40 to 75 years
- ≥1 CVD risk factors (e.g., dyslipidemia, diabetes, hypertension, smoking)
- a calculated 10-year risk of a CV event of ≥10%

STUDY TABLE: High- and Moderate-Intensity Statins

High Intensity	Moderate Intensity
Atorvastatin 40-80 mg	Atorvastatin 10-20 mg
Rosuvastatin 20-40 mg	Rosuvastatin 5-10 mg
	Simvastatin 20-40 mg
	Pravastatin 40-80 mg
	Lovastatin 40 mg
	Fluvastatin 40 mg

DON'T BE TRICKED

- **Simvastatin 80 mg/d is not recommended by the FDA because of the increased risk of rhabdomyolysis.**

Baseline laboratory studies and monitoring:

- baseline fasting lipid panel ALT level
- monitor ALT and CK only if a patient develops symptoms of hepatic or muscle disease

Patients with a fasting triglyceride level ≥500 mg/dL are treated to prevent pancreatitis. Fibrates are the most potent triglyceride-lowering agents.

Obesity

Diagnosis

STUDY TABLE: Obesity Definitions

Diagnosis	BMI
Overweight	25-29.9
Obese	
Class I	30-34.9
Class II	35-39.9
Class III	≥40

Treatment

A reasonable initial goal is weight loss of 0.5 kg to 1.0 kg/week to achieve a total weight loss of 10%.

A specific daily calorie limit should be prescribed (typically, 1500-1800 kcal/d for men and 1200-1500 kcal/d for women). All diets are equally effective. Exercise is helpful as an adjunct to diet change but not effective as monotherapy.

Pharmacologic therapy may be used as adjunctive therapy in patients with a BMI ≥30 or in patients with a BMI ≥27 and weight-associated comorbidities.

STUDY TABLE: Drugs for Weight Loss

Drug	Expected Weight Loss	Cautions and Contraindications
Orlistat (inhibitor of gastric and pancreatic lipases)	3 kg	Diarrhea, oily stools; must replace fat soluble vitamins
Combination phentermine (sympathomimetic) and low-dose topiramate (anticonvulsant)	8-10 kg	Contraindications: pregnancy, glaucoma, hyperthyroidism, and MAOI use
Lorcaserin (brain serotonin 2C receptor agonist)	4 kg	Caution in patients taking medications that increase serotonin levels
Combination sustained-release bupropion (norepinephrine-dopamine reuptake inhibitor) and sustained-release naltrexone (opioid receptor antagonist)	2-6 kg	Contraindications: epilepsy, uncontrolled hypertension, and opioid or opioid agonist use
Liraglutide	5.3 kg	Gastrointestinal upset, headache, nasopharyngitis

Bariatric surgery is considered for patients with a BMI >40 and also for patients with a BMI >35 with serious obesity-related comorbidities (severe sleep apnea, diabetes, severe joint disease).

Bariatric surgery outcomes are associated with:

- improved control or remission of type 2 diabetes
- improved quality of life

- reduced medication use
- reduced mortality

Commonly performed bariatric procedures include laparoscopic adjustable gastric banding, Roux-en-Y gastric bypass, and sleeve gastrectomy.

STUDY TABLE: Bariatric Surgery Complications

Surgery	Complications
Banding procedures	Intractable nausea and vomiting
	Marginal ulcers, stomal obstruction
Gastric bypass	Stomal stenosis
	Cholelithiasis
	Nephrolithiasis
	Dumping syndrome
	Anatomic stricture or ulceration
	Bacterial overgrowth
	Micronutrient deficiencies: folate; vitamins B_1, B_6, B_{12}, C, A, D, E, and K; iron; zinc; selenium; and copper
Sleeve gastrectomy	Staple-line bleeding, stenosis (dysphagia and vomiting), and staple-line leakage

TEST YOURSELF

A 41-year-old woman is evaluated for persistent nausea and vomiting after laparoscopic gastric bypass surgery 6 weeks ago for morbid obesity.

ANSWER: For management, select upper endoscopy to diagnose stomal stenosis or marginal ulcer.

Male Sexual Dysfunction

Diagnosis

The most common causes of sexual dysfunction are vascular and neurologic diseases. Testosterone deficiency, hyperprolactinemia, diabetes, and thyroid disorders can also cause erectile dysfunction. Rapid onset of sexual dysfunction suggests psychogenic causes or medication effects, whereas a more gradual onset suggests the presence of medical illnesses. Decreased libido suggests hormonal deficiencies, psychogenic causes, or medication effects. Also look for alcohol, tobacco, cocaine, opiate, or marijuana use.

Testing

The role of routine hormonal evaluation is unclear (see Endocrinology and Metabolism, Male Hypogonadism).

Suspect androgen steroid abuse in patients with infertility, muscular hypertrophy, testicular atrophy, and acne; laboratory data show elevated hemoglobin and suppressed LH and FSH levels.

Treatment

First-line therapy for erectile dysfunction is oral PDE-5 inhibitors (sildenafil, vardenafil, or tadalafil). These drugs are contraindicated in men who receive nitrate therapy in any form and in men with a history of nonarteritic anterior ischemic optic neuropathy. They should be used with caution in men taking α-blockers because of the risk of hypotension.

Intraurethral or intracavernous alprostadil is a second-line therapy for men who cannot take PDE-5 inhibitors.

Testosterone therapy is reserved for patients with confirmed hypogonadism.

TEST YOURSELF

A 72-year-old man cannot maintain an erection. He has diabetes mellitus, peripheral vascular disease, and CAD with stable angina, for which he takes aspirin, atenolol, isosorbide dinitrate, and glipizide.

ANSWER: For management, choose intraurethral or intracavernous alprostadil initiation.

Benign Prostatic Hyperplasia

Diagnosis

BPH leads to irritative symptoms (urinary urgency, frequency, and nocturia) and obstructive symptoms (decreased urinary stream, intermittency, incomplete emptying, and straining). BPH is diagnosed primarily by medical history and is supported by digital rectal examination. When a diagnosis of BPH has been established, the American Urological Association Symptom Index quantifies symptom severity and guides treatment decisions.

Treatment

For most patients, conservative treatment is sufficient (reduce fluid intake, stop contributing medications [diuretics, anticholinergics]). The two major BPH drug classes include:

- α-adrenergic blockers (terazosin, tamsulosin, doxazosin, alfuzosin, and prazosin)
- 5-α reductase inhibitors (finasteride, dutasteride)

α-Adrenergic blockers are superior to 5-α reductase inhibitors. α-Adrenergic blockers plus finasteride are more effective than either drug alone but are associated with increased adverse effects.

Tadalafil, a PDE-5 inhibitor, improves lower urinary tract symptoms and may be used in patients with concomitant BPH and erectile dysfunction.

Transurethral resection of the prostate or transurethral needle ablation is indicated in patients with severe urinary symptoms, urinary retention, persistent hematuria, recurrent UTIs, or kidney disease clearly attributable to BPH.

Acute Scrotal Pain

Diagnosis

Patients with **testicular torsion** have severe acute pain and may have nausea and vomiting. Absence of the cremasteric reflex on the affected side is nearly 99% sensitive for torsion. The testis is usually high within the scrotum and may lie transversely. Doppler flow ultrasonography demonstrates diminished blood flow to the affected testicle. Testicular elevation will not relieve pain.

Epididymitis causes pain localizing to the posterior and superior aspects of the testicle. Pain onset is subacute and may be accompanied by dysuria, pyuria, and fever. The scrotum may be edematous and erythematous. Pain may decrease with testicular elevation.

Orchitis is usually caused by viral infection (mumps) or extension of a bacterial infection from epididymitis or UTI. The testicle is diffusely tender. In epididymitis and orchitis, ultrasonography demonstrates normal or increased blood flow to the testicle and epididymis.

Treatment

Treatment of testicular torsion is immediate surgical exploration and reduction.

In men younger than 35 years with epididymitis, treat for gonorrhea and chlamydial infection (ceftriaxone and doxycycline). In men older than 35 years or those engaging in anal intercourse, treat with ceftriaxone and a fluoroquinolone.

Acute Prostatitis

Diagnosis

Symptoms of acute prostatitis include fever, chills, dysuria, pelvic pain, cloudy urine, obstructive symptoms, and blood in the semen. Septic shock may be a presenting feature in some men. The diagnosis is established by finding a tender prostate on physical examination and a positive urine culture.

Treatment

Begin empiric antibiotics that cover gram-negative organisms (trimethoprim-sulfamethoxazole, fluoroquinolone) for 4 to 6 weeks. For patients who appear toxic, hospitalize and add gentamicin to a fluoroquinolone.

Female Sexual Dysfunction

Diagnosis and Testing

Female sexual dysfunction describes sexual difficulties that are persistent and distressing to the patient. Abnormalities in female sexual response fall into three categories:

- sexual interest/arousal disorder (lack of sexual interest and responsiveness)
- orgasmic disorder (absence of orgasm following normal excitement phase)
- genitopelvic pain/penetration disorder (difficulty or pain with penetration)

A pelvic examination is helpful in identifying specific areas of pain or tenderness, vulvovaginal atrophy, decreased lubrication, or tissue friability. Screening for concurrent depression is indicated because sexual dysfunction and depression often coexist.

Laboratory testing is recommended only if an underlying disorder is suspected.

Treatment

Treat underlying contributing causes (e.g., vaginitis, interstitial cystitis, pelvic adhesions, infections, or endometriosis).

Use lubricants as first-line therapy to alleviate dyspareunia from vaginal atrophy. Low-dose vaginal estrogen is second-line therapy for women without contraindications to estrogen.

Use CBT for depression or anxiety.

Flibanserin may be used to treat women with low sexual desire; however, its use is limited by side effects.

DON'T BE TRICKED

- **Do not treat female sexual dysfunction with low-dose testosterone or phosphodiesterase inhibitors.**

Breast Cancer Prevention and Screening

Prevention

The Gail Model Risk Assessment Tool is used to estimate any woman's 5-year and lifetime breast cancer risk. Women age >35 years with a 5-year breast cancer risk of ≥1.7% or with lobular carcinoma in situ are candidates for breast cancer prophylaxis:

- tamoxifen before menopause
- tamoxifen and raloxifene, or exemestane after menopause

Testing for the *BRCA* gene is recommended for women whose family history suggests increased risk for mutations in the *BRCA1* or *BRCA2* gene (one or more first-degree relatives on the same side ≤50 years with breast cancer or invasive ovarian cancer; two or more relatives at any age with breast, prostate, or pancreatic cancer).

Expert opinion recommends women with *BRCA1/2* mutations should undergo:

- breast cancer screening with MRI beginning at age 25 years, then mammography beginning at age 30 years
- ovarian cancer screening with pelvic examinations, ultrasonography, and CA-125 measurement

Surgical prophylaxis options for carriers of *BRCA1/2* mutations include prophylactic bilateral mastectomy and prophylactic bilateral salpingo-oophorectomy (after childbearing).

Screening

Screening recommendations vary depending on the organization. The USPSTF recommends biennial screening mammography for average-risk women beginning at age 50 years. Individualize screening decisions in women aged 75 or older based on breast cancer risk, overall prognosis and comorbid conditions, and personal patient preferences.

Breast Mass

Diagnosis

Most breast lumps are benign, but clinical examination cannot distinguish between benign and malignant.

STUDY TABLE: Evaluation of Breast Mass

Breast Finding	Diagnostic Testing
Palpable lump or mass and age <30 years	Consider observation to assess resolution within 1 or 2 menstrual cycles If persistent, choose ultrasonography If simple cyst on ultrasound, aspirate and repeat clinical breast examination in 4-6 weeks If complex cyst on ultrasound, perform mammography and fine-needle aspiration or core-needle biopsy If aspirate fluid is bloody or a mass persists following aspiration, choose mammography and biopsy If solid on ultrasound, choose mammography and obtain tissue diagnosis (core biopsy or surgical excision)
Palpable lump or mass and age ≥30 years	Mammography: If BI-RADS category 1-3 (benign or close follow-up recommended), obtain ultrasonography and follow protocol above; if BI-RADS category 4-5 (suspicious or highly suspicious), obtain tissue diagnosis
Nipple discharge, no mass, any age	Bilateral, milky: Pregnancy test (if negative, choose endocrine evaluation) Persistent, spontaneous, unilateral, one duct, or serous/bloody: Cytology is optional; choose mammography and surgical referral for duct exploration
Skin changes (erythema, peau d'orange, scaling, nipple excoriation, eczema) and age <30 years	Consider mastitis and treat with antibiotics if appropriate and reevaluate in 2 weeks. Otherwise, evaluate as below
Skin changes (erythema, peau d'orange, scaling, nipple excoriation, eczema) and age ≥30 years	Perform bilateral mammography: If normal, obtain skin biopsy; if abnormal or indeterminate, obtain needle biopsy or excision (also consider skin punch biopsy)

BI-RADS = Breast Imaging Reporting and Data System.

DON'T BE TRICKED

- **Do not stop the evaluation of a breast mass if mammogram is normal.**
- **On mammography, an irregular mass with microcalcifications or spiculation is suspicious for malignant disease, and biopsy is mandatory.**
- **Evidence is lacking that breast self-examination offers benefit in screening for breast cancer in average-risk asymptomatic women; self-examination may be associated with a higher rate of breast biopsy.**

Cervical Cancer Screening

Screening

The USPSTF recommends cervical cancer screening in women aged 21 to 65 years with cytology (Pap test) every 3 years. The screening interval can be increased to every 5 years in women aged 30 to 65 years by either performing high-risk HPV testing (preferred) or combining cytology and high-risk HPV testing. High-risk HPV is defined as genotypes 6 and 18, which are responsible for approximately 70% of all cervical cancers worldwide.

The USPSTF recommends against routine screening in women younger than 21 years and in women older than 65 years (provided previous screenings yielded normal results, and the patient is not otherwise at high risk).

DON'T BE TRICKED

- **Do not screen women following a hysterectomy with cervix removal for benign disease (e.g., fibroids).**
- **HPV vaccine does not protect against all HPV infections and does not treat existing HPV.**
- **HPV vaccine can be given to patients who are HIV positive and otherwise immunosuppressed.**

Contraception

Available contraceptive methods include:

- hormonal contraception including intrauterine devices
- barrier contraceptives
- sterilization

STUDY TABLE: Comparison of Contraceptive Options

Agent	Advantages	Disadvantages
Combination estrogen-progestin preparations (oral, patch, vaginal ring)	Decreased incidence of endometrial, ovarian cancers Decreased dysmenorrhea, menorrhagia, symptomatic ovarian cysts Less iron-deficiency anemia	Increased risk of cancers of the cervix, liver, breast Increased risk of MI, ischemic stroke, VTE, hypertension Breakthrough bleeding
Progestin-only preparations (mini-pill)	For use when estrogen is contraindicated	Irregular bleeding, breakthrough bleeding Must maintain precise daily dosing schedule
Long-acting reversible preparations (depot medroxyprogesterone [IM or SQ], progestin implants)	Decreased risk of endometrial cancer, PID Improves endometriosis Decreased menstrual frequency	Irregular bleeding, amenorrhea, decreased bone mineral density (especially in adolescents) Delayed return to ovulation (10 months)
Intrauterine devices (copper, levonorgestrel)	Least dependence on user adherence Nonhormonal Effective for 5-10 years	Bleeding, pain, expulsion (rare) No protection from STIs
Barrier methods (cervical cap, diaphragm, male condom, female condom, vaginal sponge)	Only use when needed Protection from STIs	Most dependent on user adherence May require use of spermicide
Sterilization		
Female (tubal ligation)	May reduce ovarian cancer risk	Surgical complications Regret
Male (vasectomy)	Lower costs, more effective than tubal ligation	Surgical complications

SQ = subcutaneous.

Contraindications to combination hormonal products include:

- uncontrolled hypertension
- breast cancer
- VTE
- liver disease
- migraine with aura

Estrogen-containing preparations are contraindicated in women >35 years who smoke more than 15 cigarettes per day.

Emergency contraception is postcoital hormonal contraception used to prevent pregnancy after inadequately protected coitus. Options include:

- over-the-counter levonorgestrel
- prescription ulipristal

Menopause

Diagnosis

Menopause describes the cessation of menses and fertility and is definitive when a woman has experienced amenorrhea for 12 months. Major symptoms of menopause include vasomotor symptoms (hot flushes, night sweats) and genitourinary symptoms (vaginal dryness, dyspareunia).

DON'T BE TRICKED

- **Do not order hormone levels to diagnose menopause.**

Treatment

Vasomotor symptoms generally resolve spontaneously within a few years, and treatment should be based on symptom severity. In patients with severe symptoms, the most effective treatment is systemic hormone therapy, which can be used in healthy women <60 years and within 10 years of menopause. Keep these treatment points in mind when using estrogen:

- Contraceptive needs must be addressed during perimenopause.
- Transdermal estrogen may be associated with less VTE risk than oral estrogen.
- All women with an intact uterus must receive progesterone.
- Duration of treatment >5 years is associated with increased risk of breast cancer.
- The need for continued treatment should be reevaluated annually.

In the absence of systemic estrogen therapy, genital symptoms can be treated with vaginal lubricants or topical estrogen. Topical estrogen may be no more effective than vaginal lubricants.

Nonhormonal options for women with vasomotor symptoms and contraindications to hormone therapy include low-dose antidepressant agents (venlafaxine, desvenlafaxine, paroxetine, citalopram, and escitalopram) and gabapentin.

DON'T BE TRICKED

- **Data regarding black cohosh are inconclusive, as are studies of other herbs, soy, and other phytoestrogens.**
- **The USPSTF and other guidelines recommend against using hormonal therapy for the primary prevention of chronic conditions (such as osteoporosis) in postmenopausal women.**

Abnormal Uterine Bleeding

Diagnosis

First, exclude pregnancy, then classify bleeding as either ovulatory or anovulatory.

Ovulatory bleeding occurs at regular intervals, but the menstrual flow is excessive. Common causes:

- thyroid disease
- bleeding disorder
- structural abnormalities (uterine fibroids or polyps)

Anovulatory cycles are characteristically irregular in terms of flow and cycle duration because lack of ovulation and the resultant lack of cyclic progesterone cause endometrial hyperplasia and irregular bleeding. Common causes:

- PCOS
- hypothyroidism or hyperthyroidism
- hyperprolactinemia
- chronic liver or kidney disease
- medications (antidepressants, antipsychotics, chemotherapy)

Pelvic ultrasonography is indicated to assess for structural abnormalities in the uterus and to determine endometrial thickness. In postmenopausal women, endometrial biopsy is indicated if the endometrial thickness is >4 mm on ultrasound.

Treatment

Management of abnormal uterine bleeding is aimed at the underlying cause.

- Structural abnormalities may be surgically resected.
- Treat endocrine disorders (thyroid disease, PCOS).

For women with anovulatory cycles who wish to preserve fertility:

- medroxyprogesterone acetate used for the second half of the menstrual cycle will restore cyclic withdrawal bleeding.

For women interested in contraception:

- combined oral contraceptive pills or
- levonorgestrel intrauterine device may be used.

DON'T BE TRICKED

- **Pregnancy, including ectopic pregnancy, should always be considered in the differential diagnosis of abnormal uterine bleeding.**
- **Postmenopausal bleeding is always abnormal and requires evaluation.**

Dysmenorrhea

Diagnosis

Symptoms of dysmenorrhea include abdominal cramps, backache, headache, nausea, vomiting, and diarrhea. Symptoms coincide with the onset of menses and last 2 to 3 days.

Dysmenorrhea is classified as primary or secondary. Primary dysmenorrhea, which occurs in 90% of patients, is associated with normal ovulatory cycles and no pelvic pathology.

A secondary cause, such as endometriosis, fibroids, or uterine pathology, is found in 10% of patients.

Dysmenorrhea is sometimes associated with other cyclic symptom complexes such as PMS and premenstrual dysphoric disorder (PMDD). These disorders include physical and psychological symptoms that begin approximately 1 week before menses and cease with menstruation. PMDD is characterized by significant depressive symptoms that interfere with daily activities.

Initial evaluation includes a thorough history, with attention to risks for infection and possible physical, sexual, or emotional abuse.

Treatment

Primary dysmenorrhea is treated symptomatically without further testing with NSAIDs and cyclooxygenase-2 inhibitors. Second-line therapy includes combined hormonal contraceptive therapy.

Fluoxetine, sertraline, and paroxetine are effective first-line treatments for PMS and PMDD.

Chronic Pelvic Pain

Chronic pelvic pain is ongoing pelvic pain that has been present for 3 to 6 months in the absence of pregnancy.

STUDY TABLE: Differential Diagnosis of Chronic Pelvic Pain

If you see this...	Diagnose this...
Pelvic heaviness, abnormal uterine bleeding, infertility, and enlarged uterus on bimanual examination or ultrasonography	Uterine fibroids
Chronic pelvic pain worse before and during menses, associated with dysmenorrhea	Endometriosis
History of sexual abuse and normal physical examination and ultrasonography	Chronic pelvic pain syndrome
Urinary frequency, urgency, nocturia, and dysuria; suprapubic pain possibly relieved with voiding; and examination that shows vestibular and suprapubic tenderness	Interstitial cystitis

Testing

A urine pregnancy test and pelvic/transvaginal ultrasonography are used to evaluate women with chronic pelvic pain.

DON'T BE TRICKED

- Additional evaluation is warranted in a patient with chronic pelvic pain who has a sudden increase in pain intensity, which may indicate a superimposed acute process such as appendicitis.

Endometriosis

Endometriosis is characterized by ectopic endometrial implants, usually in the pelvis, but they can be found anywhere and cause cyclic bleeding, such as in the lungs (hemoptysis), CNS (catamenial headache), and rectum (rectal bleeding during menses).

Physical examination findings may be normal or may include abdominal masses and tenderness and abnormalities of the cervix, uterus, and adnexa. Also look for abnormalities of uterosacral ligaments on bimanual examination.

The lesions can be visualized by laparoscopy, the gold standard for diagnosis, but it is not required for medical treatment when other causes of pelvic pain have been ruled out.

DON'T BE TRICKED

- Endometriosis does not cause fever or vaginal discharge.

Treatment

NSAIDs are first-line therapy for endometriosis, followed by oral contraceptives (if pregnancy is not desired) if NSAIDs are ineffective.

Vaginitis

Diagnosis

Vaginitis is characterized by vaginal irritation, pruritus, pain, malodor, or unusual discharge. The three most common infectious causes of acute vaginitis are bacterial vaginosis, vulvovaginal candidiasis, and *Trichomonas*. Trichomoniasis is the only cause of vaginitis that is sexually transmitted.

STUDY TABLE: Diagnosis of Vaginitis

Test	Characteristics
Physical examination	Bacterial vaginosis: Thin, white discharge with "fishy" odor but without irritation or pain
	Candidiasis: External and internal erythema with itching and irritation; nonodorous; white, curd-like discharge
	Trichomoniasis: Frothy, yellow discharge; erythema of the vagina and cervix ("strawberry cervix")
Vaginal pH (normal <4.5)	Bacterial vaginosis and trichomoniasis: >4.5
	Candidiasis: <4.5
"Whiff" test	Bacterial vaginosis: "Fishy" odor after adding KOH
Microscopic examination of vaginal fluid	Bacterial vaginosis: Squamous epithelial cells covered with bacteria that obscure edges ("clue cells")
	Candidiasis: Budding yeast and pseudohyphae
	Trichomoniasis: Motile trichomonads
Other testing	Nucleic acid testing is available for bacterial vaginosis and trichomoniasis (gold standard for trichomoniasis)

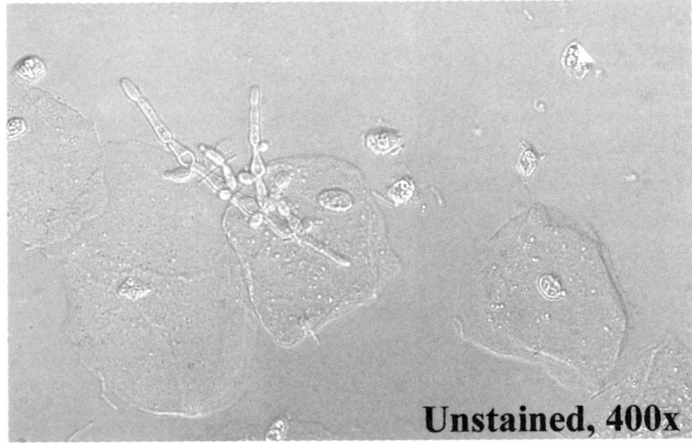

***Candida albicans*:** This wet mount specimen exhibits the typical filaments and spores associated with candidal vaginitis.

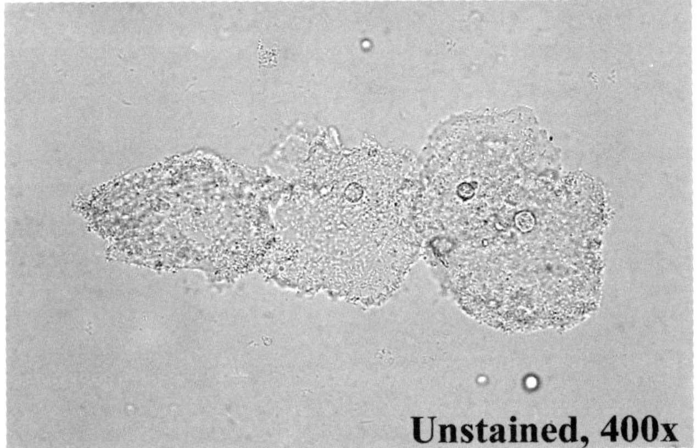

Clue Cell: This image shows clue cells (epithelial cells with borders obscured by small bacteria) on saline microscopy that is consistent with bacterial vaginosis.

DON'T BE TRICKED

- Do not order vaginal cultures to diagnose the cause of vaginitis.
- Treatment of vulvovaginal candidiasis can be initiated empirically if symptoms are accompanied by characteristic findings.

Treatment

STUDY TABLE: Treating Vaginitis	
If the diagnosis is...	**Treat with...**
Vaginal candidiasis	Topical (e.g., fluconazole, miconazole, clotrimazole) Single dose of oral fluconazole (contraindicated during pregnancy); less effective in complicated conditions (e.g., diabetes, HIV infection)
Recurrent vaginal candidiasis	Combination topical therapy and oral fluconazole.
Bacterial vaginosis	Oral or topical metronidazole or clindamycin (safe during pregnancy)
Trichomoniasis	Oral metronidazole and also for male partner (safe during pregnancy). Test for other STIs. Retest within 3 months of treatment.

DON'T BE TRICKED

- Because vaginal yeast is found in 10% to 20% of healthy women, the identification of *Candida* species in patients without symptoms does not require treatment.

TEST YOURSELF

A 21-year-old woman has a vaginal discharge and odor. Pelvic examination shows a thin, white homogeneous vaginal discharge with a normal cervix and normal vaginal mucosa. Wet mount is negative for ***Trichomonas*** and ***Candida***. Vaginal pH is 6.0.

ANSWER: For diagnosis, choose bacterial vaginosis.

Eye Disorders

Red Eye

Red eye consists of categories of entities with or without ocular pain and/or visual loss. The combination of red eye, ocular pain, and visual loss warrants emergent referral to an ophthalmologist. Select Snellen visual acuity testing for all patients.

STUDY TABLE: Causes and Treatment of Red Eye		
If you see this...	**Diagnose this...**	**Do this...**
Unilateral then bilateral purulent discharge without pain or visual disturbance	Bacterial conjunctivitis	Topical fluoroquinolones or bacitracin-polymyxin; culture not needed
Conjunctivitis associated with herpes zoster rash involving ophthalmic division of fifth cranial nerve	Herpes zoster conjunctivitis	Emergency ophthalmology referral
Acute hyperpurulent discharge in a sexually active adult	*Neisseria gonorrhoeae* conjunctivitis	Topical and systemic antibiotics and emergency ophthalmology referral
Unilateral then bilateral conjunctivitis with daytime watery or mucoid discharge	Viral conjunctivitis	Supportive care
Itching and tearing of the eyes, nasal congestion	Allergic conjunctivitis	Topical vasoconstrictors, NSAIDs, ocular antihistamines, cromolyn
Pain, photophobia, inflammation confined to corneal limbus, corneal irregularity, edema	Iridocyclitis or keratitis	Consider associated spondyloarthropathies, sarcoidosis, and herpes zoster; emergency ophthalmology referral
Unilateral deep ocular pain, nausea, vomiting, fixed nonreactive pupil, shallow anterior chamber	Acute angle-closure glaucoma	Emergency ophthalmology referral
Severe ocular pain that worsens with eye movement and light exposure; a raised hyperemic lesion that may be localized or diffuse and obscures the underlying vasculature	Scleritis	Commonly associated with collagen vascular and rheumatoid diseases; emergency ophthalmology referral
Nonpainful red, flat, superficial lesion that allows visualization of the underlying vasculature	Episcleritis	Self-limited; no treatment required
Red eye with scales and crusts around the eyelashes or dandruff-like skin changes and greasy scales around the eyelashes	Blepharitis	*Staphylococcus* (crusting) or seborrheic dermatitis (greasy scales, dandruff); warm compresses, washing with mild detergent, topical antibiotics

DON'T BE TRICKED

- Do not treat a red eye with topical glucocorticoids.

TEST YOURSELF

A 39-year-old man has bilateral red eyes and pain for 2 days. He has arthritis and chronic low back pain. Visual acuity is 20/40 bilaterally. Eyes are intensely injected, with prominent circumcorneal erythema.

ANSWER: For diagnosis, choose acute iritis associated with ankylosing spondylitis. For management, select emergent referral to an ophthalmologist.

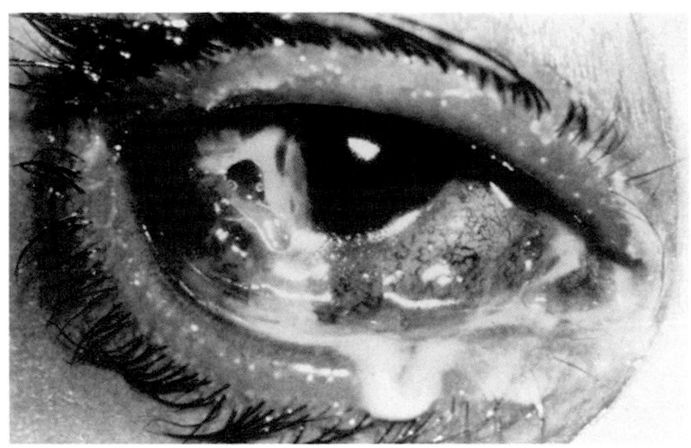

Bacterial Conjunctivitis: The conjunctiva is diffusely erythematous with mucopurulent discharge consistent with bacterial conjunctivitis. Consider gonorrhea in sexually active adult.

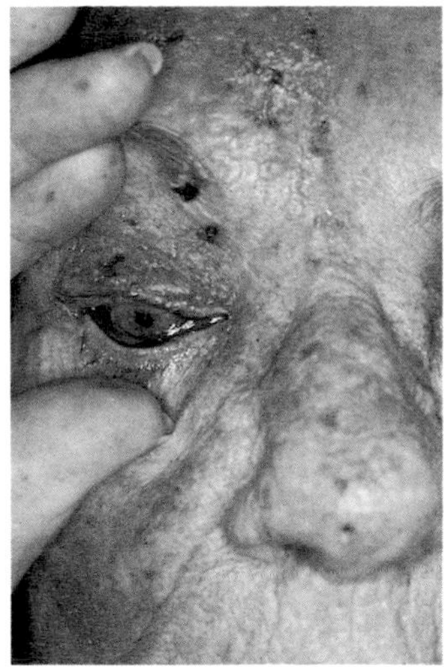

Herpes Zoster: Herpes zoster infection involving the forehead, top of the head, and eye, with evident hyperemic conjunctivitis. Corneal ulceration, episcleritis, and lid droop can occur.

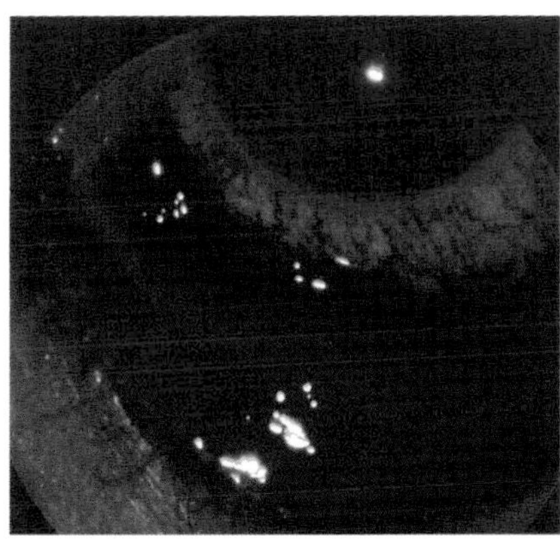

Viral Conjunctivitis: Acute adenovirus conjunctivitis is characterized by diffuse injection of the palpebral and bulbar conjunctivae and pseudomembrane formation involving the palpebral conjunctiva.

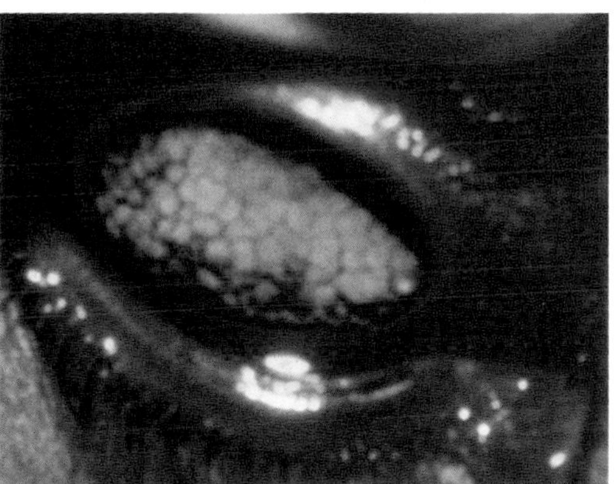

Allergic Conjunctivitis: Allergic conjunctivitis with prominent cobblestoning of the palpebral conjunctiva is shown.

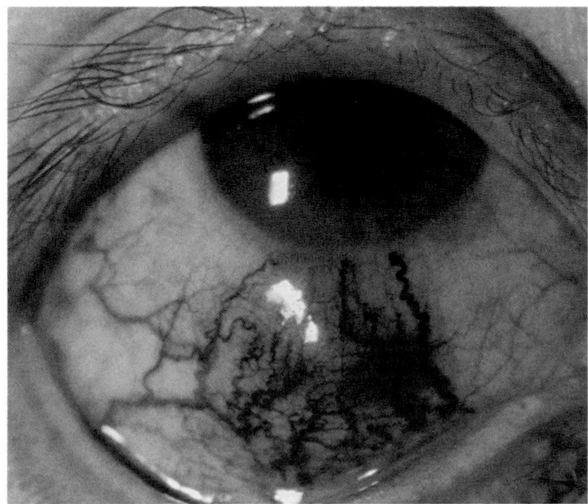

Episcleritis: The nontender, prominent, superficial dilated blood vessels of episcleritis are shown.

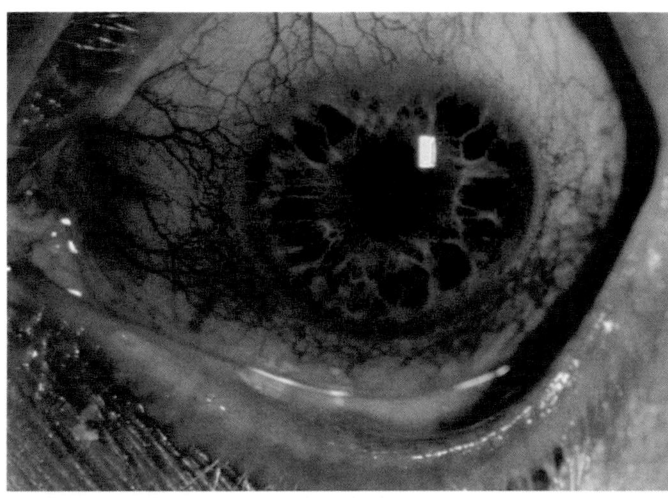

Iritis: Intense ciliary flush around the corneal-scleral junction and an irregularly shaped pupil is characteristic of iritis.

Age-Related Macular Degeneration

Dry AMD involves the deposition of extracellular material (drusen) in the macular region of one or both eyes and may cause diminished visual acuity. Smoking cessation is imperative. Progression of advanced dry AMD may be slowed with the use of zinc or antioxidants supplements.

A small percentage of patients with dry AMD will progress to develop new vessel growth under the retina (wet AMD). Bleeding and exudation results in sudden (or rapid onset over weeks), painless blurring or warping of central vision. Laser photocoagulation and intraocular injection of VEGF inhibitors is recommended for wet AMD.

Retinal Detachment

Retinal detachment occurs mainly in myopic patients. Symptoms are floaters, flashes of light (photopsias), and squiggly lines, followed by a sudden, peripheral visual field defect that resembles a black curtain and progresses across the entire visual field. Emergent ophthalmology referral is crucial, as prognosis depends on the time to surgical treatment.

Central Retinal Artery Occlusion

CRAO is caused by thrombi or emboli. Patients are usually elderly and present with profound and sudden painless vision loss.

Funduscopic examination reveals an afferent pupillary defect and cherry red fovea that is accentuated by a pale retinal background. Treatment may include measures to lower the intraocular pressure and emergent ophthalmology consultation.

Central Retinal Vein Occlusion

CRVO is usually caused by occlusion of the central retinal vein by a thrombus. Patients with CRVO present with sudden, painless, unilateral visual loss. Funduscopic examination may reveal afferent pupillary defect, congested retinal veins, scattered retinal hemorrhages, and cotton wool spots in the region of occlusion. Immediate ophthalmologic consultation is necessary.

Hearing Loss

Diagnosis

Appropriate initial tests for healing loss include the whispered voice test and finger rub test. The Weber and Rinne tests help distinguish conductive from sensorineural hearing loss.

STUDY TABLE: Conductive and Sensorineural Hearing Loss

Condition	Weber Test Result (Tuning fork to forehead)	Rinne Test Result (Tuning fork to mastoid then in front of ear)	Differential Diagnoses
Conductive hearing loss	Louder in the affected ear	Decreased in the affected ear (bone conduction > air conduction)	Cerumen impaction, foreign body, otitis media, otosclerosis, perforated tympanic membrane
Sensorineural hearing loss	Louder in the good ear	As loud or louder in the affected ear (air conduction > bone conduction)	Presbyacusis, Meniere disease, acoustic neuroma, sudden sensorineural hearing loss

In patients with a conductive hearing loss, a nonmobile tympanic membrane may indicate fluid or a mass in the middle ear or retraction from negative middle ear pressure. Sudden sensorineural hearing loss occurs acutely, usually within 12 hours of onset, and is unilateral in 90% of cases. It has many causes, including viral, vascular, autoimmune, and, most commonly, idiopathic.

Testing

Select audiography for all patients with unexplained hearing loss. For patients with progressive asymmetric sensorineural hearing loss, select MRI or CT to evaluate for acoustic neuroma.

Treatment

Treat otitis or cerumen impaction if present. Select urgent referral to an ENT specialist for sudden, unexplained hearing loss. The evidence for treatment with glucocorticoids is weak but frequently provided. For presbyacusis, hearing aids that amplify sound are often helpful.

TEST YOURSELF

A 35-year-old previously healthy man has had difficulty hearing in his right ear since last night. He has rhinorrhea and nasal congestion. His external auditory canals and tympanic membranes are normal; a 512-Hz tuning fork is placed on his forehead, and he hears the tone louder in his left ear than in his right ear.

ANSWER: For diagnosis, choose sudden sensorineural hearing loss. For management, select emergent ENT referral.

Otitis Media

Diagnosis

Acute otitis media is characterized by fluid and inflammation in the middle ear accompanied by symptoms of infection. Many patients first present with viral URI symptoms. Otitis media with effusion is characterized by fluid in the middle ear without signs of infection.

Treatment

Evidence on treatment in adults is lacking. However, analgesic therapy and decongestants are the mainstays of treatment. No evidence favors one antibiotic over another; amoxicillin is often selected. Complications include hearing loss, tympanic membrane perforation, meningitis, and mastoiditis.

External Otitis

Diagnosis

Patients with typical external otitis present with otalgia, ear discharge, pruritus, and conductive hearing loss. Be aware of the several other varieties of external otitis:

- Malignant external otitis is characterized by systemic toxicity and evidence of infection spread beyond the ear canal (mastoid bone, cellulitis) and is typically found in older adult patients with type 2 diabetes or patients who are immunocompromised. Most commonly caused by *Pseudomonas aeruginosa*.
- Ramsay Hunt syndrome is caused by varicella-zoster viral infection and characterized by facial nerve paralysis, sensorineural hearing loss, and vesicular lesions on and in the ear canal.

Treatment

Select combination antibiotic and glucocorticoid drops for typical external otitis, systemic antipseudomonal antibiotics and hospitalization for malignant external otitis, and antiviral agents for Ramsay Hunt syndrome.

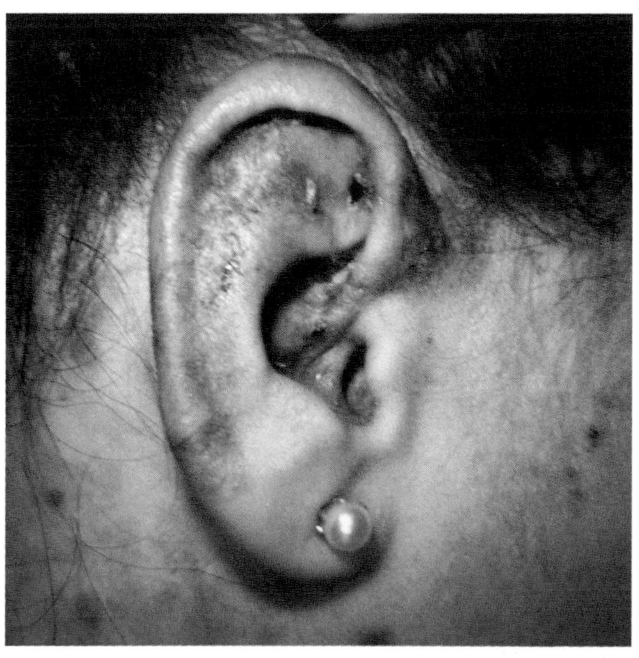

Ramsay Hunt Syndrome: These vesicular lesions on and in the ear canal are characteristic of Ramsay Hunt syndrome caused by varicella-zoster virus infection.

TEST YOURSELF

A 70-year-old man with type 2 diabetes mellitus has had a severe left earache since yesterday. He has a fever and tachycardia, and his left external ear canal is swollen. Moist white debris and granulation tissue are visible.

ANSWER: For diagnosis, choose malignant external otitis. For management, select hospitalization and IV ciprofloxacin.

Sinusitis

Diagnosis

Viral infection causes most cases of sinusitis. Bacterial sinusitis is more likely if the following are present:

- persistent symptoms (lasting >10 days)
- severe symptoms or fever (lasting 3-4 days)
- "double-sickness" characterized by worsening symptoms following a period of improvement over 3 to 4 days

Complications of acute sinusitis are unusual but deadly. Patients with cavernous sinus thrombosis have fever, nausea, vomiting, headache, orbital edema, or cranial nerve involvement. Other complications include brain abscess, bacterial meningitis, and osteomyelitis.

Testing

Imaging, including CT, should be considered in patients with AIDS or in other immunocompromised patients to evaluate for fungal infection or other atypical infections, but is not otherwise indicated.

Treatment

The first-line choice for suspected bacterial sinusitis is amoxicillin-clavulanate. Doxycycline is recommended for patients allergic to penicillin.

Allergic Rhinitis

Diagnosis

Rhinitis is an inflammation of the nasal mucosal membranes that causes rhinorrhea, nasal itching, sneezing, nasal congestion, and postnasal drainage.

Allergic rhinitis can be seasonal or perennial. Diagnosis of allergic rhinitis is usually made by history and confirmed with empiric treatment. If empiric treatment fails, diagnostic allergy testing may be appropriate to guide allergen avoidance or immunotherapy. Allergy skin testing is preferred to in vitro specific IgE antibody assay (or RAST).

In allergic rhinitis, the nasal mucosa is edematous and pale.

STUDY TABLE: Mimics of Allergic Rhinitis

Look for...	Diagnose...
Systemic illness with saddle nose deformity, nasal ulceration, or chronic sinusitis	Granulomatosis with polyarteritis
Nasal polyposis, asthma, eosinophilia, mononeuritis, petechial skin lesions	Eosinophilic granulomatosis with polyangiitis
Young person, nasal polyposis, chronic sinusitis, malnourishment, infertility, and chronic or recurrent bronchitis	Cystic fibrosis
Nonseasonal rhinitis with negative skin tests	Chronic nonallergic rhinitis (vasomotor rhinitis)
Refractory congestion after chronic use of topical nasal decongestants	Rhinitis medicamentosa
Nasal congestion in the last 6 or more weeks of pregnancy	Pregnancy rhinitis
Rhinitis, nasal polyps, asthma, and aspirin intolerance (respiratory symptoms)	Aspirin-exacerbated respiratory disease (triad asthma or Samter syndrome)

Treatment

Treatment includes the select removal of pets, animals, and carpet; allergy encasements for bedding; and small-particle filters for air conditioning.

Intranasal glucocorticoids are first-line therapy. Second-line agents include: intranasal antihistamines, oral combination antihistamines/decongestants, oral montelukast, or intranasal cromolyn. Ipratropium bromide is effective for severe rhinorrhea.

Choose skin testing and allergen immunotherapy if symptoms are not well controlled by intranasal glucocorticoids with supplemental antihistamines or decongestants.

The most consistently effective treatments for chronic nonallergic rhinitis are topical intranasal glucocorticoids, topical intranasal antihistamines, and topical ipratropium bromide. Patients with chronic rhinitis, nasal polyps, asthma, and aspirin intolerance may improve following aspirin desensitization.

DON'T BE TRICKED

- **Do not refer patients with allergic rhinitis for skin testing/immunotherapy without a trial of empiric therapy.**

TEST YOURSELF

For the past 2 months, a 30-year-old man has had nasal congestion that began with rhinorrhea, coughing, and sore throat. He has used oxymetazoline nasal spray since his symptoms started.

ANSWER: For diagnosis, select rhinitis medicamentosa. For management, choose to stop the topical decongestant and select a short course of prednisone or intranasal glucocorticoid.

Pharyngitis

Diagnosis

Use the 4-point Centor criteria to stratify adult patients according to risk of group A streptococcal pharyngitis:

- fever (subjective)
- absence of cough
- tender anterior cervical lymphadenopathy
- tonsillar exudates

Management is based on the number of Centor criteria present:

- <3: neither test nor treat with antibiotics
- ≥3: obtain a rapid antigen detection test (RADT); management is based on results

Fusobacterium necrophorum infection should be considered in adolescents and young adults with a negative RADT and an unusually prolonged and severe pharyngitis. *F. necrophorum* is the causative agent of Lemierre syndrome, septic thrombophlebitis of the internal jugular vein resulting in metastatic pulmonary infections.

Treatment

Select oral penicillin for 10 days. Choose a macrolide for patients allergic to penicillin. *F. necrophorum* is treated with ampicillin-sulbactam.

Depression

Screening

Routine screening is recommended for all adults, including postpartum women and older adults, utilizing the two-question model:

- "Over the past 2 weeks, have you felt down, depressed, hopeless?"
- "Over the past 2 weeks, have you felt little interest or pleasure in doing things?"

If screening is positive, further evaluation for depression is warranted.

Diagnosis

Major depressive disorder is diagnosed when at least five of the following symptoms are consistently present during the same 2-week period, at least one of which is depressed mood or loss of interest or pleasure:

- depressed mood
- loss of interest in daily activities
- weight loss or gain
- insomnia or hypersomnia
- psychomotor agitation or retardation
- fatigue
- feelings of worthlessness or guilt
- diminished ability to concentrate
- recurrent thoughts of death or suicide

Refer patients with a suicide plan or psychotic features to a psychiatrist, and hospitalize any patient (even against the patient's wishes) who is in imminent danger of harming himself or herself or others.

DON'T BE TRICKED

- **Select bipolar disorder if depression is accompanied by previous or current manic symptoms.**

Mimics of major depressive disorder:

- Situational adjustment reaction with depressed mood: depression with a clear precipitant. Usually resolves without medication following resolution of the acute stressor.
- Bipolar disorder: one or more manic or mixed manic and depressive episodes, usually accompanied by major depressive disorder.
- Seasonal affective disorder: a subtype of major depression, with onset during fall or winter and seasonal remission. Responds to phototherapy and SSRIs.
- Grief reaction: transient major depression may be present, but sadness without complete depression is more common. Pervasive and generalized guilt and persistent vegetative signs and symptoms are not consistent with normal grief. Loss of self-esteem is a symptom of depression rather than grief.
- PMDD: characterized by the cyclical recurrence of ≥5 symptoms of depression, anxiety, and emotional lability having their onset within 1 week before menstruation and resolution within 1 week after menstruation.
- Medical conditions: consider substance abuse, hypothyroidism, Cushing syndrome, Parkinson disease, and medications (interferon, glucocorticoids). Routine laboratory testing for these conditions is not warranted unless suggested by history and physical examination findings.

Treatment

For initial acute therapy, the 2016 clinical guideline from ACP recommends CBT or second-generation antidepressants. Any second-generation antidepressant can be used to treat major depressive disorder. Guide selection of an antidepressant by differences in side-effect profiles and personal or family history of response to a specific agent. Commonly tested treatment principles include:

- Sertraline is safe for patients with cardiovascular disease.
- Bupropion has fewer effects on sexual function and weight gain.
- Mirtazapine causes sedation and weight gain (useful for patients with insomnia or weight loss).
- Paroxetine is classified as pregnancy category D (do not use).

For patients in whom treatment with a single SSRI is unsuccessful, response does not differ whether patients receive a different SSRI, a non-SSRI antidepressant, a combination of two antidepressants, augmentation with lithium, or cognitive therapy. Therefore, in nonresponding patients, modify treatment (increase dose, switch, or add another drug) if the patient does not have ≥50% reduction in symptom score to pharmacotherapy within 6 to 8 weeks.

STUDY TABLE: Managing Duration of Antidepressant Therapy

Indications	Therapy
First episode of depression	Initiate treatment and continue at the dosage required to achieve remission for an additional 4-9 months.
First recurrence of depression	Increase maintenance treatment to one to two times the inter-episode interval (for example, choose 18-36 months if the second episode occurs 18 months after the first episode).
Three or more recurrences of depression, recurrence within 1 year of successful treatment, or suicide attempt	Select lifetime maintenance therapy.

Be alert for serotonin syndrome in patients taking SSRIs, particularly with concurrent use of other SSRIs, MAOIs, St. John's wort, trazodone, dextromethorphan, linezolid, tramadol, or buspirone. Mild symptoms include nausea, vomiting, flushing, and diaphoresis. Severe symptoms include hyperreflexia, myoclonus, muscular rigidity, and hyperthermia.

DON'T BE TRICKED

- Always ask about episodes of mania or hypomania before starting antidepressant therapy.
- Antidepressant drugs should not be stopped abruptly.
- Bereavement does not usually require pharmacologic treatment.

Bipolar Disorder

Diagnosis

Bipolar disorder features episodes of depression as well as periods of mania or hypomania. Manic findings include elevated, expansive, or irritable mood; hypersexuality; spending sprees; grandiosity; decreased need for sleep; and disruption of social or occupational functioning. Mimics of bipolar disorder include thyrotoxicosis, partial-complex seizures, SLE, and glucocorticoid side effects.

Treatment

Lithium is the most effective mood stabilizer, but long-term therapy carries significant side effects, including kidney disease, hypothyroidism, and DI. Anticonvulsants and second-generation antipsychotics are alternative first-line treatments. Monotherapy with SSRIs can unmask mania in patients with untreated bipolar disorder.

TEST YOURSELF

A 27-year-old woman requests thyroid medication to make her "stronger" because she wants to run for the senatorial position for the state of California. She is sleeping 2 to 3 hours per night and has not been eating. She spends her time writing her political action plan and shopping and has exceeded the limit on her credit card.

ANSWER: For diagnosis, choose mania.

Generalized Anxiety Disorder

Diagnosis

Generalized anxiety disorder is characterized by pervasive and excessive anxiety about a variety of events or activities, restlessness, difficulty concentrating, irritability, functional impairment, and sleep disturbance. Patients commonly have a comorbid psychiatric disorder.

Treatment

Cognitive behavioral therapy, with or without pharmacologic therapy, is first-line treatment for generalized anxiety disorder. SSRIs and SNRIs are effective. Benzodiazepines are acceptable for short-term use while titrating antidepressant doses, but dependence and tolerance complicate long-term use. Benzodiazepines should be avoided in patients with a history of substance abuse.

Social Anxiety Disorder

Diagnosis

Diagnostic criteria for social anxiety disorder include severe fear of social or performance situations resulting in symptoms such as blushing, dyspnea, palpitations, and emotional distress. Anxiety may be generalized or specific to a single activity.

Treatment

Treat social anxiety disorder with CBT and SSRIs.

Panic Disorder

Diagnosis

Diagnose panic attacks when ≥4 of the following are present:

- palpitations, sweating, and shortness of breath
- fear of dying
- chest pain
- nausea or abdominal distress
- unsteadiness, lightheadedness, faintness, paresthesias
- self-detached feeling

Panic disorder involves recurrent, unexpected attacks and persistent worry about future attacks.

Treatment

Cognitive behavioral therapy and SSRIs are first-line treatment. Long-acting benzodiazepines can be used as short-term therapy for disabling disorders until first-line treatments become effective.

DON'T BE TRICKED

- **Do not prescribe benzodiazepines as first-line, long-term treatment for panic disorder.**

Somatic Symptom and Related Disorders

Diagnosis

Diagnostic criteria for somatic symptom disorder are as follows:

- at least one somatic symptom causing distress or interference with daily life
- excessive thoughts, behaviors, and feelings related to the somatic symptom(s)
- persistent somatic symptoms for at least 6 months

Patients attribute their symptoms to an undiagnosed disorder despite multiple negative evaluations and are often not reassured despite repeated evaluations.

Treatment

The principles of therapy include regular office appointments with one physician. The patient should be reassured that life-threatening conditions have been ruled out and should be given a plausible explanation for the symptoms. Among all treatments, CBT has the broadest evidence of benefit.

DON'T BE TRICKED

- Choose malingering if a patient adopts a physical symptom for the purpose of gain.
- Choose factitious disorder if a patient adopts symptoms to remain in the sick role.
- Choose conversion disorder if a patient has abnormal sensation or motor function (such as limb weakness) that is not explained by a medical condition and is inconsistent with physical examination findings.
- Choose illness anxiety disorder (previously hypochondriasis) if the patient has excessive worry about general health and preoccupation with health-related activities.

Posttraumatic Stress Disorder

Diagnosis

Indicators suggesting PTSD include:

1. history of exposure to trauma
2. persistent re-experiencing of the traumatic event
3. avoidance of stimuli associated with the trauma
4. increased arousal

Assess for coexisting psychiatric disorders and domestic abuse.

Treatment

CBT is the treatment of choice for PTSD. Sertraline and paroxetine are adjuvant treatments.

DON'T BE TRICKED

- Do not prescribe benzodiazepines for PTSD.

Obsessive-Compulsive Disorder

Diagnosis

Obsessions are defined as persistent ideas, thoughts, impulses, or images that are intrusive and inappropriate and associated with significant anxiety or distress.

Compulsions are repetitive behaviors (handwashing, checking, and ordering) or mental acts (counting or repeating words silently) performed to try to decrease the anxiety or stress associated with the obsessions. The person must recognize that the obsessions or compulsions are excessive or unreasonable.

Treatment

Obsessive-compulsive disorder is treated with CBT and often with an SSRI.

Eating Disorders

Diagnosis

Anorexia nervosa consists of two types:

- restricting, in which patients restrict intake (anorexia nervosa)
- binge eating/purging, in which patients binge and purge to control weight (bulimia nervosa)

Diagnostic clues for the restricting type of anorexia include:

- low BMI
- fear of weight gain
- distorted body image
- amenorrhea

The medical complications include anemia, osteopenia, hypotension, electrolyte abnormalities, and arrhythmias. During the first few weeks of eating, patients are at risk for the refeeding syndrome, which can include cardiac arrest and delirium caused by exacerbation of hypophosphatemia and hypokalemia.

Diagnostic clues for **bulimia nervosa** are episodes of binging with loss of control followed by purging (vomiting, diuretic or laxative abuse), fasting, or excessive exercise. Patients usually have normal weight. Medical complications may be the presenting problem and can include acid-induced dental disease, esophageal tears, electrolyte derangements (low chloride and potassium), and metabolic alkalosis.

Treatment

For anorexia nervosa, CBT is considered first-line treatment. Psychotropic drugs do not work.

Patients with bulimia respond to CBT and antidepressants (fluoxetine or imipramine).

DON'T BE TRICKED

- **Do not choose bupropion for eating disorders because of the increased incidence of tonic-clonic seizures.**

TEST YOURSELF

A 24-year-old woman has reflux esophagitis, recurrent sore throat, and a dry cough. She exercises regularly and is "always dieting" because of her "weight problem." BMI is 25. On physical examination, the posterior pharynx and soft palate are injected without exudate. The tooth enamel is eroded.

ANSWER: For diagnosis, choose bulimia nervosa. For management, choose to begin CBT and fluoxetine.

Schizophrenia

Diagnosis

The following usually begin in mid to late adolescence:

- unusual perceptual experiences
- false beliefs
- illogical thoughts
- disorganized speech, such as frequent derailment or incoherence
- grossly disorganized or catatonic behavior
- negative symptoms, such as affective flattening, alogia (concrete replies to questions and restricted spontaneous speech), or avolition (inability to initiate and persist in goal-directed activities)

Treatment

Begin a second-generation antipsychotic agent (olanzapine, risperidone, quetiapine, aripiprazole), and refer patients to a psychiatrist.

Attention-Deficit/Hyperactivity Disorder

Diagnosis

ADHD usually first manifests in childhood and is characterized by inattention, hyperactivity, and impulsivity with functional impairment in at least two settings (home, work, school). ADHD is more prevalent in patients with mood disorders and substance abuse.

Treatment

Treat ADHD with stimulants (e.g., amphetamine or methylphenidate) but beware of the potential for abuse and use with caution in patients with hypertension or cardiovascular disease. Atomoxetine is an SNRI approved for treatment of ADHD in adults. Cognitive behavioral therapy may be used as an adjunctive therapy.

Falls

Diagnosis

Patients with a history of one fall in the last year or those who feel unsteady or unbalanced should be evaluated for balance or gait disturbance with a Timed Up and Go test. A time of longer than 12 s is abnormal, and the patient should be referred for full fall evaluation. Medications associated with fall risk (psychotropics, sedative/hypnotics) should be removed if possible.

Treatment

Multidisciplinary treatment programs that include assessment for risk factors (review of medications, sensory deficits), physical therapy, and risk factor modification are the most effective nonpharmacologic interventions for older patients.

Specific interventions for community-dwelling older adults:

- Prescribe exercise programs that emphasize balance, gait, and strength training (physical therapy or tai chi).
- Prescribe appropriate adaptive equipment (canes, walkers).
- Reduce polypharmacy (particularly psychoactive medications).
- Treat orthostasis and visual impairments.

DON'T BE TRICKED

- The USPSTF recommends against vitamin D supplementation to prevent falls in community-dwelling adults ≥65 years who are not known to have osteoporosis or vitamin D deficiency.
- Hip protectors in older people who fall are ineffective in preventing hip fractures.

TEST YOURSELF

An 80-year-old woman presents after a mechanical fall at home. Her medications are calcium, clonazepam, amlodipine, levothyroxine, and pantoprazole.

ANSWER: For management, choose to discontinue clonazepam and provide risk factor modification.

Urinary Incontinence

STUDY TABLE: Diagnosis and Treatment of Urinary Incontinence

If you see this...	Diagnose this...	Choose this...
Daytime frequency, nocturia, bothersome urgency	Urge incontinence	First-line therapy is bladder training; second-line therapy is anticholinergic drugs (oxybutynin, tolterodine)
Involuntary release of urine secondary to effort or exertion (sneezing, coughing, physical exertion)	Stress incontinence	First-line therapy is pelvic floor muscle training for women (Kegel exercises)
Urgency and involuntary release of urine	Mixed incontinence (urge and stress incontinence)	Bladder training and pelvic floor muscle training
Unable to get to bathroom on time because of mental or physical limitations	Functional incontinence	Portable commode, regular prompted urination with physical assistance to commode, treatment of underlying disorders
Nearly constant dribbling of urine, incomplete emptying of bladder, high postvoiding residual urine	Overflow incontinence	Timed urination, intermittent bladder catheterization

Obese women with either urge or stress incontinence will benefit from weight loss and exercise.

DON'T BE TRICKED

- Do not prescribe systemic estrogen-progestin therapy because it can worsen stress and urge incontinence.
- Do not order urodynamic testing because outcomes are no better than those associated with management based on clinical evaluation alone.

TEST YOURSELF

A 78-year-old woman has urinary urgency, nocturia, and urine loss with coughing and sneezing. Her medical history includes HF and glaucoma.

ANSWER: For diagnosis, select mixed incontinence. For management, choose initiation of pelvic muscle exercises and bladder training techniques.

Chronic Venous Insufficiency

Diagnosis

Characteristic symptoms and findings of chronic venous insufficiency include:

- leg heaviness, tiredness
- dependent leg edema

- hyperpigmentation, especially at medial ankle
- pruritus and eczema
- venous ulceration
- varicose or reticular veins

Treatment

First-line therapy includes compression (stockings, wraps, pumps) and leg elevation. Emollients are used for dry, itchy skin; topical glucocorticoids can be added for eczema.

DON'T BE TRICKED

- **Loop diuretic therapy is not recommended as first-line therapy for edema from chronic venous insufficiency.**

Pressure Injury

Diagnosis

Pressure injuries are ischemic soft tissue injuries resulting from pressure, usually over bony prominences. The external appearance may underestimate the extent of the injury.

Treatment

Advanced static mattresses and overlays (such as foam, gel, or air mattresses/overlays) help prevent pressure injuries in at-risk individuals.

STUDY TABLE: Pressure Injury Staging and Therapy

Ulcer Stage	Therapy
Stage 1: The skin is intact with nonblanchable redness	For all stages: positioning and support to minimize tissue pressure
Stage 2: Shallow ulcer with a red-pink wound bed or serum-filled blister	Occlusive or semipermeable dressing that will maintain a moist wound environment
Stage 3: Subcutaneous fat may be visible	Pain control, correction of identified nutritional deficiencies (supplements, tube feeding, or hyperalimentation if necessary), debridement, topical or systemic antibiotics
Stage 4: Exposed bone, tendon, or muscle	Same as Stage 3

Basic rules for treating pressure injuries:

- Air-fluidized beds enhance healing of pressure injuries compared with standard hospital mattresses.
- Dressings should maintain a moist wound environment and manage exudates.
- Restrict systemic antibiotics for cellulitis treatment (surrounding erythema, warmth, pain).
- Debride eschars and nonviable tissue.

DON'T BE TRICKED

- **Nutritional supplementation to enhance wound healing remains controversial.**
- **Hyperbaric oxygen therapy is not effective in the treatment of pressure injuries.**
- **Always consider the possibility of underlying osteomyelitis.**

Involuntary Weight Loss

Diagnosis

Causes of involuntary weight loss vary according to age (malignancy is most common in the young) and venue (depression, medications, dehydration, and issues related to dementia are most common in extended care facilities).

Weight loss is commonly associated with depression and dementia. Socioeconomic and functional problems, such as difficulty obtaining food, lack of financial resources, and social isolation, cause or exacerbate weight loss. Initial diagnostic testing is limited to basic studies (such as TSH level, HIV testing, age-appropriate cancer screening) unless the history and physical examination suggest a specific cause.

DON'T BE TRICKED

- **Imaging of the thorax and abdomen with CT or MRI in the absence of supporting history, physical examination, or laboratory findings is not helpful.**

Treatment

Treat the specific underlying disorder. The proven benefit of oral nutritional supplementation for weight loss is limited. Appetite stimulants have been shown to promote weight gain, but a survival benefit has never been demonstrated.

STUDY TABLE: Selected Nutritional Deficiencies

Finding	Deficiency
Hair loss, brittle hair	Biotin, protein, vitamin B_{12}, folate, iron
Petechiae, perifollicular hemorrhage, gingival bleeding	Vitamin C
Ecchymosis	Vitamins C and K
Skin pigmentation, cracking, and crusting	Niacin
Acro-orificial dermatitis (erythematous, vesiculobullous, and pustular)	Zinc
Angular stomatitis and cheilosis	Vitamin B complex, iron, and protein
Glossitis	Niacin, folate, and vitamin B_{12}
Ophthalmoplegia and foot drop	Thiamine
Paresthesia	Thiamine, vitamin B_{12}, and biotin
Depressed vibratory and position senses	Vitamin B_{12}
Memory disturbance	Vitamin B_{12}
Wernicke-Korsakoff syndrome	Severe thiamine deficiency

Perioperative Medicine

Preoperative Testing

Routine diagnostic testing is not indicated preoperatively. Do not obtain:

- routine preoperative laboratory studies in healthy patients undergoing elective or low-risk surgery
- preoperative chest radiography in the absence of cardiopulmonary symptoms
- repeat laboratory studies within 6 months of surgery in the absence of a clinical change

Cardiovascular Risk Assessment

Patients with an elevated risk of a major adverse cardiac event ≥1% and an estimated functional capacity of <4 METs should undergo pharmacologic stress testing if the results will change management.

Activities requiring the equivalent of ≥4 METs:

- climbing a flight of stairs
- walking up a hill without stopping
- running a short distance
- lifting or moving heavy furniture
- participating in moderate-exertion sporting activities such as bowling or golf

Obtain an ECG within 1 to 3 months of surgery (except low-risk surgery) in any patient with:

- CAD
- significant arrhythmias
- cerebrovascular disease (stroke or TIA)
- PAD

DON'T BE TRICKED

- Patients with a functional capacity ≥4 METS can undergo surgery.
- If a patient has no history, symptoms, or risk factors for CAD, no preoperative coronary evaluation is necessary, including ECG.
- Low-risk surgeries (cataract extraction, carpal tunnel release, breast biopsy, inguinal hernia repair) do not require cardiac testing even if a calculated risk score is elevated.
- Do not obtain troponin and BNP levels or CTA to assess cardiac risk.
- No survival benefit is associated with revascularization in stable patients with CAD unless they otherwise meet the general requirements for revascularization.

Cardiovascular Risk Management

Patients with a known recent major adverse cardiac event should not undergo surgery within:

- 60 days of an MI
- 30 days of a bare-metal coronary stent implantation
- 6 months of a drug-eluting coronary stent placement

Continue perioperative β-blockade in patients who are already on a β-blocker.

Continue statins to reduce perioperative cardiac risk reduction.

DON'T BE TRICKED

- Do not choose routine postoperative surveillance with ECG or cardiac biomarkers unless symptoms of an ACS are present.

Pulmonary Perioperative Management

Screen all surgical patients for OSA with a validated tool such as the STOP BANG survey. Obtain polysomnography for patients with presumed OSA and initiate CPAP for patients with severe OSA undergoing high-risk elective surgical procedures.

The greatest benefit from smoking cessation comes from quitting >8 weeks before surgery.

Select lung expansion maneuvers (deep breathing exercises, incentive spirometry, intermittent positive pressure breathing, CPAP) to prevent pulmonary complications.

DON'T BE TRICKED

- Do not order spirometry for risk assessment in the absence of dyspnea or hypoxia of uncertain cause.

Perioperative Management of Anticoagulant Therapy

Anticoagulation must be stopped for most surgical procedures except those with minimal expected blood loss (cataract surgery, dermatologic procedures, endoscopic procedures without biopsy).

- Stop warfarin 5 days before surgery.
- Stop apixaban, rivaroxaban, dabigatran 1 to 2 days before surgery if eGFR >50 mL/min/1.73 m^2. Stop earlier if eGFR is lower.

Bridging anticoagulation is providing heparin during the perioperative period until an oral anticoagulant is resumed.

- Low-risk patients do not receive bridging anticoagulation (bileaflet mechanical aortic valve, AF with $CHADS_2$ score <2, VTE >12 months ago).
- High-risk patients receive bridging anticoagulation (mitral or caged ball valve or aortic tilting disc aortic mechanical valve, AF with $CHADS_2$ score >4, rheumatic heart disease, recent CVA or TIA, VTE within the past 3 months)

Stopping and restarting perioperative anticoagulation:

- Start heparin 36 hours after the last dose of warfarin.
- Stop UFH 4 to 6 hours before surgery.
- Stop LMWH 12 hours before surgery.
- Restart heparin 24 hours after surgery.
- Restart warfarin 12 to 24 hours after surgery.
- Restart dabigatran, rivaroxaban, and apixaban 24 hours after surgery.

Hematology

Aplastic Anemia and Paroxysmal Nocturnal Hemoglobinuria

Diagnosis

Aplastic anemia is a disorder in which hematopoietic stem cells are severely diminished, resulting in hypocellular bone marrow and pancytopenia. All cell lines are involved. Autoimmune attack on stem cells is the most common identifiable cause. Other causes include toxins, ionizing radiation, drugs, nutritional deficiencies, and infections. Some patients have an associated thymoma. Patients with aplastic anemia are at increased risk of developing acute leukemia and MDS.

Aplastic anemia, PNH, and MDS are all acquired defects of hematopoietic stem cells, so clinical overlap is considerable. PNH results from a genetic mutation of membrane proteins that ameliorate complement-mediated destruction of erythrocytes. PNH is characterized by:

- chronic hemolytic anemia
- iron deficiency through urinary losses
- venous thrombosis (including Budd-Chiari syndrome)
- pancytopenia

Testing

The basic evaluation of patients presenting with pancytopenia includes:

- bone marrow aspirate and biopsy (hypocellular with increased fat content)
- cytogenetic analysis to exclude other bone marrow disorders (e.g., MDS)
- PNH screening flow cytometry with cell surface markers CD55 and CD59 absent
- vitamin B_{12} and folate levels, hepatitis serologies, and HIV testing

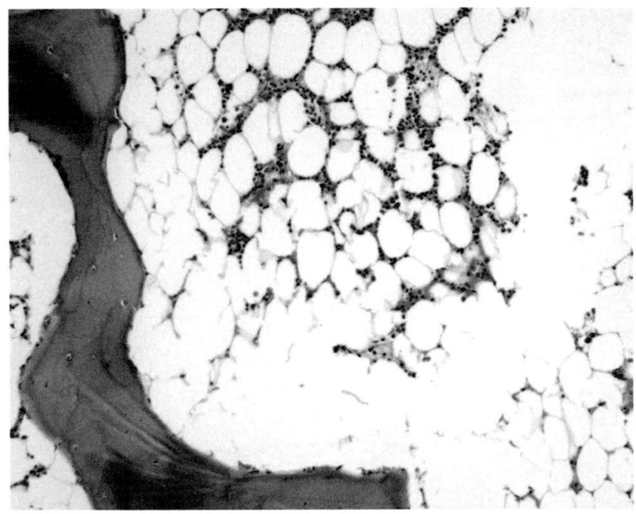

Aplastic Anemia: Profoundly hypocellular bone marrow is characteristic, with the marrow space composed mostly of fat cells and marrow stroma.

Treatment

Initial treatment of **aplastic anemia** involves withdrawal of any potentially causative agents. Immunosuppression with cyclosporine and antithymocyte globulin is first-line therapy and leads to disease control in 70% of adult patients.

Allogeneic HSCT is a potentially curative therapy and should be considered for those younger than 50 years.

In symptomatic patients with PNH, eculizumab reduces intravascular hemolysis, hemoglobinuria, and the need for transfusion. Allogeneic HSCT can lead to long-term survival. Prophylactic anticoagulation and supplementation with iron and folic acid are indicated in all patients.

DON'T BE TRICKED

- Treatment of aplastic anemia with hematopoietic growth factors is ineffective.
- PNH may present as a DAT-negative hemolytic anemia or as aplastic anemia.

Pure Red Cell Aplasia

Diagnosis

Acquired chronic pure red cell aplasia is characterized by the absence or a marked decrease of erythrocyte production with normal leukocyte and platelet counts. The cause is predominately T cell autoimmunity (pregnancy, thymoma, malignancy) or direct toxicity to erythrocyte precursors (viral infection, drug toxicity).

Testing

Bone marrow shows profound erythroid hypoplasia. Clonal CD57-positive T cells consistent with large granular lymphocytosis are often found.

The basic evaluation is similar to that for pancytopenia but includes CT of the chest to rule out thymoma.

Treatment

Patients with pure red cell aplasia are treated with:

- transfusion support and immunosuppressive drugs (prednisone, cyclosporine, antithymocyte globulin)
- thymectomy for thymoma
- IV immune globulin for patients with AIDS and chronic parvovirus B19 infection
- methotrexate or cyclosporine for large granular lymphocytosis

Neutropenia

Diagnosis

Isolated neutropenia usually has a hereditary, immune, infectious, or toxic cause.

- acute HIV, CMV, EBV
- Rickettsial infection
- cytotoxic chemotherapies
- NSAIDs, carbamazepine, phenytoin, propylthiouracil, cephalosporins, trimethoprim-sulfamethoxazole
- SLE, RA

Large granular lymphocytes may be identified in Felty syndrome (RA, splenomegaly, neutropenia).

Treatment

Remove the offending drug.

Granulocyte colony-stimulating factor can shorten the duration of neutropenia associated with chemotherapy, although it is not used routinely unless neutropenia is complicated by infection.

Treat immune-associated neutropenia (e.g., Felty syndrome) with immunosuppressive therapy (antithymocyte globulin, cyclosporine, prednisone).

Myelodysplastic Syndromes

Diagnosis

MDS are clonal disorders of the hematopoietic stem cells that occur predominantly in patients older than 60 years and are characterized by ineffective hematopoiesis and peripheral cytopenias. The differential diagnosis includes vitamin B_{12} or folate deficiency, alcohol- or drug-induced cytopenias, acute leukemia, and myeloproliferative syndromes.

Most patients eventually progress to acute leukemic syndromes or die of complications of bone marrow failure.

Testing

Bone marrow findings show a hypercellular marrow with dysplastic erythroid precursors. Look for cytopenia in at least two lines (anemia, leukopenia, thrombocytopenia) and morphologic abnormalities of erythrocytes (macrocytosis with nucleated erythrocytes and teardrop cells).

Patients may present only with anemia, an elevated MCV, and normal vitamin B_{12} and folate levels.

Detection of clonal abnormalities commonly involving chromosomes 3, 5, 7, 8, and 17 supports the diagnosis. Look for −5q syndrome, a subtype of MDS that has a specific therapy.

Treatment

Many patients with low-risk MDS (by IPSS-R score) require no treatment at all or infrequent transfusions.

In some patients needing frequent transfusions, erythropoiesis-stimulating agents (ESAs) can decrease transfusion burden.

Patients considered high or very high risk by IPSS-R criteria require treatment to prevent AML.

Allogeneic HSCT is offered to fit younger patients and azacytidine and decitabine to persons at high or very high risk for AML transformation who are not bone marrow transplant candidates.

Use lenalidomide for the specific treatment of −5q syndrome, because more than two thirds of patients with this syndrome will respond.

TEST YOURSELF

A 74-year-old man has a hemoglobin concentration of 7.5 g/dL, leukocyte count of 2200/µL, and platelet count of 87,000/µL. The peripheral blood smear shows a few nucleated erythrocytes. Bone marrow shows hypolobulated neutrophils.

ANSWER: For diagnosis, choose MDS.

Myeloproliferative Neoplasms

The MPNs are caused by acquired genetic defects in myeloid stem cells and are characterized by deregulated production of leukocytes, eosinophils, erythrocytes, or platelets. Although each disorder is named according to the dominant cell line affected, all can cause an elevation in several cell lines.

The MPNs may present with unusual thromboses, massive splenomegaly, or systemic symptoms. Each has a chronic phase that may progress to AML, although the degree of risk varies.

Chronic Myeloid Leukemia

Diagnosis: CML is characterized by myeloid proliferation associated with translocation of chromosomes 9 and 22 [t(9;22), the Philadelphia chromosome]. Patients usually present in the chronic phase. CML may transform into acute leukemia. The transformation may be recognized as an accelerated phase or as blast crisis (AML).

Characteristic findings in asymptomatic patients are splenomegaly, an elevated leukocyte count, and an increased number of granulocytic cells in all phases of maturation on the peripheral blood smear. When blasts represent more than 10% of the leukocytes, accelerated (10%-20%) or blast phase (>20%) is diagnosed.

Testing: The diagnosis is confirmed by the presence of the Philadelphia chromosome in molecular testing for *BCR-ABL* gene in the peripheral blood or cytogenetic analysis of the bone marrow. The *BCR-ABL* gene produces a mutant, activated tyrosine kinase that leads to constant downstream proliferative signaling.

STUDY TABLE: Treatment for CML

Treatment	Goal
Hydroxyurea	Palliative, only to alleviate leukocytosis and splenomegaly
Tyrosine kinase inhibitors: imatinib mesylate, dasatinib, and nilotinib	Disease control with lifelong treatment
Allogeneic HSCT	Potential cure for some patients with accelerated disease or blast crisis

DON'T BE TRICKED

- **All tyrosine kinase inhibitors can prolong the QT interval; periodic ECG monitoring is recommended.**

TEST YOURSELF

An asymptomatic 54-year-old man has an enlarged spleen. The hemoglobin concentration is 13 g/dL, leukocyte count is 170,000/µL, and platelet count is 470,000/µL, with mostly segmented and band neutrophils and circulating metamyelocytes and myelocytes. Eosinophilia and basophilia are present.

ANSWER: For diagnosis, choose CML. For management, order cytogenetic analysis of bone marrow cells or *BCR-ABL* gene detection in the peripheral blood.

Essential Thrombocythemia

Diagnosis: Essential thrombocythemia, the most common MPN, is characterized by thrombotic and hemorrhagic complications. It is marked by a predominant increase in megakaryocytes and platelet counts greater than 450,000/µL in the absence of secondary causes for reactive thrombocytosis, including iron deficiency, bleeding, cancer, infection, and chronic inflammatory disease. Many patients are asymptomatic. When they occur, symptoms include:

- vasomotor disturbances such as erythromelalgia (red and painful hands or feet with warmth and swelling)
- livedo reticularis
- headache
- vision symptoms
- arterial or venous thromboses

Splenomegaly (up to 50%) may be present. The *JAK2* mutation is found in about half of patients and helps distinguish essential thrombocythemia from secondary thrombocythemia.

Treatment: Low-risk patients (age <60 years, no previous thrombosis, leukocyte count <11,000/µL) may be treated with low-dose aspirin, which reduces vasomotor symptoms.

High-risk nonpregnant patients are treated with hydroxyurea in addition to aspirin.

Plateletpheresis is used when the platelet count must be reduced quickly in life-threatening situations such as TIA, stroke, MI, or GI bleeding.

DON'T BE TRICKED

- **The most common causes of thrombocythemia are iron deficiency anemia and infection and will improve within a couple of weeks following iron replacement or resolution of the infection, respectively.**
- **A negative *JAK2* test does not exclude the diagnosis of essential thrombocythemia.**

TEST YOURSELF

A 67-year-old man is evaluated because of red, warm, painful feet and a platelet count of 975,000/µL.

ANSWER: For diagnosis, choose essential thrombocythemia. For management, prescribe hydroxyurea. Low-dose aspirin can be used to treat the erythromelalgia.

Polycythemia Vera

Diagnosis: PV causes erythropoietin-independent (low erythropoietin level) proliferation of erythrocytes. PV is suspected when the hemoglobin level is >16.5 g/dL in men or >16 g/dL in women after secondary causes are excluded. Most causes of secondary erythrocytosis are associated with an elevated erythropoietin level, although a markedly elevated erythropoietin level suggests ectopic production by a renal cell cancer or other kidney disease. Causes of secondary polycythemia include hypoxemia (most common), volume contraction because of diuretics, use of androgens, and secretion of erythropoietin by kidney or liver carcinoma.

Characteristic findings are thrombosis or bleeding, facial plethora, erythromelalgia, pruritus exacerbated by bathing in hot water, and splenomegaly. Serious complications may include TIA, MI or stroke, DVT, and Budd-Chiari syndrome.

Testing: Patients with PCV have a low serum erythropoietin level in the setting of erythrocytosis.

An activating mutation of *JAK2* is present in 97% of patients with PV.

Microscopic hematuria may be the only sign of an erythropoietin-producing hypernephroma as the cause of an elevated hemoglobin and erythrocyte count.

Treatment: Therapeutic phlebotomy should be instituted with the goal of lowering the hematocrit level to <45%.

Hydroxyurea in addition to phlebotomy is often the treatment of choice for patients at high risk for thrombosis (e.g., >60 years, previous thrombosis, leukocytosis).

Low-dose aspirin is indicated unless strong contraindications exist.

DON'T BE TRICKED

- **Hepatic vein thrombosis (the Budd-Chiari syndrome) or portal vein thrombosis should prompt consideration of PV.**
- **Do not prescribe high-dose aspirin, which may cause increased bleeding.**

TEST YOURSELF

A 67-year-old man has intolerable pruritus. He does not smoke and takes no medications. The hematocrit value is 60%, and he has splenomegaly.

ANSWER: For diagnosis, choose PV. For management, order PCR for *JAK2* mutation, and measure the erythropoietin level.

Primary Myelofibrosis

Diagnosis: Primary myelofibrosis is the result of clonal proliferation of abnormal hematopoietic stem cells that release fibrosis-promoting cytokines. The disorder is characterized by massive splenomegaly, normocytic anemia, circulating erythroblasts and myeloid precursors, giant platelets, teardrop erythrocytes, and bone marrow fibrosis. Splenomegaly and hepatomegaly result from extramedullary hematopoiesis, and patients can develop portal hypertension. Death commonly results from bone marrow failure, transformation to acute leukemia, or portal hypertension complications.

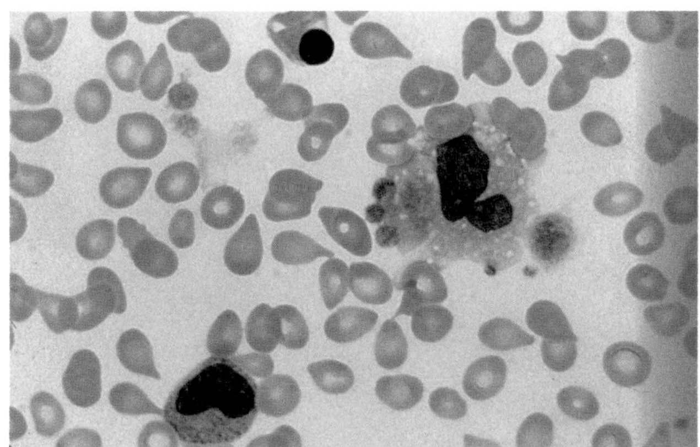

Myelofibrosis: Peripheral blood smear showing teardrop erythrocytes, nucleated erythrocytes, and giant platelets characteristic of myelofibrosis.

Treatment is usually supportive.

Hydroxyurea and ruxolitinib (a *JAK2* inhibitor) may alleviate splenomegaly and constitutional symptoms.

Allogeneic HSCT is indicated for patients <60 years of age.

DON'T BE TRICKED

- **Splenectomy should be avoided because it is associated with hemorrhagic and thrombotic complications, increased risk of progression to leukemia, and no effect on survival.**

Eosinophilia and Hypereosinophilic Syndromes

HES are characterized by eosinophil counts greater than 1500/µL; eosinophilic infiltrates of the liver, spleen, heart, and lymph nodes; and systemic symptoms. HES may have a reactive or primary cause. Primary HES is an MPN with molecular activation of platelet-derived growth factor receptor (PDGFR) α or β.

For patients with activating mutations of PDGFR, imatinib leads to durable responses. Otherwise, glucocorticoid therapy is used.

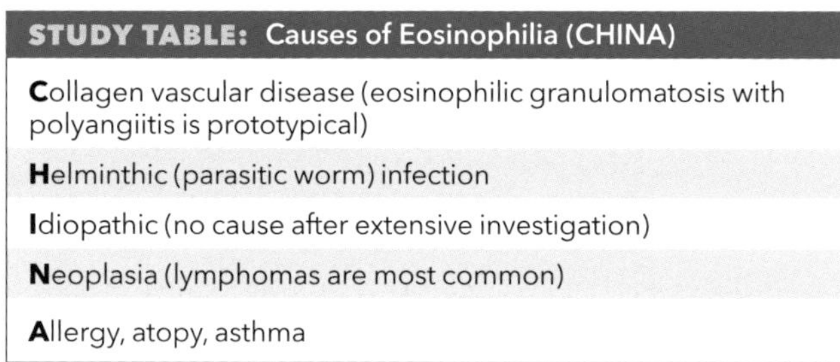

STUDY TABLE: Causes of Eosinophilia (CHINA)
Collagen vascular disease (eosinophilic granulomatosis with polyangiitis is prototypical)
Helminthic (parasitic worm) infection
Idiopathic (no cause after extensive investigation)
Neoplasia (lymphomas are most common)
Allergy, atopy, asthma

Acute Lymphoblastic Leukemia

Diagnosis

ALL is an extremely aggressive disease of precursor T or B cells. The usual presenting clinical features include rapidly rising blast cells in the blood and bone marrow, bulky lymphadenopathy (especially in the mediastinum), a younger age at onset, and cytopenia secondary to bone marrow involvement. Up to 30% of patients with ALL have CNS involvement.

Treatment

Induction therapy involves intensive combination chemotherapy often followed by allogeneic HSCT.

CNS prophylaxis (intrathecal chemotherapy with or without radiation) is also indicated.

Patients who are positive for the Philadelphia chromosome [t(9;22)] can be treated with the tyrosine kinase inhibitor dasatinib, in addition to chemotherapy and allogenic HSCT.

Acute Myeloid Leukemia

Diagnosis

AML is a malignant clonal proliferation of myeloid cells that do not fully mature. AML can appear de novo; arise after exposure to radiation, benzene, or chemotherapy; or occur as a result of transformation of an MPN.

Of all the leukemias, AML will most likely involve significant thrombocytopenia with bleeding, bruising, petechiae, and infection. Patients with AML seldom develop lymphadenopathy or hepatosplenomegaly; if present, these findings suggest an alternative or concomitant diagnosis. When the leukocyte count is very high, patients may present with leukostasis syndrome characterized by CNS manifestations, hypoxia, and diffuse infiltrates on chest x-ray.

The diagnosis of AML is suggested by an elevated leukocyte count, anemia, thrombocytopenia, and blasts on peripheral blood smear.

Gingival hypertrophy and leukemia cutis (violaceous, nontender cutaneous plaques) are commonly encountered. Pathognomonic Auer rods may be seen on a peripheral blood smear.

Testing

The diagnosis is confirmed by bone marrow aspiration and biopsy showing >20% myeloblasts.

Cytogenetic studies can classify patients into risk (for relapse) and prognostic categories:

- favorable risk: t(8;21), inv(16), t(15;17)
- high risk: complex genetic abnormalities (≥5 abnormalities); -5, -7, -5q, or 3q abnormalities

Acute promyelocytic leukemia is a special case marked by the t(15;17) translocation, which disturbs a retinoic acid receptor. Patients with acute promyelocytic leukemia have significant bleeding because of fibrinolysis and DIC.

Tumor lysis syndrome may develop in treated patients and causes a release of intracellular urate, potassium, and phosphorus.

DON'T BE TRICKED

- **In older patients, acute leukemia may present with pancytopenia, but bone marrow examination will demonstrate a hypercellular marrow with 20% or more blasts.**

Treatment

Platelet transfusion is indicated for patients with hemorrhage or a platelet count <10,000/µL.

All-*trans* retinoic acid (ATRA) is the backbone of treatment for acute promyelocytic leukemia. Patients taking ATRA or arsenic trioxide are at risk for developing differentiation syndrome. Characteristic findings are fever, pulmonary infiltrates, hypoxemia, and, occasionally, hyperleukocytosis. Treatment is dexamethasone.

Because of the high rate of early mortality in patients with acute promyelocytic leukemia, it is critical to start ATRA therapy as soon as the diagnosis is suspected.

Chemotherapy is used for non-promyelocytic leukemia (e.g., cytarabine and an anthracycline, azacitidine, or decitabine for older and frail patients).

Leukapheresis is used for symptoms of leukostasis syndrome (typical leukocyte count >50,000/µL).

Allogeneic and autologous HSCT is used for high-risk patients in first complete remission, first relapse, or second complete remission.

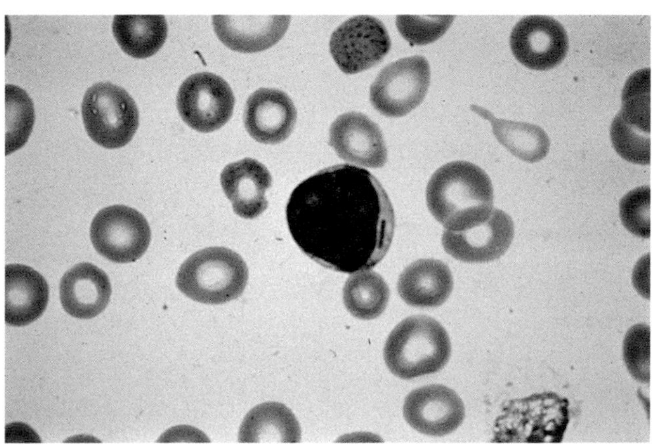

Auer Rod: This myeloblast has findings associated with AML: a large nucleus, displaced nuclear chromatin, azurophile cytoplasmic granules, and a rod-shaped inclusion (Auer rod).

DON'T BE TRICKED

- **Tumor lysis syndrome may be the first manifestation of AML.**

Plasma Cell Dyscrasias

Plasma cell dyscrasias consist of abnormal clonal proliferation of immune globulin–secreting differentiated B lymphocytes and plasma cells. Multiple myeloma is the most common malignant plasma cell dyscrasia. Other plasma cell dyscrasias include monoclonal gammopathy of undetermined significance (MGUS), Waldenström macroglobulinemia, and light-chain–associated amyloidosis (AL amyloidosis).

Multiple Myeloma

The CRAB mnemonic encompasses most myeloma-related signs and symptoms:

- C (hyper**C**alcemia)
- R (**R**enal failure)
- A (**A**nemia)
- B (**B**one disease: lytic lesions, fractures, or osteoporosis)

Testing: Diagnostic tests for multiple myeloma include CBC; serum chemistries; SPEP; 24-hour UPEP; serum and urine immunofixation assays; serum free light chain testing; and serum IgG, IgA, and IgM measurements. Think of multiple myeloma in patients with a low anion gap.

For non-IgM gammopathies, a skeletal survey (plain x-rays of the skeleton) assesses for the presence of lytic bone lesions or osteopenia.

IgM gammopathies are more likely associated with B-cell lymphomas, and CT of the chest, abdomen, and pelvis should be performed in patients with unexplained fevers or weight loss, sweats, lymphadenopathy, or hepatosplenomegaly.

MGUS and multiple myeloma are characterized by a serum monoclonal protein. Patients with MGUS should be periodically reassessed after initial diagnosis for development of asymptomatic myeloma, multiple myeloma, or AL amyloidosis.

STUDY TABLE: Diagnosis of Multiple Myeloma and MGUS

Multiple Myeloma/MGUS	Findings
MGUS	Serum monoclonal protein <3 g/dL Bone marrow clonal plasma cells <10% No end-organ damage
Monoclonal gammopathy of renal significance	See Nephrology; Monoclonal Gammopathies and Cryoglobulinemia
Smoldering multiple myeloma	Serum monoclonal protein ≥3 g/dL Bone marrow clonal plasma cells ≥10% No end-organ damage
Multiple myeloma requiring therapy	Serum monoclonal protein present Bone marrow clonal plasma cells ≥10% End-organ damage present (see CRAB mnemonic)

Most smoldering multiple myeloma progresses to multiple myeloma requiring therapy or AL amyloidosis.

DON'T BE TRICKED

- **In patients with back pain, MRI should also be performed to assess for spinal cord impingement.**
- **Do not use bone scans in patients with suspected myeloma because they are not as sensitive as a skeletal survey.**

Treatment: Treat multiple myeloma requiring therapy with induction chemotherapy, including some combination of:

- a proteasome inhibitor (bortezomib)
- an immunomodulatory agent (thalidomide or lenalidomide)

- a glucocorticoid (prednisone or dexamethasone)
- an alkylating agent (melphalan or cyclophosphamide) for nontransplant candidates

Following induction chemotherapy, autologous HSCT followed by high-dose melphalan may be considered.

DON'T BE TRICKED

- Do not treat MGUS.
- Do not use melphalan induction therapy in candidates for HSCT.
- Bortezomib and thalidomide are associated with a high risk of peripheral neuropathy.
- Patients taking thalidomide, lenalidomide, or pomalidomide are at increased risk of VTE.

AL Amyloidosis

Diagnosis: AL amyloidosis is found in 10% of patients with multiple myeloma but may be diagnosed in patients who lack other myeloma findings.

Findings in AL amyloidosis include:

- nephrotic syndrome with enlarged kidneys on ultrasonography
- delayed gastric emptying, intestinal pseudo-obstruction, malabsorption
- hepatomegaly, elevated aminotransferase levels, and portal hypertension
- distal sensorimotor polyneuropathy
- restrictive cardiomyopathy with granular appearance on echocardiography, low voltage ECG
- bleeding diathesis, periorbital purpura, factor X deficiency with prolonged PT and aPTT
- macroglossia

Testing: Confirmation of AL amyloidosis requires:

- abdominal fat pad aspirate or bone marrow biopsy demonstrating apple green birefringence under polarized light with Congo red staining
- κ/λ light-chain detection and typing
- presence of an M protein on serum or urine testing or clonal plasma cells in the marrow

Treatment: Treatment algorithms for AL amyloidosis are similar to those for multiple myeloma.

DON'T BE TRICKED

- **Abdominal fat pad or bone marrow biopsy has a high yield and is safer than liver, kidney, or heart biopsy in establishing the diagnosis.**

Waldenström Macroglobulinemia

Diagnosis: WM is a neoplastic infiltrate consisting of:

- clonal lymphocytes, plasmacytoid lymphocytes, plasma cells, and immunoblasts comprising >10% of the bone marrow cellularity ***or***
- M-protein level >3 g/dL ***and***
- presence of disease-related signs, symptoms, or organ dysfunction

Lymphadenopathy, hepatomegaly, and splenomegaly are found on physical examination. One third of patients will have hyperviscosity symptoms including headache, blurred vision, hearing loss, dizziness, altered mental status, and nasal and mucosal bleeding. Funduscopic evaluation may reveal hyperviscosity-related findings (dilated retinal veins, papilledema, flame hemorrhages).

Treatment: Waldenström macroglobulinemia hyperviscosity syndrome is a medical emergency treated with plasmapheresis.

Normocytic Anemia

Diagnosis

Normocytic anemia is associated with a normal MCV of 80 to 100 fL. The reticulocyte count can help differentiate the cause.

Increased reticulocyte count: Normocytic anemia with an increased absolute reticulocyte count (>100,000/µL) reflects either erythrocyte loss (bleeding or hemolysis) or response to therapy (iron, folate, or cobalamin).

Decreased reticulocyte count: Normocytic anemia with a lower than expected reticulocyte count indicates underproduction anemia:

- inflammation with deficient erythropoietin (most frequent cause)
- nutritional deficiencies (iron, folate, cobalamin)
- hypometabolism (hypothyroidism, testosterone deficiency)
- a primary hematopoietic disorder (pure red cell aplasia or myelodysplasia)

Iron deficiency and inflammatory anemia are often confused (see Study Table). A serum ferritin level >100 ng/mL rules out iron deficiency.

STUDY TABLE: Differentiating Iron Deficiency and Inflammatory Anemia

Test	Iron Deficiency Anemia	Inflammatory Anemia
Serum iron	Low	Low
Ferritin	Low	High
TIBC	High	Low
Transferrin saturation	Low (<10%)	Low/Normal

Testing

STUDY TABLE: Diagnostic Studies for Normocytic Anemia

Test	Comments
FOBT/FIT	Indicated for all patients; 33% of patients with iron deficiency have a normal MCV
Peripheral blood smear	Used to detect spherocytes, fragmented erythrocytes (schistocytes), or blister cells with associated hemolysis
DAT	If spherocytes are found
Hemoglobin electrophoresis	If target or sickle cells are found
Lead level	If basophilic stippling is found
Bone marrow aspiration and biopsy	If leukopenia, thrombocytopenia, myelocytes, or nucleated erythrocytes (in normocytic, microcytic, or macrocytic anemias) are found; if patient has lymphadenopathy or splenomegaly

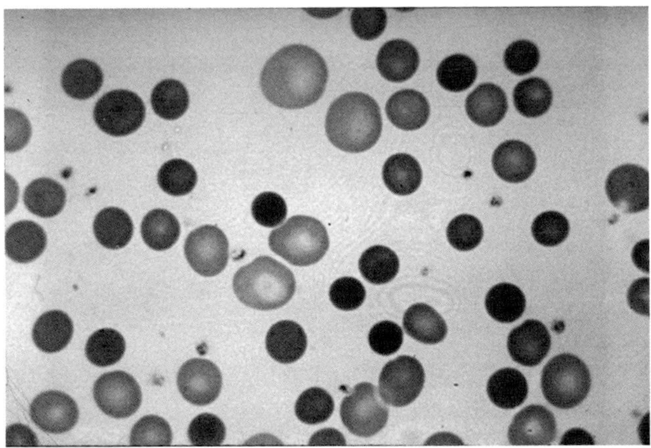

Spherocytes: This peripheral blood smear shows small erythrocytes with loss of usual central pallor. Consider acquired immune hemolytic anemia and hereditary spherocytosis.

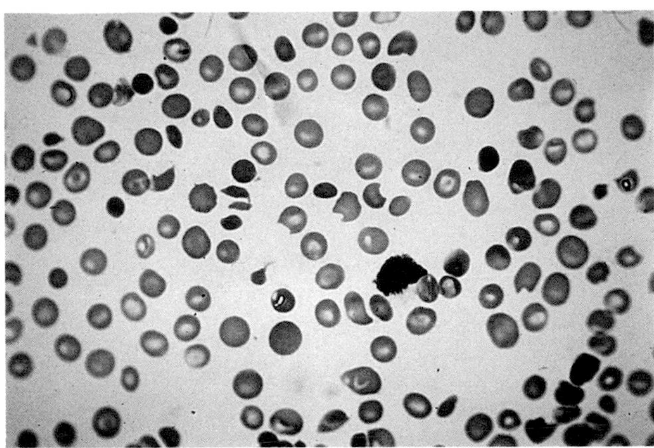

Erythrocyte Fragmentation: The erythrocytes show marked anisocytosis and poikilocytosis with prominent fragmentation. Consider DIC, TTP, mechanical heart valve, or malignant hypertension.

Treatment

Treat the underlying condition resulting in normocytic anemia.

Inflammatory anemia is usually not severe and rarely requires therapy.

Microcytic Anemia

Microcytic anemia is associated with an MCV of <80 fL.

The most common cause of microcytic anemia is iron deficiency, usually related to menstrual or GI blood loss or malabsorption syndromes (celiac disease). Other causes include inflammatory disorders and lead intoxication. Patients with microcytic anemia since childhood should be evaluated for the thalassemia trait, other hemoglobinopathies (thalassemia), or ineffective erythropoiesis (hereditary sideroblastic anemia).

Iron Deficiency Anemia

Diagnosis: The hallmark of iron deficiency is a microcytic hypochromic anemia. Signs and symptoms of iron deficiency include restless legs syndrome, hair loss, and spoon nails (koilonychia).

As hemoglobin levels decline, erythrocytes become heterogeneous in size (anisocytosis) and shape (poikilocytosis).

An elevated platelet count (usually not >1 million/µL) may be found in early disease.

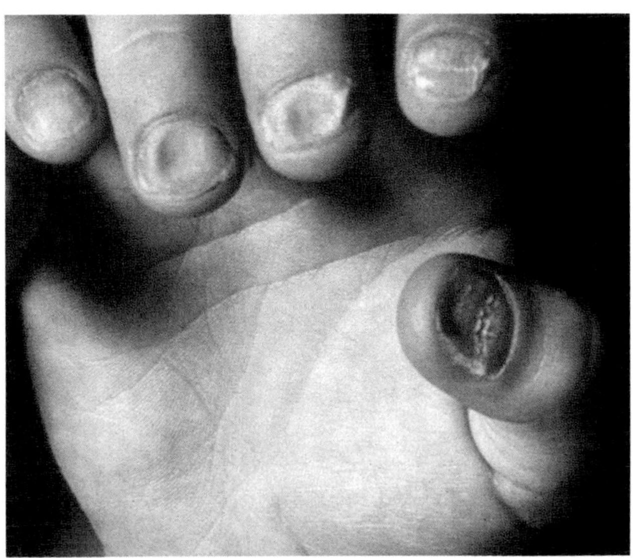

Koilonychia: Koilonychia is the upward curving of the distal nail plate, resulting in a spoon-shaped nail. Koilonychia is associated with iron deficiency anemia and other systemic conditions and may be idiopathic.

Testing

Diagnostic studies:

- serum iron and ferritin levels and TIBC
- hemoglobin electrophoresis if iron studies are normal
- endoscopy studies, starting with colonoscopy, if unexplained positive FOBT/FIT or iron deficiency is present

Serum ferritin levels are the most useful test in the diagnosis of iron deficiency. However, because ferritin is an acute-phase reactant, it has less diagnostic value in patients with infection or inflammatory disorders.

Virtually all patients with serum ferritin levels <14 ng/mL are iron deficient.

Treatment

The least expensive oral iron replacement, iron sulfate, is as effective as any of the more expensive oral preparations.

Oral iron every other day for 6 months is the standard treatment. Parenteral iron preparations are indicated only for patients who cannot tolerate or absorb oral iron or who are receiving hemodialysis.

Transfusion is reserved for severely symptomatic anemia.

DON'T BE TRICKED

- **In iron deficiency, abnormalities in iron studies typically occur first, followed by anemia and then morphologic changes in the cell.**

TEST YOURSELF

A 20-year-old woman with iron deficiency anemia does not respond to oral iron therapy. Review of systems is remarkable for IBS.
ANSWER: For diagnosis, test for celiac disease.

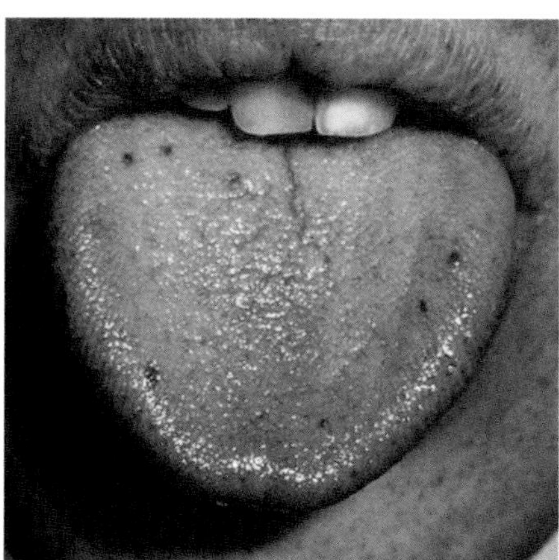

Hereditary Hemorrhagic Telangiectasia: Hereditary hemorrhagic telangiectasia can be associated with mucocutaneous telangiectasias that occur on the face, lips, tongue, buccal mucosa, fingertips, and dorsum of the hand, and are associated with GI bleeding in up to one third of patients.

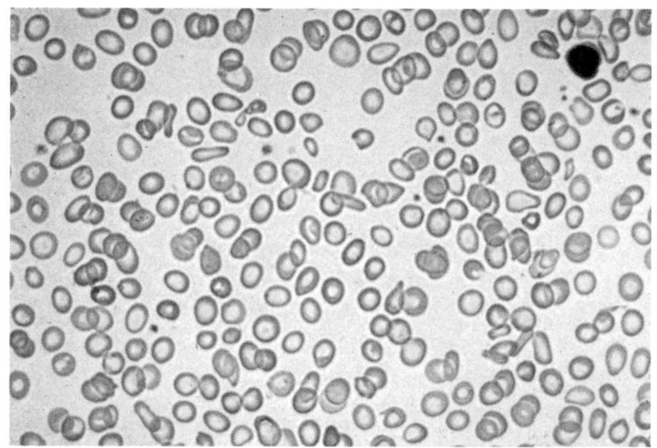

Microcytic Anemia: The erythrocytes show hypochromia, anisocytosis, and poikilocytosis. Erythrocytes in thalassemia have less variability in size and shape, and target cells are seen.

Macrocytic Anemia

Diagnosis

Macrocytic anemia is associated with an MCV of >100 fL. Macro-ovalocytes and hypersegmented neutrophils (>5 lobes) may also be present. Causes include:

- folate and/or cobalamin deficiencies
- drugs affecting folate metabolism and/or DNA synthesis (alcohol, zidovudine, hydroxyurea, methotrexate)
- acquired causes of megaloblastic maturation such as the MDS

Anemia associated with an MCV >115 fL is almost always a result of megaloblastic disorders. Because megaloblastic causes of anemia affect trilineage hematopoiesis, leukopenia and thrombocytopenia may accompany anemia.

Macrocytic anemia may also be caused by nonmegaloblastic disorders.

- Large target cells (MCV 105-110 fL) and echinocytes (burr cells with multiple undulating spiny erythrocyte membrane projections) signify membrane changes associated with liver disease.
- Diminished splenic function (hyposplenism or asplenia) results in large target cells, acanthocytes (erythrocytes with only a few rather than many spiny membrane projections), Howell-Jolly bodies, and variable numbers of nucleated erythrocytes.

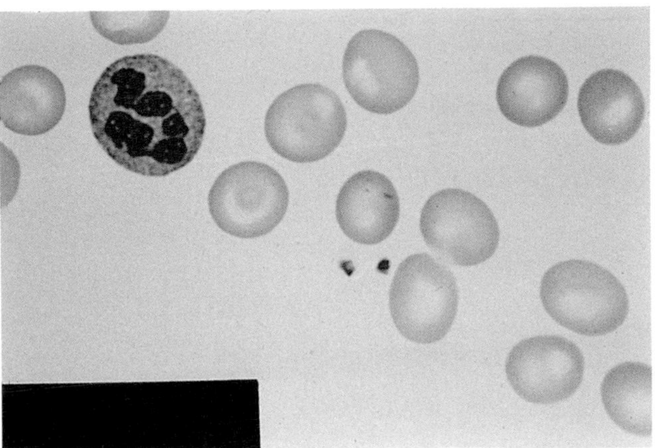

Hypersegmented Polymorphonuclear Cell: The erythrocytes are large ovalocytes, and a single PMN cell has more than 5 nuclear lobes. Consider vitamin B_{12} or folate deficiency (megaloblastic anemia).

Testing

If serum vitamin B_{12} levels are borderline low (200-300 pg/mL), measure serum methylmalonic acid and homocysteine levels. Elevated levels confirm vitamin B_{12} deficiency; elevated homocysteine and normal methylmalonic acid levels are associated with folate deficiency.

Treatment

High-dose oral vitamin B_{12} supplementation of 1000 to 2000 µg/d is usually as effective as parenteral administration and should be the initial therapy for most patients.

Patients with severe anemia, neurologic dysfunction, or those not responding to oral replacement require parenteral B_{12} injections.

Malabsorption syndromes always require parenteral vitamin B_{12}.

Folate deficiency can be treated with oral folic acid, 1 to 5 mg/d, until complete hematologic recovery; oral therapy is effective even in malabsorption conditions.

DON'T BE TRICKED

- **Reticulocytosis (e.g., secondary to hemolysis) can increase the MCV.**
- **Vitamin B_{12} deficiency can present with subacute combined degeneration of the spinal column (weakness, paresthesias, ataxia) without anemia or macrocytosis.**
- **Folate supplementation can improve the anemia of B_{12} deficiency but not prevent the associated neurologic sequelae.**

Hemolytic Anemia

Diagnosis

Characteristic findings are anemia, splenomegaly, elevated reticulocyte count, elevated LDH and indirect bilirubin, decreased haptoglobin, and elevated MCV (caused by reticulocytosis).

Hemolytic anemia can be either congenital or acquired.

Congenital hemolytic anemias include hemoglobinopathies (sickle cell), disorders of the erythrocyte membrane (hereditary spherocytosis), enzyme defects (glucose-6-phosphate dehydrogenase deficiency), and thalassemia syndromes.

In **acquired hemolytic anemia**, hemolysis can occur secondary to medications (fludarabine, bendamustine, quinine, penicillins, α-methyldopa); can be immune in nature; or can occur secondary to micro- or macroangiopathic processes, infections, or physical agents.

Examining the peripheral blood smear is central to identifying erythrocyte morphologies that implicate certain hemolytic mechanisms.

STUDY TABLE: Peripheral Blood Smear Findings in Hemolytic Anemia

Finding	Diagnosis
Schistocytes and thrombocytopenia	TTP HUS, DIC, HELLP
Schistocytes in a patient with a prosthetic heart valve	Valve leak
Erythrocyte agglutination	Cold agglutinin hemolysis (*Mycoplasma* infection, lymphoproliferative diseases, CLL)
Spherocytes	Autoimmune hemolytic anemia or hereditary spherocytosis
Target cells	Thalassemia, other hemoglobinopathy, or liver disease
Sickle cells	Sickle cell anemia
Bite cells	G6PD deficiency (suggested by eccentrically located hemoglobin confined to one side of the cell)

STUDY TABLE: Tests for Hemolytic Anemia

Test	Condition
DAT (Coombs test)	Warm autoimmune hemolytic anemia
Cryohemolysis test and eosin-5-maleimide binding test	Hereditary spherocytosis
Cold agglutinin measurement	Cold agglutinin disease
Hemoglobin electrophoresis	Thalassemia or other hemoglobinopathy
G6PD activity measurement	Test 2-3 months after hemolytic event to detect deficiency (normal enzyme concentration after a hemolytic episode)
Flow cytometry for CD55 and CD59 proteins	PNH

Treatment

All patients with sickle cell anemia or other hemolytic anemias require pneumococcal (both 23- and 13-valent), *Haemophilus influenzae* type B, influenza, and meningococcal vaccinations.

All patients with chronic hemolytic anemia require folic acid supplements.

Severe symptomatic anemia: transfusion even if fully matched erythrocytes are not available.

Warm autoimmune hemolytic anemia: initial therapy is glucocorticoids. Alternative agents are available for patients unresponsive to glucocorticoids or splenectomy.

Cold agglutinin disease: primary therapy is cold avoidance or rituximab for persistent symptoms; glucocorticoids or splenectomy are usually ineffective.

TTP: emergent plasma exchange.

Hereditary spherocytosis and transfusion-dependent thalassemias: splenectomy.

Severe thalassemia: HSCT is standard therapy.

Severe PNH: eculizumab or HSCT.

DON'T BE TRICKED

- A personal or family history of anemia, jaundice, splenomegaly, or gallstones suggests hereditary spherocytosis.

TEST YOURSELF

A previously healthy 28-year-old woman with a negative family history has weakness and a palpable spleen. Hemoglobin concentration is 7.2 g/dL and the reticulocyte count is 9.8%. Peripheral blood smear shows an occasional spherocyte.

ANSWER: For diagnosis, choose DAT to establish diagnosis of autoimmune hemolytic anemia. For management, select glucocorticoids.

Sickle Cell Disease

Diagnosis

The sickle cell syndromes can be diagnosed by hemoglobin electrophoresis.

Most clinical findings in sickle cell disease are related to vaso-occlusion from sickled erythrocytes. Characteristic findings include elevated reticulocyte, platelet, and leukocyte counts, and sickle cells on a peripheral blood smear.

Aplastic crisis is common and may result from coexisting infection, especially parvovirus B19 infection.

Several complications of sickle cell disease mimic other diseases. Keep the following diagnostic points in mind:

ACS (acute chest syndrome) vs. pneumonia, fat embolism, and PE:

- ACS is usually characterized by pulmonary infiltrates, fever, chest pain, tachypnea, and hypoxemia (and is often treated empirically as pneumonia).
- Fat embolism presents with chest pain, fever, dyspnea, hypoxia, thrombocytopenia, and multiorgan failure, and may be associated with fat bodies in bronchial washings or sputum.
- Presence of lower extremity thrombophlebitis may help differentiate PE from ACS, but pulmonary CT arteriography may be needed.

Cholecystitis vs. hepatic crisis:

- Chronic hemolysis may result in gallstones and acute cholecystitis.
- Fever, RUQ pain, and elevated aminotransferase levels may also be caused by ischemic hepatic crisis; abdominal ultrasonography can differentiate between the two.

Sickle cell anemia vs. aplastic crisis:

- Anemia that decreases by ≥2 g/dL during a painful crisis could be caused by aplastic crisis.
- Aplastic crisis could be caused by parvovirus B19 infection or cytotoxic drugs or be idiopathic.
- The reticulocyte count is decreased with aplastic crisis.

STUDY TABLE: Long-Term Complications of Sickle Cell Disease

If you see this...	Think this...
Chronic pain involving hips and shoulders	Osteonecrosis (avascular necrosis)
CVAs	Ischemic infarction in children and hemorrhage in adults
Chronic exertional dyspnea	HF or pulmonary hypertension
Infection with encapsulated organisms	Functional asplenia
Liver disease	Viral hepatitis, iron overload from transfusions, or ischemic-induced hepatic crisis
Impotence	Prolonged or repeated episodes of priapism
Proteinuria	CKD
Isosthenuria (inability to concentrate urine)	CKD
Decreased visual acuity	Retinopathy

Treatment

Vaso-occlusive crisis is managed with hydration, supplemental oxygen for hypoxemia, treatment of any precipitating event, and opioids.

The three common disease-altering strategies are hydroxyurea therapy, prophylactic exchange transfusion, and HSCT.

- **Hydroxyurea** is used for patients with more than two pain crises each year or for those with ACS.
- **Exchange transfusion** is indicated for patients with an acute stroke, fat embolism, or ACS. Use prophylactic exchange transfusion for patients with a history of ischemic stroke.
- **HSCT** should be considered for patients with severe symptoms unresponsive to transfusions and hydroxyurea or end-organ damage.

Because of transfusion-related complications, persons with sickle cell disease should not receive transfusion unless they have significant symptoms from their anemia or signs of end-organ failure (acute neurologic symptoms, ACS, multiorgan failure). The transfusion target is hemoglobin level <10 g/dL (hemoglobin A level >70%). Do not transfuse patients with simple vaso-occlusive pain.

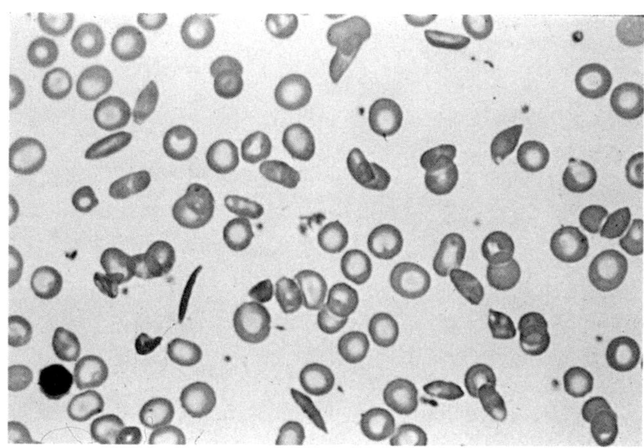

Sickle Cells: Erythrocyte anisocytosis and poikilocytosis involving several sickle cells.

Simple transfusion to a hemoglobin level of 10 g/dL has been shown to be equivalent to exchange transfusions in low- to medium-risk surgeries (e.g., adenoidectomy, inguinal hernia repair, cholecystectomy, joint replacement).

Erythropoietin is used for patients with severe anemia, low reticulocyte counts, and CKD.

DON'T BE TRICKED

- Hydroxyurea is contraindicated in pregnancy and kidney failure.
- Do not use meperidine to treat painful crises because the accumulation of the metabolite normeperidine can lead to seizures.
- Iron overload resulting from multiple transfusions may require chelation therapy.

TEST YOURSELF

A 32-year-old woman with sickle cell disease has a low-grade fever and exertional dyspnea. Hemoglobin concentration is 4.2 g/dL, and the reticulocyte count is 0.2%.

ANSWER: For diagnosis, choose aplastic crisis caused by parvovirus B19 infection.

Thalassemia

Diagnosis

Hemoglobin is a tetrameric molecule. The two α-globin chains and two β-globin chains are linked to heme (iron and protoporphyrin) and reversibly bind one molecule of oxygen. The thalassemic syndromes result from defects in synthesis of α or β chains and lead to ineffective erythropoiesis and hemolysis. Patients with α-thalassemia or β-thalassemia have microcytosis and target cells on the peripheral blood smear and may have splenomegaly.

STUDY TABLE: α-Thalassemia		
Gene Deletion	**Clinical Syndrome**	**Treatment**
(-α/αα) [single-gene deletion]	Silent carrier state that is clinically normal	None
(- -/αα; or -α/-α) [two-gene deletion]	α-Thalassemia trait; mild microcytic anemia; normal or elevated erythrocyte count; normal hemoglobin electrophoresis	None
(- -/-α) [three-gene deletion]	Hemoglobin H (β_4); severe anemia and usually early death	Intermittent transfusion
(- -/- -) [four-gene deletion]	Hydrops fetalis; fetal death	In utero transfusion

β-Thalassemia is most common among persons from the Mediterranean, Southeast Asia, India, and Pakistan. β-Thalassemia results from several abnormalities in the β-gene complex. Decreased β-chain synthesis leads to impaired production of hemoglobin A ($\alpha_2\beta_2$) and resultant increased synthesis of hemoglobin A_2 ($\alpha_2\delta_2$) and/or hemoglobin F ($\alpha_2\gamma_2$).

STUDY TABLE: β-Thalassemia		
Condition	**Characteristics**	**Treatment**
β-Thalassemia major (Cooley anemia)	Two-gene deletion leading to either no production or severely limited production of β-globin	Transfusion, iron chelation; consider splenectomy and HSCT
β-Thalassemia minor (β-thalassemia trait)	A single β-gene leading to reduced β-globin production with no or mild anemia	None
β-Thalassemia intermedia	Intermediate severity, such as in those who are compound heterozygotes of two thalassemic variants	Intermittent transfusion, iron chelation

β-Thalassemia trait and α-thalassemia trait are most commonly confused with iron deficiency anemia.

STUDY TABLE: Iron Deficiency Anemia and β-Thalassemia Trait		
Iron Deficiency Anemia	**α-Thalassemia Trait**	**β-Thalassemia Trait**
Low serum ferritin level	Normal serum ferritin level	Normal serum ferritin level
Low erythrocyte count	Normal or high erythrocyte count	Normal or high erythrocyte count
High RDW	Normal RDW	Normal RDW
Normal hemoglobin electrophoresis	Normal hemoglobin electrophoresis	Elevated hemoglobin A_2 and fetal hemoglobin

RDW = red cell distribution width.

DON'T BE TRICKED

- **β-Thalassemia can be associated with iron overload even in the absence of transfusion therapy.**

Treatment

Treatment of β-thalassemia varies with the type of disease:

- β-Thalassemia minor requires no treatment.
- β-Thalassemia major requires early-onset, lifelong transfusion therapy.
- Iron chelation therapy may be indicated if serum ferritin concentrations exceed 1000 ng/mL.
- Allogeneic HSCT is indicated for severe β-thalassemia major.

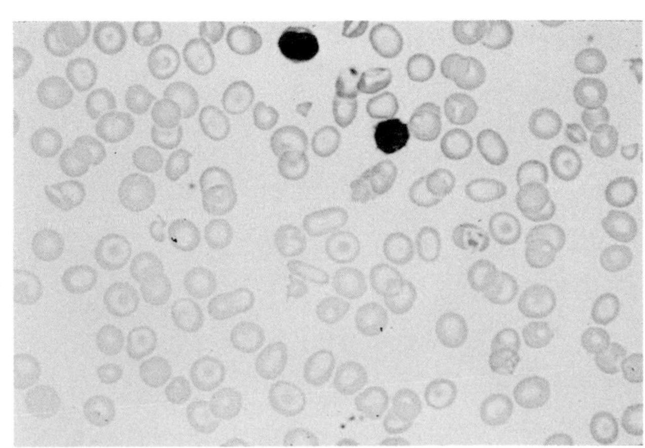

Thalassemia: Microcytosis, hypochromia, and target cells consistent with thalassemia.

TEST YOURSELF

An asymptomatic 18-year-old man has a hemoglobin concentration of 13 g/dL, an MCV of 64 fL, and a reticulocyte count of 4.0%.

ANSWER: The diagnosis is β-thalassemia or α-thalassemia trait. For management, select serum ferritin measurement and hemoglobin electrophoresis.

Approach to Bleeding Disorders

Diagnosis

Bleeding disorders are characterized by defects in primary and secondary hemostasis. Primary hemostasis involves the formation of a platelet plug at the site of vascular disruption. Secondary hemostasis is initiated by the exposure of tissue factor at the site of vascular damage and the initiation of the coagulation cascade.

- A mucocutaneous bleeding pattern (epistaxis, gingival bleeding, easy bruising, and menorrhagia) is the hallmark of primary hemostasis failure.
- Secondary hemostasis failure is characterized by bleeding into muscles and joints as well as delayed bleeding.
- Excessive bleeding after childbirth, surgery, or trauma can occur in either category.

The following tests are used when evaluating bleeding disorders:

- **The PT and aPTT** monitor for factor deficiencies and factor inhibitors.
- **A mixing study** differentiates factor deficiency from factor inhibitor by mixing patient plasma with normal plasma and retesting the PT and aPTT.
- **Bleeding time** identifies platelet disorders and vessel-wall integrity; the commercially available Platelet Function Analyzer-100 (PFA-100) also assesses platelet function.
- **Thrombin time** tests the conversion of fibrinogen to fibrin.
- **Fibrinogen, fibrinogen degradation products, and D-dimer** are used to identify excessive fibrinolysis.

Common Acquired Bleeding Disorders

Diagnosis and Treatment

Liver disease: Patients with liver failure have prolonged PT and aPTT values owing to decreased levels of coagulation factors. Despite this, patients are not protected against thrombosis, because protein C and S levels and antithrombin levels are low as well. Fibrinogen levels are low, and the fibrinogen may be dysfunctional. Patients experiencing bleeding may require vitamin K, cryoprecipitate, FFP, or platelets.

Vitamin K deficiency: Patients with liver disease and a prolonged PT require oral or subcutaneous vitamin K. Active bleeding because of vitamin K deficiency is treated with FFP. Depending on the severity of the bleeding and urgency, other options include prothrombin complex concentrate and FFP or 4f-PCC.

Factor inhibitors: Bleeding mimics hemophilia A and B. A factor inhibitor is diagnosed with a mixing study that fails to correct the coagulation abnormality. This disorder may be associated with an underlying condition such as SLE or malignancy (either lymphoproliferative or solid tumor) but is more commonly idiopathic. Bleeding is treated with activated factor concentrate, and the patient should receive immunosuppression to decrease the inhibitor levels.

DIC: Characteristic findings are thrombocytopenia, prolonged PT and aPTT, decreased plasma fibrinogen level, and elevated serum D-dimer. Schistocytes are seen on a peripheral blood smear. Treatment for active bleeding is platelet and coagulation factor replacement and management of the underlying disorder.

STUDY TABLE: Management Strategy for Elevated INRs and Bleeding in Patients Taking Warfarin			
INR	**Bleeding**	**Risk Factors for Bleeding**	**Intervention**
<5	No	N/A	Lower or omit next VKA dose(s) Reduce subsequent dose(s)
5-9	No	No	Omit next VKA dose(s) Reduce subsequent dose(s)
5-9	No	Yes	Vitamin K 1-2.5 mg PO
>9	No	N/A	Vitamin K 2.5-5 mg PO
Serious bleeding at any INR	Yes	N/A	Vitamin K 10 mg IV + 4f-PCC (or 3f-PCC + FFP or rfVIIa)

STUDY TABLE: Differential Diagnoses for Patients Experiencing Bleeding	
Clotting Assay Abnormality	**Differential Diagnoses**
Prolonged PT, normal aPTT	Factor VII deficiency or inhibitor DIC Liver disease Vitamin K deficiency Warfarin ingestion
Normal PT, prolonged aPTT	Deficiency of factors VIII, IX, XI, or XII vWD (if severe and factor VIII level is quite low) Heparin exposure
Prolonged PT and aPTT	Deficiency of factors V, X, II, or fibrinogen Severe liver disease, DIC, vitamin K deficiency, or warfarin toxicity Heparin overdose
Normal PT and aPTT	Platelet dysfunction (acquired and congenital) vWD (if mild and factor VIII level is not too low) Scurvy Ehlers-Danlos syndrome Hereditary hemorrhagic telangiectasia Deficiency of factor XIII

Hemophilia

Diagnosis

Factor VIII (hemophilia A) and factor IX (hemophilia B) deficiencies

- are X-linked disorders with clinical manifestations seen almost exclusively in men.
- should be considered in patients with a personal or family history of spontaneous, excessive posttraumatic or unexpected surgical bleeding.
- can be missed until adulthood when mild.

Up to one third of patients with hemophilia A may develop factor VIII inhibitor antibody. The presence and quantity of inhibitor are measured with the Bethesda assay, and the level of the assay determines therapy.

Factor XI deficiency

- is rare and is most prevalent in persons of Ashkenazi Jewish descent.
- typically does not cause excessive bleeding; patients have a prolonged aPTT but normal PT, thrombin time, and bleeding time.

Inherited factor XII deficiency is also rare and usually does not cause excessive bleeding; it is associated with a prolonged aPTT.

Testing

The PT is normal and the aPTT is prolonged in hemophilia A and B.

The results of a mixing study will normalize in a patient with a factor deficiency but will remain abnormal if an inhibitor is present.

Treatment

Transfusions and factor VIII or factor IX replacement are indicated for patients with hemophilia A or B, respectively, and severe bleeding or hemarthrosis.

Patients with mild hemophilia A should be given desmopressin for acute bleeding or before undergoing minimally invasive procedures (e.g., dental procedures).

Prophylactic factor replacement has been proven to reduce the incidence of arthropathy in patients with severe hemophilia.

If factor VIII inhibitor is present in low quantities (<5 Bethesda units), factor VIII replacement can overcome the inhibitor and control bleeding.

Higher levels of inhibitor may require activated prothrombin complex concentrate to control bleeding.

TEST YOURSELF

A 57-year-old man has a large left-sided ecchymosis. The hemoglobin concentration is 8 g/dL, platelet count is 220,000/µL, PT is 12 s, and aPTT is 67 s. The abnormal aPTT does not correct with a mixing study.

ANSWER: For diagnosis, choose acquired factor VIII inhibitor.

von Willebrand Disease

Diagnosis

The most common inherited bleeding disorder is vWD, an autosomal codominant disorder.

Clinically, patients have mild-to-moderate bleeding evidenced by nosebleeds, heavy menstrual flow, gingival bleeding, easy bruising, and bleeding associated with surgery or trauma.

vWF adheres platelets to injured vessels and acts as a carrier for factor VIII.

Secondary hemostatic dysfunction can occur because of concomitantly low factor VIII levels in vWD. This distinction is important for treatment purposes.

Testing

Diagnostic testing includes a prolonged bleeding time and a normal or prolonged aPTT.

Definitive diagnosis is based on the vWF antigen level, vWF activity assay, factor VIII level, and a multimer study used to diagnose subtypes of vWD.

Treatment

For mild symptoms, estrogen-containing oral contraceptives can regulate menstrual bleeding and increase vWF levels in women.

DDAVP is used for mild-to-moderate bleeding or before minor invasive procedures (e.g., dental procedures).

Intermediate-purity factor VIII concentrates, which contain vWF, can also be given for more severe bleeding.

DON'T BE TRICKED

- **Do not use cryoprecipitate to treat vWD because of its increased transfusion infection risk.**

TEST YOURSELF

A 33-year-old man is evaluated for continued bleeding following a tooth extraction. His mother has easy bruising, and his sister required a transfusion following the birth of her first child. The hemoglobin concentration is 13 g/dL, and the platelet count is 210,000/µL.

ANSWER: The diagnosis is vWD. For management, select an aPTT and bleeding time as initial diagnostic studies.

Thrombocytopenia

Thrombocytopenia is caused by decreased platelet production, accelerated destruction from consumptive disorders (such as TTP) or autoimmune-mediated destruction, or sequestration of platelets in conditions causing splenomegaly. Disorders associated with decreased bone marrow production often affect other cell lines, causing additional cytopenias. Common causes of nonimmune thrombocytopenia include:

- toxins (alcohol)
- idiosyncratic drug reactions
- metastatic cancer
- infections
- vitamin B_{12} or folate deficiency
- acute leukemia
- MDS
- aplastic anemia

Consumptive thrombocytopenia: Thrombocytopenia and the presence of schistocytes on the peripheral blood smear suggest DIC, TTP, and HUS.

Immune thrombocytopenia occurs when antibodies targeting platelet antigens mediate accelerated destruction. The characteristic finding is isolated thrombocytopenia in a patient without other apparent causes for the reduced platelets. Antibodies arise in three distinct clinical settings: drug induced, disease associated, and idiopathic.

- **Drug-induced ITP** is most often linked to heparin and certain antibiotics, but any new drug, supplement, or herbal remedy could be causative. Discontinuation of the offending drug should result in platelet recovery.
- **Disease-associated immune thrombocytopenia** causes include HIV, hepatitis C infection, hyperthyroidism, hypothyroidism, SLE, and lymphoproliferative malignancy.
- **Idiopathic immune thrombocytopenia** (immune thrombocytopenic purpura) is suggested by a peripheral blood smear that shows reduced numbers of large platelets and normal erythroid and myeloid cells in the absence of other identifiable causes. A bone marrow biopsy/aspiration is usually not necessary to make the diagnosis but should be performed if abnormalities are present in two cell lines, in older patients with new-onset ITP, or if the peripheral blood smear is abnormal.

DON'T BE TRICKED

- **Anemia does not exclude a diagnosis of ITP if the anemia can be explained by bleeding.**
- **Measurement of platelet-associated antibody is not helpful because the test lacks both sensitivity and specificity.**

STUDY TABLE: Thrombocytopenia Associations	
If you see this...	**Think this...**
Schistocytes	DIC, TTP-HUS, HELLP
Platelet clumps	Pseudothrombocytopenia caused by EDTA-dependent agglutinins leads to falsely decreased platelet counts. Repeat count using a citrated or a heparinized tube.
Teardrop (erythrocyte) cells, disorders in two cell lines	MDS
Anemia, leukopenia, lymphocytosis	Aplastic anemia
Pancytopenia, macrocytosis, macro-ovalocytes, hypersegmented neutrophils	Vitamin B_{12} or folate deficiencies
Thrombocytopenia following heparin administration or thrombocytopenia and thrombosis	HIT
Thrombocytopenia 5-10 days after blood transfusion	Posttransfusion purpura
Cirrhosis and thrombocytopenia	Splenic sequestration

Treatment

At the time of diagnosis, initiate therapy when the platelet count is <30,000/µL or with evidence of bleeding.

- Glucocorticoids are first-line therapy for ITP.
- IV immune globulin or anti-D immune globulin in persons who are Rh(D)-positive is indicated for glucocorticoid-resistant ITP or the management of severe bleeding.
- Splenectomy or rituximab is indicated for patients who are unresponsive to drug therapy or who relapse after glucocorticoids are tapered.
- Thrombopoiesis-stimulating agents (romiplostim, eltrombopag) may be attempted in refractory illness.

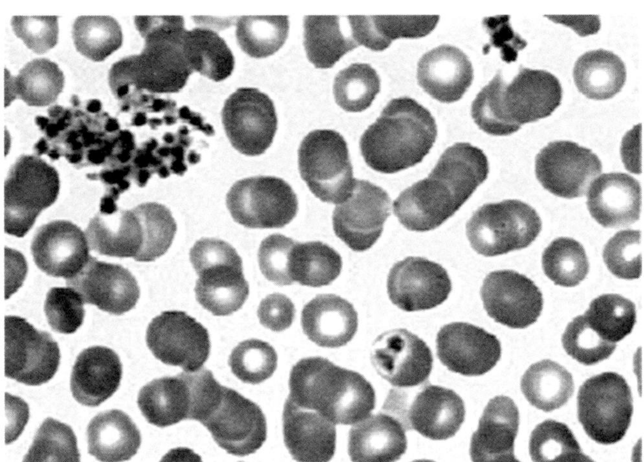

Pseudothrombocytopenia: Platelet clumps on peripheral blood smear associated with pseudothrombocytopenia.

Thrombotic Thrombocytopenic Purpura-Hemolytic Uremic Syndrome

Diagnosis

TTP and HUS are difficult to differentiate and are sometimes considered as an overlap syndrome.

TTP-HUS is a clinical diagnosis. Patients with TTP-HUS develop consumptive thrombocytopenia and microangiopathic hemolytic anemia from platelet thrombi that form throughout the microvasculature. Fever, kidney disease, and fluctuating neurologic abnormalities also occur but are seldom all present during earlier phases of the illness. Patients with TTP have been found to have unusually large multimers of vWF in their plasma and also have ADAMTS13 (vWF-cleaving protease) deficiency.

TTP can also occur by other mechanisms in patients with cancer, in transplant recipients, and following administration of chemotherapeutic agents and other drugs (quinine, clopidogrel, ticlopidine, cyclosporine, gemcitabine).

Escherichia coli O157:H7 or *Shigella* infections are more common in patients with HUS. Infection leads to the development of abdominal pain and bloody diarrhea. As many as 20% of patients with infection-related bloody diarrhea progress to HUS microangiopathic hemolytic anemia and AKI, generally within 6 days after diarrhea onset.

Testing

Laboratory studies show fragmented erythrocytes on peripheral blood smear and elevated serum bilirubin and LDH levels.

DON'T BE TRICKED

- Do not wait to initiate therapy until ADAMTS13 activity and inhibitor results are available if clinical features suggest TTP; results may not be available for several days, and these tests have poor sensitivity and specificity in the diagnosis of TTP.

Treatment

TTP caused by immune-mediated drug hypersensitivity requires immediate discontinuation of the causative drug.

Treat TTP with plasma exchange.

HUS is typically managed with supportive therapy. Antibiotics for underlying enterotoxigenic *E. coli* infection are not indicated.

DON'T BE TRICKED

- Do not order platelet transfusion in TTP-HUS because it can exacerbate the microvascular occlusion.
- PT, aPTT, D-dimer, and fibrinogen levels are normal in TTP-HUS and abnormal in DIC.
- Plasma exchange is superior to simple plasma infusion for TTP.

Heparin-Induced Thrombocytopenia and Thrombosis

Diagnosis

The characteristic findings of HIT and HITT are a platelet decrease of >50% in a patient taking heparin or a thromboembolic event 5 to 10 days after starting heparin.

A syndrome of delayed-onset HIT may develop up to 3 weeks after discontinuing heparin.

Patients with recent exposure to heparin may experience the onset of HIT more rapidly after re-exposure to heparin.

Testing

Diagnostic testing for HIT includes ELISA for heparin/PF4 antibodies and the functional assays, of which the serotonin release assay is the gold standard.

Treatment

Therapy is instituted before the results of diagnostic testing are returned if clinical suspicion is high. Heparin must be discontinued immediately.

Use a nonheparin anticoagulant (e.g., argatroban, fondaparinux, bivalirudin) to stabilize the patient.

DON'T BE TRICKED

- For HIT or HITT, warfarin or LMWH cannot be substituted for UFH.

TEST YOURSELF

A 75-year-old man who has been hospitalized multiple times for ischemic heart disease is admitted with increasing chest pain. The morning after admission, he has a painful, cold left lower leg. The platelet count is 30,000/µL.

ANSWER: For diagnosis, choose HITT. For management, stop heparin and begin argatroban.

Transfusion Medicine

Transfusions

Erythrocytes, platelets, plasma, cryoprecipitates, and (rarely) whole blood may be used for transfusion.

- Each unit of packed red blood cells results in a hemoglobin level increase of 1 g/dL.
- Each unit of platelets transfused results in a 20,000 to 25,000/µL increase in platelets.
- Platelet transfusion refractoriness is defined as an increase in the platelet count of <10,000/µL, measured 10 to 60 minutes after transfusion on at least two separate occasions. Nonimmune causes of platelet transfusion refractoriness include sepsis, DIC, drugs, and splenic sequestration. Alloimmunization is an important cause of platelet transfusion refractoriness because of the development of antibodies to antigens expressed on platelets.

In emergencies:

- Group O erythrocytes can be transfused to anyone.
- Group AB plasma and platelets can be transfused to anyone.
- Rh(D)-positive patients can safely receive either D-positive or D-negative blood, but Rh(D)-negative patients must receive D-negative blood and platelets.

Replacement of Coagulation Factors

FFP is used to replace coagulation factors. FFP is not needed for treating mild coagulopathies characterized by an INR of <1.9.

Cryoprecipitates (factor VIII, fibrinogen, vWF) are an adjunct to FFP replacement therapy and are used mainly for their fibrinogen content in patients with DIC.

Inactivated 4f-PCCs contain factors II, VII, IX, and X and are indicated for the treatment of major warfarin-associated bleeding in conjunction with vitamin K.

STUDY TABLE: Threshold Values for Prophylactic Transfusion

Condition	Threshold to Transfuse
Platelet transfusion; no other risk factors for bleeding	10,000-20,000/µL
Platelet transfusion for intracranial bleeding	100,000/µL
Hemoglobin for most medical and surgical patients	7-8 g/dL
Platelet transfusion; bleeding or planned surgery	50,000/µL

Transfusion Complications

An acute hemolytic transfusion reaction results from ABO incompatibility. Characteristic findings are:

- fever and chills
- flank and abdominal pain
- dyspnea
- hypotension and tachycardia
- red plasma and urine
- free hemoglobin in the plasma
- positive DAT (Coombs test)

Treatment of acute hemolytic transfusion reaction consists of transfusion discontinuation, IV hydration, and appropriate cardiovascular support.

A delayed hemolytic transfusion reaction results from delayed emergence of an alloantibody that causes rapid extravascular clearance of transfused erythrocytes 2 to 10 days after transfusion. Characteristic findings are an unexplained drop in hemoglobin concentration, elevated serum bilirubin and LDH levels, increased reticulocyte count, decreased haptoglobin concentration, and the presence of a new alloantibody.

A febrile nonhemolytic transfusion reaction can occur during or after a transfusion; it is caused by donor leukocyte cytokines or recipient alloantibodies directed against donor leukocytes. The transfusion should be stopped, hemolytic transfusion reaction ruled out, and antipyretic agents given.

Transfusion-related acute lung injury (TRALI) is a rare, severe reaction caused by donor antileukocyte antibodies reacting with recipient leukocytes and causing leukocyte aggregation in the pulmonary capillary bed, usually during or within 6 hours of transfusing erythrocytes, platelets, or FFP. Characteristic findings are hypoxemia and noncardiogenic pulmonary edema. The transfusion should be stopped and respiratory support provided.

Transfusion-associated circulatory overload (TACO) is the most common serious complication of blood transfusion and is more likely in patients with underlying heart or kidney disease but should be considered in any patient with new respiratory symptoms during or within 6 hours of transfusion. Management is the same as cardiogenic pulmonary edema.

An allergic transfusion reaction occurs when donor plasma constituents react with a recipient's IgE on mast cells. Characteristic findings are rash, hives, wheezing, and mucosal edema. Treatment includes antihistamines and glucocorticoids. Patients with IgA deficiency are at high risk because of the presence of anti-IgA antibodies.

Transfusion-associated graft-versus-host disease (GVHD) is a rare but fatal complication in which donor lymphocytes engraft in an immunocompromised or HLA-similar recipient and cause reactions that affect the bone marrow, liver, skin, and GI tract. Patients at risk are immunosuppressed.

STUDY TABLE: Cellular Transfusion Product Modifications

Modification	Notes
Leukoreduction	Reduces the number of leukocytes present in the transfused product. Reduces platelet transfusion refractoriness, febrile nonhemolytic transfusion reactions, and transmission of CMV.
Irradiation	Used to prevent transfusion-associated GVHD, which is mediated by donor lymphocytes.
Washing	Removes the proteins residing in the small amount of plasma in erythrocyte and platelet transfusions and is used in patients with a history of allergic reactions, IgA deficiency, or complement-dependent autoimmune hemolytic anemia.

Thrombophilia

Thrombophilia, characterized by an increased risk for VTE, can be acquired or inherited.

Inherited Thrombophilia

Prothrombin gene mutations and protein C deficiency, in addition to factor V Leiden mutation, account for 50% to 60% of causes of inherited thrombophilia. **Factor V Leiden mutation** is the most common hereditary thrombophilia in white populations.

Screening asymptomatic patients for thrombophilia is not recommended, even if a family history of thrombophilia is present.

Diagnosis: Testing patients with VTE for thrombophilic disorders is not recommended, because identification of inherited abnormalities does not alter the length of recommended anticoagulation or reliably predict the risk of recurrence.

- Heterozygosity for factor V Leiden and for prothrombin mutation modestly increases the risk of first-time VTE. Recurrent VTE is only slightly increased by factor V Leiden and is not increased by prothrombin gene mutation. Therefore, extended anticoagulation to prevent a recurrence of VTE is not indicated in these patients.
- **Protein C deficiency** is a risk factor for primary VTE, recurrent VTE, and arterial thromboembolism.

If testing is warranted, it should not be performed in the setting of an acute thrombotic event but rather weeks or months after it has occurred and when anticoagulant therapy has been discontinued, because active thrombosis and anticoagulation may alter the levels of some proteins.

STUDY TABLE: Genetic Mutations and Diagnostic Tests	
Genetic Mutation	**Testing**
Factor V Leiden	Clotting assay to determine resistance to activated protein C followed by confirmation of a positive result by genetic analysis
Prothrombin gene mutation	Molecular genetic test to identify the prothrombin *G20210A* mutation

Acquired Thrombophilia

Causes of acquired thrombophilia include immobilization or recent surgery, presence of a central venous catheter, pregnancy, oral contraceptives, kidney disease (particularly nephrotic syndrome), primary or secondary antiphospholipid antibody syndrome, and malignancy. Skin necrosis can occur in patients receiving large doses of warfarin without heparin because of the rapid depletion of protein C and the development of a hypercoagulable state.

Antiphospholipid antibody syndrome is an important cause of acquired thrombophilia. It can be a primary disease with no underlying comorbidity or a secondary disorder associated with autoimmune diseases, malignancy, or drugs. The APLA is an antibody to a protein bound to an anionic phospholipid identified as β_2-GPI.

APLAs are detected and measured in numerous ways.

- Lupus anticoagulants (LACs) are APLAs that prolong clotting times (aPTT) and are not corrected with a mixing study. Confirmation is made with the Russel viper venom time or kaolin clotting time.
- Anticardiolipin antibodies are antibodies that react with proteins associated with cardiolipin and may be measured directly (IgM and IgG).

A positive result should be confirmed later to rule out transient abnormalities from viral infection or even thrombosis itself. Positivity of LAC, anticardiolipin antibody, and anti–β_2-GPI antibodies are associated with the highest risk for thrombosis and pregnancy loss.

STUDY TABLE: Diagnosis of Antiphospholipid Syndrome	
Clinical Criteria	**Laboratory Criteria**
Presence of at least one of the following:	Presence of at least one of the following:
vascular thrombosis	LAC
≥1 fetal deaths before 34th week gestation	anticardiolipin antibody
≥3 spontaneous abortions before 10th week gestation	anti-β_2-GPI antibody

DON'T BE TRICKED

- **LACs are most commonly associated with thrombosis, not bleeding.**

Treatment

The treatment of patients with an inherited thrombophilia and VTE is generally the same as for those patients without an inherited thrombophilia.

For persons with antiphospholipid syndrome and a thromboembolic event, long-term oral anticoagulant therapy is indicated.

TEST YOURSELF

A 23-year-old woman with a history of two miscarriages develops a VTE. Before beginning heparin, the aPTT is found to be prolonged.

ANSWER: The diagnosis is antiphospholipid antibody syndrome.

Deep Venous Thrombosis and Pulmonary Embolism

Screening

Routine extensive screening for underlying cancer in all patients with unprovoked VTE is not recommended.

Prevention

Pharmacologic prophylaxis is recommended in most hospitalized patients without a contraindication. VTE prophylaxis with graduated compression stockings is not recommended. In the absence of increased bleeding risk, intermittent pneumatic compression devices are not recommended as the only prophylaxis. VTE prophylaxis is often only given during a patient's hospitalization with the exception of postdischarge prophylaxis (up to 5 weeks) following hip fracture, hip and knee replacement, and major cancer surgery.

Diagnosis

Use the Wells DVT or PE scores for all patients.

- In patients with low pretest probability for DVT (score ≤1) or PE (score ≤4), obtain a D-dimer blood test.
- If the D-dimer is negative, no further testing is needed.
- If the D-dimer is positive or the Wells score indicates that a DVT or PE is likely (Wells DVT score >1; Wells PE score >4), obtain an imaging study. Duplex ultrasonography and CTA are the diagnostic tests of choice for DVT and PE, respectively.
- PEs are categorized as "low risk" if cardiac enzyme levels and echocardiography are normal.

Treatment

Hospital admission is unnecessary for most patients with DVT; therapy can be initiated with a NOAC or LMWH for 5 days with transition to warfarin.

STUDY TABLE: Duration of Anticoagulant Therapy for VTE

Type of Thrombotic Event	Duration of Anticoagulant Therapy
Distal leg DVT	
Provoked or unprovoked, mild symptoms	No anticoagulation, but monitor with serial duplex ultrasonography for 2 weeks
Provoked or unprovoked, moderate-severe symptoms	3 months
Proximal leg DVT or PE	
Provoked (by surgery, trauma, immobility)	3 months
Unprovoked	Extended
Recurrent	Duration of therapy depends on whether VTE events were provoked or unprovoked
Upper extremity DVT, proximal	At least 3 months
Cancer-associated DVT or PE	As long as the cancer is active or being treated
	LMWH is the preferred anticoagulant
CTEPH	Extended

For PE with hypotension, systemic thrombolytic therapy is appropriate.

Anticoagulant treatment options include initial parenteral administration of LMWH, UFH, or fondaparinux followed by oral administration of dabigatran, edoxaban, or warfarin, or monotherapy (oral anticoagulant started without initial parenteral anticoagulant) with apixaban or rivaroxaban.

The only clear indication for an IVC filter is in patients with acute pelvic or proximal leg DVT who cannot be anticoagulated because of active bleeding or a very high risk for bleeding.

DON'T BE TRICKED

- If DVT is diagnosed, a CTA is not needed because the treatment is the same.
- Do not select thrombolytic therapy for most patients with DVT.
- Parenteral anticoagulant administration must overlap with warfarin for at least 5 days and until the INR is >2 for 24 hours.
- Do not use a NOAC (dabigatran, edoxaban, rivaroxaban, apixaban) if BMI >40 or GFR <30 mL/min/1.73 m^2.

Anemia and Thrombocytopenia in Pregnancy

Diagnosis

Anemia: Pregnancy results in a normal dilutional anemia. However, hemoglobin values less than 11 g/dL in the first trimester or less than 10 g/dL in the second and third trimesters should prompt a search for other causes of anemia; iron and folate deficiency are the most common causes.

Thrombocytopenia: The most common cause is gestational thrombocytopenia. HELLP syndrome, preeclampsia, and AFLP can cause thrombocytopenia and are part of a spectrum of disorders referred to as the "thrombotic microangiopathy of pregnancy." Symptoms and laboratory features for each overlap. Making the distinction between the disorders may not be critical, because the most effective therapy for each is emergent delivery of the fetus.

STUDY TABLE: Thrombocytopenia During Pregnancy

Disorder	Characteristic
Gestational thrombocytopenia	Benign thrombocytopenia typically >70,000/µL; second or third trimester; no schistocytes on peripheral blood smear No treatment needed
Preeclampsia	Hypertension, proteinuria, and thrombocytopenia developing at >20 weeks' gestation Treatment is delivery
HELLP syndrome	Microangiopathic hemolytic anemia; AST >70 U/L, platelet count <100,000/µL developing at >20 weeks' gestation Treatment is delivery
AFLP	Microangiopathic hemolytic anemia, hepatic failure, hypoglycemia, and coagulopathy at >20 weeks' gestation Treatment is delivery
TTP-HUS	See TTP-HUS section; develops at >20 weeks' gestation; not affected by pregnancy termination
ITP	May present early in pregnancy Treatment the same as for nonpregnant patients
DIC	In setting of obstetric emergency, elevated levels of fibrin degradation products and/or D-dimers, decreased fibrinogen level, possible prolongation of the PT and aPTT, and thrombocytopenia

Infectious Disease

Bacterial Meningitis

Diagnosis

Symptoms and signs of bacterial meningitis include fever, nuchal rigidity, photophobia, and altered mental status.

Testing

CT of the head is indicated before proceeding with LP if signs or symptoms of increased intracranial pressure are present (papilledema, focal neurologic deficits, altered mental status, new-onset seizures, previous CNS lesions, immunocompromise).

STUDY TABLE: Typical CSF Findings in Patients with Viral and Bacterial Meningitis

CSF Parameter	Viral Meningitis	Bacterial Meningitis
Opening pressure	≤250 mm H_2O	200-500 mm H_2O
Leukocyte count	50-1000/µL	1000-5000/µL
Leukocyte differential	Lymphocytes	Neutrophils
Glucose	>45 mg/dL	<40 mg/dL
Protein	<200 mg/dL	100-500 mg/dL
Gram stain	Negative	Positive in 60%-90%
Culture	Negative	Positive in 70%-85%

CSF Gram stain and cultures obtained before antibiotic initiation are usually diagnostic for the infecting organism.

The two most common organisms causing bacterial meningitis are *Streptococcus pneumoniae* and *Neisseria meningitidis*, accounting for >80% of cases.

Treatment

STUDY TABLE: Empiric Antibiotic Management of Bacterial Meningitis

Clinical Characteristics	Empiric Antibiotic Regimen
Immunocompetent host with community-acquired bacterial meningitis	IV ceftriaxone **or** cefotaxime **plus** IV vancomycin
Patient >50 years or those with altered cell-mediated immunity	IV ampicillin (*Listeria* coverage) **plus** IV ceftriaxone **or** cefotaxime **plus** IV vancomycin
Allergies to β-lactams	IV moxifloxacin **instead of** cephalosporin
	IV trimethoprim-sulfamethoxazole **instead of** ampicillin
Hospital-acquired bacterial meningitis	IV vancomycin **plus either** IV ceftazidime, cefepime, or meropenem
Neurosurgical procedures	IV vancomycin **plus either** IV ceftazidime, cefepime, or meropenem

In patients with suspected or confirmed pneumococcal meningitis, adjunctive dexamethasone should be given approximately 15 minutes before administration of antimicrobial agents and continued for 4 days.

Treatment of viral meningitis is symptomatic and supportive. Empiric antimicrobial agents may be initiated in viral meningitis until bacterial meningitis is excluded.

Brain Abscess

Diagnosis

Brain abscess can occur from hematogenous spread, from an ENT source, from penetrating trauma, or after neurosurgery. Clinical presentation typically includes severe headache; fever and neck stiffness may not always be present.

Testing

CNS imaging is the cornerstone of diagnosis; MRI is more sensitive than CT.

Treatment

Empiric antimicrobial treatment should be based on the suspected source and Gram stain results. A narrowed regimen is based on culture results and is continued for 4 to 8 weeks. Abscesses >2.5 cm should be excised or drained stereotactically.

DON'T BE TRICKED

- **LP is contraindicated because of the potential for increased intracranial pressure and risk of herniation.**

Herpes Simplex Encephalitis

Diagnosis

Infection with HSV-1 is the most common cause of sporadic encephalitis in the United States. Fever, altered mental status, headache, seizure, and focal neurologic deficits suggest HSE.

Testing

CSF testing shows lymphocytic pleocytosis and, when necrosis is extensive, erythrocytes. Temporal lobe abnormalities on imaging and periodic lateralizing epileptiform discharges on EEG suggest HSE.

HSV PCR of the CSF allows rapid diagnosis of HSE.

DON'T BE TRICKED

- **Order HSV PCR in all suspected cases of encephalitis, even if not typical for HSV encephalitis.**
- **Do not order CSF culture for HSV or serologic testing for HSV.**

Treatment

High-dose IV acyclovir should be started within 24 hours of symptom onset and continued for 14 to 21 days.

West Nile Neuroinvasive Disease

Diagnosis

Mosquitoes serve as the primary vector, and most human infections occur during the summer and early fall. WNND may present with meningitis, encephalitis, or myelitis. Older adults and immunocompromised patients in particular are at high risk for neuroinvasive disease.

Severe disease may manifest as acute asymmetric flaccid paralysis and may progress to respiratory failure.

Diagnosis is established by detecting serum and CSF IgM antibody to WNV.

DON'T BE TRICKED

- Don't order viral culture for WNND because it is rarely positive.

Treatment

Treatment is limited to supportive care. Monitor patients with significant muscle weakness for respiratory failure in an intensive care setting.

Autoimmune Encephalitis

Diagnosis and Testing

Anti-NMDA receptor antibody encephalitis is associated with ovarian teratomas in >50% of patients. Clinical findings include choreoathetosis, psychiatric symptoms, seizures, coma, and autonomic instability. CSF antibody testing is specific and sensitive for anti-NMDA receptor encephalitis.

Treatment

Treatment includes removal of the teratoma, when present, and immunosuppression with glucocorticoids, rituximab, cyclophosphamide, or IV immune globulin.

Cellulitis and Soft Tissue Infection

Diagnosis

Folliculitis is recognized as erythematous papules and pustules that are centered on a follicle on the face, chest, back, or buttocks. Infection is most often caused by *Staphylococcus aureus*, although pseudomonas folliculitis secondary to hot tub exposure and gram-negative folliculitis secondary to acne therapy can be seen.

A **carbuncle** is a superficial inflammatory mass consisting of several inflamed hair follicles and multiple sites of drainage.

A **furuncle** is an infection centered on a hair follicle with pus extending into the dermis forming a small abscess.

Impetigo, a streptococcal or staphylococcal infection of the epidermis, is characterized by yellow or golden-colored crusted pustules.

Erysipelas affects the superficial skin layers, including the upper dermis and dermal lymphatics. It classically involves the malar region. The key clinical finding is a sharply raised border and orange-peel texture. It is usually caused by streptococcal infection.

Cellulitis, an infection of the dermis and deeper subcutaneous tissue, features a well-demarcated area of warmth, swelling, tenderness, and erythema.

Deep tissue infection is indicated by violaceous bullae, necrosis, rapidly increasing extent of infection, massive swelling, and pain out of proportion to apparent injury. Loss of sensation may indicate compartment syndrome (increased tissue pressure within a closed muscle compartment) secondary to deep tissue infection and may be present even if peripheral pulses are palpable. Infection can be monomicrobial or polymicrobial.

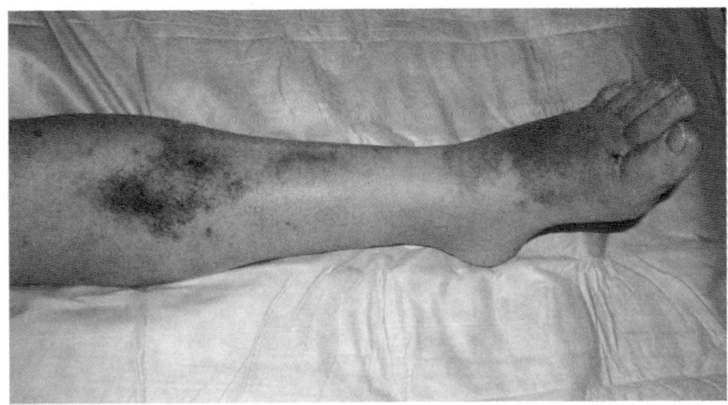

Cellulitis: Cellulitis is characterized by well-demarcated areas of tender erythema.

Most diagnoses are based on clinical findings alone. Choose blood cultures in the presence of signs and symptoms of systemic toxicity.

STUDY TABLE: Skin and Soft Tissue Infection	
If you see...	**Think...**
Honey-colored, crusted pustules	Impetigo caused by β-hemolytic *Streptococcus* or *Staphylococcus*
Sepsis, cellulitis, and hemorrhagic bullae after exposure to saltwater fish or shellfish in patients with cirrhosis or chronic illnesses such as diabetes mellitus, rheumatoid arthritis, or CKD	*Vibrio vulnificus* infection
Skin ulcer with necrotic center in a patient with neutropenia	Ecthyma gangrenosum from *Pseudomonas* or other bacterial infections
Chronic nodular infection of distal extremities with exposure to fish tanks or marine environments	*Mycobacterium marinum*
Chronic nodular infection of distal extremities with exposure to plants/soil	*Sporotrichosis* and *Nocardia*
Sepsis following a dog bite in a patient with asplenia	*Capnocytophaga canimorsus*
Swelling and erythema with pain out of proportion to physical examination findings	Necrotizing (deep) soft tissue infection (surgical emergency)
Acute, tender, well-delineated, purulent lesions	Abscess caused by *S. aureus*
Follicle-centered pustules in the beard and pubic areas, axillae, and thighs	*S. aureus* folliculitis
Follicle-centered erythematous papules and pustules on the trunk, axillae, and buttocks 1-4 days after hot tub or whirlpool exposure	*Pseudomonas* folliculitis
Symmetric, pink-to-brown patches with thin scale in intertriginous areas (axillae, groin, inframammary)	Erythrasma caused by *Corynebacterium minutissimum.* Erythrasma will fluoresce to a coral red color with a Wood lamp

Treatment

STUDY TABLE: Drug Treatment for Cellulitis and Soft Tissue Infection	
Diagnosis	**Treatment**
Nonpurulent cellulitis	Empiric treatment for β-hemolytic streptococci and MSSA Dicloxacillin, cephalexin, clindamycin (all oral); IV antibiotics for unsuccessful outpatient treatment or patients with signs of toxicity
Purulent cellulitis, mild to moderate severity	Empiric treatment for MRSA Clindamycin, trimethoprim-sulfamethoxazole, doxycycline
Purulent cellulitis with extensive disease or signs of systemic toxicity	Vancomycin (IV) or linezolid (oral or IV), daptomycin, telavancin, ceftaroline
Impetigo	Extensive disease, treat as nonpurulent cellulitis; limited disease, mupirocin (topical)
Erysipelas	With systemic symptoms, ceftriaxone (parenteral); if mild/asymptomatic, penicillin or amoxicillin (oral)
Folliculitis (staphylococcal and pseudomonal)	Spontaneous resolution is typical. Topical mupirocin or clindamycin lotion can be used
Human bites (clenched fist injury)	Ampicillin-sulbactam (IV)
Animal bites	Ampicillin-sulbactam (IV) or amoxicillin-clavulanate (oral)
Neutropenia	Vancomycin and cefepime
Necrotizing fasciitis, compartment syndrome, myonecrosis on imaging, purple bullae, or sloughing of skin	Imipenem, clindamycin, vancomycin, and prompt debridement
Erythrasma	Topical erythromycin, clarithromycin, or clindamycin

Treat risk factors for recurrent cellulitis, such as lymphedema, tinea pedis, and chronic venous insufficiency.

DON'T BE TRICKED

- Skin abscesses may have higher cure rates when incision and drainage is accompanied by antibiotic treatment with MRSA coverage.

TEST YOURSELF

A 60-year-old woman has a temperature of 38.8 °C (101.8 °F). Her right thigh is swollen and extremely tender to palpation, with a 5-cm red patch in the middle of the tender area. She requires morphine for pain.

ANSWER: For diagnosis, choose myonecrosis. For management, select urgent MRI followed by surgical debridement.

A 20-year-old college football player has a fever, furuncles, and associated cellulitis.

ANSWER: For diagnosis, choose MRSA infection. For management, select treatment with trimethoprim-sulfamethoxazole.

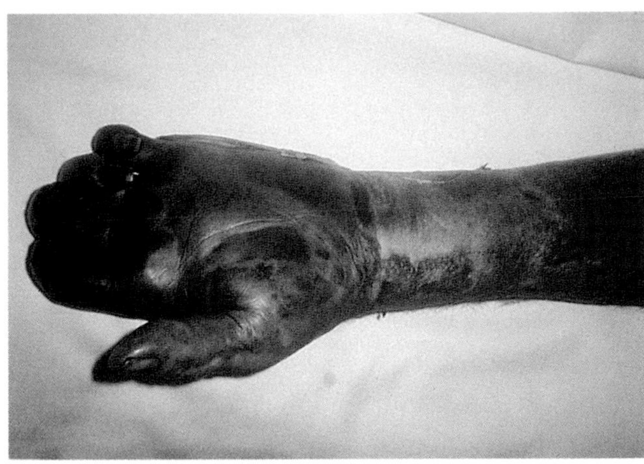

***Vibrio vulnificus* Infection:** Deep tissue infection associated with hemorrhagic bullae caused by *V. vulnificus* in a patient with cirrhosis.

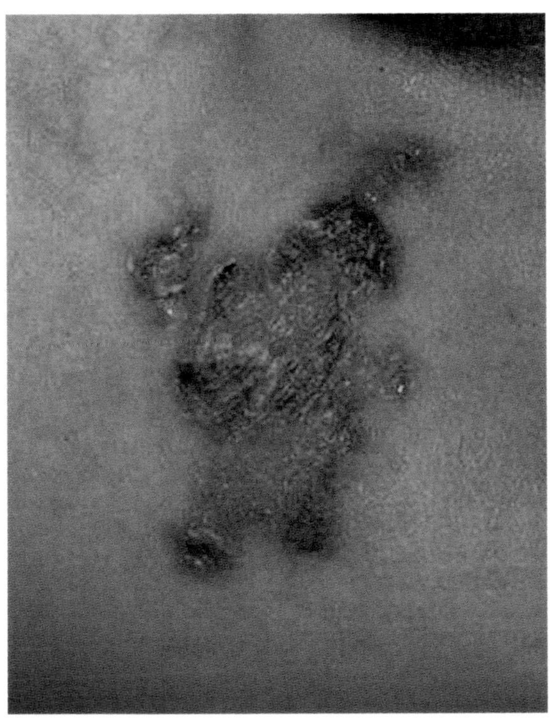

Impetigo: Erosions with golden-yellow crusts confirm the presence of impetigo.

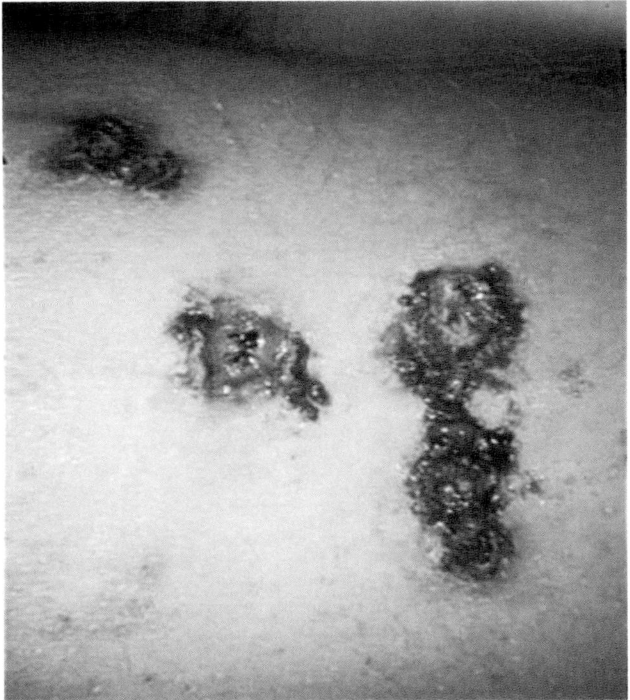

Ecthyma Gangrenosum: Ecthyma gangrenosum is characterized by single or multiple cutaneous ulcers evolving from painless nodular lesions, with surrounding erythema progressing to central hemorrhage, ulceration, and necrosis; it is caused by *Pseudomonas* or other bacteria, such as *S. aureus*, typically in a patient with neutropenia.

Diabetic Foot Infections

Diagnosis

Mild infections do not extend deeper than the skin and subcutaneous tissues; may be associated with purulent discharge, warmth, tenderness, or swelling; and erythema is ≤2 cm beyond the ulcer.

Moderate infections are associated with either:

- erythematous infection >2 cm around the ulcer
- infection deeper than the skin and subcutaneous tissues

Severe infections are associated with systemic signs of infection (hypotension, confusion, vomiting, acidosis, severe hyperglycemia, AKI).

Testing

Cultures are obtained from deep tissue curettage or biopsy. Assess all patients for arterial insufficiency (using ABI). Obtain foot imaging for all new diabetic foot infections.

Treatment

STUDY TABLE: Treatment of Diabetic Foot Infections

Category of Infection	Empiric Antibiotic Selection
Mild (nonpurulent)	Single oral antibiotic, such as cephalexin, dicloxacillin, amoxicillin-clavulanate, or clindamycin
Mild (purulent and at risk for MRSA)	Clindamycin, doxycycline, or trimethoprim-sulfamethoxazole
Moderate	Two-drug therapy, such as trimethoprim-sulfamethoxazole plus amoxicillin-clavulanate or clindamycin plus ciprofloxacin, levofloxacin, or moxifloxacin
Severe	β-lactam/β-lactamase inhibitor (e.g., ampicillin-sulbactam), a carbapenem (e.g., imipenem-cilastin), and a fluoroquinolone (e.g., moxifloxacin) and surgical debridement

Toxic Shock Syndrome

Diagnosis

TSS is characterized by fever, vomiting, diarrhea, hypotension, and rash. Exfoliation (peeling) of the skin occurs several days after the onset of the infection.

Look for:

- menstruation history and tampon use
- abscess, nasal packings, and gauze-packed wounds
- fever >38.9 °C (102.0 °F) and hypotension (SBP <90 mm Hg)
- diffuse sunburn-type rash or erythema, vaginal and oropharyngeal erythema
- multisystem organ failure: kidney (elevated serum creatinine), liver (elevated aminotransferase levels), GI tract (vomiting and diarrhea), ARDS, coagulopathy

Causes

TSS is caused by bacterial exotoxins that act as superantigens.

Staphylococcus aureus and group A β-hemolytic streptococci are the usual causative microorganisms.

Treatment

Remove sources of infection and toxin production and begin IV fluid resuscitation (up to 10-20 L/d). Start broad-spectrum antibiotics with a carbapenem or penicillin with a β-lactamase inhibitor plus clindamycin; narrow to clindamycin plus nafcillin if MSSA is identified. If TSS is associated with MRSA, vancomycin plus clindamycin or linezolid can be used. IV immune globulin may be helpful.

DON'T BE TRICKED

- Do not select glucocorticoids to treat TSS.

TEST YOURSELF

A 25-year-old man has three episodes of epistaxis that are stopped by packing his nares with petrolatum-covered cotton balls. The next day, he is confused, his temperature is 39.0 °C (102.2 °F), and BP is 90/82 mm Hg. Erythema of his face, shoulders, and palms is present. The nasal packing is still in place.

ANSWER: For diagnosis, select TSS; for management, choose removal of the nasal packing and initiation of antibiotics.

Community-Acquired Pneumonia

Diagnosis

Symptoms and Signs

Look for poor dentition and aspiration risk (anaerobic pneumonia) owing to gastrointestinal or neurologic disease, episodes of altered consciousness (e.g., alcohol use), injection drug use (*Staphylococcus aureus* pneumonia), and antibiotic therapy during the past 3 months. Pay attention to travel and occupational history.

Causes

Streptococcus pneumoniae is the most commonly identified bacterial cause of CAP in patients of all ages. CAP caused by *Moraxella* and *Haemophilus* species occurs mainly in patients with chronic pulmonary disease. Atypical microorganisms that cause CAP include *Mycoplasma pneumoniae* and *Chlamydophila pneumoniae* and are more common in persons aged 20 to 40 years.

STUDY TABLE: Possible Microbial Causes of CAP

Clinical Presentation	Commonly Encountered Pathogens
Aspiration	Gram-negative enteric pathogens, oral anaerobes
Cough >2 weeks with whoop or posttussive vomiting	*Bordetella pertussis*
Lung cavity infiltrates	Community-associated MRSA, oral anaerobes, endemic fungal pathogens, *Mycobacterium tuberculosis*, nontuberculous mycobacteria
Epidemiology or Risk Factor	**Commonly Encountered Pathogens**
Alcoholism	*S. pneumoniae*, oral anaerobes, *Klebsiella pneumoniae*, *Acinetobacter* species, *M. tuberculosis*
COPD and/or smoking	*Haemophilus influenzae, Pseudomonas aeruginosa, Legionella* species, *S. pneumoniae, Moraxella catarrhalis, C. pneumoniae*
HIV infection (early)	*S. pneumoniae, H. influenzae, M. tuberculosis*
Influenza epidemic in the community	Influenza virus, *S. pneumoniae, S. aureus, H. influenzae*
Poor dental hygiene; aspiration; presence of a lung abscess	Oral anaerobes
Residence in a nursing home; underlying cardiopulmonary disease; multiple medical comorbidities; recent antibiotic therapy	Enteric gram-negative bacteria
Structural lung disease (bronchiectasis); glucocorticoid therapy (prednisone >10 mg/d); broad-spectrum antibiotic therapy for >7 days in the past month; malnutrition	*P. aeruginosa*, *Burkholderia cepacia*, Stenotrophomonas, *Staphylococcus aureus*
Travel or residence in southwestern United States	*Coccidioides* species, *Hantavirus*
Travel or residence in Southeast and East Asia	*Burkholderia pseudomallei* (melioidosis)
Exposure to bat or bird droppings	*Histoplasma capsulatum*
Exposure to birds	*Chlamydophila psittaci*
Exposure to rabbits	*Francisella tularensis*
Exposure to farm animals or parturient cats	*Coxiella burnetii*
Exposure to rodent excreta	Hantavirus

Testing

Fever and a chest x-ray demonstrating one or more focal pulmonary infiltrates are diagnostic of pneumonia. Sputum cultures and blood cultures are indicated for inpatients and those with severe disease (ICU admission), complications (pleural effusions, cavitary lesions), underlying lung disease, active alcohol abuse, or ineffective outpatient antimicrobial therapy; blood cultures are indicated for those with asplenia, liver disease, or leukopenia.

Sputum Gram stain and sputum and blood cultures are not recommended for ambulatory patients.

Legionella and pneumococcal urinary antigen testing are also recommended when confirmation of a microbiologic diagnosis is indicated, when ICU admission is being considered, and when outpatient antimicrobial therapy fails. However, *Legionella* urinary antigen testing only detects *Legionella pneumophila* type 1 and is, therefore, not sensitive.

DON'T BE TRICKED

- Do not use chest CT for diagnosing CAP.
- The presence of cavities with air-fluid levels suggests abscess formation (staphylococci, anaerobes, or gram-negative bacilli), whereas the presence of cavities without air-fluid levels suggests TB or fungal infection.

Treatment

Severity of illness scores such as the CURB-65 criteria (Confusion, Uremia, Respiratory rate, low BP, and age ≥65 years) may help predict a complicated course. Scoring 1 point for each positive criterion, patients with a score of 0 to 1 can be managed as outpatients, those with a score of 2 should be admitted to a hospital, and those with a score of 3 or higher often require ICU care.

Also consider hospitalization for patients who do not respond to outpatient therapy or have decompensated comorbid illness, complex social needs, or require IV antibiotics or oxygenation.

General rules for antibiotic administration:

- Switch from parenteral to oral agents when 1) temperature ≤37.8 °C (100.0 °F), 2) HR ≤100/min, 3) respiration rate ≤24/min, 4) SBP ≥90 mm Hg, and 5) arterial oxygen saturation ≥90% or breathing ambient air.
- Total duration of antimicrobial therapy in patients who respond clinically within the first 2 to 3 days of treatment is generally not longer than 7 days.
- Treat severe infections, empyema, lung abscess, meningitis, or documented infection with pathogens such as *P. aeruginosa* or *S. aureus* for ≥10 days.
- Treat bacteremic *S. aureus* pneumonia for 4 to 6 weeks and obtain TEE to rule out endocarditis.
- Follow-up chest x-ray is not routine; consider in adults >50 years 2 to 3 months after antimicrobial treatment.

STUDY TABLE: IDSA/ATS Recommendations for Empiric Antibiotics in Community-Acquired Pneumonia

Site of Treatment	Patient or Epidemiologic Considerations	Regimens(s)
Outpatient	Healthy patient without antibiotics in preceding 3 months	Macrolide OR Doxycycline
	Healthy patient from region with >25% macrolide resistance among *S. pneumoniae*	Respiratory quinolone OR β-lactam plus a macrolide
	Comorbidities[a] or antibiotic use in preceding 3 months	Respiratory quinolone OR β-lactam plus a macrolide
Inpatient, non-ICU		β-lactam plus a macrolide OR Respiratory quinolone

(Continued on the next page)

STUDY TABLE: IDSA/ATS Recommendations for Empiric Antibiotics in Community-Acquired Pneumonia *(Continued)*		
Site of Treatment	**Patient or Epidemiologic Considerations**	**Regimens(s)**
ICU treatment		Parenteral β-lactam plus either azithromycin or a respiratory quinolone OR If penicillin allergic, a respiratory quinolone plus aztreonam
Any	Risk factor for *Pseudomonas*	Antipseudomonal β-lactam plus an antipseudomonal quinolone OR If penicillin allergic, a respiratory quinolone plus aztreonam
Any	Risk factor for CA-MRSA	Standard therapy PLUS vancomycin OR linezolid

[a]Comorbidities include chronic heart, lung, liver, or kidney disease; diabetes mellitus; alcoholism; asplenia; malignancies; and immunosuppression.

Reproduced with permission from Mandell LA, Wunderink RG, Anzueto A, Bartlett JG, Campbell GD, Dean NC, Dowell SF, File TM Jr, Musher DM, Niederman MS, Torres A, Whitney CG; Infectious Diseases Society of America; American Thoracic Society. Infectious Diseases Society of America/American Thoracic Society consensus guidelines on the management of community-acquired pneumonia in adults. Clin Infect Dis. 2007 Mar 1;44 Suppl 2:S27-72. [PMID: 17278083]

DON'T BE TRICKED

- Antimicrobial treatment duration for CAP is typically 5 days in outpatients.
- For inpatients, administer antibiotic while in emergency department.
- Do not select the same class of antibiotics that patients have received in the past 3 months.

Lyme Disease

Prevention

The risk of Lyme disease following a tick bite is low. Watchful waiting is preferred to giving a prophylactic antibiotic under most circumstances.

The Infectious Diseases Society of America recommends antibiotic prophylaxis with doxycycline only when the attached tick is identified as an adult or nymphal deer tick, attachment is estimated at 36 hours or longer, prophylaxis is begun within 72 hours of tick removal, the tick bite occurred in an endemic area, the patient is not pregnant or lactating or <8 years of age, and no other contraindications to doxycycline exist.

Diagnosis

Lyme disease is transmitted by the black-legged deer tick and is endemic to the northeast, mid-Atlantic, and Midwest United States. It has three stages (early, disseminated, and late) based on the time that has elapsed after exposure. The clinical presentation differs for each stage of the disease.

STUDY TABLE: Common Manifestations of Lyme Disease by Stage		
Stage	**Findings**	**Management**
Acute, localized	Within 30 days of exposure: erythema migrans, fever, fatigue, headache, arthralgia, myalgia	Treat without serologic confirmation
Acute, disseminated	Weeks to months after exposure: multiple erythema migrans lesions, heart conduction block, cranial neuropathy, radiculoneuropathy, lymphocytic meningitis, acute attacks of monoarticular or oligoarticular arthritis	Treat if ELISA is positive Obtain Western blot if ELISA is indeterminate
Late	Months to years after exposure: attacks of monoarticular or oligoarticular arthritis and/or chronic monoarthritis or oligoarthritis, peripheral neuropathy, or encephalomyelitis	Treat if ELISA is positive Obtain Western blot if ELISA is indeterminate

DON'T BE TRICKED

- **Serologic test results are often negative in acute localized Lyme disease so treat empirically.**
- Do not test for Lyme disease in patients with nonspecific symptoms of fatigue, myalgia, arthralgia, or fibromyalgia in the absence of exposure history or appropriate clinical findings.

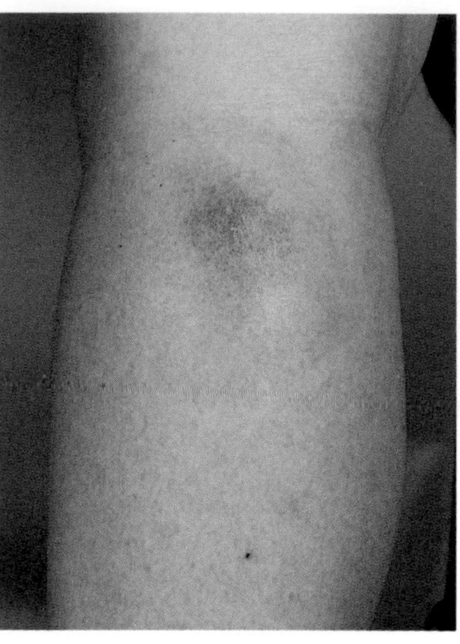

Erythema Migrans: A large erythematous ring characterizes erythema migrans and early Lyme disease.

Treatment

In patients with erythema migrans and early disease, begin doxycycline (10-21 days, preferred), amoxicillin, or cefuroxime for 14 to 21 days without laboratory confirmation of *Borrelia burgdorferi*. Manage late carditis or neurologic disease with IV penicillin or IV ceftriaxone for 28 days, and manage arthritis and facial nerve palsy with doxycycline.

DON'T BE TRICKED

- **Do not select the diagnosis "chronic Lyme disease."**
- **Do not treat post-Lyme disease syndrome (fatigue, arthralgia, myalgia, memory disturbance) with antibiotics.**
- **Do not rely on serologic test results to decide on the adequacy of treatment.**
- **Do not prescribe doxycycline for pregnant women.**

Babesiosis

Diagnosis

Babesiosis is a tick-borne (black-legged deer tick) malaria-like illness endemic to the northeast coast of the United States. Mild cases present with a febrile illness variably associated with myalgia, headache, and fatigue.

Testing

Severe hemolytic anemia, jaundice, kidney failure, and death are more common in patients that are older, immunocompromised, or have functional or anatomic asplenia. A Wright- or Giemsa-stained peripheral blood smear will show intraerythrocytic parasites in ring, or more rarely, tetrad formations (Maltese cross shape). Consider PCR for *Babesia* DNA in cases of low parasitemia.

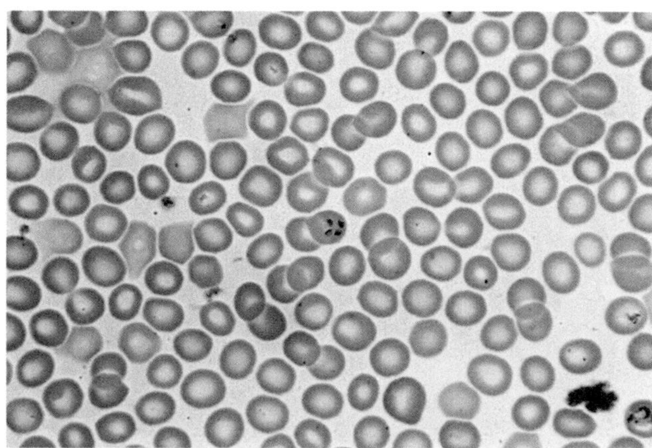

Babesiosis: Peripheral blood smear that shows intraerythrocytic parasites arranged in tetrads, resembling a Maltese cross.

DON'T BE TRICKED

- ***Babesia* trophozoites appear as ring forms inside erythrocytes and may be confused with malaria unless a thorough travel history is obtained.**

Treatment

When *Babesia* infection is detected in an asymptomatic patient, monitoring for resolution of parasitemia without treatment is recommended for 3 months. Atovaquone plus azithromycin is the treatment of choice for patients with persistent parasitemia after 3 months and for mild-to-moderate symptomatic disease. In severe disease, clindamycin plus quinine is preferable.

Ehrlichiosis and Anaplasmosis

Diagnosis

Ehrlichia chaffeensis (transmitted by the lone star tick and most prevalent in south central and southeastern United States) and *Anaplasma phagocytophilum* (transmitted by the Ixodes tick) are rickettsia-like organisms that infect leukocytes. *E. chaffeensis* causes human monocytic ehrlichiosis (HME) and *A. phagocytophilum* causes human granulocytic anaplasmosis (HGA). Ehrlichiosis and anaplasmosis are spread by ticks.

The clinical syndromes of HME and HGA are very similar:

- fever, headache, and myalgia
- multiorgan failure (AKI, ARDS, meningoencephalitis)
- fever of unknown origin (symptoms can persist for months)
- elevated aminotransferases with normal alkaline phosphatase and bilirubin levels
- leukopenia and thrombocytopenia
- presence of morulae (clumps of organisms in the cytoplasm of the appropriate leukocyte)

Testing

Whole blood PCR is the most sensitive test for diagnosis of acute infection.

DON'T BE TRICKED

- **HGA is transmitted by the same vector as Lyme disease and babesiosis so double or triple infection is possible.**

Treatment

IV or oral doxycycline is the treatment of choice for HME and HGA.

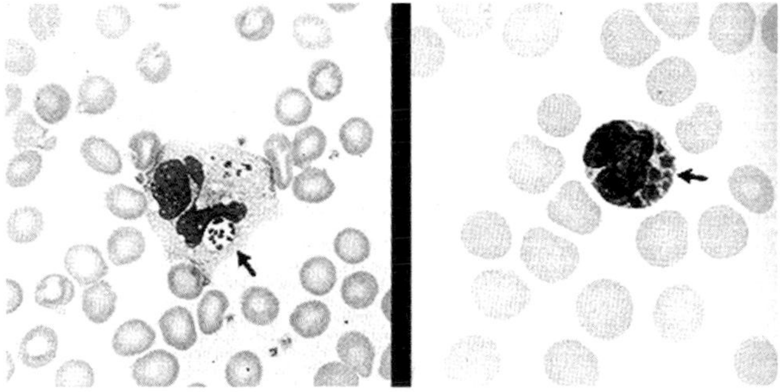

Human Granulocytic Ehrlichiosis: HME (*left*) and HGA (*right*); demonstration of morulae recognized as clumps of organisms in the cytoplasm.

Rocky Mountain Spotted Fever

Diagnosis

Rocky Mountain spotted fever is a tick-borne rickettsial infection most prevalent in the southeastern and south central states. Look for a history of tick bite and recent travel to an endemic area; febrile illness in spring and summer months; and nonspecific symptoms such as nausea, myalgia, dyspnea, cough, and headache. Also look for a macular rash starting on the ankles and wrists and often affecting the palms and soles of the feet; lesions spread centripetally and become petechial.

Testing

Thrombocytopenia and elevated aminotransferase levels are characteristic. Immunohistochemistry or PCR of a skin biopsy specimen allows diagnosis at the time of acute infection.

Treatment

Select doxycycline. In patients who are pregnant, choose chloramphenicol. Nonresponse in 72 hours suggests an alternative diagnosis.

Cystitis

Prevention

Screen for and treat asymptomatic bacteriuria only in patients who are pregnant or are about to undergo an invasive urologic procedure.

Diagnosis

Symptomatic cystitis is associated with dysuria, frequency, and urgency. Hematuria may be present.

UTIs (either cystitis or pyelonephritis) are classified as uncomplicated or complicated.

- **Uncomplicated UTI** is acute cystitis and pyelonephritis occurring in healthy, nonpregnant women with no history of urinary tract abnormalities.
- **Complicated UTI** is defined as an infection occurring in a patient with comorbid conditions or anatomic abnormalities of the urinary tract, including diabetes, pregnancy, male gender, kidney transplantation, anatomic or functional abnormalities of the urinary tract, urinary catheterization or manipulation, recent antibiotic exposure, and recent hospitalization.

Patients with complicated UTIs are at risk for infection with antibiotic-resistant microorganisms.

Testing

Patients with uncomplicated cystitis do not require a urine culture but can be diagnosed by urinalysis:

- urine dipsticks positive for leukocyte esterase and nitrites
- ≥10 WBCs/µL of unspun urine or 5 to 10 WBCs/hpf on a centrifuged specimen of urine

Obtain a culture for suspected cystitis only with:

- suspected pyelonephritis
- complicated UTI
- recurrent UTI
- suspicion of an unusual or antimicrobial-resistant microorganism or a patient who is pregnant

Treatment

For women with symptoms of uncomplicated cystitis, prescribing antibiotics over the telephone without seeing the patient or obtaining a urinalysis is acceptable.

For empiric treatment of uncomplicated cystitis in **nonpregnant women**, select one of the following:

- 3 days of oral trimethoprim-sulfamethoxazole
- 5 days of oral nitrofurantoin
- single 3-g oral dose of fosfomycin

In patients at high risk for complicated UTI, obtain a urine culture and initiate empiric treatment for 7 to 14 days with a fluoroquinolone.

For pregnant women with complicated UTI, choose 7 days of empiric therapy with amoxicillin-clavulanate, nitrofurantoin, cefpodoxime, or cefixime. Obtain a urine culture after treatment.

For recurrent uncomplicated UTIs, select one or more of the following:

- postcoital antibiotic prophylaxis, particularly if UTIs are temporally associated with coitus
- continuous antibiotic prophylaxis
- self-initiated therapy for frequent recurrent episodes

DON'T BE TRICKED

- Trimethoprim-sulfamethoxazole should not be used if it was taken in the preceding 3 months.
- Do not schedule a routine follow-up urinalysis or culture after treatment for nonpregnant women with uncomplicated cystitis.

Pyelonephritis

Diagnosis

Pyelonephritis is associated with the abrupt onset of fever, chills, nausea, and flank or abdominal pain. Urinary frequency and dysuria may precede pyelonephritis. Hypotension and septic shock may occur. Look for risk factors including obstruction, kidney stones, neurogenic bladder, and indwelling catheters.

Testing

Presence of bacteriuria and pyuria are the gold standard for the diagnosis of pyelonephritis. Gram stain of the urine sediment is particularly useful when selecting empiric antibiotic therapy. Obtain urine cultures for all patients and blood cultures for clinically ill patients. Imaging studies are indicated only for patients in whom an alternative diagnosis or a urologic complication is suspected.

Treatment

For patients with uncomplicated infection who are able to tolerate oral therapy, select an oral fluoroquinolone. Use an IV fluoroquinolone if nausea and vomiting precludes use of oral medications. Treat uncomplicated infection for 5 to 7 days and complicated infection for 14 days.

Choose broad-spectrum antibiotic coverage with an extended-spectrum β-lactam or a carbapenem in the following settings:

- suspected infection with resistant organisms
- recent antibiotic use
- urinary obstruction
- immunosuppression

Patients admitted from a long-term care facility should also receive empiric coverage for vancomycin-resistant *Enterococcus* and fluoroquinolone-resistant gram-negative rods.

Obtain ultrasonography or CT for persistent fever or continuing symptoms after 72 hours of antibiotics to evaluate for complications of pyelonephritis (e.g., perinephric abscess). CT and MRI should be considered in patients with persistent or relapsing pyelonephritis despite a negative ultrasound.

DON'T BE TRICKED

- Do not use ampicillin, nitrofurantoin, trimethoprim-sulfamethoxazole, or first-generation cephalosporins to treat pyelonephritis.

Tuberculosis

Screening

The TST or IGRA is the initial screening and diagnostic study for TB infection. IGRA is preferred in patients likely to have *Mycobacterium tuberculosis* infection, a low or intermediate risk of disease progression, or a history of bacillus Calmette-Guérin vaccination, as well as in patients unlikely to return to have their TST interpreted. Low-risk persons should not be screened, with the exception of those beginning employment in a hospital setting.

DON'T BE TRICKED

- Interpret a positive TST in a patient with a history of bacillus Calmette-Guérin vaccination the same as in a person without a history of this vaccination.
- Neither TST nor IGRA can distinguish latent from active infection.
- Do not obtain both a TST and an IGRA.

Diagnosis

Know the different TST threshold measurements for TB infection.

STUDY TABLE: Interpretation of Tuberculin Skin Test Results

Criteria for Tuberculin Positivity by Risk Group		
≥5 mm Induration	**≥10 mm Induration**	**≥15 mm Induration**
Persons who are HIV positive Recent contacts of persons with active TB Persons with fibrotic changes on chest x-ray consistent with old TB Patients with organ transplants and other immunosuppressive conditions (receiving the equivalent of ≥15 mg/d of prednisone for >4 weeks)	Recent (<5 yr) arrivals from high-prevalence countries Injection drug users Residents or employees of high-risk congregate settings: prisons and jails, nursing homes and other long-term facilities for older adults, hospitals and other health care facilities, residential facilities for patients with AIDS, homeless shelters Mycobacteriology laboratory personnel; persons with clinical conditions that put them at high risk for active disease; children aged <4 years or those exposed to adults in high-risk categories	All others with no risk factors for TB

Latent TB infection is defined by a positive TST or IGRA in the absence of any systemic manifestation of active infection and a normal chest x-ray.

Pulmonary TB accounts for 70% of active disease cases and is characterized by constitutional or pulmonary signs or symptoms that are often insidious and include:

- cough >3 weeks, chest pain, and hemoptysis
- fever, chills, and night sweats
- weight loss

Testing

Obtain acid-fast bacilli smears and cultures, chest x-ray, and IGRA in patients with suspected active TB. A false-negative test may occur in up to 25% of patients with active TB. Sputum or tissue culture is the gold standard for diagnosis, but results may be delayed for weeks. Acid-fast bacillus stains are rapid, but neither sensitive nor specific.

Nucleic acid amplification testing (NAAT) of sputum may be used to exclude TB in patients with false-positive sputum results (nontuberculous mycobacteria) or to confirm the disease in some patients with false-negative smears.

Select drug susceptibility testing on all culture isolates.

STUDY TABLE: Chest X-ray Patterns for Pulmonary TB

Syndrome	Pattern
Reactivation TB	Infiltrates in the apical-posterior segments of the upper lung and superior segments of the lower lobe
Primary progressive TB	Hilar lymphadenopathy or infiltrates in any part of the lung
Cavitary TB	Cavities without air-fluid levels; may be associated with either primary progressive or reactivation TB
Immunocompromised patients	Typical or absent radiologic findings are common
Miliary TB	Characteristic "millet seed" appearance (uniform reticulonodular infiltrate)

CT scans may identify abnormalities not yet visible on chest x-ray.

For suspected pleural TB, perform thoracentesis for analysis and culture (positive in only 50% of cases). If negative, perform pleural biopsy. Pleural fluid adenosine deaminase levels are helpful in the evaluation of suspected pleural TB in patients with a negative culture and pleural biopsy.

TB meningitis is associated with CSF showing lymphocytic pleocytosis with elevated protein and decreased glucose levels. NAAT of the CSF is highly specific.

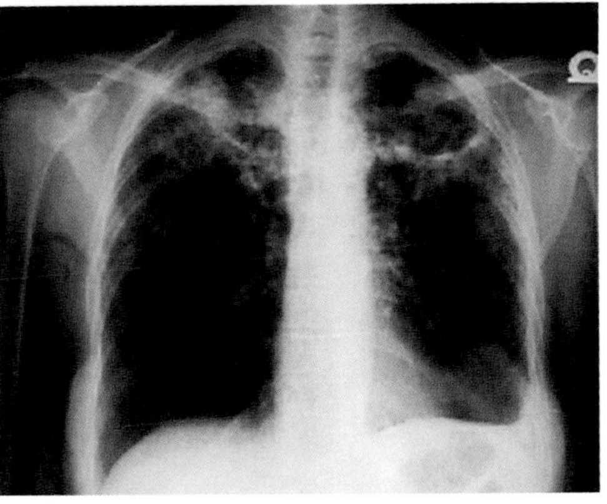

Pulmonary Tuberculosis: Upper lobe infiltrates and cavitation consistent with pulmonary TB.

DON'T BE TRICKED

- **In persons not already known to be HIV positive, test for HIV infection.**

Treatment

For latent TB: For patients without HIV, select daily isoniazid for 6 months or daily rifampin for 4 months. In patients with HIV, select daily isoniazid for 9 months. These will be the options most likely to appear on the test.

For active TB, the core first-line agents are isoniazid, rifampin, pyrazinamide, and ethambutol. These agents are administered for 8 weeks as part of the initiation phase, and then isoniazid and rifampin are continued for either 4 or 7 months as part of the continuation phase.

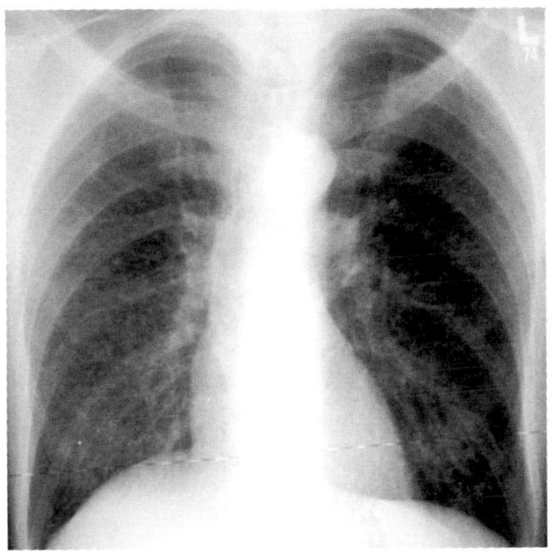

Miliary Tuberculosis: Chest x-ray reveals the bilateral presence of innumerable 1- to 3-mm nodules, predominantly seen within the lower lung fields, typical of miliary TB.

The three criteria that establish a patient as no longer infectious:

- adequate TB treatment >2 weeks
- improvement of symptoms
- three consecutive negative sputum smears

DON'T BE TRICKED

- **Drug susceptibility testing should be performed on the initial isolate in all patients.**
- **If pyrazinamide or ethambutol is used, uric acid levels or visual acuity and color vision testing are recommended, respectively.**
- **Never add a single drug to a failing TB regimen.**

TEST YOURSELF

A 40-year-old asymptomatic female hospital employee has a 10-mm TST reaction following routine screening. The employee was born in India and has lived in the United States for 10 years. She was vaccinated with bacillus Calmette-Guérin as a child. Her chest x-ray is normal.

ANSWER: For diagnosis, choose latent TB; for management, choose treatment with isoniazid or rifampin.

Mycobacterium avium Complex Infection

Diagnosis

Pulmonary disease is a classic presentation of MAC infection. It is seen in middle-aged to older adult male smokers with underlying lung disease who clinically and radiographically resemble patients with TB. Patients may present with dyspnea, cough, hemoptysis, chest discomfort, and constitutional symptoms. X-rays reveal nodular bronchiectatic disease. Another common presentation is in elderly, thin, otherwise healthy white women presenting as right middle lobe or left lingular lobe lung infection. These women often have scoliosis, pectus excavatum, or MVP suggesting an underlying connective tissue defect.

Disseminated MAC infection develops in patients with HIV who have CD4 cell counts less than 50/µL who are not receiving MAC prophylaxis. The clinical presentation often consists of fever, night sweats, weight loss, and GI symptoms.

Treatment

Clarithromycin susceptibility testing is routinely recommended for all MAC isolates. Treatment for MAC infection usually consists of clarithromycin or azithromycin with ethambutol and either rifampin or rifabutin.

DON'T BE TRICKED

- ***Mycobacterium abscessus, Mycobacterium fortuitum*, and *Mycobacterium chelonae* are causes of localized skin and soft tissue infections, usually after trauma, surgery (often associated with implanted prosthetic material), cosmetic procedures, pedicures, tattooing, and body piercing. Contaminated, nonsterile water is the source of these infections.**

Aspergillosis

Diagnosis

STUDY TABLE: Pulmonary Aspergillosis Syndromes

Condition	Characteristics
Allergic bronchopulmonary aspergillosis	Usually occurs in the setting of asthma or CF Other findings are a positive skin test, elevated IgE, and eosinophilia Presents as difficult-to-control asthma and recurrent pulmonary infiltrates
Aspergilloma (fungus ball)	Occurs in preexisting pulmonary cavities or cysts, or in areas of devitalized lung Symptoms are cough, hemoptysis, dyspnea, weight loss, fever, and chest pain
Invasive aspergillosis	Occurs in immunocompromised hosts CT scan may show the "halo sign", a target lesion with surrounding ground-glass attenuation (hemorrhage)

Neutropenic patients and organ transplant recipients are at increased risk for developing *Aspergillus* infections.

Testing

Blood cultures are rarely positive. The gold standard diagnostic test for *Aspergillus* infection is obtaining cultures from deep-body specimens. The serum galactomannan enzyme assay can support the diagnosis in the right clinical setting, and it can be followed serially to assess the response to therapy.

Treatment

Voriconazole is first-line treatment in patients with documented or suspected invasive aspergillosis. Surgical resection is indicated for aspergilloma and hemoptysis and is considered definitive therapy. Treat allergic bronchopulmonary aspergillosis with oral glucocorticoids.

DON'T BE TRICKED

- **Patients with aspergilloma who are asymptomatic and have stable x-rays do not require therapy.**

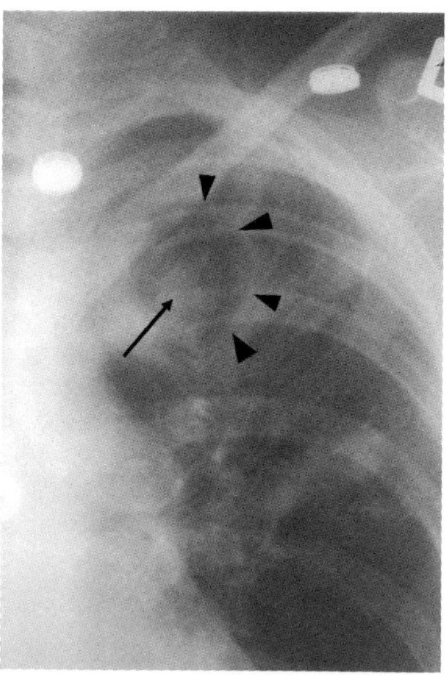

Aspergilloma: This enlarged image from a frontal chest x-ray shows a cavitary lesion (*arrowheads*) containing a round mass (*arrow*) representing a fungus ball.

Candida Infections

Diagnosis

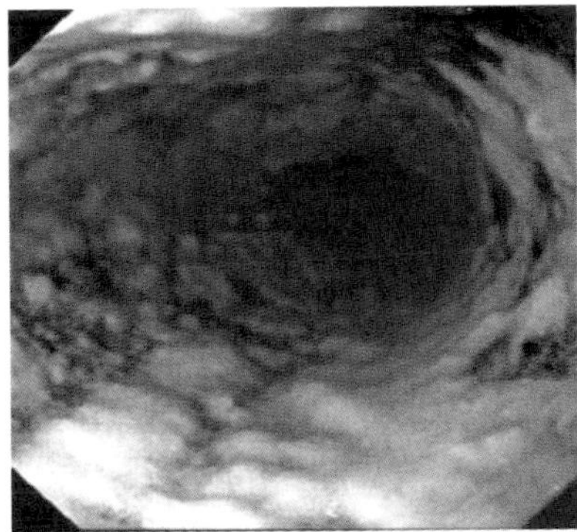

Esophageal *Candida*: White mucosal plaque-like lesions consistent with *Candida* are seen on upper endoscopy.

Mucocutaneous candidiasis may present as an erythematous intertriginous rash with satellite lesions. Oral candidiasis appears as adherent, painless white plaques on the tongue and buccal mucosa. Local invasion is most apparent in the esophagus and tends to occur in persons with reduced cell-mediated immunity or severe neutropenia.

Invasive candidiasis includes candidemia, focal organ involvement, and disseminated candidiasis, with candidemia being the most common. Candidemia occurs most frequently in the presence of an intravascular catheter.

In suspected disseminated disease, white exudates may be seen in the retina on ophthalmoscopic examination, and painless skin papules or pustules on an erythematous base may be present on the skin. Diagnosis is made by positive culture from the blood or a normally sterile body fluid or site.

DON'T BE TRICKED

- When *Candida* is isolated from the sputum, it usually reflects contamination from the oral mucosa.
- *Candida* in a blood culture is never a contaminant.

Treatment

An echinocandin (anidulafungin, caspofungin, or micafungin) is recommended as initial treatment for most patients with candidemia.

Fluconazole is effective in preventing *Candida* infections in neutropenic oncology patients, but it has limited effectiveness for preventing other fungal infections.

DON'T BE TRICKED

- Treatment is not indicated for *Candida* in the sputum of patients receiving mechanical ventilation.
- Do not treat asymptomatic candiduria except in neutropenic patients or those undergoing invasive urologic procedures.
- IV catheter removal and antifungal therapy has been associated with a shorter duration of infection and improved patient outcomes in **nonneutropenic patients** with candidemia but not in neutropenic patients.

Cryptococcal Infection

Diagnosis and Testing

The least-severe cryptococcal syndrome is characterized by lung involvement without dissemination. Disseminated disease may include fungemia and meningitis. Cryptococcal meningitis is the most common form of meningitis in patients with AIDS, who typically present with symptoms such as headache, irritability, and nausea. Most patients have a CD4 cell count of less than 100/µL. The diagnosis is based on detection of cryptococcal antigen in the CSF or culture of *Cryptococcus neoformans* in the CSF. The opening CSF pressure is typically elevated.

Treatment

Choose amphotericin B plus flucytosine for induction treatment of meningitis followed by fluconazole maintenance therapy. Maintenance therapy is indicated for patients with AIDS and cryptococcal meningitis until the CD4 cell count is ≥100/µL for ≥3 months and the viral load is suppressed. Management of elevated intracranial pressure is by serial therapeutic LPs or extraventricular drain placement.

Endemic Mycoses

STUDY TABLE: Differentiation of Endemic Mycoses

Infection	Geographic Distribution	What to Look For
Blastomycosis (*Blastomyces dermatitidis*)	Midwestern, southeastern, and south central United States (Mississippi, Missouri, and Ohio river valleys)	Symptom onset 4-6 weeks after exposure Consider in patients with primary skin lesion or concurrent pulmonary and skin or bone findings Consider in patients being evaluated for TB, malignancy
Coccidiomycosis (*Coccidioides* species)	Southern Arizona, south central California, southwestern New Mexico, west Texas	Symptom onset 1-3 weeks after exposure Consider in patients with pulmonary symptoms and erythema nodosum or erythema multiforme Consider in patients with pulmonary symptoms and prolonged constitutional symptoms (fever, fatigue) or meningitis
Histoplasmosis (*Histoplasma capsulatum*)	Midwestern states in the Ohio and Mississippi River valley regions	Symptom onset 2-3 weeks after exposure Consider in patients with complex pulmonary disease (nodular, cavitary, lymphadenopathy) Consider patients being evaluated for sarcoidosis, TB, or malignancy
Sporotrichosis (*Sporothrix schenckii*)	Occurs almost exclusively in persons who engage in landscaping or gardening	A papule appears days to weeks later at the inoculation site. Similar lesions then occur along lymphatic channels proximal to the inoculation site.

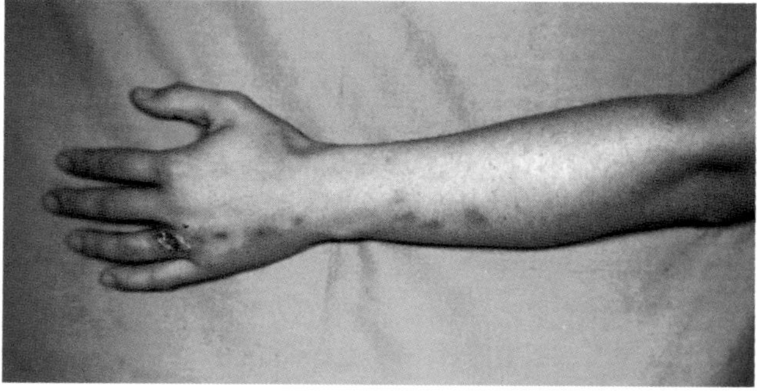

Sporotrichosis: The most common presentation of sporotrichosis is lymphocutaneous sporotrichosis. The primary lesion is located at the site of inoculation and consists of an ulcerated nodule. Similar lesions occur proximally along the lymphatics.

Chlamydia trachomatis Infection

Diagnosis and Testing

C. trachomatis is the most commonly reported STI in the United States. It may cause cervicitis, urethritis, epididymitis, and proctitis but also may be asymptomatic and lead to significant complications, including ectopic pregnancy, tubal infertility, and chronic pelvic pain syndromes.

NAAT is the preferred diagnostic test for chlamydia. NAAT can be performed on first-voided urine samples, urethral swabs from men, and vaginal or endocervical swabs from women.

Treatment

Treat chlamydial infection with azithromycin or doxycycline.

Neisseria gonorrhoeae Infection

Diagnosis

N. gonorrhoeae infection should be suspected in men with purulent or mucopurulent urethral discharge and in women with mucopurulent cervicitis. Gonorrhea and *Chlamydia trachomatis* infection are also common causes of epididymitis in sexually active men aged <35 years, proctitis in persons who engage in anal receptive intercourse, and pharyngitis in persons who engage in oral sex. Infection at any site, most notably infection of the pharynx and rectum, may be asymptomatic.

Disseminated gonococcal infection may cause two syndromes: an arthritis-dermatitis syndrome or purulent arthritis alone without skin findings. Characteristics of the dermatitis-arthritis syndrome include:

- sparse peripheral necrotic pustules
- monoarthritis or oligoarthritis (knees, hips, and wrists)
- tendon sheath inflammation

Consider terminal component complement deficiency as a possible cause of recurrent disseminated gonococcal infection.

Testing

NAAT is the preferred diagnostic test for *N. gonorrhoeae* infections. NAAT can be performed on first-voided urine, urethral swabs from men, and vaginal or endocervical swabs from women. NAAT has not been approved by the FDA for diagnosis of oropharyngeal or rectal gonorrhea, but the Centers for Disease Control and Prevention recommends its use to diagnose these infections.

STUDY TABLE: Additional Diagnostic Studies for Gonorrhea

Condition	Best Test
Arthritis	Joint fluid culture
Disseminated infection	Blood culture

DON'T BE TRICKED

- **Do not select Gram stain to diagnose gonorrheal cervicitis.**
- **Do not forget to test for chlamydia, syphilis, and HIV infection in patients with gonorrhea.**

Treatment

Because of high coinfection rates of chlamydia with gonorrheal infections, treat uncomplicated mucosal infections (cervicitis, urethritis, and proctitis) caused by gonorrhea with ceftriaxone (or other suitable third-generation cephalosporins) plus azithromycin or doxycycline. In sexually active men <35 years of age, treat epididymitis with ceftriaxone and azithromycin or doxycycline for 10 days. Treat disseminated gonococcal infection with a 7- to 14-day course of ceftriaxone.

DON'T BE TRICKED

- **Do not select fluoroquinolones to treat gonorrhea because of antibiotic resistance.**

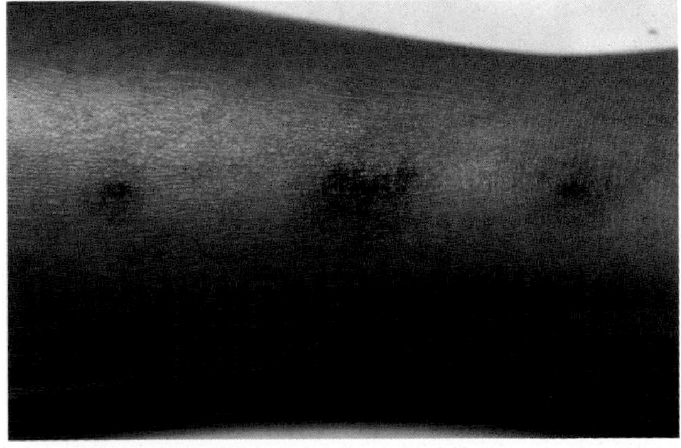

Gonorrhea: Several necrotic pustules and surrounding erythema on the leg associated with disseminated gonorrhea infection.

Pelvic Inflammatory Disease

Diagnosis and Testing

PID is a polymicrobial infection of the endometrium, fallopian tubes, and ovaries that is diagnosed by the presence of abdominal discomfort, uterine or adnexal tenderness, or cervical motion tenderness. Other criteria include:

- temperature >38.3 °C (101.0 °F)
- cervical or vaginal mucopurulent discharge
- leukocytes in vaginal secretions

PID most often occurs within 7 days of the onset of menses. Gonorrhea and chlamydia are the primary identifiable causes of PID. Order NAAT to diagnose *Neisseria gonorrhoeae* and *Chlamydia trachomatis*. All sexually active women should have a pregnancy test to rule out ectopic pregnancy. In patients with RUQ abdominal pain and elevated aminotransferase levels, consider gonorrhea or chlamydia perihepatitis (Fitz-Hugh-Curtis syndrome). Complications include infertility, ectopic pregnancy, and chronic pelvic pain.

Treatment

Outpatient treatment is as effective as inpatient treatment for women with mild-to-moderate PID. Acceptable treatment regimens include a single parenteral dose of ceftriaxone plus doxycycline with or without metronidazole for 14 days.

Choose hospitalization for the following scenarios:

- no clinical improvement after 48 to 72 hours of antibiotic treatment
- inability to tolerate oral antibiotics
- severe illness with nausea, vomiting, or high fever
- suspected pelvic abscess
- pregnancy

Inpatients are treated with parenteral cefoxitin or cefotetan and doxycycline. If the patient is nonresponsive to antibiotics in 48 to 72 hours, choose ultrasonography for evaluation of possible tubo-ovarian abscess.

DON'T BE TRICKED

- Remember to screen for other STIs such as HIV.
- Because of increasing rates of *N. gonorrhoeae* fluoroquinolone resistance, do not select fluoroquinolones for empiric treatment of PID.

Syphilis

Diagnosis

Syphilis is a sexually acquired infection caused by *Treponema pallidum*.

Primary syphilis presents as an ulcer (chancre) that develops approximately 3 weeks after inoculation. The ulcer has a clean appearance with heaped-up borders, is usually painless, and resolves spontaneously.

Secondary syphilis develops 2 to 8 weeks after the appearance of the primary chancre and is characterized by widespread hematogenous dissemination involving most often the skin, liver, and lymph nodes. Secondary syphilis resolves spontaneously.

To diagnose secondary syphilis, look for:

- fever and any type of rash (except vesicles), often with palmar or plantar involvement
- nontender generalized lymphadenopathy
- headache, cranial nerve abnormalities, altered mental status, or stiff neck
- mucous patches (a slightly elevated oval erosive lesion with surrounding inflammation) and condylomata lata lesions (grey to white, raised, wart-like lesions on moist intertriginous surfaces)

Latent (tertiary) syphilis involves the presence of serologic evidence of infection in the absence of clinical signs. Latent syphilis is divided into early latent (infection ≤1 year in duration) or late-latent (infection >1 year). If duration is unknown, it is classified as latent syphilis of unknown duration.

Manifestations of late syphilis may occur years after the initial infection. Tertiary syphilis may cause:

- meningitis and subarachnoid arteritis (a cause of stroke in a young patient)
- aortitis
- general paresis and tabes dorsalis
- gumma in any organ

Testing

Serologic testing is the mainstay of syphilis diagnosis.

Pearls about RPR and VDRL tests:

- often negative in primary infection
- positive in high titers in secondary syphilis
- lower titers are seen in latent and tertiary infection

Confirm positive RPR or VDRL with a fluorescent treponemal antibody absorption test (FTA-ABS) or *Treponema pallidum* particle agglutination (TPPA) assay.

Nontreponemal tests should decrease in titer and may become negative after treatment (but will rise again in the setting of reinfection); the FTA-ABS and microhemagglutination assay for *T. pallidum* (MHA-TP) antibodies will remain positive indefinitely. Test all patients for HIV infection.

Perform a CSF examination for patients with primary or secondary syphilis and the presence of any neurologic sign or symptom.

Diagnose neurosyphilis when any one of the following is present:

- CSF lymphocytes >5/µL
- elevated CSF protein
- positive CSF VDRL test

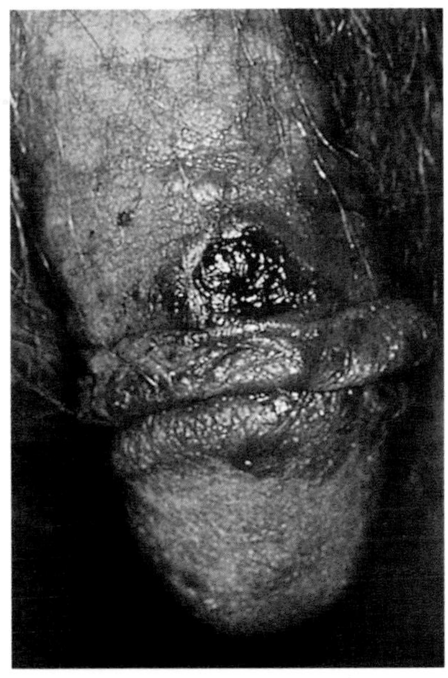

Syphilis: Primary chancre of syphilis characterized by a clean-based, nonpainful genital ulcer.

STUDY TABLE: Differential Diagnosis of Genital Ulcers

Disease	Characteristics
Herpes (HSV type 1 or 2)	Multiple 1- to 2-mm tender vesicles or erosions and tender lymphadenopathy
Syphilis (*T. pallidum*)	Single 0.5- to 1.0-cm painless indurated ulcers and nontender bilateral inguinal lymphadenopathy
Chancroid (*Haemophilus ducreyi*)	Ragged, purulent, painful ulcers with tender lymphadenopathy
Lymphogranuloma venereum (*Chlamydia trachomatis*)	Single 0.2- to 1.0-cm ulcer, sometimes painful, with tender unilateral lymphadenopathy, which may suppurate
Fixed drug eruptions (NSAIDs, phenobarbital, antibiotics)	Single or multiple blisters or erosions, 1-3 cm, frequently on the glans penis

Treatment

The preferred therapy for syphilis at all stages is parenteral penicillin, which is the only acceptable therapy for pregnant patients.

- Treat **primary or secondary or early latent syphilis** with one dose of IM benzathine penicillin.
- Treat **late latent or asymptomatic syphilis of unknown duration** with 3 weekly doses of benzathine penicillin.
- Treat **late (tertiary) nonneurosyphilis** with three weekly doses of IM benzathine penicillin.
- Treat **neurosyphilis** with continuous penicillin G infusion (or every 4 hours) for 10 to 14 days.

Doxycycline and tetracycline are alternatives for nonneurosyphilis in penicillin-allergic nonpregnant patients.

Failure of nontreponemal serologic test results to decrease fourfold in the 6 to 12 months after treatment indicates treatment failure or reacquisition.

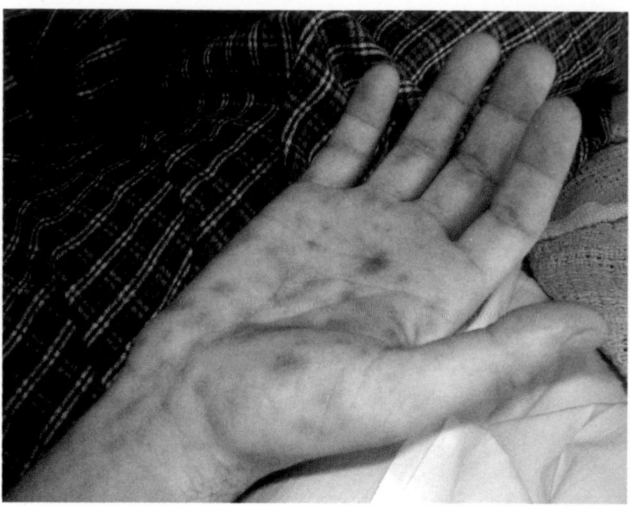

Secondary Syphilis: Pink to reddish-brown macules and papules on the palms, characteristic of secondary syphilis.

DON'T BE TRICKED

- **Pregnant patients who are allergic to penicillin must be desensitized and treated with penicillin.**
- **The Jarisch-Herxheimer reaction is an acute febrile illness occurring within 24 hours of treatment for any stage of syphilis and is not an allergic reaction to penicillin.**

Herpes Simplex Virus Infection

Diagnosis and Testing

Inoculation of HSV at mucosal surfaces or skin sites results in the sudden appearance of multiple vesicular lesions on an inflamed, erythematous base. Primary infection may also be associated with systemic symptoms, such as fever and malaise. After primary infection resolves, the virus lives in a latent state in nerve cell bodies in ganglion neurons and can reactivate.

Several herpetic syndromes are possible in the adult.

STUDY TABLE: Selected Herpes Simplex Virus Syndromes

Manifestation	Description
Oral	First-episode infections are most commonly gingivostomatitis and pharyngitis, whereas herpes labialis is the most frequent sign of reactivation disease
Herpetic whitlow	HSV infection of the finger often mistaken for bacterial infection
Genital herpes	Multiple painful vesicular or ulcerative lesions on penis or vulva Initial episode frequently associated with systemic symptoms and regional lymphadenopathy Recurrent genital herpes is usually caused by HSV-2
Keratitis	Punctate or branching epithelial keratitis
Encephalitis	Rapid onset of fever, headache, seizures, focal neurologic signs, and impaired consciousness (see Herpes Simplex Encephalitis)
Hepatitis	Rare complication of either HSV-1 or HSV-2 that is most common in immunosuppressed patients (glucocorticoid use, HIV infection, cancer, MDS, pregnancy)
Associated HIV infection	Infection can occur anywhere and often presents as extensive oral or perianal ulcers (not vesicles) or as esophagitis, colitis, chorioretinitis, acute retinal necrosis, tracheobronchitis, and pneumonia
Bell palsy	HSV is implicated in Bell palsy syndrome

PCR testing of clinical specimens obtained from ulcers and mucocutaneous sites is the most sensitive diagnostic modality available.

DON'T BE TRICKED

- A positive HSV-2 antibody test indicates only previous infection and is not a useful diagnostic test.
- Don't order a Tzanck test to diagnose HSV infection; it is neither sensitive nor specific.
- Patients with late-stage HIV are prone to frequent recurrences of genital herpes and chronic mucocutaneous ulceration (not vesicles).
- Recurrent erythema multiforme is most commonly caused by HSV recurrences.

Treatment

For the first episode of **genital herpes**, treat with acyclovir, famciclovir, or valacyclovir for 7 to 10 days. Treat recurrent disease for 3 to 5 days. Treatment decreases duration of symptoms and reduces viral shedding. Suppressive therapy may be necessary to decrease the frequency of recurrences.

Treat primary episodes of **oral HSV** infection the same as genital lesions. Recurrent disease is generally not treated. Suppressive therapy can be considered for frequent recurrences (≥6/year), particularly in immunosuppressed patients.

Treat **primary herpes keratoconjunctivitis** with topical trifluorothymidine, vidarabine, or acyclovir. Ophthalmology referral is mandatory.

For **suspected or confirmed herpes encephalitis,** use IV acyclovir.

For **Bell palsy with severe facial paralysis**, glucocorticoids may be beneficial. The role of antiviral therapy is unclear.

DON'T BE TRICKED

- Do not treat herpetic keratitis with topical glucocorticoid drops.
- Topical acyclovir is not effective for treating genital herpes.

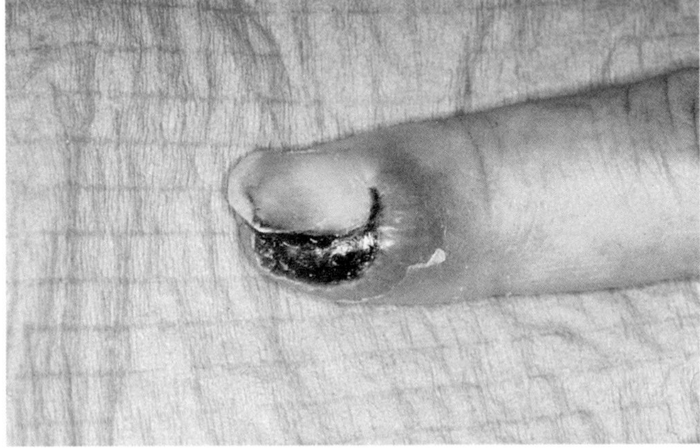

Herpetic Whitlow: Herpetic whitlow involving the lateral aspect of the index finger.

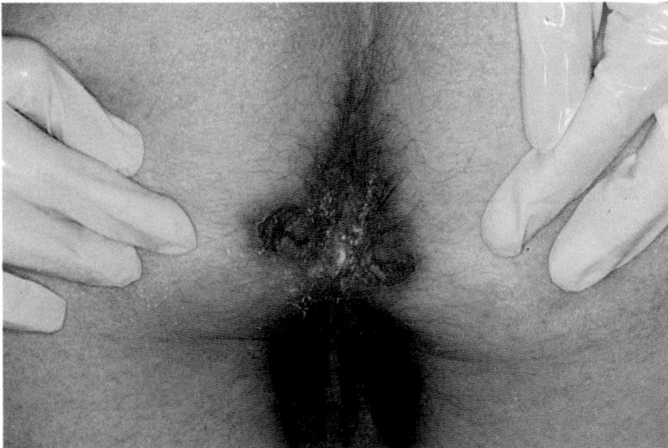

Perianal Herpes Simplex: Perianal herpes simplex in an immunocompromised patient (HIV/AIDS). In patients with HIV disease, herpes simplex may appear as painful, shallow ulcers rather than the classic vesicle.

Genital Warts

Prevention

The HPV4 and HPV9 vaccines are approved for both sexes and protect against HPV types that cause genital warts and cervical cancer.

Diagnosis

Genital warts are most commonly caused by HPV types 6 and 11. They are typically painless, flesh colored, and exophytic. Diagnosis is generally made based on clinical appearance.

Treatment

Most infections clear spontaneously. Treatment does not prevent HPV transmission. Patient-applied agents include podophylox (podophyllotoxin), imiquimod, and sinecatechins. Physician-administered treatments include podophyllin resin, trichloroacetic acid, cryotherapy, and surgical removal.

Osteomyelitis

Diagnosis

Microorganisms can reach the bone by:

- contiguous spread from adjacent soft tissue or joints
- hematogenous seeding
- direct inoculation as a result of surgery or trauma

Staphylococcus aureus is the most commonly isolated pathogen causing hematogenous osteomyelitis. Osteomyelitis associated with contiguous foci of infection, decubitus ulcers, and vascular insufficiency is often polymicrobial.

Adults with osteomyelitis usually have pain around the involved site without systemic symptoms. A draining sinus tract may be present over the area of involved bone. Patients who have undergone total joint arthroplasty and have new or unresolved joint pain may have a prosthetic joint infection.

STUDY TABLE: Categorization and Characterization of Osteomyelitis

Category	Characteristics
Acute hematogenous osteomyelitis	Infection of intervertebral disc space and two adjacent vertebrae
Contiguous osteomyelitis	Patients >50 years old with diabetes mellitus or peripheral vascular disease and a nonhealing foot ulcer despite 6 weeks of standard care
Following dog or cat bite	*Pasteurella multocida* may cause contiguous-focus osteomyelitis after dog or cat bites
Following foot puncture wound	*Pseudomonas* is frequently isolated following puncture wounds through the rubber sole of a shoe
Sternal osteomyelitis	Wound healing complications, unstable sternum, and fever after thoracic surgery
Sternoclavicular joint osteomyelitis	Pain and fever in an injection-drug user
Sickle cell disease	Bone infarcts and bone marrow thrombosis predispose to osteomyelitis most commonly caused by *Salmonella* species and *S. aureus*.

Testing

MRI is the imaging procedure of choice for patients with suspected osteomyelitis; nuclear bone scan may be chosen if MRI is contraindicated. Half of patients with acute hematogenous osteomyelitis will have positive blood cultures. Cultures are less likely to be positive with contiguous osteomyelitis.

Bone biopsy is the definitive diagnostic study for osteomyelitis. A positive blood culture obviates the need for a bone biopsy. Bone biopsy is best obtained by surgical sampling or by needle aspiration under radiographic guidance. In stable chronic osteomyelitis, antimicrobial therapy is withheld until deep bone cultures have been obtained.

The most common organism found in vertebral osteomyelitis is *S. aureus* (including MRSA); coagulase-negative staphylococci are also common. MRI is the most sensitive imaging modality to detect vertebral osteomyelitis. Patients with imaging studies suggestive of vertebral osteomyelitis but negative blood cultures should undergo a CT-guided percutaneous needle biopsy.

DON'T BE TRICKED

- Do not obtain sinus tract and wound drainage cultures.

Treatment

The pillars of treatment include:

- administration of adequate antimicrobials for a prolonged period of time (usually 6 weeks)
- surgical debridement (if warranted)
- removal of orthopedic prosthetic devices (if feasible)

Empiric antibiotic treatment may be given if a causative agent is not identified. Vancomycin or daptomycin plus ceftriaxone, ceftazidime, cefepime, or a fluoroquinolone are appropriate choices. Also consider:

- removal of orthopedic hardware for most patients with orthopedic implant-associated osteomyelitis
- a prolonged course (3-6 months) of fluoroquinolone and rifampin therapy when implant removal is not possible

For **diabetic foot infections with osteomyelitis**, surgically remove all devitalized bone and treat for 4 to 6 weeks with broad-spectrum antimicrobial therapy:

- imipenem-cilastatin
- piperacillin-tazobactam
- ampicillin-sulbactam

Vancomycin, linezolid, or daptomycin is added if MRSA coinfection is a concern.

In patients with poor arterial vascular supply, also choose revascularization.

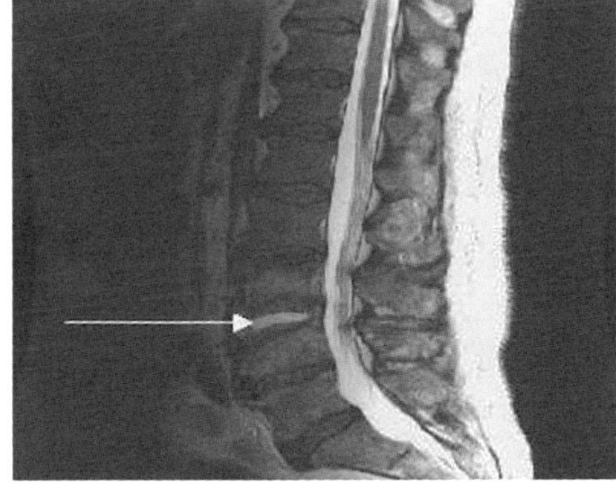

Hematogenous Osteomyelitis: MRI shows moderate destruction of the inferior L3 and superior L4 vertebral bodies compatible with osteomyelitis. Moderate narrowing of the thecal sac is seen at this level owing to retropulsion of an enhancing bony fragment.

DON'T BE TRICKED

- Surgery is not needed for uncomplicated hematogenous vertebral osteomyelitis.
- A positive MRI persists long after effective therapy for osteomyelitis; do not obtain follow-up MRI to verify clinical improvement.

TEST YOURSELF

A 60-year-old previously healthy man has nonradiating pain in his lower thoracic spine that began 10 days ago. Six weeks ago, he was unable to urinate and required an indwelling urinary catheter. Temperature is 37.9 °C (100.2 °F). Point tenderness of the lower thoracic spine is present.

ANSWER: For diagnosis, choose acute hematogenous osteomyelitis of the vertebral spine with cord compression secondary to vertebral collapse or epidural abscess formation. For management, select empiric antibiotic therapy and urgent surgical consultation.

Fever of Unknown Origin

Diagnosis

Fever of unknown origin is characterized by a temperature >38.3 °C (100.9 °F) for at least 3 weeks that remains undiagnosed after 2 outpatient visits or 3 days of inpatient evaluation.

STUDY TABLE: Categories and Common Causes of Fever of Unknown Origin

Category	Common Causes
Classic	Infection (primary CMV infection, endocarditis, TB, abscesses, complicated UTI), neoplasm, connective tissue disease, endocrine diseases
Health-care associated	Drug fever, septic thrombophlebitis, PE, sinusitis, postoperative complications (occult abscesses), *Clostridium difficile* enterocolitis, device- or procedure-related endocarditis
Neutropenic	Bacterial and fungal infections (aspergillosis, candidiasis), drug fever, PE, underlying malignancy; cause not documented in 40%-60% of cases
HIV associated	Primary HIV infection, opportunistic infections (CMV, cryptococcosis, TB and nontuberculous *Mycobacteria* infection, toxoplasmosis), lymphoma, IRIS

Drug-induced fever can occur at any time but usually appears days to weeks after initiation of a new drug. Associated features may include rash, urticaria, liver or kidney dysfunction, and mucosal ulceration. Laboratory tests may show elevated serum aminotransferases, leukocytosis or leukopenia, and eosinophilia. Look especially for anticonvulsants (phenytoin, carbamazepine), antibiotics (β-lactams, sulfonamides, nitrofurantoin), and allopurinol.

TEST YOURSELF

A 22-year-old woman begins taking phenytoin after undergoing a craniotomy for a subdural hematoma. Twelve days later, she develops a temperature of 38.3 °C (100.9 °F) and a generalized erythematous rash. The leukocyte count is 12,800/µL with eosinophilia, serum AST level is 66 U/L, and ALT level is 72 U/L.

ANSWER: For diagnosis, select DRESS, also known as hypersensitivity syndrome, as cause of fever and rash.

Primary Immunodeficiency Syndromes

Diagnosis and Testing

Consider primary immunodeficiency syndromes in patients with multiple or recurrent infections. The most common primary immunodeficiency is IgA deficiency. Most patients with isolated IgA deficiency are clinically normal, but may present with recurrent sinopulmonary infections, giardiasis, and have an increased risk for autoimmune disorders, including RA and SLE. Patients with undetectable levels of serum IgA are at high risk for transfusion reactions because of the development of anti-IgA antibodies.

CVID is the most common symptomatic primary immunodeficiency and is characterized by low levels of one or more immunoglobulin classes or subclasses. Findings include:

- hypogammaglobulinemia
- recurrent bacterial upper and lower respiratory infections (including bronchiectasis)
- predilection for infection with encapsulated bacteria (pneumococcus, *Haemophilus*)
- infectious diarrhea, specifically *Giardia lamblia* infection
- chronic diarrhea/malabsorption

Measure serum IgM, IgA, IgG (all low), and IgG subclasses (variably low), and measure the ability to mount an antibody response to tetanus toxoid (protein) and pneumococcal polysaccharide vaccine (polysaccharide) antigens.

Treatment

Choose IV immune globulin as first-line therapy for CVID. Most patients with selective IgA therapy do not require treatment.

DON'T BE TRICKED

- **Standard IV immune globulin is contraindicated in isolated IgA deficiency because these patients may have IgG or IgE antibodies directed against the transfused IgA.**

TEST YOURSELF

A 37-year-old woman has had eight episodes of documented sinusitis annually for the past 15 years. She had a single episode of pneumonia as a child.

ANSWER: For diagnosis, choose CVID. For management, choose measurement of serum immunoglobulin levels and, if low, measurement of antibody response to pneumococcal and tetanus vaccines.

Complement Deficiency

Diagnosis

Persons with deficiencies of the terminal components of the classic complement pathway (C5, C6, C7, C8, and C9) are susceptible to recurrent neisserial infections. Defects in components of the alternative complement pathway of activation and the lectin pathway may also be associated with neisserial infections. Patients with deficiencies of the early components of the complement system will have repeated infections with encapsulated bacteria and often SLE.

Testing

Obtain a CH_{50} assay. If CH_{50} is low, follow up with individual component measurements. Screen all patients with repeated episodes of disseminated gonorrhea or meningococcal infection with CH_{50} assay. Measurement of the alternative (AH_{50} assay) and lectin pathway components is indicated in patients in whom complement deficiency is suspected but CH_{50} is normal.

STUDY TABLE: Pattern Recognition Diagnosis of Repeated Infections

Presenting Pattern	Congenital Defect	Test
Invasive skin infections	Granulocyte (chronic granulomatous disease)	Dihydrorhodamine (DHR) oxidation test
Benign or intracellular viral or fungal infections	Cell mediated	CBC (lymphocyte count), CD3, CD4, and CD8 lymphocyte markers
Repeated sinopulmonary infections with encapsulated bacteria	Immunoglobulins	Quantitative serum immunoglobulins and response to tetanus and pneumococcal polysaccharide vaccines
Sinopulmonary infections, malabsorption, infertility, family history of CF	*CFTR* gene (CF)	Sweat chloride test
Recurrent *Neisseria meningitidis* infection and disseminated gonorrhea	Terminal complement components (C5, C6, C7, C8, and C9), alternative and lectin pathways	CH_{50} assay

Treatment

Patients with complement deficiency respond to standard antibiotics. Patients should maintain currency of vaccinations, especially meningococcal, pneumococcal, and *Haemophilus* b conjugate vaccine.

TEST YOURSELF

A 21-year-old male college student has meningococcal meningitis for the third time in 2 years.

ANSWER: For diagnosis, choose terminal complement deficiency. For management, select serum CH_{50} assay.

Bioterrorism

Biologic agents most likely to be used in bioterrorist events are anthrax, smallpox, plague, tularemia, botulism, and viral hemorrhagic fever. Clues suggesting a bioterrorism attack include:

- sudden onset of unusual number of cases
- increased severity or uncommon clinical presentation
- unusual geographic, temporal, or demographic clustering of cases

Smallpox

Diagnosis

The last reported case of smallpox worldwide occurred in 1977. It remains a concern because of the threat of bioterrorism and the need to distinguish smallpox from similar diseases.

To diagnose smallpox, look for:

- fever >38.5 °C (101.3 °F), fatigue, and headache and backaches
- rash beginning 2 to 3 days after onset of fever
- rash first appearing on buccal or pharyngeal mucosa, then the face and proximal arms and legs, and then spreading to the chest and distal extremities, including the palms and soles
- rash in the same stage at any one time, in any one location of the body (all papules, all vesicles, all pustules, or all crusts)

Smallpox can be confused with varicella (chickenpox).

In chickenpox, look for:

- generally mild prodrome of fever and constitutional symptoms in children and adolescents, occurring simultaneously with rash
- rash beginning on the trunk, then spreading to the face and extremities
- rash in different stages (mix of papules, vesicles, pustules, and crusts) at any one time

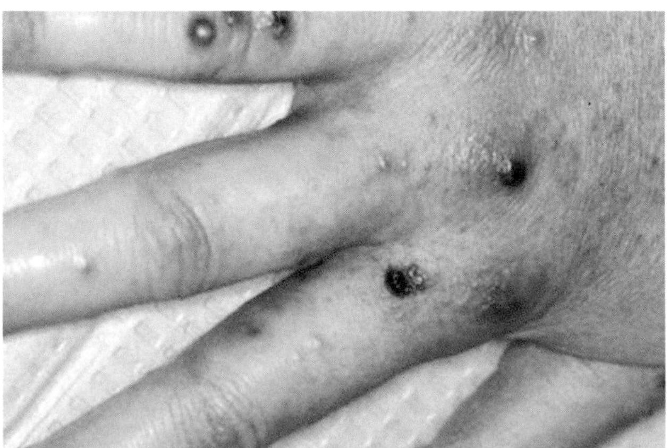

Varicella Infection: Characteristic varicella infection with rash at different stages of development (vesicles, papules, pustules, and crusts) in one region of the body.

DON'T BE TRICKED

- **Patients with smallpox remain contagious until all scabs and crusts are shed.**

Treatment

Therapy has been largely supportive, but tecovirimat has recently been approved for treatment. To prevent spread, postexposure vaccination with vaccinia within 7 days of exposure and targeting close contacts of patients with smallpox ("ring vaccination") is recommended.

Anthrax

Diagnosis

Three types of anthrax occur in humans: cutaneous, GI, and inhalational. Cutaneous anthrax is the most common type of anthrax in the United States. Look for anthrax risk factors, including:

- travel to the Middle East, Africa, South America, or Asia
- exposure to wool, hides, or animal hair from endemic countries
- bioterrorism

Select cutaneous anthrax if the patient has an enlarging, painless ulcer with black eschar surrounded by edema or large gram-positive bacilli on Gram stain. Look for inhalational anthrax if the patient has dyspnea, fever, chest pain, and a widened mediastinum on chest x-ray or CT scan.

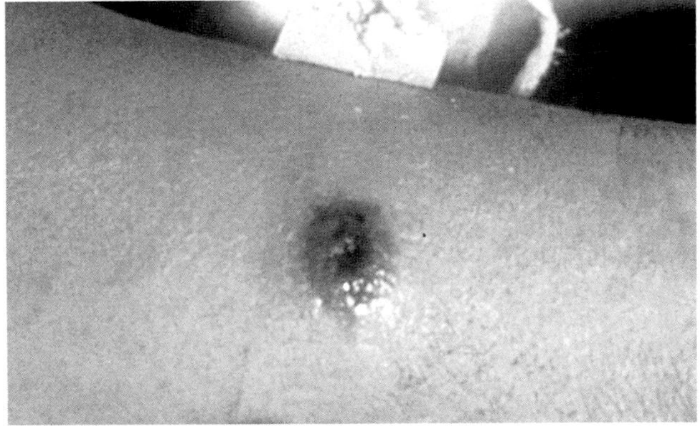

Cutaneous Anthrax: The primary lesion of cutaneous anthrax is a painless, pruritic papule. As the lesion matures, a painless ulcer develops, covered by the characteristic black eschar surrounded by nonpitting edema.

Prevention

To prevent inhalational anthrax, select postexposure vaccination and ciprofloxacin for 60 days. Raxibacumab, a monoclonal antibody that neutralizes *Bacillus anthracis* toxin, is also approved for prevention of inhalational anthrax.

Treatment

Cutaneous anthrax: Select oral ciprofloxacin.

Inhalational anthrax, anthrax meningitis, and severe cutaneous disease (involving the head and neck): Choose IV ciprofloxacin and two additional antibiotics (penicillin, ampicillin, imipenem, meropenem, clindamycin, linezolid, rifampin, vancomycin, clarithromycin). Raxibacumab, a monoclonal antibody that neutralizes *Bacillus anthracis* toxin, is also approved for the treatment of inhalational anthrax.

TEST YOURSELF

A 57-year-old male government clerk has 3 days of malaise, fever, cough, and headache. Temperature is 39.0 °C (102.2 °F), and lung crackles are heard bilaterally. A chest x-ray shows scattered pulmonary infiltrates and a widened mediastinum.

ANSWER: For diagnosis, select inhalational anthrax. For treatment, choose IV ciprofloxacin and two other antibiotics.

Plague

Diagnosis

Yersinia pestis most often is transmitted by fleas, but may also arise from inhalation.

Forms of plague:

- **Bubonic plague** follows primary cutaneous exposure and is characterized by buboes (infected, swollen lymph nodes).
- **Septicemic plague** is characterized by DIC and multiorgan system failure.
- **Pneumonic plague** most often arises secondarily through hematogenous spread from a bubo or direct inhalation.

Patients with pneumonic plague present with sudden high fever, pleuritic chest discomfort, a productive cough, and hemoptysis. The chest x-ray is nonspecific. Sputum Gram stain (and possibly blood smear) may identify the classic bipolar gram-negative staining or "safety pin" shape.

Treatment

Treat with either streptomycin or gentamicin.

Tularemia

Diagnosis and Testing

Francisella tularensis is gram-negative coccobacillus that exists mainly as a zoonotic disease but can cause significant illness through inhalation.

Pneumonic tularemia is characterized by a cough, dyspnea, and substernal or pleuritic chest pain. Respiratory failure may ensue. Typical chest x-ray findings include infiltrates (at times nodular or rounded), hilar lymphadenopathy, and pleural effusion.

A high index of clinical suspicion is necessary for diagnosis. Routine laboratory tests are nonspecific. Diagnosis is confirmed 2 or more weeks after infection with presence of IgM and IgG antibodies to *Francisella tularensis.*

Treatment

Treat mild or moderate disease with oral ciprofloxacin or doxycycline, and treat severe tularemia with streptomycin or gentamicin.

Botulism

Diagnosis and Testing

The *Clostridium botulinum* neurotoxin inhibits acetylcholine release at ganglia and neuromuscular junctions, causing bulbar palsy and symmetric flaccid paralysis beginning 12 to 72 hours after exposure. The toxin can be inhaled or ingested.

Remember the "Five D's" of botulism:

- Diplopia
- Dysphonia
- Dysarthria
- Dysphagia
- Descending paralysis (starting with facial muscles)

Disease confirmation depends on identifying botulinum toxin from samples of the patient's blood, stool, gastric contents, and wound.

Treatment

Ventilatory capacity must be monitored (often in the ICU), and respiratory support may be required. In patients with wound botulism, the wounds should be debrided. A trivalent (types A, B, C) equine serum antitoxin should be administered as early as possible to prevent progression; it cannot reverse existing paralysis.

Viral Hemorrhagic Fever

Diagnosis and Testing

Viral hemorrhagic fevers are a group of febrile illnesses caused by zoonotic RNA viruses. Ebola is the best known in this group endemic to Central Africa.

A high febrile prodrome universally occurs, accompanied by myalgia and prostration. Early signs of infection often include conjunctival injection, petechial hemorrhages, and easy bruising. As the disease advances, patients experience shock and generalized bleeding from the mucous membranes, skin, and GI tract with multiorgan failure. Virus can be transmitted in blood, urine, saliva, feces, vomit, and sweat. Isolation precautions are important to protect health care providers and limit the spread of infection.

Diagnostic confirmation requires RNA detection by reverse transcription PCR, the presence of viral protein antigens, development of IgM antibodies, or isolation of the virus.

Treatment

Treatment is primarily supportive.

Travel-Related Illness

STUDY TABLE: Travel-Associated Infections

Condition	Clinical Clues
Febrile Illnesses	
Malaria	Paroxysmal fever (every 48 or 72 hours, depending on the species and may be continuous with *Plasmodium falciparum*), intraerythrocytic parasites, thrombocytopenia
Dengue fever	Acute onset of fever with chills, biphasic fever pattern ("saddleback"), frontal headache, lumbosacral pain, extensor surface petechiae
Chikungunya fever	Fever (abrupt onset up to 40 °C [104 °F] with rigors with recrudescent episodes), rash, and small joint polyarthritis
Zika virus	Nonspecific symptoms of fever, rash, joint pain, and/or conjunctivitis (asymptomatic in up to 80% of persons)
Typhoid fever	Prolonged fever, pulse-temperature dissociation, diarrhea or constipation, faint salmon-colored macules on the abdomen and trunk ("rose spots")
Novel coronaviruses (severe acute respiratory syndrome [SARS], Middle East respiratory syndrome [MERS-CoV])	Flu-like syndrome prodrome, diarrhea, dry cough with progressive dyspnea, lymphopenia, thrombocytopenia, elevated lactate dehydrogenase
Hemorrhagic fever viruses (Ebola, Marburg, and Lassa)	Fever, malaise, myalgia, vomiting, diarrhea, coagulation disorders, and bleeding
Rabies	Paresthesias or pain at wound site, fever, nausea and vomiting, hydrophobia, delirium, agitation
Travelers' Diarrhea	
Bacterial agents: *Escherichia coli*, *Campylobacter* species, *Salmonella* species, *Vibrio* species, *Shigella* species	Abrupt onset, crampy diarrhea, blood in stools
Viral agents: rotavirus, norovirus	Closed setting (such as cruise ship or classroom) acquisition, vomiting, diarrhea, short duration
Protozoa: *Cryptosporidium* species, microsporidia, *Giardia* species, *Entamoeba histolytica*, and *Isospora* species	Gradual onset, progressive and prolonged diarrhea, foul-smelling and greasy stools, mucus or visible blood in stools

Zika Virus

Zika virus is a mosquito-borne flavivirus. Transmission can also occur through maternal-fetal transmission, sex, blood transfusion, or organ transplantation. Zika virus infection during pregnancy has been associated with microcephaly and other congenital malformations.

Prevention

Advise women who are pregnant against travel to areas where Zika virus is present. Women and men who are planning to conceive in the near future should consider avoiding nonessential travel to areas with risk of Zika infection; it is recommended that couples wait to conceive until at least 3 months (for men) or 8 weeks (for women) after last possible Zika virus exposure, onset of symptoms, or Zika infection diagnosis.

Diagnosis

Symptoms of Zika virus infection:

- fever
- rash
- joint pain
- conjunctivitis
- muscle pain
- headache

Only 18% of infected persons, however, develop symptoms.

Testing and Treatment

All pregnant women should be assessed for possible Zika exposure, and those who return from areas with outbreaks should be screened for evidence of infection.

Reverse transcriptase PCR testing on serum and urine is used for diagnostic evaluation during the initial 2 weeks after illness onset. Thereafter, IgM antibody detection is used.

No specific medications are available for treating Zika virus.

Malaria

Prevention

Select chloroquine for travelers to areas where chloroquine-resistant *Plasmodium falciparum* has not been reported (Central America, Haiti, Dominican Republic). Otherwise, select mefloquine, atovaquone-proguanil, or doxycycline.

Diagnosis and Testing

Most infections are caused by *P. falciparum* or *Plasmodium vivax*, and most deaths are because of *P. falciparum*.

Symptoms develop after an incubation period of 1 week to 3 months.

Look for:

- cyclical paroxysms of rigors
- fever, drenching sweats
- travel history and inadequate antimalarial prophylaxis
- jaundice
- splenomegaly
- coma, seizure
- headache

Select thick and thin peripheral blood smears to diagnose malaria. Parasitemia levels >2% are most consistent with *P. falciparum* or *Plasmodium knowlesi* (South and Southeast Asia) infection.

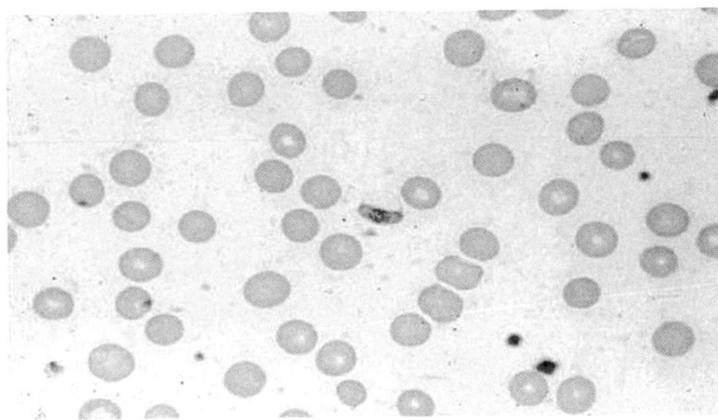

***Plasmodium falciparum* Infection:** In the center of the peripheral blood smear is a banana-shaped gametocyte diagnostic of *P. falciparum* infection.

DON'T BE TRICKED

- **Any traveler who has returned from a malaria-endemic area in the past year and has an undiagnosed febrile illness should undergo malaria evaluation.**

Treatment

Use chloroquine for malaria acquired where chloroquine resistance has not been reported. Choose artemisinin derivative combinations, atovaquone-proguanil, mefloquine, and quinine-based regimens for malaria acquired where chloroquine-resistant parasites are present.

Leptospirosis

Diagnosis

Leptospirosis is a zoonosis caused by the spirochete *Leptospira interrogans*. Most clinical cases occur in the tropics (Hawaii in the United States). Patients typically become infected following exposure to animal urine or contaminated water or soil. Most patients present with the abrupt onset of fever, rigors, myalgias, and headache. Kidney failure, uveitis, respiratory failure, myocarditis, and rhabdomyolysis can occur. A key physical sign is conjunctival suffusion, infrequently found in other infectious diseases. The diagnosis is usually made by serologic confirmation.

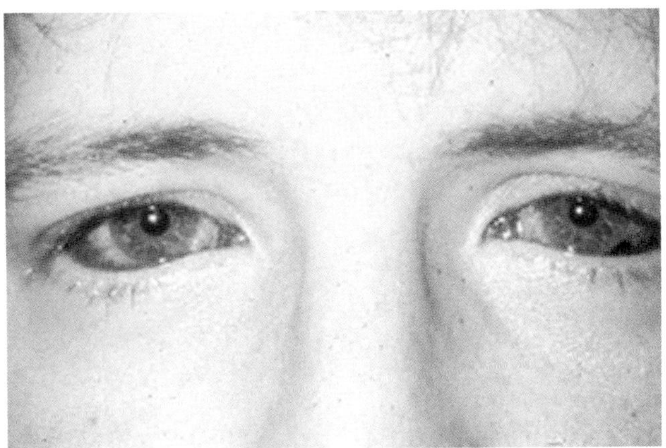

Conjunctival Suffusion in Leptospirosis: Subconjunctival suffusion typical of leptospirosis.

Treatment

Most cases are self-limited, but doxycycline and penicillin may be helpful in severe disease or shortening the duration of mild disease.

Infectious Gastrointestinal Syndromes

STUDY TABLE: Agents, Presentation, and Treatment of Infectious Gastrointestinal Syndromes

Agent	Clinical Findings	Diagnosis	Empiric Treatment
Bacterial			
Campylobacter	Fevers, chills, bloody diarrhea, abdominal pain Postinfectious IBD, reactive arthritis, Guillain-Barré	Routine stool culture	Azithromycin or erythromycin
Shigella	Dysentery Day-care center or nursing home workers Rare cause of HUS or reactive arthritis	Routine stool culture	Usually self-limited Fluoroquinolone; azithromycin for severe symptoms or positive stool cultures to reduce transmission
Salmonella (nontyphoidal)	Fever, chills, diarrhea; bacteremia in 10%-25% of cases and may result in endothelial infection, including aortitis, arteritis, mycotic aneurysm; osteomyelitis in sickle cell disease	Routine stool culture; blood cultures (with moderate to severe illness)	Do not treat mild disease; this may lead to prolonged shedding of bacteria in stool If significant comorbid illness or severe illness, treat with fluoroquinolone
STEC including *Escherichia coli* O157:H7	Bloody stools in >80% of cases; fever often absent; may be associated with HUS	*E. coli* O157:H7: stool culture with specialized media followed by serology Other STEC: stool culture with specialized media followed by Shiga toxin serology or PCR	None (antibiotic treatment of STEC may increase the risk of HUS)
Enterotoxigenic *E. coli* (travelers' diarrhea)	Nonbloody, watery stools	None	Fluoroquinolone, azithromycin, or rifaximin
Yersinia	Fever, diarrhea, RLQ pain (mimics appendicitis), pharyngitis Postinfectious reactive arthritis	Routine stool culture	Fluoroquinolone; trimethoprim-sulfamethoxazole
Vibrio cholerae	Bloody stools (>25% of cases), fever, vomiting (>50% of cases) Severe infection with sepsis in patients with hepatic dysfunction or alcoholism	Stool culture with specialized media	Fluoroquinolone; azithromycin
Clostridium difficile	Diarrhea, fever, abdominal pain, colonic distention (including toxic megacolon in severe cases), leukocytosis, sepsis	PCR or stool EIA for toxin	Oral vancomycin
Viral			
Norovirus	Watery, noninflammatory diarrhea; vomiting in >50% of cases; highly transmissible; frequent cause of outbreaks	PCR	None
Parasitic			
Giardia	Watery diarrhea, abdominal cramping, steatorrhea, weight loss Prolonged infection with IgA deficiency	Microscopy or stool antigen	Metronidazole × 5-10 days or tinidazole
Cryptosporidium	Watery diarrhea HIV-infected patients at high risk	Modified acid-fast stain, stool antigen	Supportive care Nitazoxanide for symptomatic patients
Amebiasis	Dysentery	Microscopy, stool antigen	Metronidazole, plus paromomycin for symptomatic patients
Cyclospora	Watery diarrhea, bloating, flatulence, weight loss HIV patients have more severe illness with wasting	Modified acid-fast stain	Trimethoprim-sulfamethoxazole

STEC = Shiga toxin-producing *Escherichia coli*.

Posttransplantation Infections

Diagnosis

Within the first 4 postoperative weeks, the most common infections in solid organ transplant recipients are the same as those that develop postoperatively in patients who have undergone non–transplant-related surgery. Patients with HSCT pre-engraftment (days 1-30) are neutropenic and susceptible to *Candida*, molds, and bacterial infections.

After the first month following transplantation, CMV frequently occurs, most often in the setting of a CMV-negative transplant recipient with a transplant from a CMV-positive donor. CMV is associated with:

- an increased risk for renal graft failure
- GI perforations and significant bleeding
- CMV-related pneumonia and respiratory failure
- EBV, polyomavirus BK, polyomavirus JC, and hepatitis B and C reactivation

Polyomavirus JC infection may cause progressive multifocal leukoencephalopathy. EBV infection is found in almost all patients with posttransplantation lymphoproliferative disease.

Kidney transplant patients with polyomavirus BK infection may develop nephropathy, organ rejection, or ureteral strictures. HSCT recipients with BK infection may develop hemorrhagic cystitis.

Prevention

During neutropenia, prophylaxis usually includes an antifungal such as voriconazole. Trimethoprim-sulfamethoxazole is the preferred agent for *Pneumocystis* and *Toxoplasma* prophylaxis. Prophylaxis with valganciclovir is appropriate for solid organ transplant recipients at risk for or with known CMV infection. For patients with HSCT, use acyclovir for antiviral prophylaxis to avoid myelosuppression. Patients receiving adequate anti-CMV prophylaxis have a lower incidence of polyomavirus BK and EBV reactivation.

Treatment

For treatment of CMV infection in posttransplant patients, immunosuppressive therapy may need to be reduced. IV ganciclovir, oral valganciclovir, oral foscarnet, and IV cidofovir are used for treatment. The only known effective treatment for polyomavirus JC infection is to reverse immunosuppressive therapy.

DON'T BE TRICKED

- **Preventive therapy for CMV need not be given if donor and recipient are both seronegative.**
- **Patients undergoing HSCT need revaccination with complete series after immune system reconstitution.**
- **Live vaccines are typically contraindicated for patients receiving immunosuppression after transplantation.**

TEST YOURSELF

A 63-year-old woman is evaluated for fever and hypotension 4 days after kidney-pancreas transplantation surgery. She has erythema and tenderness around the surgical wound.

ANSWER: For diagnosis, select staphylococcal wound infection as the most likely cause of an early infection in a transplant patient.

Catheter-Associated UTIs

Prevention

CAUTIs can be prevented by using a urinary catheter only when indicated and removing it as soon as possible. Maintain a closed catheter system at all times, and keep the catheter bag below the level of the bladder.

Diagnosis

Typical signs and symptoms of UTI may not be present in a catheterized patient. Obtain urine cultures in patients with symptoms attributable to the urinary tract or in patients with altered mental status or fever.

Treatment

If a CAUTI is suspected, management includes catheter removal and urine culture. Cefotaxime, ceftriaxone, ciprofloxacin, or levofloxacin is generally used for suspected gram-negative infection, and vancomycin is used for suspected staphylococcal or enterococcal infection. When culture data are available, treatment should be adjusted to the narrowest coverage spectrum possible.

DON'T BE TRICKED

- **In patients with a urinary catheter, do not obtain routine urinalysis or cultures and do not treat asymptomatic bacteriuria.**
- **Don't treat asymptomatic candiduria with antifungal therapy; do remove the catheter.**

Hospital-Acquired and Ventilator-Associated Pneumonia

Prevention

HAP is defined as pneumonia that occurs ≥48 hours after admission. VAP, a subset of HAP, is defined as occurring >48 hours after endotracheal intubation.

Procedures to reduce VAP include:

- following daily weaning protocols for timely extubation
- keeping the head of the bed elevated >30 degrees
- avoiding nasal intubation and nasogastric tubes
- using chlorhexidine mouth rinse and subglottic suction catheters

Diagnosis

The diagnosis of HAP is based on a new or progressive radiographic infiltrate plus clinical signs of pneumonia (fever, purulent sputum, leukocytosis, hypoxemia).

Treatment

Antibiotic selection is based on the risk for multidrug-resistant organisms (MDRO) as well as risk factors for MRSA. Risk factors for MDRO are:

- current hospitalization ≥5 days
- admission from a health care–related facility
- recent antibiotic therapy
- immunosuppression

Risk factors for MRSA include IV antibiotics within the last 90 days, exposure to a hospital unit with >20% of *Staphylococcus aureus* isolates resistant to methicillin, or in which methicillin resistance is unknown.

Choose cefepime, piperacillin-tazobactam, or levofloxacin for patients with no MDRO risk factors; choose one agent to treat MSSA (e.g., nafcillin) in patients with no risk factors for MRSA.

If MDRO and MRSA risk factors are present, select two antibiotics of different classes with activity against *Pseudomonas aeruginosa* (for example piperacillin-tazobactam plus gentamycin) and one drug with activity against MRSA (vancomycin or linezolid).

Narrow the empiric therapy based on culture results.

DON'T BE TRICKED

- Do not delay empiric antibiotic therapy to perform diagnostic studies.

TEST YOURSELF

A 78-year-old woman was admitted from home for treatment of a hip fracture. Four days after admission, she develops a temperature of 38.3 °C (100.9 °F) and a cough. A chest x-ray shows a new left lower lobe infiltrate.

ANSWER: For diagnosis, choose HAP; for treatment, select cefepime, piperacillin-tazobactam, or levofloxacin and nafcillin.

Clostridium difficile Antibiotic-Associated Diarrhea

Diagnosis

C. difficile antibiotic-associated colitis is produced by two toxins, A and B. The most important risk factors are antibiotic use and hospitalization, but community-acquired infection is becoming increasingly common. EIAs to detect the toxins are specific, but sensitivity using a single stool sample is 75% to 85%. PCR assays to detect the genes responsible for production of toxins A and B are more sensitive compared with EIAs.

Management of *C. difficile* infection is based on disease severity. Severe disease is defined by any one of the following:

- leukocyte count >15,000/µL
- serum creatinine level ≥1.5 times baseline level
- age >60 years

Hospitalized patients with known or suspected illness should be placed under contact isolation.

Treatment

Discontinue the offending antibiotic.

First-line treatment for an initial *C. difficile* infection is oral vancomycin or fidaxomicin. Severe disease associated with ileus may benefit from the addition of IV metronidazole and vancomycin enemas; select colectomy for fulminant or complicated disease (e.g., toxic megacolon or severe sepsis) that is unresponsive to enteral vancomycin or fidaxomicin and IV metronidazole. A first recurrence is treated with a vancomycin pulse/slow taper regimen or with fidaxomicin. Fecal microbiota transplant is used for patients with multiple relapses.

DON'T BE TRICKED

- Do not obtain stool cultures or cell culture cytotoxicity assays to diagnose *C. difficile* infection.

Intravascular Catheter-Related Infection

Prevention

Use of IV catheters should be reserved for patients with a proven need, and the catheter should be removed as soon as clinically possible.

STUDY TABLE: Prevention Strategies for Intravascular Catheter-Related Infections	
Choose...	**Do not choose...**
Maximum sterile barrier precautions and chlorhexidine for skin decontamination during catheter insertion	Routine dressing changes
Subclavian insertion	Femoral artery insertion
Catheter-care teams	Routine replacement of central venous catheters

Diagnosis

Consider catheter-related infection in any patient with fever and a central venous catheter. Purulence and cellulitis around the catheter site are specific, but not sensitive, for catheter-related infection. Begin the evaluation of suspected infection by removing the catheter and culturing the catheter tip.

- If the tip is culture positive and associated with fever or a positive peripheral blood culture, the diagnosis is catheter-related infection.
- A negative central blood culture has a good negative predictive value. However, a positive central or peripheral blood culture alone requires clinical interpretation to differentiate infection from colonization.

Treatment

Remove the catheter in the following situations:

- tunnel or pocket infection
- sepsis
- metastatic infection (septic thrombosis, endocarditis, or osteomyelitis)
- *Staphylococcus aureus* or *Pseudomonas* infection
- fungemia

IV catheter-related *S. aureus* bacteremia that clears within 72 hours without evidence of endocarditis or metastatic infection may be treated with 10 to 14 days of parenteral antibiotics. Persistent *S. aureus* bacteremia >72 hours after the start of appropriate antimicrobial therapy suggests a complicated infection. Evaluate with echocardiography, preferably transesophageal. Treat complicated *S. aureus* bacteremia for 4 to 6 weeks.

- MSSA is treated with either nafcillin (or oxacillin) or cefazolin
- MRSA is treated with vancomycin or daptomycin

Empiric treatment for neutropenic or septic patients should cover gram-negative organisms including *Pseudomonas*. Narrow antibiotic selection based on culture and susceptibility results.

DON'T BE TRICKED

- A normal TTE does not exclude endocarditis in the setting of *S. aureus* bacteremia.
- Catheter removal is not required for transient coagulase-negative staphylococcal bacteremia.

HIV Infection

Prevention

Daily use of tenofovir disoproxil fumarate-emtricitabine **preexposure prophylaxis** (PrEP) has resulted in a >90% decrease in the risk of acquiring HIV in HIV-negative adults at high risk. Condom use is advised in addition to PrEP, which does not decrease the risk of other sexually transmitted diseases.

Postexposure prophylaxis should be started as soon as possible following HIV exposure. The standard course is three drugs (typically tenofovir, emtricitabine, and raltegravir) for 4 weeks. Testing for HIV should be done immediately and at 6 weeks, 12 weeks, and 6 months.

Screening

Routinely screen all Americans aged 13 to 64 years for HIV infection. One-time testing is reasonable in persons at low risk, but persons engaged in high-risk behavior should be tested at least annually.

Screen using the following protocol:

- a fourth-generation combination immunoassay that includes an EIA for HIV antibody (HIV-1 and HIV-2) and HIV p24 antigen
- if combination immunoassay is positive, obtain immunoassay to differentiate HIV-1 from HIV-2
- detection of either HIV-1 or HIV-2 antibody confirms the diagnosis
- if differentiation immunoassay is inconclusive for either HIV-1 or HIV-2, obtain NAAT
- a positive NAAT in the setting of a negative antibody test indicates acute HIV infection

DON'T BE TRICKED

- **If a test is positive on the initial antigen/antibody combination immunoassay but negative on the antibody differentiation immunoassay and NAAT, the initial test result was a false positive.**

Diagnosis

Diagnose primary HIV infection (initial acute HIV infection) by a febrile illness that occurs within several weeks of a potential HIV exposure. Additional symptoms may include fatigue, lymphadenopathy, pharyngitis, rash, and/or headache. During the "window period" before seroconversion, the diagnosis of primary infection is confirmed with a positive NAAT.

Test for HIV in any patient with signs or symptoms of immunologic dysfunction, weight loss, generalized lymphadenopathy, fever and night sweats of more than 2 weeks' duration, or severe aphthous ulcers.

Certain diagnoses warrant HIV testing:

- severe or treatment-refractory HSV infection
- oral thrush or esophageal candidiasis
- *Pneumocystis jirovecii* pneumonitis
- cryptococcal meningitis
- disseminated mycobacterial infection
- CMV retinitis or GI disease
- toxoplasmosis
- severe seborrheic dermatitis, or new or severe psoriasis
- recurrent herpes zoster infections

Testing

Rapid HIV tests, which give results from salivary samples in about 20 minutes, are available for clinic and home use. Positive tests must be confirmed using the same HIV testing as described above.

The HIV RNA viral load is the most reliable marker for predicting the long-term risk of progression to AIDS or death. The CD4 cell count is the most reliable marker for the current risk of opportunistic complications.

AIDS is diagnosed in an HIV-infected person if the CD4 cell count is <200/µL or if an AIDS-defining illness is present.

Treatment

Consider initiating treatment in all patients motivated to start lifelong medication, regardless of CD4 cell count. Perform resistance testing on all patients before starting ART.

STUDY TABLE: Preferred Regimens for Initial Treatment of HIV Infection[a]
Abacavir/lamivudine/dolutegravir
Tenofovir alafenamide/emtricitabine/dolutegravir
Tenofovir alafenamide/emtricitabine/cobicistat/elvitegravir
Tenofovir alafenamide/emtricitabine/raltegravir

[a]Endorsed by the 2016 International Antiviral Society-USA Panel and the 2017 Department of Health and Human Services guidelines.

Check the viral load 4 weeks after ART is initiated or changed. Viral load should fall quickly and progressively and reach undetectable levels within a few months. Viral loads should remain undetectable while the patient is receiving ART. Persistent detectable levels of virus should be regarded as treatment failure, and resistance testing should be repeated.

DON'T BE TRICKED

- **Resistance testing should be done while the patient is still receiving the ineffective regimen.**

All **pregnant women** should be tested for HIV infection and, if positive, treated.

Initial treatment regimen selection in pregnant women does not typically differ from nonpregnant women; however, elvitegravir-cobicistat, bictegravir, and tenofovir alafenamide are not recommended. Additionally, dolutegravir is not recommended in the first 8 weeks of pregnancy.

Breastfeeding should be avoided in women with HIV infection.

IRIS is an intense inflammatory disorder associated with paradoxical worsening of preexisting infectious processes following the initiation of ART therapy. IRIS may occur in one of two ways:

- a preexisting subclinical infection is "unmasked" by immune system recovery
- a previously treated infection may "paradoxically" recur because of the presence of persistent antigens

The most important therapy for IRIS is treatment of the underlying infection. Glucocorticoids and NSAIDs are sometimes added to decrease the inflammatory response.

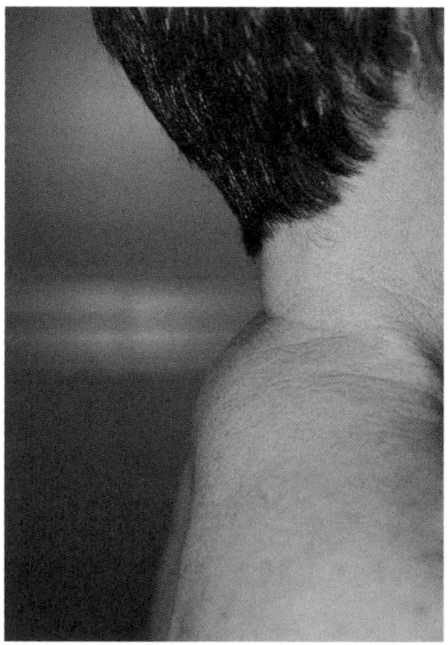

Protease Inhibitor Fat Dystrophy: Increase in subcutaneous fat at back of neck, creating a "buffalo hump" in a patient with HIV taking a protease inhibitor.

TEST YOURSELF

A 29-year-old man with recently diagnosed pulmonary TB is found to have late-stage HIV infection. Three-drug ART and four-drug TB therapy is initiated, and he quickly improves. Four weeks later, he develops recurrent fever and neck pain and swelling. He has bilateral tender cervical lymphadenopathy.

ANSWER: For diagnosis, choose IRIS. For treatment, choose to continue ART and administer antituberculous drugs.

DON'T BE TRICKED

- Do not stop ART in the setting of IRIS.

STUDY TABLE: Adverse Effects and Precautions of Commonly Used Antiretroviral Drugs

Drug	Side Effects	Precautions
Emtricitabine	Well-tolerated, minimal toxicity Skin discoloration or hyperpigmentation	Lactic acidosis, severe hepatomegaly Acute exacerbations of hepatitis B when discontinued
Tenofovir	Well-tolerated Nausea, diarrhea, asthenia, headache May cause kidney injury (Fanconi syndrome), decreased bone density	Lactic acidosis, severe hepatomegaly Acute exacerbations of hepatitis B when discontinued Avoid combining with didanosine
Efavirenz	CNS adverse effects that may diminish after 2 weeks (such as dizziness, insomnia, sleep disturbance, mood or psychiatric alterations, vivid dreams, hallucinations), rash	Avoid with pregnancy CYP3A4 drug interactions (including protease inhibitors)
Darunavir	Rash, diarrhea, nausea, LFT elevations, hepatotoxicity, hyperlipidemia, hyperglycemia	Substrate and inhibitor of CYP3A Caution with sulfonamide hypersensitivity
Atazanavir	Nausea, abdominal pain, headache, prolonged PR interval Jaundice or scleral icterus resulting from indirect hyperbilirubinemia	Caution with conduction abnormalities CYP3A4 drug interactions
Ritonavir	Paresthesias, nausea, vomiting, headache, diarrhea, insulin resistance, lipodystrophy, hyperlipidemia, hepatic dysfunction Liquid has unpleasant taste	Drug interactions Substrate and potent inhibitor of CYP3A4
Raltegravir	Well-tolerated Nausea, diarrhea, headache, elevated creatine phosphokinase Rash possible (including hypersensitivity reactions, SJS, TEN)	
Abacavir	Potentially fatal hypersensitivity reaction	Screen all abacavir-naïve patients for the presence of HLA-B*5701 (associated with a higher risk of AHR). Rechallenge with abacavir is contraindicated in patients having previous AHR.

STUDY TABLE: Prophylaxis for Patients with HIV Infection

Preventable Condition	When	Agent
P. jirovecii pneumonitis	CD4 cell count <200/µL	Trimethoprim-sulfamethoxazole
Toxoplasmosis	CD4 cell count <100/µL and positive IgG for toxoplasmosis	Trimethoprim-sulfamethoxazole
MAC infection	CD4 cell count <50/µL	Azithromycin
Active TB	TST ≥5 mm or positive IGRA	Isoniazid for 9 months
Influenza	Annual vaccination for all HIV-infected patients	Inactivated influenza vaccine
Pneumococcal pneumonia	Upon diagnosis	Pneumococcal conjugate vaccine (PCV13) and pneumococcal polysaccharide vaccine (PPSV23) See General Internal Medicine, Screening and Prevention
Hepatitis A and B	Completion of series	Hepatitis A and B vaccine

Discontinue *Pneumocystis jirovecii*, toxoplasmosis, and MAC prophylaxis when ART therapy produces CD4 cell counts >200/µL and the viral load is undetectable for at least 3 months.

DON'T BE TRICKED

- **Live vaccines are contraindicated in immunocompromised patients, but the MMR and varicella vaccines can be given to HIV patients with CD4 cell counts >200/µL.**

Pneumocystis jirovecii Pneumonia

Prevention

Select prophylaxis (usually with trimethoprim-sulfamethoxazole) for patients with HIV infection and a CD4 cell count <200/µL. In patients treated with HIV antiretroviral medications, discontinue prophylaxis when the CD4 cell count is >200/µL for 3 months.

Diagnosis

In patients infected with HIV, *P. jirovecii* pneumonia is gradual in onset and characterized by nonproductive cough and progressive dyspnea. Other findings may include:

- fever, chills, night sweats, and weight loss
- tachypnea and crackles on lung examination
- typical chest x-ray findings include diffuse bilateral, interstitial infiltrates

Testing

An elevated LDH level may be present in HIV-infected patients with *P. jirovecii* pneumonia. The diagnosis is established by immunofluorescent monoclonal antibody stain or silver stain examination of induced sputum or a bronchoscopic sample showing characteristic cysts.

DON'T BE TRICKED

- **The most common cause of a pneumothorax in a patient with AIDS is *P. jirovecii* pneumonia.**
- ***P. jirovecii* pneumonia can occur in patients not infected with HIV, typically in association with immunosuppressant drug therapy.**

Treatment

Select 3 weeks of treatment with:

- oral trimethoprim-sulfamethoxazole for mild to moderate pneumonia
- IV trimethoprim-sulfamethoxazole for moderate to severe pneumonia
- glucocorticoids within 72 hours for A-a ≥35 mm Hg or arterial Po_2 <70 mm Hg
- IV pentamidine or IV clindamycin plus oral primaquine for patients with sulfa allergy

TEST YOURSELF

A 45-year-old man with HIV and a CD4 cell count of 100/µL has had 3 weeks of dry cough and progressive dyspnea on exertion, now present at rest. On examination, his temperature is 38.3 °C (100.9 °F) and Po_2 is 67 mm Hg breathing ambient air. His chest x-ray shows diffuse bilateral infiltrates.

ANSWER: For diagnosis, choose presumed *P. jirovecii* pneumonia; for management, choose empiric treatment with IV trimethoprim-sulfamethoxazole and glucocorticoids.

Toxoplasmosis

Diagnosis and Testing

Toxoplasmosis is caused by an intracellular protozoan parasite, *Toxoplasma gondii*. Immunocompetent persons with primary infection are usually asymptomatic, but latent infection can persist, and reactivation of the infection is a risk if the person becomes immunocompromised. Look for:

- encephalitis, chorioretinitis, or pneumonitis in immunocompromised patients
- any focal neurologic syndrome, acute or subacute
- mononucleosis-like syndrome

Select IgG serologic testing in patients with suspected toxoplasmosis and brain MRI or head CT for neurologic signs and symptoms. Typical findings on imaging include multiple ring-enhancing lesions.

STUDY TABLE: Differential Diagnosis of Cerebral Toxoplasmosis in Immunocompromised Patients

Diagnosis	Characteristics
Lymphoma (primary CNS, B-cell lymphoma)	Often a solitary lesion is located in the periventricular or periependymal area or in the corpus callosum Neither clinical nor neuroradiologic findings reliably distinguish lymphoma from toxoplasmosis Brain biopsy is diagnostic
Progressive multifocal leukoencephalopathy	Dementia is often the presenting symptom CD4 cell counts are usually <50/µL and PCR of CSF can show JC virus Brain biopsy is diagnostic
Cryptococcus neoformans	Headache, fever, and altered mental status are present CD4 cell counts are usually <100/µL CSF culture for *Cryptococcus* or cryptococcal antigen tests on CSF and serum are diagnostic; elevated CSF opening pressure is characteristic
Mycobacterium tuberculosis	Basilar meningitis with cranial nerve abnormalities Culture and PCR of CSF are diagnostic
CMV	Diffuse encephalitis and fever are characteristic CD4 cell counts are <50/µL; CSF PCR is positive, and brain biopsy is diagnostic
Neurosyphilis	Atypical and accelerated neurosyphilis is seen in HIV infection Lymphocytic pleocytosis and elevated CSF protein Positive serum RPR or VDRL test, FTA-ABS, and MHA-TP; positive CSF VDRL

Treatment

Select empiric treatment with sulfadiazine, pyrimethamine, and folic acid in patients with multiple ring-enhancing lesions, positive *T. gondii* serologic test results (IgG), and immune suppression (CD4 cell count <200/µL). Treat patients with persistent immunosuppression indefinitely. Biopsy lesions that fail to respond to 2 weeks of empiric therapy.

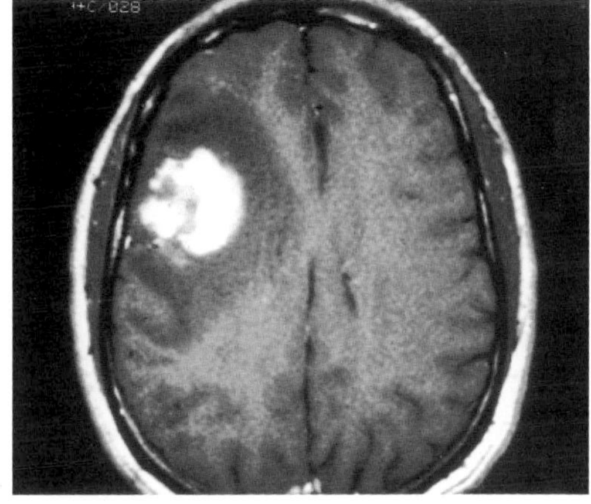

Intracerebral Toxoplasmosis: MRI showing a single ring-enhancing brain lesion associated with edema consistent with toxoplasmosis. Most patients with AIDS with cerebral toxoplasmosis have multiple ring-enhancing brain lesions.

Influenza Virus

Prevention

See General Internal Medicine, Screening and Prevention. For institutional outbreaks, vaccinate staff members and residents not already immunized and give chemoprophylaxis with zanamivir or oseltamivir for at least 2 weeks following immunization.

DON'T BE TRICKED

- Do not administer live attenuated influenza vaccine to persons who have close contact with immunocompromised patients.

Diagnosis and Testing

During November through April, look for acute onset of high fever, headache, fatigue, nonproductive cough, sore throat, nasal congestion, rhinorrhea, and myalgia. Use diagnostic testing (rapid antigen tests) in patients for whom results would influence management (e.g., initiating antiviral treatment, performing other diagnostic testing, or inpatient infection control measures). The most common complications of influenza are primary influenza pneumonia and secondary bacterial pneumonia (*Streptococcus pneumoniae, Staphylococcus aureus*).

Treatment

In addition to standard precautions in hospitalized patients, droplet precautions should be used for all patients with suspected influenza. Treat all hospitalized patients with confirmed infection and outpatients at high risk for severe disease. Select zanamivir or oseltamivir, both of which are active against influenza A and B. Peramivir is available for IV administration.

Risk factors for severe disease:

- immunosuppression (highest risk)
- chronic pulmonary disease (highest risk)
- age >64 years
- pregnancy (or delivery within 2 weeks)
- diabetes
- significant cardiovascular, kidney, liver, or hematologic disease
- BMI ≥40

DON'T BE TRICKED

- Do not administer amantadine or rimantadine to prevent or treat influenza virus because of the high rate of resistance.
- Zanamivir (inhaled) has been associated with bronchospasm and is contraindicated in patients with pulmonary or cardiovascular disease.

TEST YOURSELF

A 68-year-old woman with diabetes is admitted to the hospital in November with the acute onset of fever, chills, nonproductive cough, and fatigue. Her 6-year-old granddaughter has had similar symptoms for 3 days.

ANSWER: For diagnosis, choose influenza; for treatment, select immediate initiation of oseltamivir.

Varicella-Zoster Virus

Epidemiology, Clinical Features, and Diagnosis

Primary varicella infection (chickenpox) from infection with VZV (human herpesvirus type 3) presents with a febrile pruritic vesicular rash affecting the skin and mucocutaneous surfaces; most children recover without sequelae, but adults may develop pneumonia, encephalitis, hepatitis, and cerebellar ataxia.

Herpes zoster (shingles) results from a reactivation of latent VZV within sensory ganglia, especially in adults >60 years or in immunosuppressed patients. It typically causes a painful vesicular rash following a dermatomal distribution that does not cross the midline. Young patients presenting with herpes zoster should be tested for HIV. Immunosuppressed patients can present with multiple dermatomes affected or with disseminated disease.

Postherpetic neuralgia is defined as neuropathic pain lasting more than 1 month after resolution of the vesicular rash. Other complications include herpes zoster ophthalmicus with visual loss, Ramsay Hunt syndrome (vesicular rash in external ear associated with ipsilateral peripheral facial palsy and altered taste), pneumonia, hepatitis, and CNS complications such as meningitis, encephalitis, myelitis, and stroke caused by vasculitis.

Testing

Varicella or herpes zoster can be diagnosed clinically by the typical vesicular rash and confirmed with VZV PCR testing of the base of a vesicular lesion. VZV is underdiagnosed in the absence of a rash (zoster sine herpete); in such cases, serologic tests (VZV IgM and IgG) and VZV PCR testing of CSF can be used to diagnose the infections.

Treatment

Antiviral therapy (acyclovir, valacyclovir, and famciclovir) speeds recovery and decreases the severity and duration of neuropathic pain if begun within 72 hours of VZV rash onset.

Intravenous acyclovir should be used for immunosuppressed or hospitalized patients and those with neurologic involvement.

First line treatment for postherpetic neuralgia includes tricyclic antidepressants, gabapentin, and pregabalin.

Prevention

For **prevention of primary varicella infection**, immunization with varicella vaccine is recommended by the Advisory Committee on Immunization Practices (ACIP) for immunocompetent children beginning at age 12 to 15 months and for adults without evidence of previous infection.

For **prevention of herpes zoster**, the ACIP recommends the recombinant zoster vaccine for all adults ≥50 years, including those who have previously had herpes zoster infection or have been vaccinated with the live attenuated vaccine.

Postexposure prophylaxis should be provided to susceptible persons (VZV IgG negative); postexposure varicella vaccination is appropriate in immunocompetent persons, and varicella-zoster immune globulin should be used in immunocompromised adults and in pregnant women.

Epstein-Barr Virus

Diagnosis

EBV is the primary agent of infectious mononucleosis and is associated with the development of B-cell lymphoma, T-cell lymphoma, Hodgkin lymphoma, and nasopharyngeal carcinoma. Another EBV manifestation is oral hairy leukoplakia that characteristically affects the lateral portions of the tongue as white corrugated painless plaques. Oral hairy leukoplakia is most commonly associated with underlying HIV infection.

Typical symptoms in patients with acute infectious mononucleosis include:

- severe fatigue, headache, and sore throat
- fever associated with posterior cervical lymphadenopathy
- splenomegaly
- reactive lymphocytosis

Consider EBV infection in all patients with aseptic meningitis or encephalitis, hepatitis, hemolytic anemia, and thrombocytopenia.

DON'T BE TRICKED

- **The morbilliform rash appearing in patients with infectious mononucleosis following the administration of ampicillin is not an allergic reaction; patients can subsequently use ampicillin without rash recurrence.**

Testing

Select a Monospot test (heterophile antibody test), which is specific but not very sensitive early in disease. If the Monospot test is negative, repeat in 2 weeks or select EBV serology. Infectious mononucleosis syndrome can also be caused by CMV or HIV infection; it is often not possible to make a clinical diagnosis, and serologic testing is necessary.

STUDY TABLE: Epstein-Barr Virus Serology

Condition	Antibody
Acute primary infection	Elevated VCA IgM, VCA IgG, and EA IgG
	Low or undetectable EBNA-1 IgG
Past infection	Undetectable VCA IgM and EA IgG
	Elevated VCA IgG and EBNA-1 IgG

EA = early antigen; EBNA = Epstein-Barr nuclear antigen; VCA = viral capsid antigen.

Treatment

Supportive care is typically sufficient. Select glucocorticoids only if airway obstruction or other life-threatening conditions such as hemolytic anemia is present.

DON'T BE TRICKED

- **Do not prescribe antiviral drugs for treatment of infectious mononucleosis.**

TEST YOURSELF

An 18-year-old female soccer player has malaise, anorexia, and a sore throat for 3 days. She has exudative pharyngitis, tender anterior and posterior cervical lymph nodes, and fullness in her left upper abdominal quadrant. Leukocyte count is 8500/µL with moderate atypical lymphocytes.

ANSWER: For diagnosis, choose infectious mononucleosis. For management, select contact sport avoidance because of the risk of splenic rupture in the setting of splenomegaly.

Nephrology

Glomerular Filtration Rate

At high levels of GFR, small changes in the serum creatinine may reflect large changes in GFR. At low levels of GFR, large changes in the serum creatinine reflect relatively smaller changes in GFR.

In patients who become functionally anephric, the serum creatinine increases 1.0 to 1.5 mg/dL per day.

Serum cystatin C is an alternative marker of GFR less influenced than serum creatinine by age, gender, muscle mass, and body weight; it is more sensitive in identifying milder decrements in kidney function than serum creatinine.

Three equations to estimate GFR are commonly used: the Cockcroft-Gault equation, the Modification of Diet in Renal Disease (MDRD) study equation, and the Chronic Kidney Disease Epidemiology (CKD-EPI) Collaboration equation.

- MDRD study performs best when GFR is <60 mL/min/1.73 m^2
- CKD-EPI equation performs better at near normal GFR values
- Cockcroft-Gault is the least accurate

For drug-dosing purposes, the Cockcroft-Gault equation functions as well the CKD-EPI and MDRD study equations.

Conditions that decrease kidney perfusion, such as hypovolemia or HF, are associated with increased reabsorption of BUN in the proximal tubules and a disproportionate increase in the BUN-creatinine ratio, typically to 20:1 or higher.

DON'T BE TRICKED

- **A reduction or loss of muscle mass because of advanced age, liver failure, or malnutrition may cause a disproportionately low serum creatinine concentration, which results in overestimation of the GFR.**
- **When the MDRD study equation is used to estimate GFR, higher levels of GFR are reported only as >60 mL/min/1.73 m^2, but this does guarantee an absence of structural kidney disease.**

Urinalysis

Proteinuria

Albumin is the only protein that is detected on dipstick urinalysis.

The sulfosalicylic acid (SSA) test can detect the presence of albumin and other proteins such as urine light chains or immunoglobulins but is not widely used. Protein detected by urine dipstick should always be quantified with either a 24-hour urine collection or protein-creatinine or albumin-creatinine ratio on random urine samples.

Levels of proteinuria are diagnostically helpful:

- >150 mg/g but <200 mg/g = tubulointerstitial disease or glomerular disease
- >3500 mg/g = glomerular disease

The albumin-creatinine ratio measures only albumin in the urine and is used to evaluate diabetic kidney disease:

- 30 to 300 mg/g, previously termed *microalbuminuria*, is now referred to as *moderately increased albuminuria*.
- >300 mg/g, previously known as *macroalbuminuria* or *overt proteinuria*, is now referred to as *severely increased albuminuria*.

A protein-creatinine ratio can be used to measure proteinuria (abnormal protein-creatinine ratio defined as >0.2 mg/mg).

Proteinuria is a marker of renal parenchymal and glomerular disease and an independent predictor of progressive kidney disease, cardiovascular disease, and peripheral vascular disease.

DON'T BE TRICKED

- **Dipstick urinalysis does not detect immunoglobulin light chains associated with multiple myeloma.**
- **Positional (orthostatic) proteinuria, a benign cause of isolated proteinuria, is diagnosed by obtaining split daytime (standing) and nighttime (supine) urine collections.**

Hematuria

Hematuria is classified as glomerular and extraglomerular. Erythrocyte casts and dysmorphic erythrocytes (acanthocytes, erythrocytes with "Mickey Mouse" ears) in the urine indicate glomerular disease (see Nephritic Syndrome following). Coexisting proteinuria supports glomerular causes of hematuria, even in the absence of casts.

Hematuria with preserved erythrocyte morphology in the urine, often without proteinuria or casts, is consistent with extraglomerular bleeding (GU cancer, kidney stones, trauma, infection, and medications) and requires additional diagnostic studies to locate the extraglomerular source. The proper evaluation is directed by findings in the history and physical examination.

Consider the following sequenced evaluation of extraglomerular bleeding:

- urinalysis or urine culture to exclude infection, and if normal...
- noncontrast helical CT to detect calculi and contrast CT to detect renal cell carcinoma, and if normal...
- urine cytology, then stop evaluation if normal and patient is at low risk for malignancy (age <35 years, female sex, no other risk factors), otherwise...
- cystoscopy for patients with positive urine cytology, aged >35 years, male, or if risk factors for malignancy are present (cigarette smoking, analgesic abuse, benzene exposure, or voiding abnormalities)

DON'T BE TRICKED

- **Evaluate hematuria even in patients taking anticoagulants.**

Leukocytes and Other Formed Elements

Leukocytes in the urine may be caused by glomerular or tubulointerstitial inflammation, infection, or an allergic reaction.

Remember:

- Sterile pyuria (pyuria and a negative urine culture) suggests ***Mycobacterium tuberculosis***, interstitial cystitis, or interstitial nephritis.
- Eosinophiluria suggests AIN, postinfectious GN, atheroembolic disease of the kidney, septic emboli, or small-vessel vasculitis.

DON'T BE TRICKED

- **Absence of eosinophiluria does not rule out AIN, postinfectious GN, atheroembolic disease of the kidney, septic emboli, or small-vessel vasculitis.**

Patients with hemolysis and rhabdomyolysis test positive for blood on dipstick urinalysis in the absence of intact erythrocytes on urine microscopy. Urine lipids and fat are almost always associated with heavy proteinuria or the nephrotic syndrome. These may appear as free lipid droplets, round or oval fat bodies, or fatty casts.

Casts are cylindrical aggregates of Tamm-Horsfall mucoproteins that trap the intraluminal contents and appear in the urine.

Different types of casts are associated with specific disorders:

- Erythrocyte casts and acanthocytes indicate glomerular disease.
- Leukocyte casts indicate inflammation or infection of the renal parenchyma.
- Muddy brown casts are associated with ATN.
- Broad casts are associated with CKD.

Imaging

The three main modalities of kidney imaging are ultrasonography, CT, and MRI.

Ultrasonography is used to look for:

- nephrolithiasis
- kidney size and cortical thickness (increased echogenicity implies parenchymal disease)
- renal cysts and tumors
- obstruction and hydronephrosis
- bladder size, postvoid residual, and the prostate in bladder outlet obstruction

CT is used to look for:

- nephrolithiasis (noncontrast abdominal helical CT)
- renal tumors and cysts (contrast abdominal CT)
- causes of unexplained urologic/nonglomerular hematuria (CT urography)

MRI is used:

- when radiocontrast agents must be avoided (risk of nephrogenic systemic fibrosis in patients with CKD)
- to characterize renal masses, cysts, and renal vein thrombosis
- to look for renal artery stenosis using MRA with gadolinium contrast

Kidney Biopsy

Kidney biopsy should be considered in patients with:

- glomerular hematuria
- severely increased albuminuria
- acute or CKD of unclear origin
- kidney transplant dysfunction

Common contraindications to kidney biopsy include bleeding diatheses, severe anemia, UTI, hydronephrosis, uncontrolled hypertension, renal tumor, and atrophic kidneys.

Hyponatremia

Diagnosis

The first step in assessing low serum sodium is to determine if true hyponatremia is present by measuring serum osmolality.

Pseudohyponatremia is a laboratory artifact caused by severe hyperlipidemia or hyperproteinemia. In pseudohyponatremia, the measured osmolality is normal.

If **true hyponatremia** exists, classify it as hyperosmolar or hypo-osmolar.

Hypertonic (hyperosmolar) hyponatremia is caused by the presence of an osmotically active substance such as:

- glucose (most common)
- BUN
- alcohols
- mannitol
- sorbitol
- glycine (bladder irrigation during urological procedures)

Hypo-osmolar hyponatremia is the most common form of hyponatremia and is further classified based on the patient's volume status.

STUDY TABLE: Evaluating Hypo-osmolar Hyponatremia

Volume Status	Laboratory Studies	Differential Diagnosis
Hypovolemia (hypotension, tachycardia)	Spot urine sodium <20 mEq/L BUN/creatinine >20:1	GI or kidney sodium losses, mineralocorticoid insufficiency
Hypervolemia (edema, ascites)	Spot urine sodium <20 mEq/L (HF and cirrhosis in absence of diuretic therapy) Spot urine sodium >20 mEq/L (acute and chronic kidney failure)	HF, cirrhosis, kidney failure
Euvolemia (normal volume)	Spot urine sodium >20 mEq/L Urine osmolality usually >300 mOsm/L	SIADH, hypothyroidism, adrenal insufficiency (Addison disease), cerebral salt wasting syndrome
Euvolemia (normal volume)	Spot urine sodium >20 mEq/L Urine osmolality 50 to 100 mOsm/L	Compulsive water drinking

Causes of SIADH include malignancy (SCLC); intracranial pathology; and pulmonary diseases, especially those that increase intrathoracic pressure and decrease venous return to the heart. Many medications can cause SIADH, including thiazides, SSRIs, tricyclic antidepressants, narcotics, phenothiazines, and carbamazepine.

Cerebral salt wasting syndrome may result from a recent neurosurgical procedure or SAH. Hypovolemia and hypotension result in hypo-osmolar hyponatremia and laboratory parameters identical to SIADH.

DON'T BE TRICKED

- Do not miss adrenal insufficiency as a cause of hypo-osmolar hyponatremia.

Treatment

IV volume replacement with normal saline is indicated for hyponatremia resulting from **volume depletion**, including hyponatremia from thiazide diuretics and cerebral salt wasting syndrome.

Acute symptomatic hyponatremia should be treated with a 100-mL bolus of 3% saline to increase the serum sodium by 2.0 to 3.0 mEq/L.

Symptomatic patients with a more chronic (>48 hours) decline in serum sodium should be treated to a target of <8 to 10 mEq/L in 24 hours.

If neurologic impairment is significant (seizures or coma), sodium can be acutely increased (2.0-4.0 mEq/L) using a bolus of 3% saline as long as the total increase remains ≤10 mEq/L in 24 hours.

Should the serum sodium concentration be overcorrected, administer desmopressin and IV 5% dextrose in water. Central pontine myelinolysis (osmotic demyelination syndrome) may occur if hyponatremia is corrected too rapidly.

Water restriction is used initially for asymptomatic or minimally symptomatic outpatients with **SIADH**. Patients who do not respond to water restriction can be treated with loop diuretics combined with oral salt supplementation. Demeclocycline can also be used for outpatients who do not respond to fluid restriction. The IV V_1 and V_2 receptor antagonist conivaptan and the oral V_2 receptor antagonist tolvaptan (vaptans) are approved for treatment of euvolemic and hypervolemic hyponatremia. Oral tolvaptan should be reserved for the management of serum sodium concentration <120 mEq/L and persistent SIADH that has failed water restriction and/or oral furosemide and salt tablets. No data show that the vaptans are associated with improved patient outcomes compared with conventional therapy, and vaptans are very expensive.

DON'T BE TRICKED

- **Vaptan agents should not be used to treat hypovolemic hyponatremia or acute symptomatic hyponatremia.**

TEST YOURSELF

A 53-year-old man has a 3-week history of increasing weakness and anorexia. On physical examination, BP is 130/70 mm Hg, and pulse rate is 80/min without orthostatic changes. Laboratory studies: BUN, 12 mg/dL; serum creatinine, 0.8 mg/dL; serum sodium, 123 mEq/L; potassium, 3.4 mEq/L; chloride, 91 mEq/L; bicarbonate, 22 mEq/L; and urine sodium, 110 mEq/L.

ANSWER: For diagnosis, choose SIADH. For management, select serum osmolality measurement to confirm the presence of hypo-osmolality. If hypo-osmolality is present, the patient likely has SIADH (most common), thyroid disease, or adrenal insufficiency.

Hypernatremia

Diagnosis

Hypernatremia is defined as a serum sodium >145 mEq/L. Severe hypernatremia indicates a defective thirst mechanism, inadequate access to water (older patients in nursing homes), a kidney concentrating defect (DI, most commonly caused by lithium), and/or impaired pituitary secretion of ADH (e.g., sarcoidosis). Most commonly, hypernatremia results from loss of hypotonic fluids (GI, kidney, skin) with inadequate water replacement.

Treatment

Treatment is directed at free water replacement and correction of the underlying problem leading to hypotonic fluid loss. The water deficit is calculated as $[(Na^+ - 140)/140] \times TBW$ where $TBW = 0.5 \times$ weight (kg) in women or $0.6 \times$ weight (kg) in men. Correct the water deficit over 48 to 72 hours.

In volume depletion, fluid resuscitation with normal saline should precede correction of the water deficit with hypotonic fluids. Neurogenic (central) DI is treated with intranasal desmopressin.

Hyperkalemia

Diagnosis

The most common causes of hyperkalemia include:

- hyporeninemic hypoaldosteronism (Type 4 RTA; commonly seen among patients with diabetes)
- acute and chronic kidney failure
- low urine flow states
- medications (ACE inhibitors, ARBs, potassium-sparing diuretics, pentamidine, trimethoprim-sulfamethoxazole, and cyclosporine)
- potassium shifts (rhabdomyolysis, hemolysis, hyperosmolality, insulin deficiency, β-adrenergic blockade, and metabolic acidosis)

The earliest ECG changes of hyperkalemia are peaking of the T waves and shortening of the QT interval. As hyperkalemia progresses, the PR interval is prolonged, a loss of P waves occurs, and eventual widening of the QRS complexes is seen with a "sine-wave" pattern that can precede asystole.

Pseudohyperkalemia is an in-vitro phenomenon caused by the mechanical release of potassium from cells during phlebotomy or specimen processing or in the setting of marked leukocytosis and thrombocytosis. In patients with pseudohyperkalemia, the plasma potassium concentration is normal.

DON'T BE TRICKED

- **Significant hyperkalemia associated with a normal ECG suggests pseudohyperkalemia.**

Treatment

If hyperkalemia is associated with ECG changes or arrhythmias, begin IV calcium gluconate to stabilize the myocardium. Use insulin and glucose or inhaled β-adrenergic agonists to shift potassium inside the cells. Remove potassium from the body with loop diuretics (particularly if the patient is volume overloaded), and institute dietary potassium restriction.

Hemodialysis is often needed to correct life-threatening hyperkalemia but is never the "first step" because of the time delay in initiating dialysis.

DON'T BE TRICKED

- **Absolute levels of potassium cannot reliably determine if a life-threatening condition exists. Only ECG can assess the effect of hyperkalemia on the cardiac membrane.**

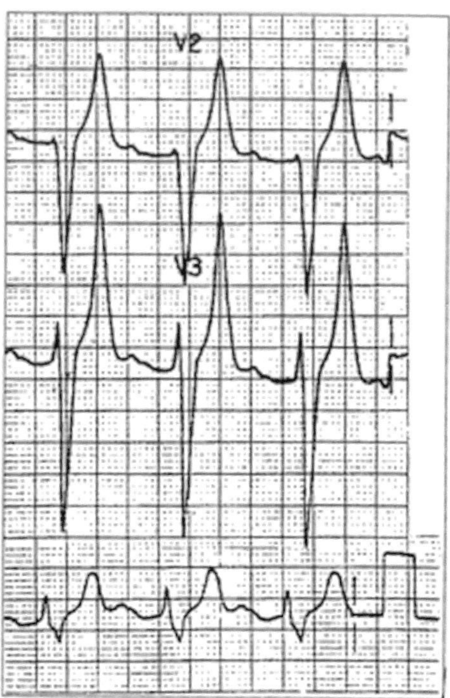

Characteristics of Hyperkalemia: ECG showing flattened P waves; prolonged PR interval; widened QRS; and tall, peaked T waves characteristic of hyperkalemia.

Hypokalemia

Diagnosis and Testing

The most common causes of hypokalemia are vomiting and diarrhea and use of diuretics. Urine potassium loss >20 mEq/24 h, a spot urine potassium >20 mEq/L, or a spot urine potassium-creatinine ratio >20 mEq/g suggests excessive urinary losses. Conversely, urine potassium loss <20 mEq/24 h suggests cellular shift, decreased intake, or extrarenal losses of potassium.

Other causes include:

- primary aldosteronism (hypertension, urine [Cl^-] >40 mEq/L, low plasma renin activity, and elevated aldosterone level)
- Bartter syndrome (normal BP, hypokalemia, metabolic alkalosis, and elevated renin and aldosterone levels)
- Gitelman syndrome (normal BP, hypokalemia, and hypomagnesemia)
- inhaled β_2-agonists (may lead to hypokalemia in certain clinical settings)
- hypokalemic periodic paralysis

Hypokalemic periodic paralysis is a rare familial or acquired disorder characterized by flaccid generalized weakness from a sudden intracellular potassium shift precipitated by strenuous exercise or a high-carbohydrate meal. The acquired form occurs with thyrotoxicosis and is found in men of Asian or Mexican descent. It is resolved with treatment of hyperthyroidism.

Characteristic findings of hypokalemia include ileus, muscle cramps, rhabdomyolysis, and hypomagnesemia. ECGs may show U waves and flat or inverted T waves.

Treatment

For severe hypokalemia, IV potassium chloride is indicated. Total body potassium deficits are typically large (200-300 mEq for a serum potassium concentration of 3 mEq/L). Hypomagnesemia and metabolic alkalosis should be corrected, if present.

Hypomagnesemia

Diagnosis and Testing

If hypomagnesemia is suspected, look for neuromuscular irritability, hypocalcemia, and hypokalemia.

The most common causes of hypomagnesemia include:

- GI losses (diarrhea, steatorrhea, intestinal bypass, pancreatitis)
- kidney losses (loop and thiazide diuretics, alcohol-induced)
- medications (cisplatin, aminoglycosides, amphotericin B, cyclosporine)
- hungry bone syndrome following parathyroidectomy

Usually the source of hypomagnesemia is obvious. If no cause is clinically apparent, GI and kidney losses can be differentiated by measuring the 24-hour urine magnesium excretion (elevated in kidney losses, low in GI losses). Hypomagnesemia is often associated with hypokalemia because of urine potassium wasting. Hypomagnesemia is also associated with hypocalcemia because of lower PTH secretion and end-organ resistance to PTH.

DON'T BE TRICKED

- **Correction of hypokalemia and hypocalcemia is difficult unless magnesium depletion is also corrected.**

Treatment

Administer oral slow-release magnesium and IV magnesium sulfate to achieve a serum magnesium level >1 mg/dL.

TEST YOURSELF

A 30-year-old woman with Crohn disease has an ileostomy. For the past week, she has noted increased ostomy output, weakness, and paresthesias. Laboratory studies show serum sodium, 129 mEq/L; potassium, 2.9 mEq/L; bicarbonate, 18 mEq/L; calcium, 5.5 mg/dL; and phosphorus, 1.3 mg/dL. After treatment with isotonic saline plus potassium chloride and sodium bicarbonate, the bicarbonate concentration is 22 mEq/L. However, the serum potassium level is still 2.9 mEq/L, and the serum calcium level is 5.3 mg/dL.

ANSWER: For diagnosis, choose hypomagnesemia. For management, measure magnesium level and, if low, begin IV magnesium replacement.

Hypophosphatemia

Diagnosis

Phosphate is primarily excreted through the kidneys and is reabsorbed mainly in the proximal tubule. The primary hormonal factors regulating phosphorus balance are PTH (which decreases phosphorus reabsorption and promotes kidney phosphate excretion) and calcitriol (which stimulates phosphate absorption in the gut). Characteristic findings in severe hypophosphatemia are HF, muscle weakness, rhabdomyolysis, hemolytic anemia, and metabolic encephalopathy.

Common causes include:

- refeeding after starvation
- insulin administration for severe hyperglycemia
- hungry bone syndrome following parathyroidectomy
- respiratory alkalosis
- chronic diarrhea
- chronic alcoholism
- hyperparathyroidism
- vitamin D deficiency

If the cause of hypophosphatemia is not evident from the history, a 24-hour urine phosphate collection or calculation of the FEPO4 from a random urine sample can help differentiate renal from extrarenal causes. The FEPO4 can be calculated as follows:

$$(\text{Urine PO4} \times \text{Serum Creatinine} \times 100)/(\text{Serum PO4} \times \text{Urine Creatinine})$$

Urine phosphate excretion >100 mg/d or an FEPO4 >5% indicates renal phosphate wasting.

Treatment

In asymptomatic patients, administer oral phosphorus replacement as a sodium or potassium salt. Parenteral therapy with either of these agents is indicated for symptomatic patients or for those whose phosphorus level is <1 mg/dL.

Approach to Acid-Base Problem Solving

You must be able to diagnose double and triple acid-base disorders.

Answer these four questions when solving acid-base problems:

1. What is the primary disturbance?
2. Is compensation appropriate?
3. What is the anion gap?
4. Does the change in the anion gap equal the change in the serum bicarbonate concentration (a value called the delta-delta)?

When diagnosing a primary acid-base disorder, remember that:

- Acidemia is defined as a pH <7.38. Metabolic acidosis = $[HCO_3]$ <24 mEq/L. Respiratory acidosis = arterial Pco_2 >40 mm Hg.
- Alkalemia is defined as a pH >7.42. Metabolic alkalosis = $[HCO_3]$ >24 mEq/L. Respiratory alkalosis = arterial Pco_2 <40 mm Hg.

STUDY TABLE: Compensatory Response to a Primary Acid-Base Disturbance

Condition	Expected Compensation	Interpretation
Metabolic acidosis	Acute: Δ arterial $Pco_2 = (1.5)[HCO_3^-] + 8 \pm 2$ Chronic: Δ arterial $Pco_2 = [HCO_3^-] + 15$	Failure of the arterial Pco_2 to decrease to expected value = complicating respiratory acidosis Excessive decrease of the arterial Pco_2 = complicating respiratory alkalosis
Respiratory acidosis	Acute: 1 mEq/L ↑ in $[HCO_3^-]$ for each 10 mm Hg ↑ in arterial Pco_2 Chronic: 3.5 mEq/L ↑ in $[HCO_3^-]$ for each 10 mm Hg ↑ in arterial Pco_2	Failure of the $[HCO_3^-]$ to increase to the expected value = complicating metabolic acidosis Excessive increase in $[HCO_3^-]$ = complicating metabolic alkalosis
Metabolic alkalosis	0.7 mm Hg ↑ in arterial Pco_2 for each 1 mEq/L ↑ in $[HCO_3^-]$	This response is limited by hypoxemia
Respiratory alkalosis	Acute: 2 mEq/L ↓ in $[HCO_3^-]$ for each 10 mm Hg ↓ in arterial Pco_2 Chronic: 4 mEq/L ↓ in $[HCO_3^-]$ for each 10 mm Hg ↓ in arterial Pco_2	Failure of the $[HCO_3^-]$ to decrease to the expected value = complicating metabolic alkalosis Excessive decrease in $[HCO_3^-]$ = complicating metabolic acidosis

Anion Gap

The anion gap = $[Na^+] - ([Cl^-] + [HCO_3^-])$. The normal anion gap is 10 ± 2 mEq/L. Acidoses can be divided into normal anion gap acidosis and increased anion gap acidosis.

Always calculate the anion gap, regardless of the metabolic disturbance.

- When the primary disturbance is a metabolic acidosis, the anion gap differentiates increased anion gap from normal anion gap acidosis.
- A reduced anion gap (<4 mEq/L) suggests multiple myeloma or hypoalbuminemia.

Increased Anion Gap Acidosis

Common causes of increased anion gap metabolic acidosis include:

- DKA
- CKD
- lactic acidosis (usually because of tissue hypoperfusion)
- aspirin toxicity
- alcoholic ketoacidosis
- methanol and ethylene glycol poisoning (also typically associated with an osmolar gap)

Normal Anion Gap Acidosis

Common causes of normal anion gap metabolic acidosis include:

- GI HCO_3^- loss (diarrhea)
- kidney HCO_3^- loss (ileal bladder, proximal RTA)
- reduced kidney H^+ secretion (distal RTA, type IV RTA)
- Fanconi syndrome (phosphaturia, glucosuria, uricosuria, aminoaciduria)
- carbonic anhydrase inhibitor use (acetazolamide and topiramate)

Urine Anion Gap

Increased acid excretion by the kidney is reflected as a marked increase in urine ammonium. Urine ammonium measurement is difficult to obtain; because chloride is excreted into the urine in amounts equal to ammonium, the amount of chloride in the urine reflects the amount of ammonium present.

The ability to excrete acid in the form of ammonia is calculated with the UAG. The UAG is defined as (urine $[Na^+]$ + urine $[K^+]$) – urine $[Cl^-]$.

- During normal anion gap metabolic acidosis resulting from extrarenal bicarbonate loss (diarrhea), the kidney will excrete increased urine ammonium (and chloride), resulting in a markedly negative (-20 to -25 mEq/L) UAG.
- During impaired urine acidification caused by type 1 RTA (distal renal tubule), urine ammonium (and chloride) excretion is impaired, with the UAG being markedly positive (20-40 mEq/L).

Renal Tubular Acidosis

Normal anion gap metabolic acidosis is seen in all three types of RTA.

STUDY TABLE: Differential Diagnosis of Renal Tubular Acidosis

Diagnosis	Metabolic Findings	Associated Findings
Distal (classic or type 1) RTA	Normal anion gap metabolic acidosis, hypokalemia, positive UAG, urine pH >5.5 (only in the setting of systemic acidosis), serum $[HCO_3] \cong$ 10 mEq/L	Nephrolithiasis and nephrocalcinosis, autoimmune disorders (SLE, Sjögren syndrome), amphotericin B use, urinary obstruction
Proximal (type 2) RTA	Normal anion gap metabolic acidosis, normal or negative UAG, hypokalemia, urine pH <5.5, serum $[HCO_3] \cong$ 16-18 mEq/L	Glycosuria, phosphaturia, uricosuria, aminoaciduria, and tubular proteinuria (Fanconi syndrome)
Type 4 RTA (hyporeninemic hypoaldosteronism)	Normal anion gap metabolic acidosis, hyperkalemia, positive UAG, urine pH <5.5	Diabetes mellitus, urinary tract obstruction

Treatment

In **distal (type 1) RTA,** administration of bicarbonate usually corrects the metabolic acidosis. The potassium deficit should be corrected before correcting the acidemia.

In **proximal (type 2) RTA**, correction of acidemia with bicarbonate therapy is often not possible. The addition of a thiazide diuretic may help by inducing volume depletion, lowering the GFR, and thereby decreasing the filtered load of bicarbonate. The addition of a potassium-sparing diuretic may limit the degree of kidney potassium wasting.

In **type 4 RTA,** the primary goal of therapy is to correct the hyperkalemia, which will treat the acid-base disturbance. These patients, often with early CKD and diabetes, may develop severe hyperkalemia following treatment with ACE inhibitors or ARBs.

Treat **alcoholic ketoacidosis** with IV normal saline, glucose, and thiamine.

See Endocrinology and Metabolism for **diabetic ketoacidosis**.

TEST YOURSELF

A 31-year-old woman with IBD passes a kidney stone. Serum sodium is 142 mEq/L, potassium is 2.9 mEq/L, chloride is 112 mEq/L, and bicarbonate is 20 mEq/L. Urine pH is 6.5.

ANSWER: For diagnosis, choose distal RTA.

Delta-Delta

In anion gap acidosis, the expected ratio between the change in anion gap (normal anion gap-measured anion gap) and the change in plasma [HCO_3] (normal HCO_3-measured HCO_3) concentration (Δ anion gap/Δ [HCO_3]) is 1 to 2.

- If (Δ anion gap/Δ [HCO_3]) is <1, consider concurrent normal anion gap acidosis.
- If (Δ anion gap/Δ [HCO_3]) is >2, consider concurrent metabolic alkalosis.

Metabolic alkalosis is often caused by upper GI loss of hydrogen chloride from vomiting or by kidney loss of hydrogen chloride during diuretic therapy. Metabolic alkalosis is maintained by extracellular fluid volume contraction, chloride depletion, hypokalemia, or elevated aldosterone activity.

You must be able to answer questions like these:

- Problem #1: pH, 7.31; arterial P_{CO_2}, 10 mm Hg; sodium, 127 mEq/L; chloride, 99 mEq/L; bicarbonate, 5 mEq/L. Answer: Mixed increased anion gap and normal anion gap metabolic acidosis and respiratory alkalosis (triple acid-base disorder)
- Problem #2: pH, 7.20; arterial P_{CO_2}, 23 mm Hg; sodium, 134 mEq/L; chloride, 80 mEq/L; bicarbonate, 8 mEq/L. Answer: Mixed increased anion gap metabolic acidosis and metabolic alkalosis (double acid-base disorder)

Alcohol Poisoning

Diagnosis

Determine the presence of an osmolal gap, which is the difference between measured and calculated osmolality. The calculated plasma osmolality = 2 × serum [Na^+] + [BUN]/2.8 + blood [glucose]/18; sodium concentration is measured as mEq/L, and BUN and glucose concentration are measured as mg/dL.

The normal osmolal gap is 10 mOsm/kg H_2O. If a larger gap exists, consider alcohol poisoning as the source of unmeasured osmoles. Ethanol is the most common cause of alcohol poisoning. Methanol, isopropyl alcohol, and ethylene glycol can also increase the osmolal gap.

STUDY TABLE: Presentation and Treatment of Alcohol Poisoning

Alcohol	Common Sources	Major Findings	Anion Gap	Osmolar Gap	Treatment
Ethanol	Alcoholic beverages	CNS depression Flank pain, hematuria, oliguria	No	Yes	Supportive care
Isopropyl alcohol	Rubbing alcohol	CNS depression ↑ Ketones	No	Yes	Supportive care
Methanol	Windshield wiper fluid De-icing solutions	CNS depression Vision loss	Yes	Yes	Fomepizole Dialysis (if severe) Folic acid
Ethylene glycol	Antifreeze De-icing solutions	CNS depression Acute kidney injury Calcium oxalate crystals in the urine	Yes	Yes	Fomepizole Dialysis (if severe)

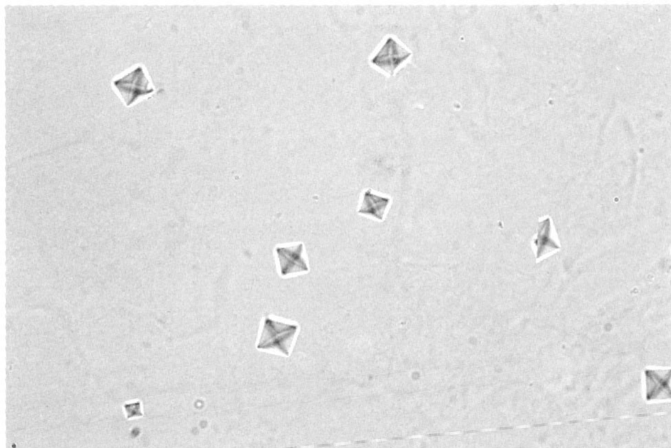

Calcium Oxalate Crystals: Characteristic envelope-shaped calcium oxalate dihydrate crystals, which may be seen in late ethylene glycol intoxication.

Hypertension

Diagnosis

Before labeling a person as having hypertension, use an average BP based on two or more readings obtained on two or more occasions. Out-of-office and self-monitoring BP measurements are recommended to confirm the diagnosis of hypertension and for titration of BP-lowering medication.

White coat hypertension. In adults with an untreated SBP >130 but <160 mm Hg or DBP >80 but <100 mm Hg, it is reasonable to evaluate for the presence of white coat hypertension using either daytime ABPM or HBPM before diagnosis of hypertension.

Masked hypertension. Masked hypertension is defined as elevated BP detected by ABPM but with a normal office BP measurement. In adults with elevated office BP (120-129/<80 mm Hg) but not meeting the criteria for hypertension, evaluating for masked hypertension with daytime ABPM or HBPM is reasonable.

Ambulatory BP measurement is the gold standard to confirm the diagnosis of hypertension and to diagnose white coat and masked hypertension.

Target BP for older adult patients. The ACC/AHA target SBP for noninstitutionalized, ambulatory, community-dwelling patients who are ≥65 years is <130 mm Hg. The ACP guideline recommends a target SBP <150 mm Hg in patients ≥60 years.

Target BP for patients with selected comorbidities. The target BP is 130/80 mm Hg for patients with hypertension and stable ischemic heart disease; heart failure with reduced ejection fraction; heart failure and preserved ejection fraction; peripheral artery disease; DM; CKD; or a history of intracerebral hemorrhage with hypertension in the outpatient setting. ACP guidelines indicate a target SBP <140 mm Hg may be reasonable in some patients ≥60 years at high cardiovascular risk, based on individualized assessment.

A target BP of <130/80 mm Hg may be reasonable in adults following recovery from stroke or TIA, although the benefit of initiating antihypertensive therapy in these patients with a BP <140/90 mm Hg is uncertain. The ACP guideline indicates it is reasonable to consider initiating or intensifying pharmacologic treatment in patients ≥60 years with a history of stroke or TIA to achieve a target SBP <140 mm Hg to reduce the risk for recurrent stroke.

Secondary hypertension. Most patients with established hypertension have primary (essential) hypertension. Consider secondary hypertension in patients who have atypical clinical features (early onset, absent family history, hypokalemia, evidence of kidney disease) or have resistant hypertension (not at target goal despite the use of three antihypertensive agents, including a diuretic).

STUDY TABLE: Selected Secondary Causes of Hypertension

Condition	Notes
Drug induced	NSAIDs, amphetamines/cocaine, sympathomimetics, oral contraceptives, glucocorticoids
CKD	Elevated BUN, serum creatinine, and potassium; most patients present at an earlier stage with minimal signs and symptoms
Renovascular disease (atherosclerotic and fibromuscular)	Onset of hypertension at young age, especially in women (fibromuscular); atherosclerotic disease often associated with cigarette smoking, flash pulmonary edema, CAD, flank bruits, advanced retinopathy, increased creatinine (usually with bilateral renovascular disease), and increased creatinine after treatment with an ACE inhibitor or ARB; notable for hypokalemia and elevated renin and aldosterone levels
Aortic coarctation	Headache, cold feet, leg pain, reduced or absent femoral pulse, delay in femoral pulse compared with radial pulse, murmur heard between scapulae, figure 3 sign and rib notching on chest x-ray
Primary hyperaldosteronism	Muscle cramping, nocturia, thirst; physical examination normal; hypokalemia and elevated plasma aldosterone-plasma renin activity ratio
Cushing syndrome	Weight gain, menstrual irregularity, hirsutism; truncal obesity, abdominal striae; hypokalemia, metabolic alkalosis
Pheochromocytoma	Sweating, heart racing, pounding headache; pallor; tachycardia; hypertension may be episodic with intervals of normal BP; increased urine or plasma catecholamines or metanephrine
Sleep apnea	Increased BMI >30, neck size >17, crowded oropharynx; snoring, witnessed apneic events

DON'T BE TRICKED

- **Do not use plasma renin activity to risk-stratify patients with hypertension or to predict response to specific drugs.**

TEST YOURSELF

A 35-year-old woman is evaluated for persistent fatigue and resistant hypertension. Serum potassium is 3.3 mEq/L.

ANSWER: For diagnosis, choose primary aldosteronism. For management, select measurement of plasma aldosterone-plasma renin activity ratio.

Testing

Hypertension evaluation includes collecting data on cardiovascular risk factors and symptoms or signs of a possible underlying secondary cause. Initial evaluation includes:

- laboratory testing for kidney function, fasting blood glucose, fasting lipid panel, serum potassium, and serum calcium
- ECG
- urinalysis and albumin-creatinine ratio

Treatment

From the list of first-line drugs, patient characteristics will influence the final choice.

STUDY TABLE: ACC/AHA Classification and Treatment of Blood Pressure			
BP Category	**Office-Based Readings (mm Hg)**	**Treatment**	**BP Target (mm Hg)**
Normal	SBP <120 and DBP <80	NA	NA
Elevated BP	SBP 120-129 and DBP <80	Nonpharmacologic therapy (NPT) if clinical CV disease or 10-year ASCVD risk <10%	SBP <120 and DBP <80
Hypertension, Stage 1	SBP 130-139 or DBP 80-89	NPT if 10-year ASCVD risk <10% NPT + first-line drugs if clinical CV disease or 10-year ASCVD risk ≥10%	<130/80
Hypertension, Stage 2	SBP ≥140 or DBP ≥90	Two first-line drugs of different classes, preferably with once daily dosing, if BP 20/10 mm Hg above target	<130/80

STUDY TABLE: Selection of an Antihypertensive Agent		
Agent	**Potential Clinical Indications**	**Potential Clinical Contraindications**
Thiazide diuretic	Isolated systolic hypertension in older adults Hypertension in black patients HF	Gout, hyponatremia, glucose intolerance, concomitant lithium use
ACE inhibitor/ARB	HF Post-MI CKD Proteinuria Diabetes mellitus/metabolic syndrome	Pregnancy,[a] hyperkalemia, bilateral renal artery stenosis
Calcium channel blocker	Isolated systolic hypertension in older adults Hypertension in black patients	HF (non-dihydropyridine)
β-Blockers	Post-MI HF Tachyarrhythmia Pregnancy Angina (NOT recommended for initial use except under these conditions)	Peripheral artery disease, COPD, glucose intolerance

[a]Absolute contraindication.

Typically, 75% of a drug's BP-lowering effect is achieved with 50% of its maximal dose. A combination of two agents at moderate dose is often more successful at achieving BP goals than one BP agent at maximal dose.

DON'T BE TRICKED

- **Thiazide diuretics are not effective in patients with kidney disease (GFR <30 mL/min/1.73 m^2); select a loop diuretic.**

Hypertensive Urgency

The treatment of hypertensive urgency (BP >180/120 mm Hg in the absence of symptoms or progressive target-organ damage) differs if the patient has previously treated hypertension or untreated hypertension.

In patients with preexisting treated hypertension:

- restart the medication(s) in nonadherent patients
- in adherent patients, either increase the dose of the medication(s) or add an additional agent

In patients with previously untreated hypertension:

- consider oral furosemide or small doses of clonidine or captopril and observe for several hours for a BP drop of 20 to 30 mm Hg (not to normal BP)
- begin a long-acting agent; discharge home with follow-up in 2 to 3 days

Hypertensive Emergency

A hypertensive emergency can be life threatening. Initial treatment is best performed in the ICU; see the Pulmonary and Critical Care Medicine chapter for information on treatment.

Hypertension in Pregnancy

Diagnosis

Chronic hypertension in pregnancy. Hypertension before the 20th week of gestation is most consistent with previously undiagnosed chronic hypertension.

Gestational hypertension is hypertension that develops after 20 weeks of pregnancy without preexisting hypertension, proteinuria, or other end-organ damage. Gestational hypertension is a risk factor for preeclampsia and the development of chronic hypertension.

Preeclampsia is new-onset hypertension after 20 weeks of pregnancy with proteinuria. Eclampsia is the presence of generalized, tonic-clonic seizures in a preeclamptic woman.

Treatment

Treatment of hypertension less than 160/110 mm Hg during pregnancy is controversial, and benefits of treatment have not been demonstrated.

Drugs that can be used during pregnancy:

- methyldopa
- labetalol
- calcium channel blockers (e.g., long-acting nifedipine)

Antihypertensive medications absolutely contraindicated during pregnancy:

- ACE inhibitors
- ARBs
- renin inhibitors

Diuretics may induce oligohydramnios if initiated during pregnancy.

Preeclampsia. Definitive treatment is delivery, including induction of labor in women at or near term.

DON'T BE TRICKED

- **Treatment of gestational hypertension does not prevent the occurrence of preeclampsia or chronic hypertension.**

Glomerular Diseases

Glomerular disease should be suspected when proteinuria and/or hematuria are seen on urinalysis.

The most common distinction is usually made between the nephrotic syndromes and the nephritic syndromes, also referred to as GN. Some conditions may present with either or both patterns, and some may progress from one pattern to the other.

The Nephrotic Syndrome

Diagnosis

The nephrotic syndrome is characterized by:

- urine protein excretion >3500 mg/24 h or a urine protein-creatinine ratio of >3500 mg/g
- hypoalbuminemia, edema, and hyperlipidemia may be present

The nephrotic syndrome may be primary or secondary to systemic diseases such as diabetes, infection, or autoimmune diseases.

STUDY TABLE: Common Causes of the Nephrotic Syndrome

Condition	Clinical Associations	Diagnosis	Treatment
Focal segmental glomerulosclerosis	Most common cause of nephrotic syndrome in blacks "Collapsing" variety associated with HIV Associated with morbid obesity	Biopsy	Glucocorticoids or calcineurin inhibitors
Membranous glomerulopathy	Most common cause of nephropathy in whites Positive antibody against phospholipase A2 receptor Secondary causes include: infection (hepatitis B and C, malaria, syphilis); SLE; drugs (NSAIDs); cancer (solid tumors, lymphoma) High propensity for thrombosis, especially renal vein thrombosis	Biopsy	33% spontaneously remit in 6-12 mo Glucocorticoids and cyclophosphamide or calcineurin inhibitors Treat concurrent hepatitis B
Minimal change glomerulopathy	Most common cause of primary nephrotic syndrome in children 10% of nephrotic syndrome in adults	Biopsy	Glucocorticoids
Diabetic nephropathy	Most common secondary cause of the nephrotic syndrome and the most common overall cause in adults Annual measurement of albumin-creatinine ratio measured beginning 5 years after diagnosis of type 1 diabetes and at time of diagnosis of type 2 diabetes	Clinical diagnosis	Excellent BP and glucose control ACE inhibitors or ARBs

DON'T BE TRICKED

- **Nephrotic range proteinuria in a patient with diabetes but without diabetic retinopathy is not caused by diabetes. Kidney biopsy is required for definitive diagnosis.**

Treatment

Treatment of the consequences of the nephrotic syndrome should occur simultaneously with treatment of the specific cause (if nephrotic syndrome is secondary to an underlying condition):

- statins for elevated lipid levels
- anticoagulation for thrombotic complications (because of urinary loss of antithrombins)
- low salt diet and loop diuretics for edema

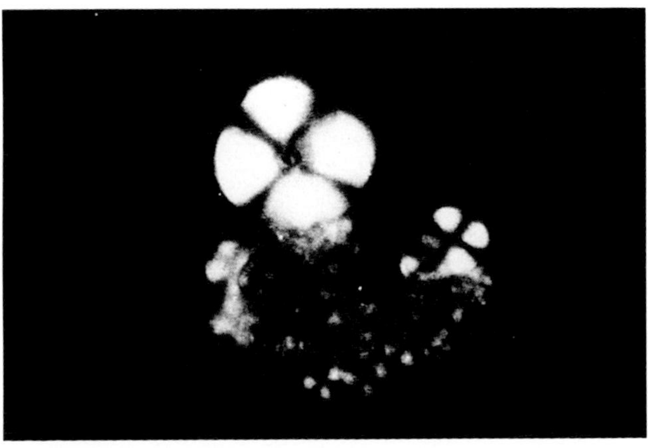

Fat Droplet: Typical "Maltese cross" appearance of a fat droplet under polarized light microscopy commonly found in the nephrotic syndrome.

The Nephritic Syndrome

Diagnosis

The nephritic syndrome is associated with glomerular inflammation resulting in hematuria, proteinuria, and leukocytes in the urine sediment. The hallmark is the presence of dysmorphic erythrocytes and erythrocyte casts. Proteinuria is variable. Systemic findings may include edema, hypertension, and kidney failure.

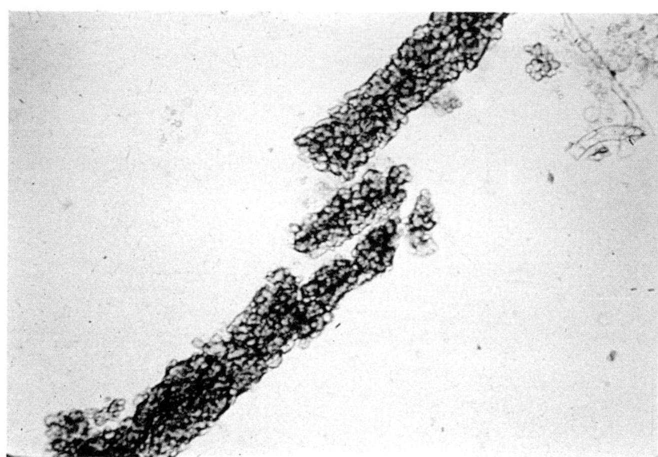

Glomerulonephritis: Erythrocyte casts consistent with glomerulonephritis.

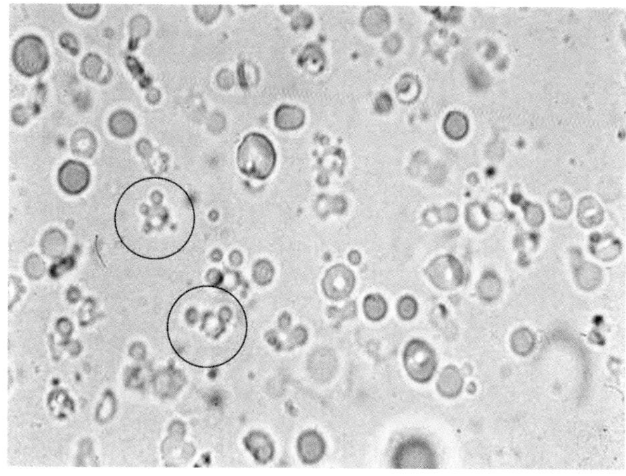

Dysmorphic Erythrocytes: Erythrocytes with abnormal morphology seen in glomerulonephritis, including those with "Mickey Mouse ears."

STUDY TABLE: Common Causes of the Nephritic Syndrome

Pathological Mechanism	Specific Diseases
Anti-GBM antibodies (normal complement)	Anti-GBM antibody disease
Pauci-immune GN (necrotizing GN with few immune deposits, normal complement)	Granulomatosis with polyangiitis
	Microscopic polyangiitis
	Eosinophilic granulomatosis with polyangiitis
Immune complex deposition (low complement with exception of IgA nephropathy)	IgA nephropathy
	IgA vasculitis (Henoch-Schönlein purpura)
	LN
	Infection-related GN
	Membranoproliferative GN
	Cryoglobulinemia (see Monoclonal Gammopathies and Cryoglobulinemia)

Rapidly progressive GN is a clinical syndrome characterized by evidence of GN with progression to kidney failure within weeks. It may be associated with any cause of GN or may be idiopathic. Rapidly progressive GN is particularly common with anti-GBM antibody disease (in younger patients) and pauci-immune small-vessel vasculitis (in older patients).

Anti-Glomerular Basement Membrane Antibody Disease

This is an autoimmune disease caused by antibodies directed against type IV collagen. If pulmonary capillaries are involved, it causes pulmonary hemorrhage (Goodpasture syndrome).

Findings include normal complement levels and elevated levels of anti-GBM antibodies. Kidney biopsy shows proliferative GN with linear deposition of immunoglobulin.

Treatment is cyclophosphamide and glucocorticoids, combined with daily plasmapheresis.

Pauci-Immune Glomerulonephritis

Kidney manifestations range from only hematuria to rapidly progressive GN. Systemic symptoms may include arthritis, leukocytoclastic vasculitis (palpable purpura), and pulmonary disease (pulmonary infiltrate to pulmonary hemorrhage).

More than 80% of patients with MPA or granulomatosis with polyangiitis are ANCA positive; granulomatosis with polyangiitis is associated with (PR3)-ANCA and MPA is associated with (MPO)-ANCA.

Complement levels are normal. Kidney biopsy shows absent or minimal staining with immunoglobulin.

Induction therapy consists of glucocorticoids and cyclophosphamide (or rituximab) with or without plasmapheresis.

IgA Nephropathy

Most commonly presents as asymptomatic microscopic hematuria (with or without proteinuria) or episodic gross hematuria coincident with a URI (synpharyngitic nephritis).

Kidney biopsy shows glomerular IgA deposits on immunofluorescence. Complement levels are normal.

Most patients have a benign course without treatment; patients with proteinuria and risk factors for progression may benefit from ACE inhibitors or ARBs.

IgA Vasculitis (Henoch-Schönlein Purpura)

Kidney involvement is similar to IgA nephropathy, and other organ involvement may occur.

Diagnosis is confirmed either by finding an IgA-dominant leukocytoclastic vasculitis or by kidney biopsy, which shows lesions similar to IgA nephropathy. Complement levels are normal.

Henoch-Schönlein purpura is typically self-limiting without treatment.

Lupus Nephritis

Patients typically have extrarenal symptoms of SLE at the time of diagnosis of LN.

ANA and anti-double-stranded antibodies are positive, and C3 and C4 complement levels are depressed.

Classification and recommended treatment of LN is made after kidney biopsy:

- Class I and II (minimal or proliferative mesangial) lesions require no specific therapy.
- Classes III and IV (focal and diffuse glomerular lesions) are treated with high-dose glucocorticoids and either IV cyclophosphamide or mycophenolate mofetil.
- Class V (membranous) LN has a course similar to idiopathic membranous glomerulopathy.

Infection-Related Glomerulonephritis

Staphylococcal infection is as common as or more common than streptococcal infection as a cause of infection-related GN. The clinical manifestations of poststreptococcal GN typically occur after a latent period of 1 to 6 weeks (check antistreptolysin O, anti-DNase titers) but occur at the time of infection with other infectious agents.

Diagnosis is clinical in nephritic patients who have an ongoing or preceding infection. Complement levels are low.

Treatment focuses on the underlying infection.

Membranoproliferative Glomerulonephritis

Membranoproliferative GN manifests in children or young adults as proteinuria or the nephrotic syndrome. It is associated with immune complex disease (SLE), infections (hepatitis C), and monoclonal gammopathy.

Complement levels are low.

Treatment of the causative infection, autoimmune disease, or monoclonal gammopathy is the primary therapy.

Causes of Glomerular Diseases Associated with Low Complement Levels

Causes include

- postinfectious GN (e.g., endocarditis, Group A streptococcal infection)
- SLE
- cryoglobulinemia
- membranoproliferative GN
- atheroembolic disease

Monoclonal Gammopathies and Cryoglobulinemia

Kidney manifestations of monoclonal gammopathies may include proteinuria (sometimes nephrotic range), tubular dysfunction, hypertension, and kidney failure.

Diagnosis of monoclonal gammopathy of renal significance usually requires kidney biopsy.

Management is focused on treatment of the underlying monoclonal disorder.

STUDY TABLE: Monoclonal Gammopathies and Cryoglobulinemia-Related Kidney Diseases

Condition	Pathology	Clinical Syndrome
Amyloidosis	Deposits that stain apple green with Congo red	Proteinuria or nephrotic syndrome
Monoclonal immunoglobulin deposition disease	Congo red-negative light or heavy chain deposits	Proteinuria or nephrotic syndrome
Multiple myeloma	Accumulation of light chains in the renal tubule (cast nephropathy) Light chains absorb and crystallize in proximal tubular cells	Acute kidney injury Acute or CKD associated with Fanconi syndrome
Cryoglobulinemia	Vasculitic syndrome with GN with membranoproliferative features	Most often associated with type II cryoglobulins (HCV infection) Proteinuria, hematuria, nephrotic syndrome, rapidly progressive GN Low C4 (sometimes C3)
Monoclonal gammopathy of renal significance	Most often caused by monoclonal antibody deposition in the kidney	The presence of MGUS with kidney abnormalities, including proteinuria, nephrotic syndrome, Fanconi syndrome, GN

Autosomal Dominant Polycystic Kidney Disease

Diagnosis

ADPKD occurs in 1 in 400 to 1 in 1000 live births. The hallmark of ADPKD is large kidneys with multiple kidney cysts resulting from genetic mutations in *PKD1* and *PKD2*. More than 90% of PKD is as an autosomal dominant trait.

Kidney ultrasonography is used to diagnose ADPKD. In patients with a family history of ADPKD, the number of cysts needed for diagnosis increases with age:

- ≥2 cysts (unilateral or bilateral) for ages 15 to 29 years
- ≥2 cysts in each kidney for ages 30 to 59 years
- ≥4 cysts in each kidney for ages >60 years

DON'T BE TRICKED

- Direct mutational analysis of the *PKD1* and *PKD2* genes is reserved for equivocal cases following imaging.

Hypertension is a common presentation. More than 50% of patients develop recurrent flank or back pain from kidney stones, cyst rupture or hemorrhage, or infection.

A ruptured intracranial cerebral aneurysm is the most serious extrarenal complication of ADPKD and occurs most commonly in patients with a family history of hemorrhagic stroke or intracranial cerebral aneurysm.

Treatment

ADPKD has no specific treatments.

- Treat hypertension with an ACE inhibitor or an ARB.
- Treat cyst infection or pyelonephritis with fluoroquinolones or trimethoprim-sulfamethoxazole.
- In a randomized clinical trial, tolvaptan has been shown to reduce the rate of increase in kidney size and loss of GFR, but poor tolerance, hepatotoxicity, and expense limit its use.

Patients with a history of ADPKD, particularly those with a family history of intracranial aneurysm, should be offered screening for aneurysm by CTA or MRA.

DON'T BE TRICKED

- Up to 25% of patients with newly diagnosed ADPKD may have a negative family history owing to mild disease in an affected parent or earlier death from other causes.

Inherited Collagen Type IV-Related Nephropathies

Two relevant inherited collagen type IV-related nephropathies:

- hereditary nephritis
- thin GBM disease

Hereditary nephritis is a rare cause of end-stage kidney disease. When the genetic mutation is X-linked (80% of patients), the condition is termed Alport syndrome. Classic Alport syndrome is accompanied by sensorineural hearing loss and characteristic ocular findings such as lenticonus. Proteinuria, hypertension, and CKD usually develop over time. End-stage kidney disease occurs between the late teenage years and the fourth decade of life. Hereditary nephritis has no specific therapy.

Thin GBM disease manifests as microscopic or macroscopic hematuria, usually first appearing in childhood. Long-term prognosis is excellent.

Acute Kidney Injury

Diagnosis and Testing

AKI is defined as an abrupt elevation in the serum creatinine concentration or a decrease in urine output. The cause may be secondary to prerenal causes, intrinsic kidney disease, or postrenal obstruction of urine outflow. Prerenal and postrenal causes must be distinguished from intrinsic renal parenchymal disease because they are often rapidly reversible.

AKI is also divided into oliguric (≤400 mL/24 h) and nonoliguric (>400 mL/24 h) forms. The lower the urine output, the worse the prognosis.

STUDY TABLE: Diagnostic Findings in AKI					
Condition	**BUN-Creatinine Ratio**	**Urine Osmolality (mOsm/kg H_2O)**	**Urine Sodium (mEq/L)**	**FE_{Na}**	**Urinalysis and Microscopy**
Prerenal	>20:1	>500	<20	<1%	Specific gravity >1.020; normal or hyaline casts
ATN	10:1	~300	>40	>2%[a]	Specific gravity ~1.010; muddy brown casts and tubular epithelial cells
AIN	Variable	Variable	Variable	Variable	Mild proteinuria; leukocytes; erythrocytes; leukocyte casts; eosinophiluria
Acute GN	Variable	Variable	Variable	Variable	Proteinuria; dysmorphic erythrocytes; erythrocyte casts
Postrenal	>20:1	Variable	Variable	Variable	Variable, bland

[a]FE_{Na} can be low in contrast nephropathy and pigment nephropathy.

FE_{Na} may be >2% in prerenal patients who are taking diuretics. In the setting of diuretics, the FE_{Urea}, calculated as $(U_{Urea} \times P_{Cr})/(U_{Cr} \times P_{Urea}) \times 100$, is more accurate in detecting volume-depleted states and prerenal AKI. An FE_{Urea} of <35% is consistent with a prerenal cause of AKI.

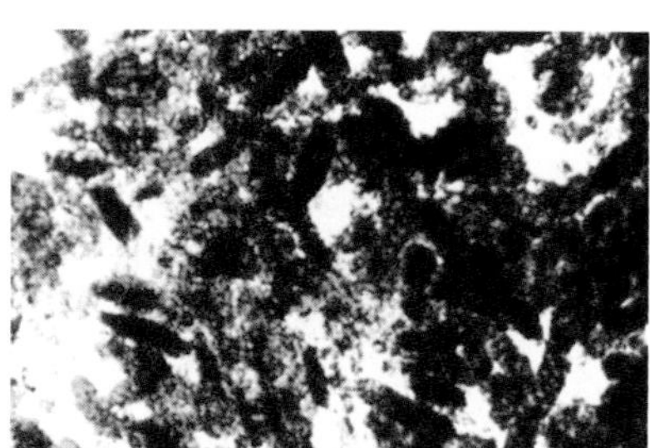

Muddy Brown Granular Casts: Muddy brown granular casts consistent with kidney injury secondary to tubular necrosis.

Knowing a few basic epidemiologic facts can help identify the cause of AKI:

- Prerenal AKI is the most common form of AKI in the outpatient setting.
- A prolonged prerenal state can lead to ATN.
- The most common cause of hospital-acquired AKI is ATN.
- Hospital-acquired ATN is most commonly caused by toxins such as radiocontrast and antibiotics (i.e., gentamicin).
- Obstruction of the upper tract (ureters or renal pelvis) must be bilateral to cause AKI.

STUDY TABLE: Differential Diagnosis of AKI		
When You See This...	**Think of...**	**And Select...**
Minimal proteinuria, no hematuria or pyuria; presence of muddy brown casts	ATN	FE_{Na} and/or spot urine sodium
Erythrocytes, erythrocyte casts, or dysmorphic erythrocytes	GN	As appropriate: Titers for ANA; anti-dsDNA antibodies; and antistreptolysin O antibodies; C3, C4, and CH_{50}; hepatitis and HIV serologies and cryoglobulins; p-ANCA/c-ANCA and anti-GBM antibodies
Pyuria	Pyelonephritis AIN	Urine culture Review of medication list
Eosinophilia, eosinophiluria, and rash	AIN Cholesterol emboli	Review of medication list Investigation for previous vascular procedure (angiography)
Livedo reticularis (violaceous reticular rash)	Cholesterol emboli Vasculitis	Investigation for previous vascular procedure (angiography) Consideration for cryoglobulinemia
Hypercalcemia and anemia	Multiple myeloma	Serum and urine protein electrophoresis, quantitative immunoglobulins
Nephrotic syndrome	Diabetes mellitus Renal vein thrombosis	Plasma glucose Renal vein Doppler study

(Continued on the next page)

STUDY TABLE: Differential Diagnosis of AKI *(Continued)*		
When You See This...	**Think of...**	**And Select...**
Obstruction on kidney ultrasound	BPH Nephrolithiasis Obstructing malignant mass Retroperitoneal fibrosis	Residual bladder volume, noncontrast CT or MRI
Complete anuria	Renal cortical necrosis	Kidney ultrasonography
Large kidneys on ultrasound	Amyloidosis, diabetes (early), HIV nephropathy	SPEP, blood glucose, HIV serologic studies
Kidney failure following colonoscopy	Phosphate-containing bowel prep (acute calcium phosphate crystal deposition in the kidneys)	Supportive care (fluids, stop ACE inhibitors, ARBs, NSAIDs)
Recent abdominal surgery, hemorrhage, or acute pancreatitis	Abdominal compartment syndrome	Intravesicular pressure >20 mm Hg
Peripheral blood smear schistocytes, thrombocytopenia	Thrombotic microangiopathy (HUS/TTP, DIC, scleroderma renal crisis)	As indicated, CBC, coagulation parameters
Urine dipstick positive for blood, no erythrocytes on urinalysis	Hemolysis, rhabdomyolysis	Serum CK, serum haptoglobin, reticulocyte count, peripheral blood smear
AKI associated with acute leukemia or lymphoma or its treatment	Tumor lysis syndrome	Uric acid, phosphorus, potassium (all elevated)
Worsening kidney function in the setting of diuretic-resistant HF	Cardiorenal syndrome	Diuretics, ACE inhibitors or ARBs, vasodilators, and inotropes for improved cardiac function
Worsening kidney function in setting of cirrhosis and ascites	Hepatorenal syndrome	IV albumin and intravascular volume repletion. Liver transplantation (See Gastroenterology and Hepatology, Cirrhosis)

TEST YOURSELF

A 65-year-old man develops eosinophilia, AKI, and a net-like rash on his lower extremities following a cardiac catheterization.

ANSWER: For diagnosis, choose atheroembolic disease with cholesterol emboli to the skin and kidney.

A 35-year-old woman with necrotizing pancreatitis and tense ascites develops AKI.

ANSWER: For diagnosis, choose abdominal compartment syndrome; for management, choose measurement of intravesicular pressure.

Treatment

Begin IV normal saline for patients with volume depletion. Stop potential nephrotoxic drugs and look particularly for aminoglycoside antibiotics, ACE inhibitors, loop diuretics, cyclosporine, and NSAIDs.

Select dialysis for:

- refractory hyperkalemia, acidemia, or volume overload
- signs or symptoms of uremia (altered mentation, asterixis, pericardial friction rub, vomiting)
- certain drug intoxications

Generally, intermittent hemodialysis is used for stable patients with AKI, and continuous renal replacement therapy or prolonged intermittent renal replacement therapy is used for critically ill patients with unstable hemodynamics, multiorgan failure, or high catabolic states.

For urinary obstruction, choose a catheter to relieve bladder outlet obstruction. If the obstruction is above the bladder, select retrograde or antegrade nephrostomies.

DON'T BE TRICKED

- Do not withhold dialysis until BUN, creatinine, or both reach "threshold" values.

STUDY TABLE: AKI Treatment Protocol

Indication	Treatment
Severe acidemia (pH <7.20)	IV bicarbonate or hemodialysis
Severe hypertension	Vasodilators, β-blockers, calcium channel blockers
Rapidly progressive GN, granulomatosis with polyangiitis, and severe IgA nephropathy	Cyclophosphamide, glucocorticoids
Scleroderma renal crisis	ACE inhibitor, regardless of serum creatinine level
Hydronephrosis on ultrasound	Depending on cause, bladder catheter or nephrostomy tube
Abdominal compartment syndrome	Surgical decompression

DON'T BE TRICKED

- Do not select loop diuretics (without evidence of volume overload), dopamine, or mannitol to treat AKI.

Contrast-Induced Nephropathy

Prevention

In patients at high risk requiring imaging with contrast, avoid volume depletion and NSAIDs. Use the smallest possible dose of a low-osmolar or iso-osmolar contrast agent, and treat with isotonic saline or bicarbonate before and immediately after the procedure.

DON'T BE TRICKED

- Contrast-induced nephropathy is not prevented by dialysis immediately after contrast media administration.
- Do not use oral or intravenous acetylcysteine to prevent AKI secondary to radiocontrast.

Nephrolithiasis

Diagnosis

Kidney stones are predominantly composed of calcium but may be formed by other substrates such as uric acid, struvite, or cystine.

Important risk factors for stone formation include:

- insufficient fluid intake
- increased dietary sodium and protein intake
- hypercalciuria, hyperuricemia, hyperoxaluria
- low urine citrate levels (citrate inhibits crystal formation)
- primary hyperparathyroidism with hypercalciuria
- metabolic syndrome and type 2 diabetes mellitus
- recurrent UTIs with urease-splitting organisms such as *Klebsiella* and *Proteus* (struvite stones)
- sarcoid (hypercalciuria/hypercalcemia)

Patients with suspected nephrolithiasis should be asked about:

- a personal or family history of stone disease
- polycystic kidney disease, medullary sponge kidney, distal RTA
- high-risk medical illness (Crohn disease, ileostomy)

- high-risk medications (indinavir, acetazolamide)
- diets with increased protein (Atkins diet)
- repeated UTIs, high urine pH, and staghorn calculi (*Proteus* infections)

The classic symptoms of nephrolithiasis are acute flank pain with radiation to the groin and hematuria. Urinalysis usually reveals blood, and the urine sediment has intact, nondysmorphic erythrocytes. Ultrasonography or noncontrast CT is the preferred imaging choice.

DON'T BE TRICKED

- **The absence of erythrocytes on urinalysis does not rule out nephrolithiasis.**

Treatment

Treatment varies according to the specific findings. Kidney stones <5 mm in diameter typically pass spontaneously. Stones >10 mm often require invasive measures. Patients with stones 6 to 10 mm in size will benefit from expulsive therapy with either tamsulosin or nifedipine. These drugs induce ureteral dilatation and relaxation.

Urgent urologic consultation is indicated for patients with:

- pyelonephritis or urosepsis
- AKI
- large stones requiring surgical removal
- bilateral obstruction
- obstruction of a solitary kidney

Urologic referral is also indicated for ambulatory patients who do not pass stones with conservative management or who have stones >10 mm in diameter.

Chronic treatment:

- 2 L fluid intake per day
- calcium composite stones: thiazide diuretic, allopurinol, or citrate
- large struvite stones: percutaneous nephrostolithotomy and long-term prophylactic antibiotics

DON'T BE TRICKED

- **Asymptomatic kidney stones found on imaging studies do not require urgent stone removal.**
- **Do not select a low-calcium diet for patients with kidney stones. Calcium restriction does not prevent stones and may actually increase stone formation and contribute to bone demineralization.**

TEST YOURSELF

A 35-year-old woman is evaluated in the emergency department for right flank pain and hematuria. She has a long history of Crohn disease and has had multiple operations to remove portions of her ileum and colon.

ANSWER: For diagnosis, select calcium oxalate stones secondary to increased oxalate absorption in the GI tract and subsequent hyperoxaluria.

Chronic Kidney Disease

Diagnosis

CKD, characterized by an alteration in kidney function or structure for ≥3 months, occurs most often in patients with diabetes and hypertension. Characteristic findings of uremia are asterixis, loss of appetite, nausea, vomiting, and a pericardial rub.

Differential diagnosis of CKD:

- Diabetic kidney disease: Look for early moderately increased albuminuria (spot albumin-creatinine ratio, 30-300 mg/g), followed by overt proteinuria, declining GFR, and a bland urine sediment. The presence of retinopathy strongly suggests coexisting diabetic nephropathy.
- Glomerular disease: Look for glomerular hematuria, proteinuria, and hypertension, often with other systemic manifestations (LN and postinfectious GN). If nephrotic syndrome is present, look for focal segmental glomerulosclerosis, membranous nephropathy, and minimal change disease. Kidney biopsy is often needed to make a specific diagnosis and guide therapy.
- Tubulointerstitial disease: Look for proteinuria, glycosuria, concentrating defect, sterile pyuria, and leukocyte casts, as well as papillary necrosis on ultrasound. Consider analgesic nephropathy (medication use, papillary necrosis), infection (TB, legionnaires disease, leptospirosis), allergic drug reaction (eosinophilia, eosinophiluria), autoimmune disorder (SLE, sarcoidosis, Sjögren syndrome), and lead nephropathy (occupational exposure).
- Vascular disease: Look for hematuria, proteinuria, and associated systemic illness. Vasculitis often presents with rapidly progressive GN and palpable purpura (leukocytoclastic vasculitis).
- After transplantation: CKD in the kidney transplant recipient may be caused by chronic allograft nephropathy, drug toxicity (cyclosporine), polyomavirus BK infection, or recurrence of disease.
- Structural disease (polycystic kidney disease): Look for hypertension, hematuria, palpable kidneys (advanced disease), and family history of CKD.

DON'T BE TRICKED

- **If the kidneys are markedly scarred and small (<9 cm), do not select aggressive diagnostic or therapeutic measures.**

Complications

Many patients with CKD are asymptomatic. Cardiovascular disease is the leading cause of death in patients with CKD. Chronic anemia and metabolic acidosis are also common complications.

Renal osteodystrophy refers to alteration of bone morphology in patients as a result of CKD.

STUDY TABLE: Renal Osteodystrophy

Condition	Mechanism	Characteristics
Osteitis fibrosa cystica	Secondary hyperparathyroidism	Subperiosteal resorption of bone, most prominently at the phalanges
Adynamic bone disease	Suppressed levels of PTH because of chronic illness or aggressive treatment with vitamin D analogues	Increased risk of fractures; made worse with bisphosphonate therapy
Osteomalacia	Vitamin D deficiency	Bone pain, fractures

Treatment

Avoid exposure to kidney toxins (contrast agents, NSAIDs). Avoid gadolinium-enhanced MRI because of the risk of nephrogenic systemic fibrosis (greatest risk in patients receiving dialysis). Begin restriction of sodium, potassium, and phosphorus. Avoid significant protein restriction. Drug and alkali therapy is based on specific findings.

In patients with CKD stages 3a to 5 not receiving dialysis:

- elevated phosphorus levels should be lowered toward the normal range but not into the normal range
- avoid hypercalcemia; mild and asymptomatic hypocalcemia can be tolerated
- restrict or do not use calcium-based phosphate binders
- avoid routine use of calcitriol and vitamin D analogues to lower PTH levels

In patients receiving dialysis:

- calcimimetics, calcitriol, or vitamin D analogues, or their combination, should be used to lower PTH levels

STUDY TABLE: Drug Therapy for CKD	
If You See This...	**Select...**
Hypertension	BP target <130/80 mm Hg
	Initial treatment in black patients with proteinuria is an ACE inhibitor or ARB; in black patients without proteinuria, options include a diuretic, calcium channel blocker, ACE inhibitor, or ARB
	Beneficial effect of ACE inhibitors or ARBs is limited to patients with albuminuria >300 mg/g
	Use a loop diuretic rather than a thiazide for GFR <30 mL/min/1.73 m^2
Hyperlipidemia	Treat patients >50 years with CKD with statins
	Do not treat patients receiving dialysis with statins (no benefit)
Anemia	Erythropoietin to maintain hemoglobin levels of 10-11 g/dL and iron to maintain iron stores (always check iron levels before starting erythropoietin)
Metabolic acidosis	Alkali therapy to maintain [HCO_3] between 23-28 mEq/L

DON'T BE TRICKED

- **The anemia of CKD is a diagnosis of exclusion.**
- **Do not use ACE inhibitors in combination with ARBs or renin inhibitors to treat CKD patients with proteinuria.**

TEST YOURSELF

A 55-year-old woman with chronic lower back pain, polyuria, and nocturia is found to have CKD. Urinalysis shows no protein or erythrocytes, 5 to 10 leukocytes/hpf, and no casts. Urine culture shows no growth. Kidney ultrasound shows only papillary necrosis.

ANSWER: For diagnosis, choose tubulointerstitial disease secondary to analgesic abuse.

Nephrogenic Systemic Fibrosis: This patient with CKD developed nephrogenic systemic fibrosis after an MRI with gadolinium injection. The skin demonstrates erythema, edema, and a peau d'orange appearance.

Kidney Replacement Therapy

Remember these points regarding kidney replacement therapy:

- Clinical outcomes are equivalent for patients receiving peritoneal dialysis compared with hemodialysis.
- Peritoneal dialysis catheters are placed approximately 1 month before therapy is initiated.
- Patients who opt for hemodialysis should be referred for arteriovenous fistula placement 2 months or more before their eGFR drops below 15 mL/min/1.73 m^2 to allow sufficient time for arteriovenous fistula maturation.
- Kidney transplantation is associated with superior quality of life and improved survival and is less expensive compared with long-term dialysis.
- All patients with end-stage kidney disease are considered candidates for kidney transplantation unless they have systemic malignancy, chronic infection, severe cardiovascular disease, or neuropsychiatric disorders.
- Transplantation is particularly beneficial in young patients.
- Suitable candidates for kidney transplantation should be referred for evaluation when their eGFR is <20 mL/min/1.73 m^2.

Patients with kidney transplants must receive immunosuppressive medications to prevent their immune system from rejecting the kidney allograft.

STUDY TABLE: Common Adverse Effects of Immunosuppressants		
Class	**Medication**	**Common Side Effects**
Calcineurin inhibitor	Cyclosporine	Hypertension, decreased GFR, dyslipidemia, hirsutism
	Tacrolimus	Diabetes, decreased GFR, hypertension
Antimetabolite	Mycophenolate	Leukopenia, anemia
	Azathioprine	Leukopenia
mTOR inhibitor	Sirolimus; everolimus	Proteinuria, dyslipidemia, diabetes, anemia, leukopenia
Glucocorticoid receptor agonist	Prednisone	Osteopenia, hypertension, edema, diabetes

Immunosuppression increases the risk for infections and cancers (see Infectious Disease section on Posttransplantation Infections).

- The most common malignancy in kidney transplant recipients is cutaneous SCCs.
- Kaposi sarcoma is much more common in kidney transplant recipients; reduce the immunosuppression and switch to sirolimus-based immunosuppression.
- Posttransplant lymphoproliferative disease is associated with EBV infection; reduce immunosuppression and administration of rituximab in patients with CD20+ tumors.

DON'T BE TRICKED

- Do not use magnesium-containing antacids in patients with end-stage kidney disease.

Neurology

Primary Headaches

More than 90% of headaches are primary headaches, including migraine, tension-type headaches, and trigeminal autonomic cephalgias.

Migraine Headache

Migraine is the most common headache in clinical practice and is frequently missed or misdiagnosed as another type of headache (tension-type or sinus headache).

Diagnosis

Approximately 30% of patients with migraine experience aura during or within the hour before the headache. An aura may manifest as visual loss, hallucinations, flashing lights, numbness, tingling, aphasia, or confusion, with a typical duration of 5 to 60 minutes. Migraine with brainstem aura is defined by the presence of vertigo, ataxia, dysarthria, diplopia, tinnitus, hyperacusis, or alteration in consciousness. Any aura complex that involves some degree of motor weakness is categorized as hemiplegic migraine.

STUDY TABLE: POUND Mnemonic to Diagnose Migraine
Pulsatile quality
One-day duration (between 4 and 72 hours)
Unilateral in location
Nausea or vomiting
Disabling intensity (patient goes to bed)

Four or more features are 90% predictive of migraine headache. Rule out medication overuse headache. Patients with this diagnosis (see Study Table) must be weaned off headache medications.

DON'T BE TRICKED

- **Ninety percent of patients with "sinus headache" have migraine headache that will respond to triptan medications.**
- **Neuroimaging is indicated only for atypical headache features or for headaches that do not meet the strict definition of migraine.**

STUDY TABLE: Differential Diagnosis of Migraine

Disease	Considerations
Tension-type headache	30 minutes to 7 days Typically bilateral location Pressure or tight quality Does not prohibit activity Not associated with nausea Treat acute headache with NSAIDs A tricyclic antidepressant may be needed for prophylaxis

(Continued on the next page)

STUDY TABLE: Differential Diagnosis of Migraine *(Continued)*	
Disease	**Considerations**
Trigeminal neuralgia	Brief paroxysms of unilateral lancinating pain in the V_2 or V_3 distribution of the trigeminal nerve, often triggered by light touch of the affected area Obtain an MRI to exclude intracranial lesions and MS Select carbamazepine for treatment
Medication overuse headache	Chronic headache that occurs ≥10 days per month in patients using combination analgesics, ergotamine products, or triptans; chronic headache that occurs >15 days per month in patients using simple analgesics Must withdraw all pain medications
Chronic migraine headache	Headache occurring ≥15 days per month for >3 months Headache possessing the features of migraine ≥8 days per month Risk factors include migraine headache frequency or acute medication use >10 days per month

DON'T BE TRICKED

- **Avoid butalbital and opioid analgesics in headache management.**
- **Muscle relaxants, benzodiazepines, and botulinum toxin A have no role in the acute or prophylactic treatment of tension-type headache.**

Treatment

Migraine treatment is categorized as acute, prophylactic, and rescue. First-line treatment for acute mild-to-moderate migraine is aspirin or NSAIDs. A triptan or dihydroergotamine may be used for severe acute migraine or for poor response to first-line treatment. Migraine that is present on awakening, is associated with vomiting, or is found to escalate rapidly may be best treated by nasal triptans or subcutaneous sumatriptan. Metoclopramide and prochlorperazine are also effective for migraine-associated nausea and enhance the efficacy of the abortive medication.

Choose migraine prophylaxis when:

- migraines do not respond to therapy
- headache occurs ≥10 days per month
- disabling headache occurs ≥4 days per month
- use of acute migraine medications is >8 days per month

Evidence-based migraine prophylaxis (in nonpregnant patients) includes amitriptyline, metoprolol, propranolol, timolol, topiramate, valproic acid, and venlafaxine. Onabotulinum toxin A is indicated in chronic migraine.

DON'T BE TRICKED

- **Do not choose oral medications for patients with severe nausea and vomiting.**
- **Triptans are contraindicated in the presence of CAD and cerebrovascular disease, brainstem aura, and hemiplegic migraine.**
- **Do not use acute therapies more than 2 to 3 days per week to avoid medication overuse headaches.**
- **Estrogen-containing contraceptives must be avoided in women experiencing aura with migraine because of the increased risk of stroke.**

TEST YOURSELF

A 39-year-old woman has chronic headaches that occur daily and do not respond to analgesics. Medications are zolmitriptan, naproxen, acetaminophen with codeine, and amitriptyline.

ANSWER: For diagnosis, choose chronic daily headache from medication overuse. For management, select taper of all acute headache medications.

Trigeminal Autonomic Cephalgias

These primary headache disorders are characterized by severe unilateral pain in the first division of the trigeminal nerve (periorbital, frontal, temporal) accompanied by ipsilateral autonomic symptoms. These headaches are differentiated from each other by the duration of pain and frequency of attacks.

STUDY TABLE: Trigeminal Autonomic Cephalgias

Diagnosis	Characteristics
Cluster headache	Pain usually periorbital, duration 15-180 minutes, several times per day. Repeating over weeks then disappearing for months or years. Unilateral tearing and nasal congestion or rhinorrhea, eyelid edema, miosis and/or ptosis. Treat acute headache with a triptan (or oxygen) and verapamil for long-term prevention.
Chronic paroxysmal hemicranias	Occurs at least five times daily lasting 2-30 minutes. Responds completely to indomethacin.
SUNCT	Dozens to hundreds of times per day, with durations of 1 to 600 seconds. Typically resistant to treatment.
Hemicrania continua	Persistent strictly unilateral headache that responds to indomethacin.

SUNCT = Short-lasting Unilateral Neuralgiform headaches with Conjunctival injection and Tearing.

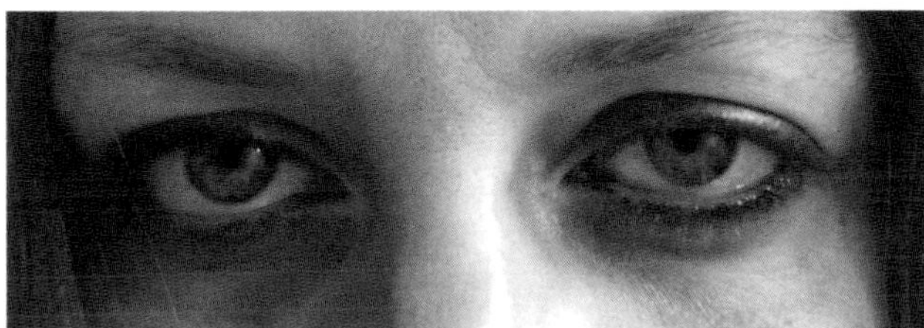

Cluster Headache: Ptosis, miosis, and increased tears in the left eye in a patient with cluster headache. Reprinted from Hale N, Paauw DS. Diagnosis and treatment of headache in the ambulatory care setting: a review of classic presentations and new considerations in diagnosis and management. Med Clin North Am. 2014 May;98(3):505-27. [PMID: 24758958], with permission from Elsevier.

Selected Secondary Headache Disorders

Diagnosis

Secondary headache disorders typically display "red flags":

- first or worst headache
- abrupt onset or thunderclap attack
- progression or fundamental change in headache pattern
- abnormal physical examination findings
- neurologic symptoms lasting >1 hour
- new headache in persons >50 years old
- new headache in patients with cancer, immunosuppression, or pregnancy
- association with alteration in or loss of consciousness
- headache triggered by exertion, sexual activity, or Valsalva maneuver

Testing

Order as appropriate:

- MRI over CT in nonemergency situations
- CT for suspected acute ICH

- ESR or CRP for suspected giant cell arteritis
- LP for suspected infectious or neoplastic meningitis or disorders of intracranial pressure

DON'T BE TRICKED

- EEG has no role in the assessment of headache disorders.

Thunderclap Headaches

An important category of secondary headaches is "thunderclap" headaches defined as reaching maximum intensity within 1 minute.

STUDY TABLE: Important Thunderclap Headaches

Headache Type	Clues	Treatment
Subarachnoid hemorrhage (SAH)	Sudden onset of "worst headache of my life" Many patients have warning "sentinel" headaches before SAH	Neurosurgery in selected cases (85% of nontraumatic cases caused by ruptured aneurysm)
Carotid or vertebral dissection	Neck pain and ipsilateral headache; neurologic findings in territory of involved vessel	Aspirin, heparin, or oral anticoagulation
Thrombosis of cerebral vein or dural sinus	Exertional headache, papilledema, neurologic findings Consider in hypercoagulable states, pregnancy, use of oral contraceptives	LMWH followed by warfarin
Reversible cerebral vasoconstriction syndrome	Recurrent thunderclap headache syndrome, more frequent in women. Associated with pregnancy, neurosurgical procedures, exposure to adrenergic or serotonergic drugs. Imaging shows strokes, hemorrhages, or cerebral edema	Normalization of BP and elimination of any triggering drug or substance; glucocorticoids may worsen outcomes

Idiopathic Intracranial Hypertension

Idiopathic intracranial hypertension (pseudotumor cerebri) is characterized by increased intracranial pressure without identifiable structural pathology. Patients are typically female, obese, and of child-bearing age. Papilledema is nearly always present.

Diagnosis is confirmed by a CSF pressure >250 mm H_2O with normal fluid composition. MRI may be normal or show small ventricles, widened optic nerve sheaths, or a partially empty sella.

First-line treatment is acetazolamide.

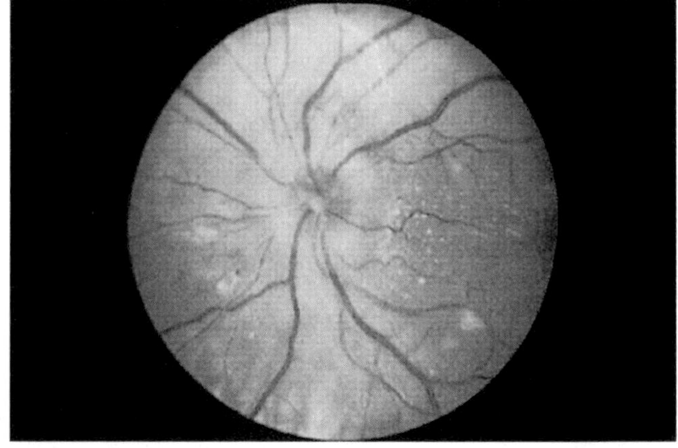

Papilledema: Fully developed papilledema is often present in patients with idiopathic intracranial hypertension. On funduscopic examination, loss of disc margins, cotton wool spots, and flame-shaped hemorrhages may be seen. Funduscopic findings are usually bilateral.

Traumatic Brain Injury

Diagnosis

Mild TBI presents as loss of consciousness or alteration in awareness ("dazed" after a head injury), amnesia near the time of the event, or focal neurologic deficit. Postconcussion syndrome describes the persistence of symptoms of mild TBI beyond a typical recovery period of several weeks.

Head injury may result in epidural or subdural hematomas presenting with headache and mental status abnormalities. Rapid neurologic decline with ipsilateral pupillary dilatation and brain herniation can occur. Some patients with epidural hematoma exhibit loss of consciousness followed by a brief "lucid interval" before subsequent precipitous decline. The tempo of clinical deterioration of subdural hematoma is slower, over days to weeks. It is often impossible to clinically distinguish between epidural and subdural hematoma.

DON'T BE TRICKED

- **Subdural hematomas can occur in the absence of significant trauma, particularly among older persons and those taking anticoagulant drugs.**

Testing

Neuroimaging is recommended for patients with worsening headache, repeated vomiting, drowsiness, persistent confusion, focal neurologic findings, seizure, suspected substance intoxication, and "dangerous" causes of injury (fall from a height >3 feet or 5 steps, ejection from a vehicle, being struck by a vehicle as a pedestrian).

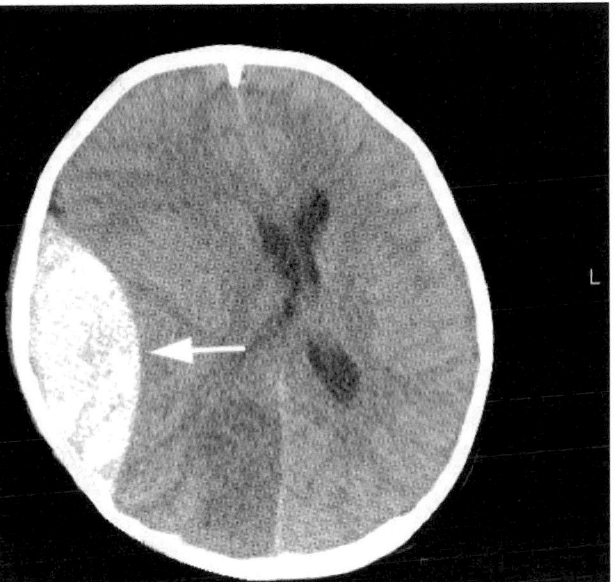

Epidural Hematoma: CT scan of an epidural hematoma shows biconvex lens appearance between the skull and outer margin of the dura (*arrow*).

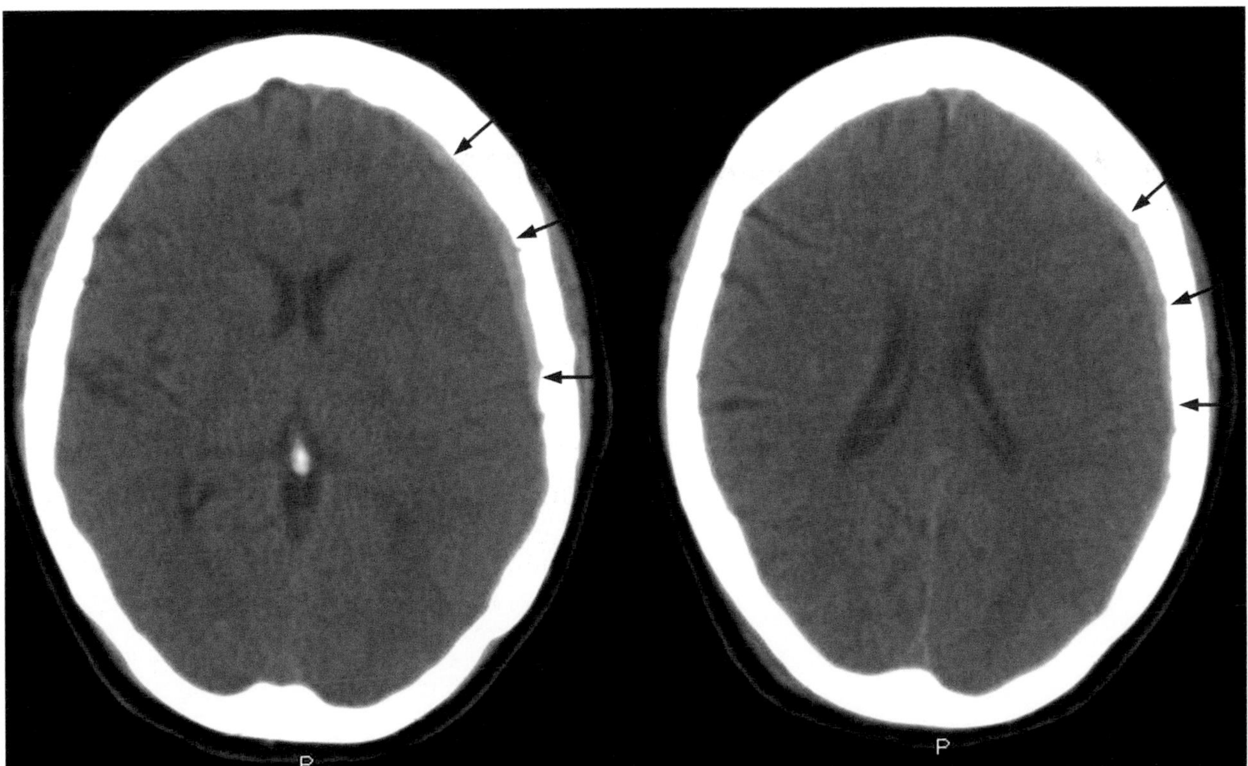

Subdural Hematoma: CT scan of a subdural hematoma shows the crescent shape of blood separating the dura from the arachnoid membrane (*arrows*).

Treatment

Athletes suspected of having a mild TBI should be immediately removed from play and should undergo sideline assessment. Participation in sports must be prohibited until the patient returns to cognitive baseline and is asymptomatic without taking any medication.

Management of postconcussion syndrome is supportive and rehabilitative. NSAIDs and triptans may be useful in treating posttraumatic headache. Tricyclic antidepressants, SSRIs, and SNRIs can also manage posttraumatic headache, as well as mood and anxiety disorders.

The treatment for epidural hematoma is emergent evacuation of blood to prevent death. The treatment of subdural hematoma depends on clinical circumstances; observation is appropriate in stable, asymptomatic patients.

Epilepsy

Diagnosis

Epilepsy is characterized by two or more unprovoked seizures occurring more than 24 hours apart or one unprovoked seizure with a significant ongoing risk of further unprovoked seizures. Focal seizures result from an electrical discharge that originates in a focal region of the brain. Primary generalized seizures are caused by an electrical discharge that involves all areas of the brain simultaneously. The electrical discharge in secondarily generalized seizures is focal in onset but rapidly spreads to involve the entire cerebral cortex. Clinical clues to identifying a focal seizure that has progressed to a generalized seizure include:

- unilateral shaking
- head turning (versive) to one side
- aura
- postictal (temporary) weakness

Common epilepsy comorbidities include mood disorders, sleep disorders, metabolic bone disease, and hyperlipidemia.

STUDY TABLE: Seizure Classifications

Seizure Type	Characteristics
Focal seizure without alteration of awareness (formerly simple partial seizures)	Normal consciousness and awareness Single neurologic modality (sensory, motor, olfactory, visual, gustatory) involving a single region of the body, such as the hand or arm
Focal seizure with alteration of awareness (formerly complex partial seizure)	Conscious but unresponsive or staring Automatism (lip smacking, swallowing, or manipulating objects) Postictal confusion
Primary generalized seizure	Loss of consciousness or awareness at onset No prodromal or localizing symptoms Whole-body stiffening (tonic) and/or jerking (clonic) seizures

STUDY TABLE: Common Epilepsy Syndromes

Temporal lobe epilepsy	Focal seizures with alteration of awareness preceded by an aura before losing consciousness. Often unaware that they have become impaired and may have no recollection of the seizure. Medial temporal sclerosis is a characteristic finding on MRI.
Frontal lobe epilepsy	Nocturnal complex seizures that awaken patients from sleep. Often associated with underlying structural pathology (e.g., tumor, vascular malformations).
Idiopathic (genetic) generalized epilepsy	Any combination of tonic-clonic seizures, absence seizures, and myoclonic seizures. MRI typically normal. EEG may show generalized spike-wave abnormality.
Myoclonic seizure	A generalized seizure associated with brief, lightning-like jerks of the arms, not associated with loss of consciousness (misdiagnosed as "jitteriness").
Convulsive status epilepticus	Characterized by continuous seizure for ≥5 minutes. Most common cause is low AED level. Complications include aspiration pneumonia, fever, hemodynamic instability, acidosis, PE, and rhabdomyolysis; associated with a mortality rate of approximately 20%.

Several medical conditions can provoke seizures, including metabolic disturbances, drug intoxication or withdrawal, or infection. Single seizures that are provoked should be addressed by correcting the underlying condition or removing the offending agent; single seizures usually do not require treatment with an antiepileptic drug.

DON'T BE TRICKED

- **Consider drugs (alcohol and cocaine) as cause of first-time seizure.**
- **Diagnostic evaluation may not be needed for a provoked seizure if the patient has normal findings on neurologic examination.**

Psychogenic nonepileptic spells (PNES) are a type of conversion disorder. Some of the characteristic features include:

- forced eye closure
- long duration
- hypermotor activity that starts and stops
- pelvic thrusting

Testing

Initial evaluation for a first unprovoked seizure:

- EEG (although a normal EEG does not rule out a seizure)
- CBC, electrolyte and glucose levels, and toxicology screen
- brain MRI (or head CT in an emergency)
- CSF examination if the patient has fever, prolonged altered mental status after the seizure, is immunosuppressed, or has a severe headache

Inpatient video EEG monitoring is required to make the diagnosis of PNES because of the difficulty in distinguishing between PNES and epileptic seizures. PNES is strongly associated with PTSD in military veterans.

If the patient is not returning toward baseline mental status by 15 minutes after a seizure, obtain continuous EEG monitoring to rule out nonconvulsive status epilepticus.

DON'T BE TRICKED

- **Syncope may be associated with brief loss of consciousness and occasional tonic-clonic jerking, but recovery is quick and complete, unlike a seizure.**
- **Do not choose absence seizure in an adult.**

Treatment

For most adults who have had a first seizure, the risk for a second event is about 50%, and antiepileptic drug (AED) therapy reduces the risk of a second seizure by only 50%. Start anticonvulsant therapy after ≥2 unprovoked seizures. Start AEDs after a single high-risk unproved seizure characterized by focal findings on neuroimaging, focal findings on EEG, or significant risk factors for epilepsy such as severe head trauma or after brain tumor resection.

Choose single-agent therapy and increase the dosage until seizures are controlled or the patient develops adverse medication effects. If unsuccessful, discontinue the first drug, and initiate a second drug as a single agent. Although serum drug level monitoring may be helpful, targeting a clinical response is more important than achieving a specific serum level. Adding new medications that alter the metabolism of anticonvulsants may result in a loss of seizure control.

Guide to initiating AED:

- lamotrigine, levetiracetam, topiramate, valproic acid, and zonisamide can be used to treat both generalized and focal epilepsy syndromes
- valproic acid may be superior to other AEDs for treating generalized epilepsy

- carbamazepine is a cost-effective option for focal seizures
- levetiracetam has few drug-drug interactions, is typically well-tolerated, and can be used during pregnancy

AED important side effects:

- carbamazepine: interactions with other hepatically metabolized drugs and increased risk for osteoporosis and hypercholesterolemia
- valproic acid: weight gain, hypercholesterolemia, PCOS, teratogenicity, hepatotoxicity
- topiramate and zonisamide: increased risk of kidney stones
- carbamazepine and oxcarbazepine: hyponatremia, pancytopenia
- all AEDs: drug hypersensitivity syndrome, SJS, and suicidal ideation

Patients not responding to either their first or their second AED (in sequence or combination) have refractory epilepsy and are candidates for epilepsy surgery. The most common surgical procedure is resection of mesial temporal lobe sclerotic lesions associated with focal seizures.

AEDs may be effectively withdrawn in many patients who have been seizure-free for 2 to 5 years.

Most women require continued drug therapy during pregnancy. Lamotrigine (requires upward dose adjustment during pregnancy for patients already taking drug) and levetiracetam are good options. Valproic acid and topiramate should be discontinued (pregnancy risk category D drugs).

Convulsive status epilepticus: Thiamine and glucose are administered if alcohol abuse is suspected or the cause of the status epilepticus is unknown. Emergent head imaging should be obtained in the absence of a known underlying cause but should not delay treatment.

The most common cause of convulsive status epilepticus is a low AED blood level. First-line treatment is IV lorazepam, IV diazepam, or IM midazolam. Patients not taking AEDs should then be treated with phenytoin or fosphenytoin, administered after 5 minutes of continuous seizing. All patients with convulsive status epilepticus who stop seizing but do not return to baseline within 30 minutes should be monitored with continuous EEG monitoring for nonconvulsive seizures.

For patients with **PNES**, referral to appropriate psychological resources provides the best chance of a good outcome.

DON'T BE TRICKED

- Primary prophylaxis with AEDs is not indicated for a new stroke or tumor.
- Patients with juvenile myoclonic epilepsy require lifelong medication.
- Carbamazepine, oxcarbazepine, phenytoin, and topiramate clobazam, inactivate many forms of hormonal contraception.

TEST YOURSELF

A 33-year-old woman has "spells" during which she is conscious but unresponsive and unaware of her environment. She has repetitive hand movements that last approximately 1 minute followed by several minutes of mild confusion.

ANSWER: For diagnosis, choose temporal lobe seizure. For management, select carbamazepine.

Ischemic Stroke and Transient Ischemic Attack

Prevention

Risk factor modification is mandatory for all patients (diabetes, hypertension, hyperlipidemia, tobacco use).

Revascularization with either stenting or endarterectomy is for patients with >80% or rapidly progressive stenosis and low cardiovascular risk, if the operative complication rate is <3%.

Begin warfarin (or a NOAC) in most patients with nonvalvular AF. Start aspirin therapy in patients with nonvalvular AF who are at low risk of stroke.

Surgical clipping or endovascular coiling of aneurysms are indicated for patients with aneurysms ≥7 mm in the posterior circulation or ≥12 mm in the anterior circulation.

DON'T BE TRICKED

- **Warfarin is the only approved drug for AF associated with valvular heart disease.**

Diagnosis

Stroke is a sudden focal neurologic deficit caused by ischemia (85%) or hemorrhage (15%). Ischemic stroke may be further characterized by the causative mechanism (large-artery atherosclerosis, cardioembolic, small-vessel disease, cryptogenic). Hemorrhagic stroke is classified as either subarachnoid or intracerebral (intraparenchymal).

TIA is a transient focal neurologic deficit resulting from ischemia rather than infarction. TIA is defined by the absence of infarction on neuroimaging, independent of symptom duration, which typically lasts 5 to 60 minutes.

All patients with stroke or TIA require:

- emergent head CT without contrast (to rule out intracranial hemorrhage)
- ECG and telemetry or event monitoring (to rule out AF)
- vascular studies (cerebrovascular ultrasonography or cerebrovascular MRA, CTA)
- echocardiography (to rule out LV or valvular thrombus)

Patients with TIA have an elevated risk of subsequent stroke, particularly in the next 48 hours. Decision to admit patients to the hospital is based upon risk stratification. The most widely used risk stratification is the $ABCD^2$ score.

STUDY TABLE: $ABCD^2$ Scoring System

Patient Characteristics	Score
Age ≥60 y	1
Blood pressure ≥140/90 mm Hg	1
Clinical Symptoms	
• focal weakness with the TIA	2
• speech impairment without weakness	1
Duration of TIA	
• ≥60 min	2
• 10-59 min	1
Diabetes mellitus present	1

Hospital admission for TIA is recommended for all patients with an $ABCD^2$ score of ≥3.

DON'T BE TRICKED

- **Routine evaluation for thrombophilia is not indicated for patients with TIA or stroke.**
- **Patients with cryptogenic stroke should undergo prolonged cardiac rhythm monitoring to rule out AF.**
- **Consider vertebral-basilar stroke in older adults with persistent, acute-onset vertigo.**

Treatment

Select intubation and mechanical ventilation for patients with a decreased level of consciousness.

Administer rtPA to all patients with ischemic stroke within 3 hours of stroke onset (if unknown onset, then within 3 hours of the last time the patient was seen to be well). rtPA may rarely be administered up to 4.5 hours after onset in selected patients who do not possess any of the following exclusionary criteria:

- age >80 years
- severe stroke
- diabetes mellitus with a previous infarct
- anticoagulant use

Additional exclusionary criteria for thrombolysis in general include any increased risk of bleeding, diagnosis of ICH, or SBP >185 mm Hg and DBP >110 mm Hg.

In patients with suspicion of a thrombolysis-induced intracranial hemorrhage manifesting as neurologic deterioration, stop ongoing infusion of rtPA and evaluate with another CT.

Additional therapy in patients with stroke:

- treat temperature >38.0 °C (100.4 °F) with acetaminophen
- administer normal saline to maintain euvolemia
- give aspirin, 325 mg, unless thrombolysis is planned
- start DVT prophylaxis within 48 hours

Do not begin antihypertensive treatment within the first 48 hours unless:

- SBP is >220 mm Hg, DBP is >120 mm Hg, or MAP is >140 mm Hg
- thrombolytic therapy is planned, and SBP >185 mm Hg or DBP >110 mm Hg
- ACS, aortic dissection, or end-organ damage is present

If the patient is eligible for thrombolysis, BP must be lowered to <180 mm Hg systolic and <105 mm Hg diastolic and maintained below these levels for at least 24 hours after therapy. Preferred antihypertensive agents include IV labetalol and IV nicardipine.

A swallowing assessment is recommended for patients with strokes before they start to eat or drink. Early stroke rehabilitation improves clinical outcomes.

STUDY TABLE: Secondary Prevention of Stroke

Intervention	Indication
Antiplatelet therapy	In the acute setting, begin aspirin immediately or within 24 hours after giving thrombolytic agents. In the chronic setting, aspirin plus dipyridamole is superior to aspirin alone. Clopidogrel is equivalent to aspirin and dipyridamole.
Anticoagulation therapy	After 48 hours, treat high-risk cardioembolic causes of stroke and TIA with warfarin (or a NOAC), including in patients with AF, left atrial appendage thrombus, LV thrombus, and dilated cardiomyopathy with reduced EF.
Revascularization	Endarterectomy or stenting is recommended within 2 weeks after a nondisabling stroke or TIA if ipsilateral carotid stenosis is >70% provided the patient is likely to live 5 years.
Statins	Begin high-intensity statin therapy for all patients regardless of cholesterol level.
Hypertension	Maintain BP <130/80 mm Hg after recovery from the acute event.
Depression	Prevalent in the acute and chronic setting and identification and treatment improve recovery.
Device closure of PFO plus aspirin	To prevent second stroke in patients with thoroughly investigated cryptogenic stroke

DON'T BE TRICKED

- If the patient is unable to report the time of onset, and no other person witnessed the onset, rtPA treatment is contraindicated.
- Do not select heparin for most patients with ischemic stroke.
- Do not select anticonvulsant medications after stroke unless the patient has had a seizure.
- Do not select carotid endarterectomy for 100% carotid artery stenosis

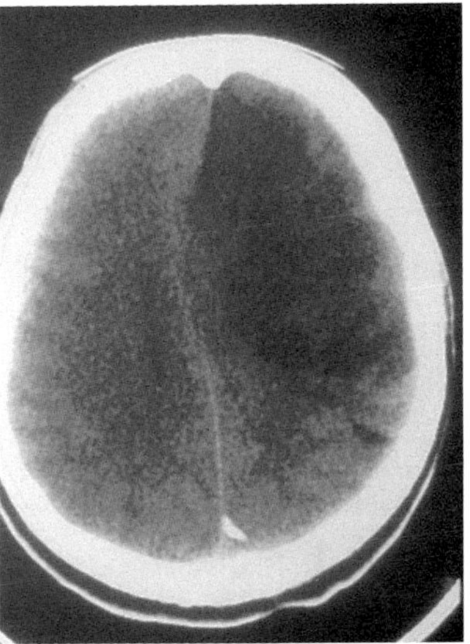

Ischemic Stroke: CT scan of the brain without contrast shows a large wedge-shaped hypodensity with mass effect 24 hours after symptom onset.

Subarachnoid Hemorrhage

Prevention

Patients with small (<7 mm posterior or <12 mm anterior circulation) unruptured aneurysms can be followed with MRI; those with larger aneurysms are candidates for surgery. The risk of rupture increases with size and location of the aneurysm in the posterior circulation.

Diagnosis

The most common symptom associated with SAH is altered consciousness. Spontaneous SAH most commonly results from the rupture of saccular ("berry") aneurysms of the circle of Willis. SAH less commonly results from rupture of an AVM, arterial dissection, coagulopathy, or cocaine abuse. Most patients present to the emergency department with sudden onset of the "worst headache of my life" or "thunderclap headache" (reaches maximal intensity in 60 minutes). However, up to 40% of patients with SAH experience a "sentinel hemorrhage" characterized as severe headache during the previous 2 to 3 weeks. Focal neurologic deficits occur from aneurysms that compress a cranial nerve (third nerve palsy and dilated pupil), bleed into brain parenchyma, or cause focal ischemia because of vasospasm.

Testing

Noncontrast CT establishes the diagnosis of SAH in >90% of patients. Cerebral angiography identifies the aneurysm and determines management. Other causes of abrupt severe headache include arterial dissection and venous sinus thrombosis, both of which may be detected with vascular imaging, pituitary apoplexy, hypertensive emergency, and ICH.

DON'T BE TRICKED

- If the CT scan is normal, always select CSF examination to look for erythrocytes or xanthochromia.

Treatment

The three main neurologic complications for a patient with a SAH are rebleeding, delayed brain ischemia from vasospasm, and hydrocephalus. To manage these complications, do the following:

- Treat ruptured aneurysms with surgical clipping or endovascular coiling within 48 to 72 hours.

- Maintain BP <140/80 mm Hg to prevent rebleeding.
- Select oral nimodipine for 21 days to prevent vasospasm and improve neurologic outcomes.

Any change in mental status should prompt emergency CT to evaluate for repeat bleeding and for signs of hydrocephalus, which is treated with ventricular drainage. Screening transcranial ultrasonography or CTA is used to detect cerebral vasospasm.

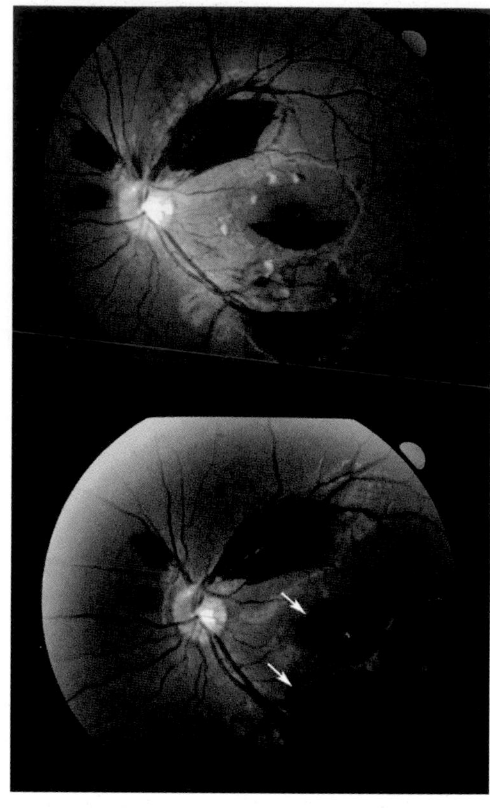

Subhyaloid Hemorrhage: Bleeding under the vitreous membrane (subhyaloid hemorrhage) is a finding associated with SAH.

TEST YOURSELF

A 44-year-old woman comes to the emergency department reporting "the worst headache of my life." She has meningismus but no focal neurologic findings. CT scan is normal.

ANSWER: For diagnosis, choose SAH. For management, select CSF examination.

Intracerebral Hemorrhage

Diagnosis

The most common risk factor for ICH is hypertension. Other risk factors include amyloid angiopathy (primarily in older adult patients with lobar hemorrhage), coagulopathy, vascular malformations, and the use of cocaine or alcohol.

ICH, with symptoms similar to those of ischemic stroke, cannot be reliably distinguished by clinical criteria alone. CT without contrast establishes the diagnosis. Cerebral angiography is indicated for patients <45 years of age with ICH related to cocaine use (which is associated with a high incidence of vascular anomalies).

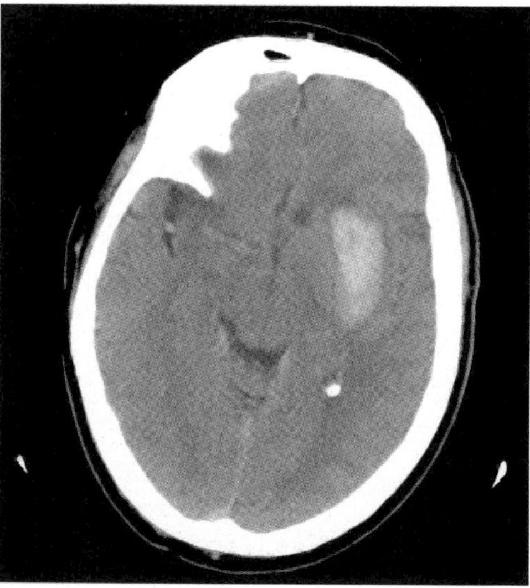

Intracerebral Hemorrhage: CT scan of the brain shows a hemorrhage in the left basal ganglia.

Treatment

Identify and reverse anticoagulation. Mannitol, barbiturate coma, and hyperventilation may be used to reduce intracranial pressure. IV nicardipine, or labetalol, is indicated to maintain SBP between 140 and 160 mm Hg (MAP between 70 and 130 mm Hg). Intraventricular hemorrhage requires prompt ventricular drainage to reduce intracranial pressure. Cerebellar hemorrhages require surgical posterior fossa decompression.

For warfarin-associated ICH, IV vitamin K and prothrombin complex concentrates are recommended.

DON'T BE TRICKED

- Do not select nitroglycerin or nitroprusside to lower BP because they can increase intracerebral pressure.
- Platelet transfusions or glucocorticoids are not recommended for intracranial hemorrhage.

Dementia

Diagnosis

Dementia is an acquired chronic impairment of memory and other aspects of intellect that impedes daily functioning.

Mild cognitive impairment (MCI) describes cognitive decline greater than expected for age but without interference with daily functioning and is a risk factor for dementia.

DON'T BE TRICKED

- **No test can predict the likelihood that an individual patient with MCI will develop dementia.**
- **No treatments delay the onset of Alzheimer disease in patients with MCI.**

Alzheimer disease is the most prevalent neurodegenerative dementia, accounting for 60% to 80% of cases.

Characteristic findings of Alzheimer disease are memory loss; getting lost; difficulty finding words; and difficulty with dressing, grooming, and doing housework.

A score <24 on the Mini-Mental State Examination is compatible with dementia. Other diagnostic tools include the Montreal Cognitive Assessment and "Mini-Cog" test.

Testing

Routinely obtain brain imaging with CT or MRI to detect nondegenerative causes that would alter management, such as cerebrovascular disease, neoplasm, subdural hematoma, or hydrocephalus. **Screen all patients for depression.** Consider LP and CSF examination in the following situations:

- rapidly progressive dementia
- age of onset <60 years
- history of malignancy or paraneoplastic disorders
- suspicion for acute or subacute infection; immunosuppressed or immunodeficiency state
- positive syphilis or Lyme serology
- systemic autoimmune disease; suspected CNS autoimmune or inflammatory disorder

Creutzfeldt-Jacob disease is the most common cause of rapidly progressive dementia. Early-onset or rapidly progressive dementia requires early brain MRI, CSF analysis, and EEG.

STUDY TABLE: Differential Diagnosis of Dementia

When you see this...	Choose this...
Acute onset, fluctuating course, inattention, disorganized thinking, and altered consciousness	Delirium
Evidence of objective memory impairment in the absence of other cognitive deficits and intact activities of daily living	MCI
Gradual memory loss, aphasia, apraxia, agnosia, inattention, and decrease in executive function	Alzheimer disease
Imaging or history positive for stroke responsible for impairment of at least one cognitive domain Common findings include focal neurologic findings, depression, pseudobulbar palsy, gait abnormalities, and urinary difficulties	Vascular neurocognitive disorder
Mild parkinsonism characterized by postural instability and gait difficulty, fluctuating cognition, delusions, and visual hallucinations	Dementia with Lewy bodies

(Continued on the next page)

STUDY TABLE: Differential Diagnosis of Dementia *(Continued)*	
When you see this...	**Choose this...**
Early and prominent personality changes, behavioral disturbances including disinhibition and impulsivity, diminished frontal and/or temporal lobes on MRI, onset before age 60 years	Frontotemporal dementia, behavioral variant
Dementia, shuffling gait, urinary incontinence, and ventriculomegaly in the absence of past history of meningitis, SAH, or trauma	Normal-pressure hydrocephalus
Choreoathetosis and dementia, autosomal dominant pattern of inheritance	Huntington disease
Prominent myoclonus, characteristic EEG pattern of triphasic sharp waves, CSF protein 14-3-3, rapidly progressive onset at early age	Creutzfeldt-Jakob disease
Early postural instability and falls, apathy, parkinsonism poorly responsive to levodopa, and vertical gaze palsy	Progressive supranuclear palsy
History of head injury followed by delayed development (10 years) of impaired concentration, short-term memory, executive dysfunction, and judgment; aggression, depression, irritability, violent behaviors, and suicidality; and parkinsonism, unsteady gait, shuffling gait, and slurred speech	Chronic traumatic encephalopathy

DON'T BE TRICKED

- **Do not order apolipoprotein E genotyping in patients with suspected Alzheimer disease.**
- **Relative sparing of memory and visuospatial function (not getting lost) are characteristic of early frontal temporal dementia differentiating it from Alzheimer disease.**
- **Vascular neurocognitive disorder can mimic normal-pressure hydrocephalus but is suggested by the presence of diabetes mellitus, dyslipidemia, hypertension, ischemic infarctions, and ischemic heart disease.**

Treatment

Select acetylcholinesterase inhibitors (donepezil, rivastigmine, and galantamine) to slow intellectual decline in patients with mild to moderate Alzheimer disease. Acetylcholinesterase inhibitors can have prominent cholinergic side effects, including bradycardia, diarrhea, heart block, nausea and vomiting, and syncope. Memantine delays cognitive decline in patients with moderate to advanced Alzheimer disease (Mini-Mental State Examination score of 3-14).

Also choose:

- acetylcholinesterase inhibitors for dementia with Lewy bodies
- risk factor modification and acetylcholinesterase inhibitors for vascular cognitive impairment
- large-volume LP with symptom assessment before and after to evaluate response to shunting for normal-pressure hydrocephalus

Nonpharmacologic interventions are first-line treatment for behavioral symptoms. Atypical antipsychotics can treat agitation, aggression, delusions, and hallucinations but have a black box warning for increased mortality; they are used when patient safety is jeopardized.

Treat depression with SSRIs.

DON'T BE TRICKED

- **Combination therapy with an acetylcholinesterase inhibitor and memantine is no more effective than a cholinesterase inhibitor alone.**
- **No drug is beneficial for frontotemporal dementia.**
- **Benzodiazepines are not recommended for the treatment of behavioral symptoms in patients with dementia.**
- **Do not select tricyclic antidepressants in patients with dementia because they can exacerbate confusion.**

Delirium

Diagnosis

Diagnosis of delirium is based on the Confusion Assessment Method diagnostic algorithm, which provides greater accuracy than laboratory tests or imaging studies. Diagnose delirium if the first two points and either point 3 or point 4 are present:

1. Acute onset and fluctuating course
2. Inattention
3. Disorganized thinking
4. Altered level of consciousness

Look for triggers of delirium, particularly alcohol, medications known to cause delirium, and polypharmacy. Pay particular attention to alcohol, anticholinergics, anticonvulsants, antidepressants, antihistamines, antipsychotics, barbiturates, opioid analgesics, sedative-hypnotics, fluoroquinolones, and antiparkinsonian agents. Also consider fluid and electrolyte abnormalities, uncontrolled pain, hypoxemia, anemia, infections, immobility, visual and hearing impairment, sleep cycle disruption, and catheters and other "tethers" (ECG leads, IV lines, and restraints).

DON'T BE TRICKED

- **Brain imaging is usually not helpful in diagnosing delirium unless a history of falls or evidence of focal neurologic impairment is present.**

Treatment

Treat or eliminate precipitating factors. Achieve behavior control with environmental or social measures rather than pharmacologic or physical restraints. In severe cases and especially when safety is a concern, newer generation antipsychotic agents may help control behavior.

All atypical antipsychotics (aripiprazole, clozapine, olanzapine, quetiapine, risperidone, and ziprasidone) and older antipsychotics (haloperidol) are associated with an increased risk of mortality in patients with dementia and psychosis or behavioral disturbances.

DON'T BE TRICKED

- **Always select behavioral interventions first and order a "sitter" instead of using restraints or drugs.**
- **Benzodiazepines can worsen delirium and are not recommended, except in the management of alcohol withdrawal.**

Parkinson Disease

Diagnosis

Parkinsonism refers to any cause of parkinsonian symptoms and signs. Parkinson disease, caused by the degeneration of dopaminergic neurons in the substantia nigra of the midbrain, is characterized by at least two of the following conditions:

- bradykinesia (slowed movement and decreased amplitude of repetitive movement)
- rigidity (cogwheel type)
- resting tremor (or with movement)
- postural reflex abnormality (falling)

Patients with parkinsonism are at increased fall risk and may present for evaluation of frequent falls.

Neurologic signs and symptoms are asymmetric at onset. Diminished sense of smell, constipation, and acting out dreams may precede the onset of motor symptoms by years. Early dementia within the first year of the appearance of parkinsonism is a hallmark of dementia with Lewy bodies.

Seborrheic dermatitis is a well-recognized Parkinson disease cutaneous association.

Parkinson disease is a clinical diagnosis. Brain imaging may be obtained to exclude other disease processes such as hydrocephalus, vascular disease, and other degenerative diseases that may mimic Parkinson disease.

DON'T BE TRICKED

- **Early symmetric symptoms or signs, early falls, rapid progression, poor or waning response to levodopa, early autonomic failure or dementia, and ataxia suggest a diagnosis other than Parkinson disease.**

STUDY TABLE: Differential Diagnosis of Parkinson Disease

Disease	Considerations
Multiple system atrophy	Severe orthostatic hypotension and ataxia MRI showing "necrosis" of the putamen and cerebellar atrophy
Progressive supranuclear palsy	Unexplained falls (typically backward), inability to move eyes vertically, and parkinsonian features
Dementia with Lewy bodies	Early dementia, parkinsonism, and hallucinations
Medication-induced parkinsonism	Antiemetics (prochlorperazine, metoclopramide), antipsychotics (haloperidol), reserpine, lithium, and methyldopa

DON'T BE TRICKED

- **Drug-induced parkinsonism is distinguished from Parkinson disease by the symmetry of symptoms and the absence of typical nonmotor features.**

Treatment

Levodopa is the most effective medication used in the treatment of Parkinson disease but is associated with motor fluctuations, including dyskinesias, and a "wearing-off" effect (enhanced parkinsonian symptoms). Initiating therapy with a dopamine agonist (pramipexole, ropinirole) in patients younger than 65 years avoids the early appearance of these side effects. Levodopa is the drug of choice in older patients. Levodopa is administered in combination with carbidopa, which prevents the peripheral conversion of levodopa to dopamine.

Side effects of dopamine agonists include sedation and an increase in compulsive behaviors such as gambling, shopping, and hypersexuality.

Increasing the dose or frequency of levodopa or using a sustained release formulation is indicated to treat the symptoms of wearing off.

Deep brain stimulation is indicated for patients who have sustained motor benefit from levodopa but are limited by disabling medication-related adverse effects refractory to medical management.

DON'T BE TRICKED

- **Begin drug therapy for Parkinson disease when symptoms begin to interfere with function.**
- **Failure to respond to dopamine therapy is the most important red flag indicating atypical parkinsonism.**

TEST YOURSELF

A 68-year-old woman has a 2-year history of falls and imbalance. She has a staring facial expression and impaired upward gaze.

ANSWER: For diagnosis, choose supranuclear palsy.

Hyperkinetic Movement Disorders

Diagnosis

Hyperkinetic movement disorders include:

- tremors (rhythmic oscillation)
- dystonia (sustained contraction of opposing muscles, resulting in repetitive movements or abnormal posture)
- myoclonus (nonrhythmic jerking movements of the extremities)
- tics (stereotyped, brief, rapid movements)
- chorea (random, nonrepetitive, flowing dance-like movements)

STUDY TABLE: Hyperkinetic Movement Disorders

Condition	Key Manifestations	Treatment
Essential tremor	Typically slowly progressive or stable over time Bilateral postural or kinetic tremor; improves with alcohol Family history positive in 50%	Propranolol, primidone, or topiramate
Huntington disease	Most common neurodegenerative cause of generalized chorea Also progressive dementia and psychiatric manifestations Autosomal dominant	Symptomatic treatment with tetrabenazine and deutetrabenazine
Drug-induced dystonia	Tardive dyskinesia associated with choreiform and dystonic craniofacial movements Can be caused by neuroleptic, antiemetic, and serotoninergic medications	Stop the offending drug Valbenazine, clonazepam, tetrabenazine, anticholinergic agents, and clozapine
Cervical dystonia (torticollis)	Cervical muscle contractions resulting in abnormal posture of the head and neck	Botulinum toxin (first line)
Tourette syndrome	Childhood onset, multiple complex motor tics, and presence of vocal tics (e.g., echolalia)	Reassurance or cognitive behavioral therapy
Myoclonus	Rapid, shock-like, jerky movements of isolated body parts Underlying metabolic disorder, serotonin syndrome, postanoxic, Creutzfeldt-Jakob disease, corticobasal degeneration	Treat the underlying metabolic disorder

DON'T BE TRICKED

- **Rigidity and resting tremor are not features of essential tremor.**
- **Screen patients <40 years with "essential tremor" or dystonia for Wilson disease with serum ceruloplasmin and 24-hour urine copper measurements.**

Multiple Sclerosis

Diagnosis

MS is characterized by episodes of dysfunction resulting from demyelinating lesions (plaques) in different areas of the CNS (brain, brain stem including optic nerve, or spinal cord) at different times.

Clinical course follows one of three patterns:

- **Relapsing-remitting:** Clinical episodes of neurologic dysfunction, typically lasting weeks before improving, that may lead to the accumulation of disability.

- **Secondary progressive disease:** Disappearance of evidence of clinical relapses in the relapsing-remitting form and by progressive disability.
- **Primary progressive disease:** Progressive disability accumulation from the time of disease onset.

Those who do not meet the full diagnostic criteria for MS after a first event have a clinically isolated syndrome. The 10-year risk of MS associated with a clinically isolated syndrome and lesions on MRI is 90%.

STUDY TABLE: Common Symptoms/Findings Associated with MS

Finding or Anatomical Involvement	Description
Optic neuritis	Subacute visual deficit in one eye along with pain with eye movement
Afferent pupillary defect	Paradoxical dilation of the pupil when light is rapidly shifted from the unaffected to the affected eye
Papillitis	Inflammatory changes in the retina causing a flared appearance of the optic disc
Myelitis	Focal inflammation within the spinal cord manifesting as sensory, autonomic, or motor symptoms below the affected spinal level
Lhermitte sign	A shock-like sensation radiating down the spine or limbs induced by neck movements
Bladder	Urinary frequency, urgency, or retention
Cerebellum	Ataxia and vertigo
Brainstem (internuclear ophthalmoplegia)	Inability to adduct one eye and nystagmus in the abducting eye
Uhthoff phenomenon	Transient worsening of baseline neurologic symptoms with elevations of body temperature

Diagnosis requires evidence of CNS demyelination disseminated in both space and time as demonstrated through a combination of documented clinical relapses, signs on physical examination, and the distribution of lesions on an MRI.

CSF may contain oligoclonal IgG bands or an elevated IgG index. CSF analysis is not necessary but can be helpful when the diagnosis remains questionable.

DON'T BE TRICKED

- **MS generally is not associated with cortical syndromes, such as aphasia and neglect.**
- **Migraine, microvascular ischemic disease, and head trauma can also cause white matter lesions on MRI.**

Treatment

IV methylprednisolone followed by oral glucocorticoids speeds recovery from acute exacerbations, most effectively in acute optic neuritis. Treat fever and look for underlying infection before beginning glucocorticoids, because fever worsens symptoms of MS (pseudorelapse), and treatment of the underlying trigger will improve symptoms.

After the first attack of a clinically isolated syndrome (optic neuritis, spinal cord syndrome, or brain stem-cerebellar syndrome), prescribe interferon beta or glatiramer acetate if imaging suggests MS. Teriflunomide may also be effective.

Prescribe interferon beta or glatiramer acetate for confirmed relapsing-remitting MS (RRMS).

MS relapses that have no or minimal impact on function may simply be observed.

Vitamin D added to interferon beta reduces the accumulation of MRI lesions and is recommended for all patients with MS. All patients should receive annual influenza vaccination and maintain their regular immunization schedule.

STUDY TABLE: Symptomatic Management in Multiple Sclerosis		
Symptom	**Nonpharmacologic Management**	**Pharmacologic Management**
Spasticity	Physical therapy, stretching, massage therapy	Baclofen, benzodiazepines, cyclobenzaprine, tizanidine
Neuropathic pain	n/a	Carbamazepine, duloxetine, gabapentin, pregabalin, topiramate
Fatigue	Proper sleep hygiene, regular exercise	Amantadine, amphetamines, armodafinil, modafinil
Depression	Individual or group counseling	Antidepressants (SNRIs, SSRIs)
Cognitive dysfunction	Cognitive rehabilitation and accommodation strategies	No proven therapy
Mobility	Physical and occupational therapy; use of braces, canes, rolling walkers, or electrostimulatory walk-assist devices	Dalfampridine
Urinary retention	Manual pelvic pressure, intermittent catheterization	None

Encourage smoking cessation because of the threefold increase in the risk of secondary progression associated with cigarette smoking.

DON'T BE TRICKED

- **Interferon agents are contraindicated in patients with liver disease or depression.**
- **Pregnancy does not cause additional permanent disability in women with MS.**
- **Combining glatiramer acetate with interferon beta provides no added benefit to either drug alone.**

TEST YOURSELF

A 25-year-old woman has a 2-week episode of new-onset gait ataxia, nystagmus, and dysarthria. Two years ago, she had optic neuritis. An MRI of the brain now shows brain lesions consistent with MS.

ANSWER: For diagnosis, choose relapsing-remitting MS. For management, select IV methylprednisolone and interferon beta.

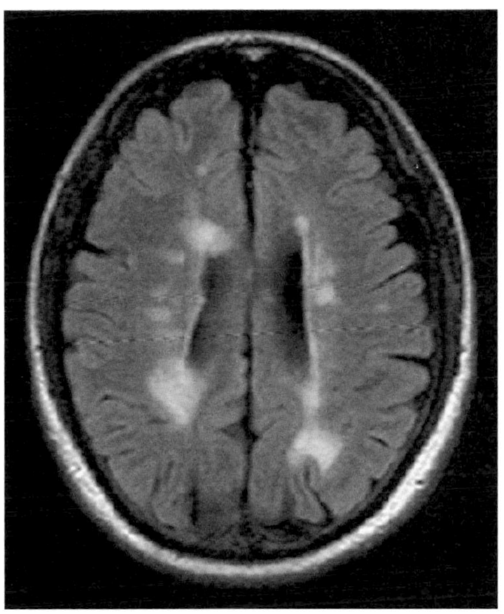

Multiple Sclerosis Lesions: Fluid-attenuated inversion recovery MRI shows MS lesions in the paraventricular white matter bilaterally.

Myelopathy

Diagnosis

Spinal cord dysfunction, or myelopathy, can occur because of a lesion arising within the spinal cord (intramedullary) or because of extrinsic compression of the spinal cord.

Injury to the corticospinal tracts manifests as weakness, hyperreflexia, muscle spasms, and extensor plantar responses.

Involvement of the distal cord and lower roots (cauda equina syndrome) manifests as lower extremity weakness with decreased muscle tone and areflexia.

Causes of noncompressive myelopathy include inflammatory or demyelinating lesions, spinal cord infarction, and copper or vitamin B_{12} deficiency.

STUDY TABLE: Selected Causes of Intramedullary Myelopathy	
Cause	**Features**
MS	See Multiple Sclerosis
Neuromyelitis optica (Devic disease)	Recurrent episodes of myelitis and optic neuritis without the brain lesions typical of MS; NMO-IgG autoantibody may be present
Idiopathic transverse myelitis	Subacute onset of weakness, sensory changes, and bowel/bladder dysfunction, typically after a viral infection Distinguished from MS by the presence of complete myelitis, no oligoclonal bands or elevated IgG index in the CSF, and no lesions on brain MRI
Vitamin B_{12} deficiency	Paresthesias, lower-extremity weakness, and gait instability Findings may include paraparesis, vibration and position sense loss, and sensory ataxia. Anemia may be absent
Copper deficiency	Mimics vitamin B_{12} deficiency May develop after bariatric surgery or from excessive zinc ingestion
Infarction of the spinal cord	Acute onset of flaccid paralysis or weakness and pinprick sensation loss below the level of the infarction Potential causes include emboli, hypotension during cardiovascular/aortic surgery, and AV malformations

Spinal cord compression most commonly presents with neck or back pain, followed by weakness, sensory changes, and bowel and bladder dysfunction associated with upper motoneuron signs (weakness, spasticity, hyperreflexia, extensor plantar responses) and occasionally lower motoneuron signs (atrophy, hyporeflexia).

Clues to the cause of compression myelopathy:

- fever – epidural abscess
- anticoagulation – epidural hematoma
- cancer – metastases
- trauma – vertebral fracture
- elderly with chronic back/leg pain – spinal stenosis

Select MRI of the spine to exclude spinal cord compression in all patients with clinical suspicion of spinal cord disorder. LP may be beneficial in patients with suspected inflammatory or demyelinating spinal cord lesions.

DON'T BE TRICKED

- **Check methylmalonic acid and homocysteine measurements for patients with borderline vitamin B_{12} values.**

Treatment

Treat spinal cord compression caused by metastatic disease emergently with high-dose glucocorticoids and subsequent surgical decompression followed by radiation for most tumor types.

Spinal cord infarction has no treatment.

For treatment of demyelinating diseases, see Multiple Sclerosis.

Treat vitamin B_{12} and copper deficiencies with supplementation.

Direct inflammatory and infectious myelopathy treatment at the underlying disorder.

Treat transverse myelitis with IV methylprednisolone.

DON'T BE TRICKED

- **Spinal cord compression caused by leukemia, lymphoma, myeloma, and germ cell tumors may be treated urgently with radiation therapy rather than surgery.**
- **Do not use glucocorticoids to treat spinal cord compression caused by infection or hematoma.**

Amyotrophic Lateral Sclerosis

Diagnosis and Testing

The defining characteristic is the combination of upper motoneuron signs (e.g., hyperreflexia, spasticity, and extensor plantar response) coexistent with lower motoneuron findings (e.g., atrophy and fasciculation). Sensory deficits are characteristically absent.

Muscle weakness in patients with ALS usually begins distally and asymmetrically, although 20% of patients have bulbar-onset ALS with difficulty speaking and swallowing. All patients with suspected ALS should undergo EMG to test for muscle degeneration and MRI of the appropriate anatomic areas to diagnose treatable neurologic disorders that may mimic ALS. Pulmonary function tests and overnight pulse oximetry studies can establish the presence of respiratory insufficiency. Patients with bulbar signs or symptoms require evaluation of swallowing function.

DON'T BE TRICKED

- **Findings not typical for ALS include predominant sensory symptoms or pain, early cognitive impairment, and ocular muscle weakness.**
- **Fasciculations in the absence of associated muscle atrophy or weakness are not caused by ALS.**
- **Weakness in the absence of fasciculations is not a result of ALS.**

Treatment

Riluzole may increase survival by about 3 months. Begin noninvasive ventilatory support for patients with respiratory insufficiency. Placement of a percutaneous endoscopic gastrostomy tube is indicated when weight loss or swallowing difficulty occurs.

Myasthenia Gravis

Diagnosis

MG is an autoimmune disease caused by antibodies directed against the acetylcholine receptor, which results in impaired neuromuscular transmission. Characteristic findings of MG include:

- ptosis or diplopia (first manifestation in most patients)
- muscle weakness, including dysphagia and dyspnea
- positive anti-acetylcholine receptor antibody titer (found in 90% of patients; negative titer does not rule out MG)
- normal deep tendon reflexes and sensation
- decremental response to repetitive stimulation on EMG

Myasthenic crisis, which may include rapidly progressive respiratory failure, can occur as part of the natural history of myasthenia or be triggered by infection, surgery, or medications. Look for aminoglycosides, quinolones, magnesium, β-blockers, or calcium channel blockers as precipitants of myasthenic crisis.

Include botulism and Lambert-Eaton myasthenic syndrome in the differential diagnosis. Botulism starts with cranial nerve involvement, including diplopia, dysphagia, and sluggish or nonreactive pupils, whereas the pupils are normal in MG.

Lambert-Eaton myasthenic syndrome involves progressive proximal weakness and diminished tendon reflexes that improve with repetitive movement of affected muscles. Diagnosis is confirmed by detection of serum anti-voltage-gated calcium channel antibodies and the EMG finding of facilitation of motor response to rapid repetitive stimulation. Most patients with this syndrome have an undetected malignancy, typically SCLC.

Testing

Single-fiber EMG can establish the diagnosis. Look for elevated serum TSH levels because of the association of MG with autoimmune thyroid disorders. Perform CT of the chest to detect thymoma.

Treatment

Pyridostigmine is the initial therapy. Thymectomy is indicated if a thymoma is found on imaging.

Myasthenic crisis and refractory disease should be treated with plasmapheresis or IV immune globulin.

DON'T BE TRICKED

- **Pyridostigmine monotherapy should be avoided in those with myasthenic crisis because the drug increases respiratory secretions.**

Peripheral Neuropathy

Diagnosis

Patients with neuropathy may present with pain, paresthesias, weakness, or autonomic dysfunction. Neuropathies can be classified by:

- distribution of sensorimotor deficits (symmetric vs asymmetric, distal vs proximal, focal vs generalized)
- pathology (demyelinating vs axonal)
- size of nerve fibers involved (large vs small fibers)
- family history
- autonomic involvement

Mononeuropathies, isolated disorders affecting a single peripheral nerve, are most frequently caused by nerve entrapment or compression (carpal tunnel syndrome).

Mononeuropathy multiplex involves multiple noncontiguous peripheral nerves, either simultaneously or sequentially. This is often the result of a systemic disease.

Polyneuropathy refers to a diffuse, generalized, and usually symmetric peripheral neuropathy. Polyneuropathy is often a manifestation of systemic disease (e.g., diabetes, vitamin B_{12} deficiency) or exposure to a toxin (e.g., alcohol) or medication (e.g., chemotherapy).

EMG and nerve conduction velocity can be helpful to characterize the type (axonal or demyelinating), severity, and distribution of the disease. Other routine tests include vitamin B_{12} level, SPEP, UPEP, ESR, and blood glucose level.

STUDY TABLE: Diagnosing and Managing Peripheral Neuropathy

If you see this...	Think this...	And choose this...
Isolated anterolateral thigh numbness without weakness	Meralgia paresthetica (a compressive neuropathy of the lateral femoral cutaneous nerve)	Locate and relieve pressure (binding clothes, excessive weight)
Sensory loss over palmar surface of first three digits and weakness with thumb abduction and opposition	Median neuropathy (carpal tunnel syndrome)	Wrist splints or glucocorticoid injections for mild disease; surgical release if severe
Numbness of the fourth and fifth fingers and weakness of interosseous muscles	Ulnar neuropathy	Elbow splinting or elbow pads; surgical release if severe
Pain, tingling, and numbness in great toe and along medial foot	Tarsal tunnel syndrome	Local glucocorticoid injection; decompression surgery if severe
Upper and lower face weakness	Bell palsy Assess for diabetes mellitus, vasculitis, Lyme disease, sarcoidosis, HIV infection, and compressive or infiltrative malignancies only if additional suggestive features are present	Prednisone if within 72 hours of onset

(Continued on the next page)

STUDY TABLE: Diagnosing and Managing Peripheral Neuropathy *(Continued)*		
If you see this...	**Think this...**	**And choose this...**
Multiple, noncontiguous nerve deficits (mononeuritis multiplex)	Consider vasculitis (especially if painful), lymphoma, amyloidosis, sarcoidosis, Lyme disease, HIV, leprosy, and diabetes	Treat underlying disorder
Distal and symmetric (stocking-glove) sensory or sensorimotor	Axonal polyneuropathies; diabetes and alcohol are the most common causes; small fiber neuropathy will present with pain only	Treat underlying disorder; treat pain and dysesthesias symptomatically
Severe unilateral leg pain, numbness, proximal weakness, atrophy, and weight loss	Diabetic lumbosacral radiculoplexus neuropathy (diabetic amyotrophy)	Treat diabetes
Acute, ascending, areflexic paralysis and paresthesias often preceded by GI illness (usually *Campylobacter* infection); CSF shows elevated protein and a normal cell count (albuminocytologic dissociation)	Guillain-Barré syndrome	Plasma exchange or IV immune globulin
Progressive proximal motor and sensory neuropathy that evolves over months. Initial EMG and CSF findings similar to Guillain-Barré syndrome	Chronic inflammatory demyelinating polyneuropathy	Prednisone, plasma exchange, or IV immune globulin
Symmetric distal sensory neuropathy in the setting of MGUS, multiple myeloma, amyloidosis, and cryoglobulinemia	Paraproteinemic neuropathy	Treat underlying disorder

Treatment

Only pregabalin, duloxetine, and tapentadol (extended release) are FDA approved for the treatment of painful neuropathy.

Glucocorticoids, but not antivirals, are effective for Bell palsy when initiated within 72 hours of onset.

DON'T BE TRICKED

- **When the presentation of Bell palsy is classic and without any additional neurologic deficits, brain imaging and routine laboratory testing are not necessary.**
- **Do not treat Bell palsy with antiviral drugs.**
- **Screening for glucose intolerance should be performed in all nondiabetic patients who have distal sensory neuropathy.**
- **Glucocorticoids are not beneficial in Guillain-Barré syndrome and may even slow the recovery.**

TEST YOURSELF

A 37-year-old woman has difficulty going up stairs. She had diarrhea and low-grade fever 2 weeks ago. Physical examination shows weakness of both lower extremities and diminished deep tendon reflexes.

ANSWER: For diagnosis, choose Guillain-Barré syndrome. For management, select plasma exchange and IV immune globulin.

Myopathy

Myopathies typically present with symmetric weakness of the proximal muscles.

- Normal sensory and reflex examination differentiates myopathy from neuropathy.
- Serum CK level is elevated and falls in response to treatment.
- EMG confirms the presence of myopathic changes (low amplitude, short duration, and polyphasic motor unit potentials).

See Rheumatology chapter for more detailed information on the inflammatory myopathies (polymyositis, dermatomyositis, inclusion body myositis).

STUDY TABLE: Myopathy Diagnostic Features	
Condition	**Diagnostic Clues**
Hypothyroid myopathy	Diffuse myalgia, proximal muscle weakness, delayed relaxation phase of deep tendon reflexes, and elevation of CK
Hyperthyroidism	Myopathy, brisk reflexes, fasciculation, and ophthalmoplegia
Vitamin D deficiency	Proximal muscle weakness, myalgia, fatigue, and osteomalacia-related bone pain
Glucocorticoid myopathy	Proximal weakness and myalgia, normal CK levels, and normal EMG findings
Statin myopathy	Subacute toxic myopathy associated with rhabdomyolysis
Myotonic dystrophies	Myotonia (manifested as delayed hand-grip release) and distal weakness

DON'T BE TRICKED

- Lipophilic statins (atorvastatin, simvastatin, and lovastatin) have a higher propensity to cause statin myopathy compared with hydrophilic statins (fluvastatin, pravastatin, and rosuvastatin).

Primary Central Nervous System Lymphoma

Diagnosis

PCNSL is a non-Hodgkin lymphoma that commonly presents as a focal supratentorial lesion. Visual symptoms are common because of frequent tumor involvement of the optic radiations. PCNSL most commonly affects immunocompromised patients but can occur in patients with intact immune systems. A brain biopsy specimen is required to make a diagnosis. Ocular involvement in the vitreous or retina may be seen in up to 20% of patients and can be detected with a slit lamp examination and confirmed by vitreal biopsy.

Treatment

In patients with PCNSL and HIV infection, start ART; for those who have undergone organ transplantation, immunosuppressive therapy should be stopped. PCNSL is sensitive to both whole brain radiation and chemotherapy.

DON'T BE TRICKED

- Resection of PCNSL is not indicated and can worsen patient outcomes.

Meningioma

Diagnosis

Meningiomas are usually benign in histology and behavior. These tumors are usually discovered incidentally during neuroimaging for unrelated symptoms. Symptomatic patients typically have progressive headache and focal neurologic lesions. CT scan of the head will show a partially calcified, homogeneously enhancing extra-axial mass adherent to the dura and an enhancing dural "tail."

Treatment

Surgical resection is the treatment of choice for symptomatic meningiomas or enlarging meningiomas. Observation is appropriate for small, asymptomatic meningiomas.

DON'T BE TRICKED

- Chemotherapy has no established role in patients with meningioma.

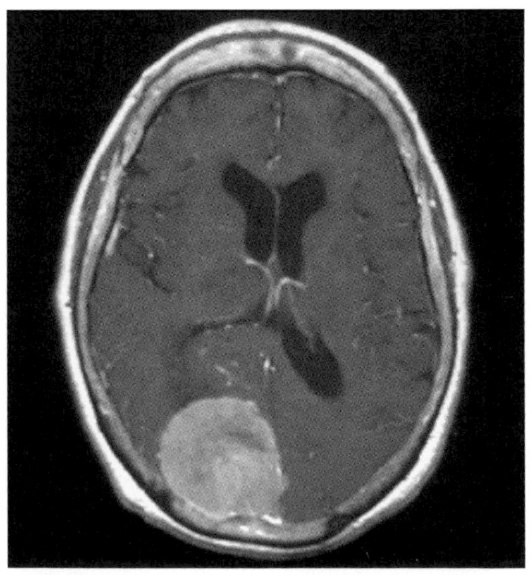

Meningioma: Coronal MRI with contrast shows meningioma with the enhancing dural "tail" inferior to the tumor's dural attachment.

Metastatic Brain Tumors

Diagnosis

Parenchymal metastases usually present as multiple, ring-enhancing, centrally necrotic lesions. These lesions have a proclivity for the junction between the gray and white matter and are typically associated with significant surrounding edema and mass effect. If a metastatic brain tumor is the first indication of malignancy, evaluate the patient for lung cancer, breast cancer, and melanoma.

Lymphoma and leukemia cause leptomeningeal metastases and may present with headache or spinal pain, cranial nerve or spinal radicular pain, weakness, and mental status changes. Communicating hydrocephalus may be present. Leptomeningeal tumors are characterized on MRI by a diffuse or patchy enhancement of the surface of the brain and spinal cord or roots.

DON'T BE TRICKED

- **MRI is required for all patients with systemic cancer and new neurologic findings.**
- **In patients with active, biopsy-proven systemic malignancy and multiple enhancing brain lesions, brain biopsy is not indicated.**

Treatment

Glucocorticoids are a first-line treatment for parenchymal and leptomeningeal tumors. Chemotherapy (methotrexate and cytarabine) is the initial therapy for patients with leptomeningeal metastases from leukemia and lymphoma. Palliative whole-brain radiation therapy is indicated for multiple parenchymal metastases from a known primary solid tumor. Resection is an option for solitary, accessible brain metastases and controlled extracranial disease.

DON'T BE TRICKED

- **Chemotherapy is not indicated for parenchymal brain metastases from most solid tumors.**

TEST YOURSELF

A 60-year-old woman with a history of adenocarcinoma of the lung has a 3-week history of diplopia, dysphagia, and foot drop. CT scan of the head shows multiple ring-enhancing lesions.

ANSWER: The probable diagnosis is metastatic cancer. For management, select glucocorticoids, and arrange for palliative brain radiation.

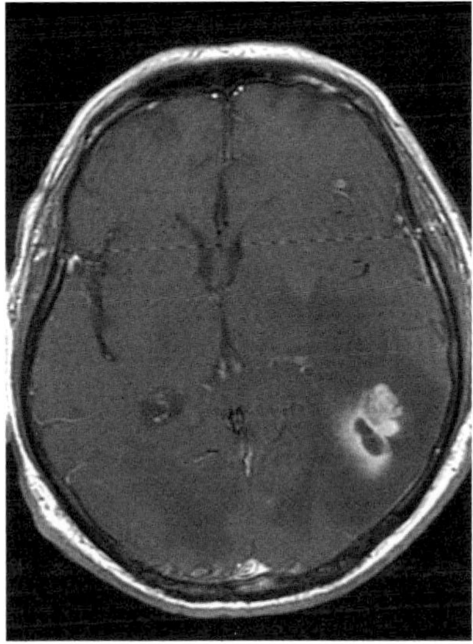

Parietal Lobe Metastatic Nodule: Axial postcontrast T1-weighted MRI shows an enhancing metastatic nodule in the left parietal lobe with surrounding edema and mass effect.

Coma

Diagnosis

Coma is a state of unarousable unresponsiveness. It can be caused by diffuse insults to the cerebral hemispheres, damage to the reticular activating system, or a combination of hemispheric and brain stem dysfunction. Unilateral hemispheric lesions do not result in coma unless edema and mass effect cause compression of the contralateral hemisphere or the reticular activating system. Coma can be caused by a variety of structural lesions and toxic, metabolic, and infectious causes.

Patients in a vegetative state are unaware of self and the environment and show no purposeful responses to stimuli. They continue to have sleep-wake cycles and brain stem function.

The three cardinal findings of brain death are coma, absence of brain stem reflexes, and apnea.

STUDY TABLE: Key Points in the Evaluation of Coma	
Finding	**Consider**
Coma without focal signs, fever, or meningism	Hypoxia or a metabolic cause, toxic reaction, drug-induced state, infection, or postictal state
Coma without focal signs but with meningismus	Meningitis, meningoencephalitis, or SAH
Coma with focal signs	Stroke, hemorrhage, tumor, or abscess
Quadriplegic, mute, but preserved vertical eye movements	"Locked-in" state caused by a pontine infarction or hemorrhage

Focal findings or any unexplained coma is an indication for emergent imaging of the brain to exclude hemorrhage or mass lesion. A CT is the appropriate test in emergency situations. LP is indicated when meningitis or SAH is suspected but neuroimaging is normal. Emergent EEG can exclude nonconvulsive status epilepticus.

DON'T BE TRICKED

- **Respiratory drive and motor posturing signs are incompatible with a diagnosis of brain death.**

Treatment

Attend to airway, breathing, and circulation first. All patients with unexplained coma should be urgently treated with thiamine and glucose (unless rapid finger stick rules out hypoglycemia). Give naloxone if an opiate overdose is suspected and flumazenil if a benzodiazepine overdose is being considered.

Oncology

Breast Cancer

Screening and Diagnosis

See General Internal Medicine, Breast Cancer Prevention and Screening.

The USPSTF recommends biennial screening mammography for asymptomatic average-risk women aged 50 to 74 years, with individualized screening decisions for patients aged 40 to 49 years. For women ≥75 years, evidence is insufficient to recommend for or against screening.

Testing

Schedule mammography (and ultrasonography as needed) in women with any new breast symptoms or abnormal findings on physical examination.

In premenopausal women, following the abnormality through one menstrual cycle instead of scheduling immediate imaging is reasonable.

Schedule biopsy for suspicious lesions noted during physical examination or screening mammography. If histopathologic studies confirm invasive breast cancer, determine estrogen/progesterone receptor and *HER2/neu* status.

Any fluid discharge from the nipple requires a cytopathologic examination. The two factors that are most prognostic are tumor size and axillary lymph node status.

DON'T BE TRICKED

- A normal mammogram or ultrasound does not rule out breast cancer.
- A breast lump should always be biopsied, even if a mammogram is normal.
- Bone scan, CT, or tumor marker tests are not routine studies for staging DCIS (stage 0) or early stage (I and II) breast cancer.

Treatment

DCIS can be treated with **breast-conserving therapy**, which consists of wide excision (lumpectomy) followed by breast radiation. In patients with estrogen-positive DCIS, tamoxifen decreases the risk of local recurrence but not survival. Lumpectomy followed by radiation therapy is equivalent to mastectomy followed by radiation therapy with comparable survival in most women with invasive breast cancer.

Mastectomy is recommended for tumors involving the skin, chest wall, or more than one quadrant of the breast, for inflammatory breast cancer, or if contraindications to radiation therapy (previous irradiation) exist. Bilateral mastectomy is an option for women with familial breast cancer syndromes.

Axillary lymph node dissection is performed if sentinel lymph node biopsy is positive or axillary lymph nodes are clinically involved.

Chest wall radiation therapy after mastectomy is recommended in patients with tumors >5 cm, positive surgical margins, skin or chest wall involvement, and inflammatory breast cancer, and for most patients with ≥4 positive axillary nodes.

Adjuvant systemic therapy is used to prevent or delay systemic recurrence for stages I to III breast cancer, stages in which the cancer is not metastatic and is potentially curable.

Most patients with hormone receptor–positive breast cancer receive adjuvant antiestrogen therapy. In premenopausal women, a 5- to 10-year course of adjuvant tamoxifen is standard of care. Premenopausal women who previously completed 5 years of tamoxifen benefit from taking an aromatase inhibitor for 5 years when they become postmenopausal.

Postmenopausal women are treated with 5 years of an aromatase inhibitor (anastrozole, letrozole, exemestane). Patients taking aromatase inhibitors should undergo DEXA scans periodically (generally every 2 years) and receive bisphosphonate therapy if T scores are less than −2.5.

Adjuvant chemotherapy is indicated for patients with hormone receptor–negative (triple-negative) tumors, *HER2*-positive tumors, high-grade tumors, extensive lymphovascular invasion, and positive lymph nodes.

Molecular prognostic profiles, such as the 21-gene recurrence score, which can be used in ER/PR positive and *HER2*-negative tumors, help determine the benefit of adjuvant chemotherapy. Patients with high-risk recurrence scores will benefit from adjuvant chemotherapy followed by antiestrogen therapy, whereas those with low-risk scores do not benefit from adjuvant chemotherapy.

For patients with *HER2*-positive breast cancer, a monoclonal antibody (e.g., trastuzumab), is used as adjuvant therapy along with chemotherapy. Patients should undergo evaluation of LV function before initiating and during trastuzumab treatment.

Inflammatory breast cancer is an aggressive and rapidly progressive type of cancer characterized by erythema and edema of the skin of the breast ("peau d'orange"). Inflammatory breast cancer is treated with neoadjuvant chemotherapy, followed by surgery, and then radiation.

Hormone receptor–positive metastatic disease can be treated with antiestrogen therapy. Patients who are hormone receptor–negative or who fail to respond to antiestrogen therapy are treated with single-agent chemotherapy. Lytic bone metastases are treated with bisphosphonates to decrease bone pain and skeletal-related events. The monoclonal antibody denosumab is an alternate option. Painful skeletal disease is treated with radiation therapy.

Follow-Up

Patients with early-stage breast cancer should receive annual mammography. MRI of the breast is reserved for patients who have an especially high risk for subsequent breast cancer from *BRCA1/2* mutations or strong family history of breast cancer. Surveillance blood tests and other imaging studies are not recommended.

DON'T BE TRICKED

- Aromatase inhibitors are contraindicated in premenopausal women.
- Ovarian ablation or suppression can be used for premenopausal women with contraindications to tamoxifen.
- Do not select mastectomy in patients with metastatic disease unless required for local cancer control.
- Pregnancy following breast cancer treatment does not increase the risk of breast cancer recurrence.

STUDY TABLE: Breast Cancer Treatment Side Effects

Drug	Side Effect
Aromatase inhibitors (anastrazole, letrozole, exemestane)	Arthralgia, bone pain, hyperlipidemia, osteoporosis
Tamoxifen	Endometrial cancer, VTE disease
Anthracyclines (doxorubicin, epirubicin)	Cardiomyopathy, acute leukemia
Trastuzumab	Cardiomyopathy, especially if used with an anthracycline
Bisphosphonates	Osteonecrosis of the jaw, particularly in patients with dental disease
Denosumab	Hypocalcemia and osteonecrosis of the jaw, particularly in patients with dental disease

DON'T BE TRICKED

- Biopsy new metastatic lesions; primary tumor and metastatic tumor estrogen receptor and *HER2* status differs in up to 15% of patients.

TEST YOURSELF

A 50-year-old premenopausal woman has a 1.5-cm moderately differentiated breast cancer. The lesion is completely excised (lumpectomy), and the surgical margins are negative. Three axillary lymph nodes are positive. The tumor is negative for estrogen/progesterone receptors and is highly positive for *HER2/neu*.

ANSWER: For diagnosis, choose stage III *HER2*-positive, hormone-receptor negative breast cancer. For management, select post-operative radiation therapy, adjuvant chemotherapy, and trastuzumab, but not tamoxifen or aromatase inhibitors.

Lung Cancer

Screening and Prevention

Smoking cessation is the most effective preventive measure for lung cancer; 90% of lung cancers are smoking related. Asbestos exposure is another risk factor.

Annual screening with low-dose CT in patients aged 55 to 74-80 years (guidelines vary) with a 30-pack-year history of smoking, including those who quit smoking in the preceding 15 years, has been associated with a decrease in lung cancer and all-cause mortality.

DON'T BE TRICKED

- Do not screen for lung cancer with chest x-ray and/or sputum cytology.
- Do not prescribe vitamin A derivatives (β-carotene and retinol) or vitamin E (α-tocopherol) to prevent lung cancer.

Diagnosis

Common symptoms include hemoptysis, pulmonary infections, dyspnea, cough, chest pain or paraneoplastic syndromes (Cushing syndrome, hypercalcemia, hyponatremia), mechanical effects of tumor (SVC syndrome), or Horner syndrome (ipsilateral ptosis, miosis, enophthalmos, anhidrosis).

Testing

The most characteristic finding is a mass lesion on chest x-ray. Radiographic abnormalities should first be compared with previous chest imaging studies. A solid lung nodule that has been stable for 2 years or longer is highly unlikely to be cancer. Histologic confirmation is necessary for diagnosis and can be obtained by percutaneous lung biopsy, peripheral lymph node biopsy, pleural fluid cytology, or transbronchial biopsy. Whenever possible, select the biopsy site that will simultaneously diagnose and stage the disease (peripheral lymph node, mediastinal node). Treatment and prognosis vary based on whether the patient has NSCLC (adenocarcinoma, SCC, large cell carcinoma) or SCLC.

Small Cell Lung Cancer

SCLC is generally viewed as a systemic (metastatic) disease at the time of diagnosis; most patients have obvious extensive disease. Limited-stage disease is confined to one hemithorax, with hilar and mediastinal lymphadenopathy that can be encompassed within one tolerable radiotherapy portal. Extensive-stage disease consists of any disease that exceeds those boundaries, including malignant pleural effusion. Typical staging studies include CT of the chest, abdomen, and pelvis; whole-body bone scintigraphy or CT/PET scan; and MRI of the brain.

SCLC characteristically produces peptide hormones, which can cause endocrine syndromes such as hyponatremia from the SIADH and hypercortisolism through secretion of ACTH. Neurologic symptoms such as the Lambert-Eaton syndrome, cortical cerebellar degeneration, limbic encephalitis, and peripheral neuropathy may also occur in patients with lung cancer, but they are rare.

Non-Small Cell Lung Cancer

In staging NSCLC, the task is to identify metastatic disease, which eliminates surgery as a therapeutic option. Perform a staging evaluation with chest and upper abdominal CT plus a PET scan (or a PET/CT) to assess for lymphadenopathy.

Measurement of the CBC and serum calcium, alkaline phosphatase, and aminotransferase levels can detect more advanced disease. PET/CT and whole-body PET are commonly used for staging, which eliminates the need for bone scan. A brain MRI is indicated in the presence of neurologic signs or symptoms or in patients being considered for surgery or combined modality (chemo-radiation) therapy for early stage lung cancer.

DON'T BE TRICKED

- Do not order routine bone scans or CT of the head in patients without bone or neurologic symptoms.
- If a patient has a lung mass and hypercalcemia, choose SCC as the likely cause.

Treatment

STUDY TABLE: Treatment of SCLC

If you see this...	Select this...
Limited-stage disease	Concurrent chemotherapy and radiation therapy
Extensive-stage disease	Chemotherapy
Complete or partial response to therapy (both limited and extensive stages)	Add prophylactic cranial irradiation
Symptomatic brain metastases	Whole-brain radiation therapy

STUDY TABLE: Treatment of NSCLC

If you see this...	Select this...
Stage I disease (solitary tumor 3-5 cm with no lymphadenopathy or metastases) or stage II disease (solitary tumor ≥5 cm, regional lymphadenopathy, pleura or chest wall involvement, tumors located near carina)	Surgical resection for cure followed by cisplatin-based adjuvant chemotherapy (only if solid tumor >4 cm) and radiation therapy for positive margins
Stage III disease (involving mediastinum or contralateral mediastinal lymph nodes)	Platinum-based chemotherapy and radiation therapy
Stage IV disease (metastatic cancer, including malignant pleural or pericardial effusion)	Chemotherapy only if good performance status; include immunotherapy with anti-PD1 and anti-PDL1 checkpoint inhibitor as first-line therapy if PDL1 expression is high or as second-line therapy in any NSCLC
Solitary brain metastasis	Surgical excision and postoperative brain radiation

Patients with *EGFR* mutations should receive erlotinib (or gefitinib, afatinib), whereas those with *ALK* translocations and *ROS1* mutations benefit from crizotinib. Maintenance chemotherapy is typically given until the patient experiences disease progression or an unacceptable level of toxicity.

Use glucocorticoids and radiation therapy for patients with multiple brain metastases. Select thoracic irradiation for pulmonary airway obstruction, SVC syndrome, and spinal cord metastases (following surgical decompression). Radiation therapy relieves pain, particularly bone pain, visceral pain secondary to capsular distention, or pain because of nerve compression. Treat symptomatic pleural effusions with thoracentesis and indwelling pleural catheter or pleurodesis if necessary.

Follow-Up

Following curative-intent treatment for NSCLC, patients should undergo follow-up monitoring with periodic history, physical examination, and CT of the chest.

DON'T BE TRICKED

- Patients with extensive-stage SCLC (extending beyond a single hemithorax) and poor performance status because of tumor burden should be offered chemotherapy because it can significantly improve symptoms and increase survival.
- Consider no chemotherapy for patients with NSCLC with poor performance status (extreme fatigue or weakness, weight loss >10%, severe symptoms).

TEST YOURSELF

A 51-year-old man presents with facial plethora, neck vein distention, shortness of breath, and a hilar mass.

ANSWER: For diagnosis, choose SVC syndrome. For management, select contrast-enhanced chest CT and obtain tissue diagnosis.

Gastric Cancer

Diagnosis

Most patients have locally advanced or metastatic disease at diagnosis. The most common symptoms are abdominal pain, anorexia, bleeding, dysphagia, nausea, and weight loss. Important physical examination findings may include periumbilical nodes (Sister Mary Joseph node) and left supraclavicular lymphadenopathy (Virchow node).

Testing

The initial diagnostic procedure is upper endoscopy. CT scans are used to identify the presence of regional and metastatic disease. Endoscopic ultrasonography is superior to CT in the evaluation of depth of tumor invasion and lymph node involvement and aids in preoperative evaluation.

DON'T BE TRICKED

- Always obtain upper endoscopy and biopsy in a patient with "achalasia" to rule out gastric cancer.

Treatment

For patients with **localized tumors**, standard therapy includes neoadjuvant chemotherapy (or chemoradiation therapy) followed by surgery.

Combination platinum-based regimens are used for **metastatic cancer**. Up to 20% of gastric cancers overexpress the *HER2* growth factor receptor. In these patients, add trastuzumab to the chemotherapy regimen.

Use antibiotic and PPI therapy for early-stage **MALT lymphoma** of the stomach and evidence of *Helicobacter pylori* infection.

Colorectal Cancer

Screening

Average risk: See General Internal Medicine chapter for USPSTF-recommended screening.

High risk: The risk for colorectal cancer is elevated in ulcerative colitis and Crohn disease of the colon. This increased risk depends on the proximal extent of mucosal involvement; patients with pancolitis are at highest risk, whereas risk is negligible in patients with proctitis. Risk is also increased with longer duration of disease, greater severity of inflammation, and the presence of coexistent PSC.

The following is a list of hereditary syndromes that commonly appear on examinations:

Familial adenomatous polyposis is an autosomal dominant disorder that requires prophylactic colectomy; duodenal and periampullary cancers are the second leading cause of cancer death in this group.

Gardner syndrome is a type of familial adenomatous polyposis with extraintestinal manifestations, including osteomas, duodenal ampullary tumors, thyroid cancers, and medulloblastomas.

Hereditary nonpolyposis colon cancer (HNPCC) is an autosomal dominant disorder. Diagnostic criteria include:

- ≥3 relatives with colorectal cancer
- one relative must be a first-degree relative of the other two
- ≥2 successive generations affected
- one cancer diagnosed before age 50 years

Lynch syndrome is diagnosed if a patient meets the criteria for HNPCC and also has an identified germline mutation in one of the four mismatch repair genes or the epithelial cell adhesion molecule (*EPCAM*). Lynch syndrome is also associated with an increased risk for extracolonic tumors, most commonly endometrial.

If an inherited colon cancer syndrome is suspected, the patient and family members should be referred for genetic counseling and more intense cancer surveillance.

STUDY TABLE: Age and Frequency of Colon Cancer Screening (for patients choosing colonoscopy)

Risk Profile	When to Initiate Colonoscopy Screening
Average risk	Age 50 years - every 10 years to age 75 years (other screening modalities are available)
First-degree relative with colon cancer at age ≥60 years	Age 50 years - every 10 years to age 75 years (other screening modalities are available)
First-degree relative diagnosed with an adenomatous polyp or colon cancer at age ≤60 years	Age 40 years, or 10 years younger than the earliest diagnosis in the family - every 5 years
Two second-degree relatives with adenomatous polyp or colon cancer at any age	Age 40 years or 10 years younger than the earliest diagnosis in the family - every 5 years
Two first-degree relatives with colon cancer	Age 40 years, or 10 years younger than the earliest diagnosis in the family - every 3-5 years
HNPCC risk	Age 20 or 25 years, or 10 years earlier than the age of youngest person in family diagnosed with colon cancer - every 1-2 years
Familial adenomatous polyposis risk	Age 10-12 years - every 1-2 years with colonoscopy or sigmoidoscopy
Pancolitis (ulcerative colitis or Crohn disease)	8 years after initial diagnosis - every 1-2 years
Primary sclerosing cholangitis	At time of diagnosis - every 1-2 years

DON'T BE TRICKED

- **A single positive FOBT finding constitutes a positive screening test and requires prompt follow-up colonoscopy.**

Adenomatous polyps are premalignant lesions defined by their glandular architecture: tubular, villous, or a combination of both. Different levels of follow-up are recommended for patients discovered to have a colonic polyp on screening colonoscopy.

STUDY TABLE: Postpolypectomy Surveillance

Adenomatous Polyps	Interval to Next Colonoscopy
1-2 tubular adenomas <10 mm	5-10 years
3-10 adenomas, ≥10 mm, villous histology, or high-grade dysplasia	3 years
≥10 adenomas on single examination	<3 years; a genetic cause of disease should be investigated

DON'T BE TRICKED

- **Patients with a few small (<10 mm), distal hyperplastic polyps should be screened according to average risk guidelines (i.e., every 10 years).**

Diagnosis

Characteristic findings are rectal bleeding or change in bowel habits. Other findings include pelvic pain or tenesmus, weight loss, rectal or abdominal mass, hepatomegaly, and iron deficiency anemia. Patients with obstruction have hypogastric abdominal pain, abdominal distention, nausea, and vomiting.

Testing

Although multiple modalities are recommended for screening, colonoscopy is the diagnostic procedure of choice when other modalities are positive. Patients with colorectal cancer should undergo molecular testing of their tumor to determine if it has evidence of defective mismatch repair gene or microsatellite instability.

Staging also consists of contrast-enhanced CT of the abdomen, chest, and pelvis and a serum CEA level.

DON'T BE TRICKED

- **Do not obtain a serum CEA level to screen for or diagnose colon cancer.**
- **Do not obtain a PET scan for initial staging of colorectal cancer.**

Treatment

General rules for colorectal cancer therapy:

- confined to colon (stage I) or local invasion (stage II) → resection for cure
- metastatic to regional lymph nodes (stage III) → resection and adjuvant chemotherapy
- distant metastases (stage IV) → resection of primary lesion for palliation (if needed) and chemotherapy
- stage II-III rectal cancer → combination radiation therapy and chemotherapy before surgery with adjuvant chemotherapy after surgery

Adjuvant chemotherapy with FOLFOX or CAPOX is associated with improvement in disease-free and overall survival for patients with stage III colon cancer.

Patients with stage II and stage III rectal cancer are treated with preoperative (neoadjuvant) radiation therapy and chemotherapy and postoperative (adjuvant) chemotherapy.

Patients with a single metastatic lesion to a single organ may be cured with surgical removal of the primary tumor and the metastasis. Surgical resection of the primary tumor and metastases in patients with ≤3 liver metastases can result in cure in about 25% of cases.

The FOLFOX and FOLFIRI regimens are equally efficacious for metastatic colon cancer. The addition of bevacizumab, a monoclonal antibody against VEGF, further increases the efficacy of chemotherapy. The anti-EGFR monoclonal antibody cetuximab or panitumumab may be useful, alone or combined with other chemotherapies. These agents are inactive in nearly half of patients with the K-*ras* and N-*ras* mutations and should not be used in these patients.

Follow-Up

Recommended follow-up includes:

- CEA measurement every 6 months for 5 years
- colonoscopy 1 year following resection in patients with preoperative colonoscopy, 3 years later, and then every 5 years
- for patients in whom preoperative colonoscopy was not possible, perioperative colonoscopy followed by the above surveillance schedule
- CT of the abdomen, chest, and pelvis annually for 5 years

DON'T BE TRICKED

- Do not treat asymptomatic, widely metastatic disease because treatment is not associated with improved outcomes and has significant treatment toxicity.
- Do not use PET scans to follow patients for recurrent colorectal cancer.
- Anti-VEGF and anti-EGFR monoclonal antibodies should not be used together.
- Do not institute therapy for metastatic disease based on CEA elevation alone.

TEST YOURSELF

A 63-year-old man has a 4-month history of increasing fatigue and a nonobstructing colon cancer metastatic to the liver and lungs. His hemoglobin level is 12.5 g/dL.

ANSWER: For management, select multiagent chemotherapy. Surgery is not indicated.

Anal Cancer

Prevention

Most anal cancers are associated with HPV infection. HPV vaccine prevents anal HPV infection and anal intraepithelial neoplasia, precursors of anal cancer.

Diagnosis

Most patients present with a perianal lesion or mass associated with rectal bleeding or anal discomfort. Biopsy is essential to establish the diagnosis. Anoscopy; digital rectal examination; inguinal lymph node palpation (with biopsy or fine-needle aspiration if enlarged); and CT of the pelvis, abdomen, and chest are performed for staging.

Treatment

Anal cancer is treated with radiation therapy and concurrent mitomycin plus 5-FU. Anal tumors may continue to regress for at least 6 months up to 1 year after completion of chemoradiation therapy.

DON'T BE TRICKED

- Do not select surgery for anal cancer.

Hepatocellular Carcinoma

Prevention

The most important preventive measure for HCC is hepatitis B vaccination.

Screening

Most guidelines recommend that all patients with cirrhosis and some patients with chronic hepatitis B without cirrhosis (patients from America who are black and patients from Asia or Africa) should be screened with abdominal ultrasonography every 6 months.

DON'T BE TRICKED

- Serum AFP measurement alone is not recommended for HCC screening or surveillance.

Testing

Order a contrast-enhanced CT or MRI of the liver when the abdominal ultrasound is abnormal. Because the radiographic findings of HCC are fairly characteristic (arterial phase enhancement), biopsy for confirmation is usually unnecessary.

Treatment

Surgical resection or liver transplantation is first-line therapy. Small single lesions in patients with cirrhosis but without portal hypertension and hyperbilirubinemia are managed with surgical resection. Patients with cirrhosis and up to three tumors ≤3 cm or one tumor ≤5 cm without vascular invasion or extrahepatic spread are treated with liver transplantation.

Percutaneous ethanol injection or radiofrequency ablation (in tumors <2 cm) is used for patients who cannot undergo surgery or liver transplantation. Chemoembolization is used for patients with advanced, multifocal HCC who are not candidates for surgical resection, liver transplantation, or ablative therapy. Sorafenib improves overall survival in patients with advanced/metastatic HCC.

STUDY TABLE: Other Hepatic Tumors and Cysts

Type	Characteristics
Cavernous hemangioma	Early peripheral nodular enhancement on contrast CT or MRI, followed by delayed fill-in toward the center of the lesion. No therapy is required.
Hepatic adenoma	Early arterial enhancement with rapid loss of enhancement and return to isointensity with the surrounding liver. Adenomas are typically heterogeneous in appearance because of regions of hemorrhage or necrosis. Patients may have a history of using oral contraceptives. Select resection if >5 cm.
Focal nodular hyperplasia	Early arterial enhancement with rapid loss of enhancement in the portal venous phase with return to isointensity with the surrounding liver. Many larger focal nodular hyperplasias have a central stellate scar. No therapy is required.
Metastatic tumors	Single or multiple hypoechoic lesions on ultrasonography that are hypovascular on contrast-enhanced CT scans. Isolated lesions may be amenable to resection.

TEST YOURSELF

A 60-year-old man with chronic hepatitis C and cirrhosis is found to have a 4-cm liver mass on screening ultrasonography. A CT scan showed the mass enhances on arterial phase.

ANSWER: For diagnosis, choose hepatocellular carcinoma. For management, select liver transplantation.

Cholangiocarcinoma

Diagnosis and Treatment

The most important established risk factor is the presence of PSC. Symptoms may include RUQ pain or jaundice. Diagnosis of extrahepatic bile duct cancers usually requires ERCP in combination with MRCP or contrast-enhanced CT. Surgical resection is the treatment of choice. Chemotherapy is reserved for nonresectable cholangiocarcinoma. Liver transplantation is an option for nonresectable, perihilar cholangiocarcinoma without extrahepatic spread.

DON'T BE TRICKED

- CA-19 measurement is not able to confirm or exclude the diagnosis of cholangiocarcinoma.
- Do not perform percutaneous biopsy of a perihilar cholangiocarcinoma in patients for whom liver transplantation may be an option.

Pancreatic Cancer

Diagnosis

Symptoms are influenced by tumor site and extent and may include:

- upper abdominal discomfort and lumbar back pain
- anorexia and weight loss
- obstructive jaundice
- marked weight loss
- vascular thromboses (Trousseau syndrome)

Physical examination findings may include a palpable gallbladder and jaundice.

Testing

Contrast-enhanced multidetector CT has 90% sensitivity for detecting pancreatic cancer. Endoscopic ultrasonography does not influence staging but is more sensitive in detecting small cancers (<2 cm) and allows tissue diagnosis by fine-needle aspiration when needed.

DON'T BE TRICKED

- **Serum tumor markers are not used to diagnose pancreatic cancer.**
- **AIP can be mistaken for pancreatic cancer; look for elevated serum levels of IgG4 in patients with AIP, and biopsy the pancreas.**

Treatment

Surgical resection is appropriate for patients with resectable pancreatic cancer. For patients with locally advanced but unresectable disease (tumor involvement of the superior mesenteric artery or the celiac trunk), treatment is controversial. Choices include:

- radiation therapy alone
- 5-FU plus radiation therapy (commonly used)
- single-agent chemotherapy (usually gemcitabine)

Palliative measures to alleviate pain in patients with unresectable or metastatic disease include optimization of analgesic medications, radiation therapy, chemical splanchnicectomy, or celiac nerve blocks. Palliation of biliary obstruction may be achieved with surgical biliary bypass, percutaneous radiology biliary stent placement, or endoscopic biliary stent placement.

Neuroendocrine Tumors

Diagnosis

NETs arising from the endocrine cells of the pancreas are called pancreatic NETs, whereas those arising from all other neuroendocrine tissues of the aerodigestive tract are called gastrointestinal NETs (formerly called carcinoid tumors).

Most NETs are hormonally nonfunctioning, but about 25% manifest a hormone. Gastrointestinal NETs can produce serotonin, which can cause diarrhea and facial flushing.

Pancreatic NETs may produce insulin, gastrin, glucagon, somatostatin, or vasoactive intestinal peptide, with resulting hormonal syndromes based on the type of hormone elaborated. This tumor may be part of the multiple endocrine neoplasia type 1 (MEN1) syndrome (primary hyperparathyroidism, pituitary tumors, enteropancreatic tumors).

Nonfunctioning tumors may be asymptomatic and develop metastatic disease many years before diagnosis. The liver is the most common and the incidental finding of hepatomegaly is the most common presentation.

Testing

Triple-phase contrast-enhanced CT and MRI with gadolinium are the preferred imaging modalities. Indium 111 pentetreotide scanning can be used to establish the presence of somatostatin receptors.

Treatment

Most NETs are indolent and can be followed until symptomatic. Surgery can be used to remove localized tumors. Hormonally active tumors with somatostatin receptors may be treated with the somatostatin analogues octreotide or lanreotide.

In pancreatic NETs, sunitinib (an anti-VEGF agent) and everolimus (an mTOR inhibitor) and chemotherapy are effective treatments.

Chemotherapy is minimally effective in gastrointestinal NETs.

Cervical Cancer

Prevention and Screening

See General Internal Medicine, Cervical Cancer Screening.

Diagnosis

Abnormal vaginal bleeding is the most common clinical presentation (postmenopausal, postcoital, and intermenstrual). Associated pain and abnormal discharge are usually signs of advanced disease.

Testing

Punch biopsy of obvious lesions or colposcopy-directed biopsy is usually required for diagnosis.

Treatment

Early (stage I) cancers may be treated with loop electrosurgical excision procedure or cervical conization to preserve childbearing; patients who have finished childbearing may undergo hysterectomy without lymph node dissection. Radiation therapy and cisplatin chemotherapy are used for patients with stage II, III, or IV disease. Treat patients with recurrent disease or distant metastases with local radiation (for local control) and chemotherapy plus bevacizumab.

Ovarian Cancer

Prevention

Oophorectomy after childbearing or at age 35 years can be offered to women with *BRCA1/2* genetic mutations or ≥2 first-degree relatives with ovarian cancer.

Screening

Screening women at average risk for ovarian cancer is not indicated. Screening with serum CA-125, pelvic examination, and transvaginal ultrasonography is a reasonable but unproven strategy for women at high risk (e.g., ovarian cancer in a first- or second-degree family member, family member with ovarian cancer at age <50 years).

Diagnosis

Patients may have a family history of breast, ovarian, or colon cancer. Characteristic findings are abdominal swelling, ascites, and pain, as well as abnormal vaginal bleeding and dyspareunia. A pelvic mass or nodularity may be present in the cul-de-sac.

Testing

If ovarian cancer is suspected, CT or MRI of the abdomen and pelvis and chest imaging are performed to assess disease extent. In patients with an adnexal mass without ascites, surgical removal of the mass without biopsy is associated with a survival benefit. In patients with advanced disease, diagnosis may be made by cytologic examination of ascites or pleural effusion or biopsy of peritoneal masses.

DON'T BE TRICKED

- Do not use CA-125 antigen to diagnose ovarian cancer.
- Women with peritoneal CUP have ovarian cancer until proven otherwise.

Treatment

Surgery is indicated to remove the ovaries and any evidence of grossly visible disease within the abdomen. Most patients with stage IA and IB disease with grade 1 (well-differentiated) histology do not receive adjuvant chemotherapy. Patients with stage IC to IV disease are treated with adjuvant platinum-based chemotherapy. Intraperitoneal chemotherapy shows a survival benefit in patients with small amounts of residual disease confined to the peritoneal cavity following surgery. Selected patients with good performance status and local recurrence of ovarian cancer may experience enhanced survival if they undergo comprehensive secondary surgical cytoreduction.

DON'T BE TRICKED

- Do not opt for "second-look surgery" following completion of chemotherapy.
- All women with ovarian cancer are candidates for *BRCA1/2* testing.

Follow-Up

Limit follow-up to physical examination with pelvic examination and serum CA-125 measurement (if initially elevated).

TEST YOURSELF

A 60-year-old woman has a 3-month history of increasing abdominal girth, constipation, and pain. Physical examination is normal except for ascites. Pelvic ultrasonography is normal. Laparoscopy shows diffuse peritoneal carcinomatosis.

ANSWER: For diagnosis, select adenocarcinoma of unknown primary site. For management, select ovarian cancer treatment.

Endometrial Cancer

Diagnosis

Characteristic findings include irregular vaginal bleeding after age 40 years or in perimenopausal women, persistent pink or brown vaginal discharge, postmenopausal bleeding, and a Pap smear revealing atypical glandular cells of undetermined significance or containing endometrial cells. The diagnosis is made by endometrial biopsy.

Treatment

Surgical resection of the uterus, cervix, and adnexa is first-line treatment; radiation therapy and/or chemotherapy may be added for higher risk disease. Radiation therapy alone is an alternative for high-risk surgical patients.

DON'T BE TRICKED

- Do not screen for endometrial cancer; screening does not reduce mortality.
- Women taking tamoxifen are at increased risk for endometrial cancer.
- Symptom monitoring and physical examination are as effective as imaging for diagnosing recurrent endometrial cancer.

Prostate Cancer

Prevention

Finasteride reduces the incidence of prostate cancer but not cancer mortality rates and is not recommended for prevention.

Diagnosis

Most patients with prostate cancer are asymptomatic at the time of diagnosis. Characteristic findings include a rapidly rising serum PSA level, a nodule or firmness on rectal examination, and obstructive symptoms, although these are more likely associated with BPH.

Testing

Obtain transrectal ultrasonography–guided prostate biopsy for a significantly elevated or rapidly rising PSA level or a nodule or firmness on digital rectal examination.

Tumors are classified according to their histology using the Gleason score. Risk stratification using serum PSA, Gleason score, and TNM cancer staging based on biopsy results and digital rectal examination is essential for determining prognosis and treatment options.

Patients in high risk and very high risk categories require a bone scan and CT of the abdomen and pelvis to evaluate for metastatic disease.

DON'T BE TRICKED

- Acute urinary retention significantly increases the PSA level regardless of the cause of obstruction.

Treatment

The NCCN has developed guidelines for the initial treatment of men with prostate cancer based on their risk score and general life expectancy. The three major treatment strategies for localized prostate cancer are surgery, radiation therapy, and active surveillance. Active surveillance is the postponement of definitive local therapy coupled with surveillance using serum PSA measurement, digital rectal examination, and repeat prostate biopsy. Men undergoing active surveillance receive referral for definitive local therapy if any disease progression is evident.

General rules for treating prostate cancer:

- Active surveillance is indicated for men with very low-risk cancer and a life expectancy >10 years.
- Options for local therapy include external-beam radiotherapy, brachytherapy, and radical prostatectomy.
- After local therapy, high-risk disease is treated with adjuvant ADT with a GnRH agonist (e.g., leuprolide, goserelin) for 2 to 3 years.
- Hormonal therapy is also used for patients with a rising serum PSA level after initial definitive therapy for prostate cancer.
- Hormonal therapy is as effective as bilateral orchiectomy (surgical castration) in treating patients with metastatic disease.

The addition of docetaxel to ADT has been shown to increase progression-free and overall survival in castration-sensitive disease, although adverse effects of docetaxel are significant. Prostate cancer that progresses despite ADT is "castrate resistant." Men who were previously treated with only a GnRH agonist may respond to the addition of an anti-androgen (such as bicalutamide). Castrate-resistant disease may also respond to ketoconazole, megestrol, glucocorticoids, and estrogens. The new anti-androgens abiraterone and enzalutamide also improve overall survival in castrate-resistant disease.

Docetaxel-based therapy improves median overall survival in patients with hormone-refractory metastatic prostate cancer. The combination of docetaxel and prednisone is recommended as a first-line approach for initial chemotherapy in men with ADT-refractory disease.

Bisphosphonates (e.g., zoledronic acid) or denosumab reverse or prevent osteopenia resulting from hormonal therapy, inhibit tumor-mediated bone resorption, and decrease morbidity from bone fractures or bone pain. External-beam radiotherapy and bone-targeted radiopharmaceutical agents treat painful bone metastases. Radiation is most appropriate for a few painful metastatic sites, and radium-223 is indicated for multiple painful sites.

DON'T BE TRICKED

- **Surgery or radiation therapy is not indicated for metastatic prostate cancer in the absence of local GU symptoms.**

Testicular Cancer

Diagnosis

Primary testicular cancer, or germ-cell tumor, is the most common solid malignant tumor in men between the ages of 15 and 35 years. Characteristic findings include a testicular mass, testicular swelling and pain, weight loss, retroperitoneal lymphadenopathy, and metastatic pulmonary lesions. Cryptorchidism is a strong risk factor for testicular cancer.

Testing

After discovery of a testicular mass, ultrasonography should be performed to confirm the presence of a solid mass. Other diagnostic studies include obtaining tissue (inguinal orchiectomy, not needle biopsy) for histopathologic examination; chest x-ray; CT of the abdomen and pelvis; and measurement of the β-hCG, LDH, and AFP levels.

- AFP is never elevated in a pure seminoma.
- An elevated serum AFP level always indicates the tumor has a nonseminomatous component.
- hCG may be present in seminomatous or nonseminomatous tumors.

Any testicular cancer that has a nonseminomatous component based on histologic examination or the presence of an elevated serum AFP level is considered a nonseminoma and is treated as such.

DON'T BE TRICKED

- Do not select testicular biopsy.

Treatment

Semen cryopreservation is common for all men before they undergo therapy for testicular cancer. Inguinal orchiectomy is the initial step in treatment for all testicular tumors. Additional treatment modalities are determined by tumor histology and clinical stage.

Seminoma

- Observation is the preferred initial approach in low-risk, early-stage seminomas (stage I disease). When treatment is recommended, one to two doses of carboplatin chemotherapy is preferred over radiation therapy to the para-aortic lymph nodes.
- Cisplatin-based chemotherapy (preferred) or radiation therapy is recommended for patients with intermediate disease (stage IIA or IIB).
- Chemotherapy (cisplatin-based) is recommended for advanced disease (stage IIC or III).
- Chemotherapy (cisplatin-based) is recommended for nonpulmonary visceral metastases.

PET/CT can be used to determine whether residual masses require resection. Residual masses that are PET scan–positive should be resected.

Nonseminoma

- Stage I disease can be managed with active surveillance, one cycle of cisplatin-based chemotherapy, or retroperitoneal lymph node dissection.
- For patients with bulky retroperitoneal lymphadenopathy identified on CT, cisplatin-based chemotherapy is recommended.
- Cisplatin-based chemotherapy is recommended for advanced disease (IIC or III).
- Patients with elevated serum tumor marker levels postoperatively but without radiographic evidence of disease also receive chemotherapy.

If tumor markers have normalized, select surgical resection of residual masses (masses may represent a teratoma).

Follow-Up

Patients with either seminoma or nonseminoma require frequent follow-up chest x-ray, serum tumor marker assays, and PET/CT of the abdomen and pelvis because of the potential for cure even in patients with recurrent disease.

TEST YOURSELF

A 28-year-old man has weight loss and abdominal pain. Evaluation reveals para-aortic lymphadenopathy. Testicular examination is normal. A lymph node biopsy shows poorly differentiated CUP.

ANSWER: For management, measure the serum AFP and β-hCG levels.

Renal Cell Carcinoma

Diagnosis

Patients with renal cell carcinoma are often asymptomatic until they have advanced disease, but possible symptoms and signs include hematuria, abdominal pain and mass, weight loss, and sudden onset of a varicocele.

Renal cell carcinoma has been associated with various paraneoplastic syndromes, including erythrocytosis, AA amyloidosis, polymyalgia rheumatica, and hepatic dysfunction (unrelated to metastatic disease).

Testing

The initial evaluation is a CT scan or ultrasound. Small lesions are biopsied whereas large lesions are removed without biopsy. CTs of the abdomen, pelvis, and chest are performed to evaluate the local disease extent and assess for metastatic disease.

Treatment

Manage early-stage localized renal cancer with partial or radical nephrectomy. Patients with metastatic disease and good functional status are candidates for debulking nephrectomy.

Targeted therapies include VEGF inhibitors and mTOR inhibitors or immunotherapy with PD1 antibodies (e.g., pembrolizumab or nivolumab).

- VEGF inhibitors include bevacizumab and various VEGF tyrosine kinase inhibitors, such as sunitinib, sorafenib, pazopanib, and axitinib.
- mTOR inhibitors include temsirolimus and everolimus.

Zoledronate decreases skeletal complications and delays progression of bone lesions.

TEST YOURSELF

A 48-year-old man has progressive, severe headaches. Physical examination is normal. Hemoglobin level is 20.2 g/dL and urinalysis shows 30-50 erythrocytes/hpf. A chest x-ray shows multiple bilateral noncalcified nodules measuring 1 to 2 cm.

ANSWER: For diagnosis, choose renal cell carcinoma. For management, select abdominal CT.

Thyroid Cancer

Diagnosis

The four main types of thyroid cancer are:

- papillary (85%)
- follicular (10%)
- medullary (3%)
- anaplastic (1%)

Characteristic findings are a very firm nodule with fixation to adjacent structures, vocal cord paralysis, and enlarged regional lymph nodes.

Consider MEN type 2A or 2B and associated medullary thyroid cancer in a patient with:

- headache, sweating, palpitations, and hypertension (pheochromocytoma)
- kidney stones and hypercalcemia (hyperparathyroidism)
- marfanoid habitus and ganglioneuromas on the tongue, lips, and eyelids (MEN type 2B)
- elevated serum calcitonin level (medullary thyroid cancer)

Testing

FNAB is the diagnostic study for thyroid nodules >1 cm. The aspirate should be analyzed for the *BRAF* gene mutation when the diagnosis is indeterminate. The *BRAF* gene mutation is specific for papillary carcinoma and more aggressive forms of thyroid cancer. Inherited forms of medullary thyroid cancer are associated with germ-line mutations in the *RET* proto-oncogene. Screen family members for disease when a patient presents with a new diagnosis of medullary thyroid cancer.

Treatment

Treat papillary thyroid cancer and follicular thyroid cancer with total thyroidectomy followed by radioiodine therapy in most cases. Medullary thyroid cancer is treated with total thyroidectomy and varying degrees of neck dissection to remove involved lymph nodes.

DON'T BE TRICKED

- **Radioiodine is not taken up by C cells and is not a treatment option for medullary thyroid cancer.**
- **Chemotherapy does not prolong or improve the quality of life for patients with metastatic thyroid carcinoma.**

TEST YOURSELF

A 37-year-old woman has a 2-cm right-sided thyroid nodule that is firm and nontender and moves when she swallows. Serum TSH is 1.8 μU/mL and serum calcium is 11.8 mg/dL.

ANSWER: For diagnosis, choose medullary thyroid cancer. For management, select serum calcitonin measurement.

Lymphoma

Patients with soft, small, freely moveable lymph nodes that are limited to one or two adjacent sites and who have no other significant history or physical examination findings can be followed over 6 to 8 weeks and require no other blood work or imaging.

Persistent or enlarging lymphadenopathy, particularly when associated with systemic symptoms such as fever, night sweats, or weight loss, requires further evaluation.

To establish a diagnosis of lymphoma, perform an excisional biopsy. Core needle biopsy can be used for deep lymph nodes, but fine-needle aspiration should be avoided.

After a diagnosis of lymphoma is made, a total-body CT scan with PET and a bone marrow biopsy are performed to complete staging.

Lymphomas are divided into Hodgkin and non-Hodgkin lymphomas. Lymphomas are further classified into three prognostic groups: indolent, aggressive, and highly aggressive.

Indolent lymphomas may not require therapy for decades but are difficult to cure. The most common indolent lymphomas are:

- follicular lymphoma
- MALT
- CLL
- hairy cell leukemia

Aggressive lymphomas require immediate therapy and often can be cured. The most common types of aggressive lymphomas are:

- diffuse large B-cell lymphoma (DLBCL)
- mantle cell lymphoma
- Hodgkin lymphoma

Follicular Lymphoma

Most patients have lymphadenopathy but no other symptoms. Diagnosis is confirmed by cytogenetic analysis identifying a translocation [t(14:18)] that causes an overexpression of the *bcl-2* oncogene.

Therapy is withheld until patients become symptomatic. Localized symptoms can be treated with involved-field radiation combined with rituximab. Symptomatic, systemic disease is treated with rituximab plus multiagent chemotherapy. Allogeneic HSCT is curative therapy but is associated with a significant morbidity and mortality.

Mucosa-Associated Lymphoid Tissue Lymphoma

The clinical course of MALT lymphoma is usually indolent, and presentation is usually localized. Gastric MALT lymphoma occurs most commonly and is caused by chronic infection with *Helicobacter pylori*. Complete remissions are achieved in most patients after completion of antimicrobial therapy directed against *H. pylori* infection (e.g., clarithromycin, amoxicillin, and omeprazole).

Chronic Lymphocytic Leukemia

Patients are usually asymptomatic and are identified by a relative lymphocytosis. Smudge cells may be seen on the peripheral blood smear. Diagnosis is confirmed by flow cytometry demonstrating cell surface antigens CD5 and CD23. Asymptomatic patients are observed without therapy. Combination therapy with rituximab and multiagent chemotherapy is used for symptomatic late stage disease. Chlorambucil and ibrutinib are first-line therapies in older patients because of their improved tolerance.

Concomitant autoimmune disease, including immune thrombocytopenia and hemolytic anemia, is common among patients with CLL. Low serum IgG levels require replacement therapy to prevent infection. Patients are at increased risk for transformation from CLL to a large cell lymphoma requiring aggressive chemotherapy.

CLL "Smudge Cell": Peripheral blood smear showing a "smudge cell," which is a lymphocyte that appears flattened or distorted and is characteristic of CLL.

Hairy Cell Leukemia

Hairy cell leukemia is characterized by pancytopenia and progressive splenomegaly without lymphadenopathy. Typically, an attempt at bone marrow aspiration is unsuccessful. The cells have the classic appearance of thread-like projections emanating from the cell surface ("hairy" cells). Treatment with cladribine results in complete and durable remission in most patients.

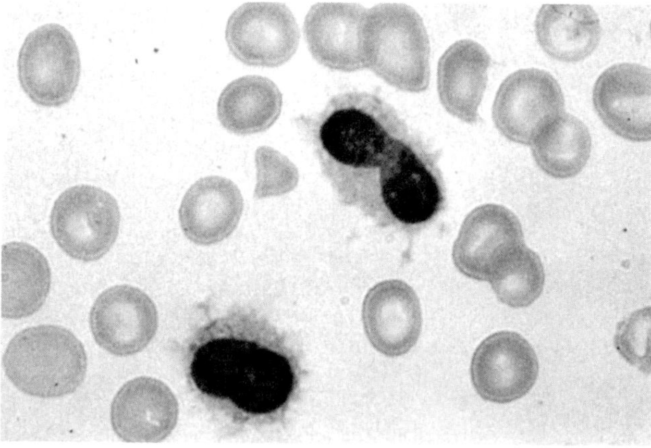

Hairy Cell Leukemia: Atypical lymphocytes with cytoplasmic projections characteristic of hairy cell leukemia.

Aggressive Large Cell Lymphomas

The most aggressive forms of large cell lymphoma are Burkitt lymphoma and lymphoblastic lymphoma. Onset of disease is acute, and patients usually present with life-threatening metabolic and structural abnormalities. Treatment is the same as that used for ALL. Treatment is associated with high response rates and is curative in nearly 50% of patients.

Mantle Cell Lymphoma

Patients present with advanced disease characterized by lymphadenopathy, weight loss, and sometimes fever, and have diffuse sites of involvement, including the GI tract, bone marrow, and blood stream. Intensive chemotherapy and autologous HSCT have increased median survival rates. Allogeneic HSCT can produce long-term remission but is associated with significant morbidity and mortality.

Hodgkin Lymphoma

Diagnosis: Hodgkin lymphoma commonly presents locally, with palpable, firm lymphadenopathy or a mediastinal mass on chest x-ray. Some patients may have B symptoms, splenomegaly, and hepatomegaly.

Hodgkin lymphoma is curable in most patients. The staging evaluation consists of PET scanning. Routine bone marrow biopsy, in the absence of unexplained blood abnormalities, is not indicated.

Treatment: ABVD followed by radiation therapy is used for all patients regardless of prognosis. Fewer chemotherapy cycles may be effective in patients with favorable prognoses.

Patients with advanced disease or those with B symptoms usually require a full course of chemotherapy.

Patients who have a negative PET scan after two to three cycles of chemotherapy have >90% likelihood of long-term disease response.

Patients with recurrent, chemotherapy-sensitive disease are candidates for autologous HSCT, whereas those with resistant disease can achieve long-term remissions with allogeneic HSCT.

Follow-up after treatment: Patients with Hodgkin lymphoma, including those cured by therapy, should be monitored for late reactivation of viruses. Patients are also at risk for secondary cancers (breast, lung, skin) and MDS. For women, begin annual mammography. In high-risk women, such as those with mantle radiotherapy treatment for Hodgkin lymphoma at a young age, the addition of MRI screening of the breasts may be appropriate.

DON'T BE TRICKED

- **All patients with Hodgkin lymphoma previously treated with mediastinal radiation who present with chest pain should be evaluated for CAD, regardless of age.**

Diffuse Large B-Cell Lymphoma (DLBCL)

DLBCL is the most common subtype of non-Hodgkin lymphoma. Most patients with DLBCL present with fever, night sweats, or weight loss ("B symptoms"), and experience rapid disease progression without therapy. Standard therapy for all patients with DLBCL, regardless of stage or prognosis, is R-CHOP. Involved-field radiation therapy is added for patients with bulky disease.

Cutaneous T-Cell Non-Hodgkin Lymphoma

Cutaneous T-cell lymphomas infiltrate skin and initially cause a rash (mycosis fungoides) and occasionally circulate in the blood (Sézary syndrome). The large, CD4-expressing malignant T cells have classic cerebriform-appearing nuclei. Disease progression manifests with raised plaques, diffuse skin erythema, and skin ulcers. In the final stages of disease progression, organ infiltration and immunodeficiency cause recurrent bacterial infections, sepsis, and death.

Early-stage disease limited to the skin is treated with topical glucocorticoids. Advanced-stage disease is often treated with electron-beam radiation therapy, photopheresis, and monoclonal antibodies. Allogeneic HSCT may be curative in young patients.

Carcinoma of Unknown Primary Origin

Diagnosis

Metastatic CUP accounts for as many as 3% to 5% of patients with solid tumors. The clinical evaluation in patients with CUP should not involve an exhaustive search for a primary site because finding an asymptomatic and occult primary site does not improve outcome. Diagnostic efforts should focus on identifying patients with CUP who have a more favorable prognosis and who can benefit from a specific treatment strategy.

Favorable subgroups include those with isolated regional lymphadenopathy, peritoneal carcinomatosis in women, and poorly differentiated non-adenocarcinoma.

STUDY TABLE: Examples of Favorable Subgroups and Management	
Axillary lymphadenopathy in women	Obtain breast MRI. If positive, treat according to stage. If negative, treat as if stage II breast cancer.
Isolated cervical lymphadenopathy	Obtain upper endoscopy, bronchoscopy, and laryngoscopy. If negative, treat with chemotherapy and radiation for head and neck cancer.
Isolated inguinal lymphadenopathy	Anorectal, genital, and perineal examination. If negative, lymph node resection or locoregional radiation.
Peritoneal carcinomatosis and ascites	Treat as ovarian carcinoma with cytoreductive surgery and chemotherapy.
Midline non-adenocarcinoma of mediastinum or retroperitoneum	Measure serum AFP and β-hCG, perform testicular exam and testicular ultrasonography; treat with platinum-containing germ cell tumor regimens.

DON'T BE TRICKED

- Do not select routine radiographic contrast studies of the GI tract.
- Do not measure CA-19-9, CA-15-3, and CA-125, because they are rarely helpful and virtually never diagnostic.
- Do not order PET scans, because the findings are rarely definitive and do not improve long-term outcome.

TEST YOURSELF

A 45-year-old woman has an axillary lymph node that is positive for adenocarcinoma. Bilateral mammogram, breast MRI, and CT scans of the chest and abdomen are normal. She has never smoked.

ANSWER: For diagnosis, choose CUP. For management, select treatment for stage II breast cancer.

Effects of Cancer Therapy

STUDY TABLE: Short- and Long-Term Effects of Cancer Therapy

Category	Potential Complications
Cardiovascular	Doxorubicin: dose-related HF (irreversible) Tamoxifen: VTE Trastuzumab: non-dose-related HF (reversible) Mediastinal radiation: myocardial, valvular, pericardial fibrosis, and premature CAD
Pulmonary	Bleomycin: pulmonary toxicity, most commonly bleomycin-induced pneumonitis Radiation: radiation-induced pneumonitis
Reproductive	Chemotherapy: premature ovarian failure, male infertility Tamoxifen: endometrial cancer
Endocrine	Radiation therapy to head and neck: hypothyroidism
Musculoskeletal	Aromatase inhibitors: osteoporosis Leuprolide, goserelin, castration: osteoporosis
Cancer	Mantle radiation: breast, lung, and esophageal cancer Chemotherapy (breast cancer): MDS and acute leukemia
Kidney and bladder	Cisplatin and ifosfamide: renal tubular damage and CKD Cyclophosphamide and ifosfamide: hemorrhage cystitis

TEST YOURSELF

A 44-year-old man is evaluated for cough and dyspnea 2 weeks after he completed his ABVD therapy for Hodgkin lymphoma. The chest x-ray shows bilateral interstitial infiltrates.

ANSWER: For diagnosis, choose bleomycin-induced lung injury.

Cancers of Infectious Origin

STUDY TABLE: Malignancies with Infectious Causes

Cancer	Associated Infection
Cervical and anal cancers	HPV Increased incidence in HIV infection Risk proportional to number of sexual partners
Kaposi sarcoma	Human herpes virus 8 Primarily in younger HIV-infected men who have sex with men May be mistaken for bacillary angiomatosis (bartonellosis)
Hodgkin lymphoma	EBV
Burkitt lymphoma	EBV t(8;14)-positive Increased incidence in HIV infection (AIDS-defining cancer) Presents as oral and nasopharyngeal cancer in China and Southeast Asia and as posttransplantation lymphoma in immunosuppressed patients
MALT lymphoma	*Helicobacter pylori* Usually involves the GI tract, particularly the stomach Treat early disease with antibiotics and PPIs (localized radiation therapy for *H. pylori*–negative disease)
HCC	Cirrhosis and hepatitis C infection or hepatitis B infection with or without cirrhosis
Non-Hodgkin lymphoma	Increased incidence in HIV infection (AIDS-defining cancer)
Head and neck (nasopharynx)	EBV
Head and neck (oropharynx)	HPV

Cancer Emergencies

Hypercalcemia

Testing: Characteristic findings are elevated serum calcium, low PTH, low or normal phosphorus, and low or normal 1,25-dihydroxyvitamin D_3 levels. PTH-related protein can be a diagnostic aid in patients with hypercalcemia of unclear cause. In these patients, an elevated level would suggest a tumor.

Treatment: All patients require immediate volume repletion with normal saline followed by forced diuresis with normal saline. Use bisphosphonates such as pamidronate and zoledronate or RANK-ligand inhibitors (e.g., denosumab) for long-term control. Add glucocorticoids in steroid-sensitive malignancies such as myeloma and lymphoma.

Hyponatremia

See Nephrology, Hyponatremia.

Treatment: Initially treat asymptomatic or mildly symptomatic patients with SIADH with fluid restriction. Give 3% sodium chloride and furosemide to symptomatic patients with altered mental status or other neurologic findings.

Deep Venous Thrombosis

Treatment: Begin long-term LMWH for initial treatment and secondary prevention of thromboembolic disease in patients with underlying cancer. Use an IVC filter if anticoagulation is contraindicated.

Metastatic Brain Tumor

See also Neurology, Metastatic Brain Tumors.

Characteristic findings:

- headache
- vomiting
- altered mental status
- focal neurologic deficits
- loss of consciousness

Testing and treatment: Obtain emergent assessment with CT or MRI.

Oral glucocorticoids are appropriate for minimally symptomatic disease; osmotic diuresis and IV glucocorticoids are used for more advanced disease. When intracranial pressure is controlled, an isolated brain metastasis can be treated with surgical excision followed by radiation. Multiple brain metastases are treated with radiation therapy (solid tumors) and chemotherapy (leukemia, lymphoma).

DON'T BE TRICKED

- **Do not treat an isolated brain mass in a young patient with HIV infection without first performing a brain biopsy to confirm lymphoma.**

Spinal Cord Compression

See also Neurology, Myelopathy.

Diagnosis: Characteristic findings include:

- localized spinal or radicular pain
- sensory loss (especially perineal)
- muscle weakness
- change in bowel or bladder function
- autonomic dysfunction

Testing: The diagnosis is established by gadolinium-enhanced MRI of the entire spine (more than one site of compression is common).

DON'T BE TRICKED

- **Do not order plain x-rays or bone scans to diagnose spinal cord compression.**

Treatment: Treat immediately with glucocorticoids and decompressive surgery followed by radiation therapy. Systemic chemotherapy is useful in patients with highly chemosensitive tumors such as lymphoma or breast cancer. Prescribe opioid therapy as needed for pain.

Superior Vena Cava Syndrome

Diagnosis: Characteristic findings are shortness of breath, cough, facial edema, plethora, swollen arms, jugular venous distention, stridor (tracheal obstruction), and prominent collateral veins on the anterior chest wall.

Testing and treatment: Mediastinal widening and pleural effusions are common radiographic findings. Tissue biopsy is essential for establishing a histologic diagnosis and guiding therapy for the specific cancer type. Mediastinoscopy is commonly used to obtain tissue and percutaneous transthoracic CT-guided needle biopsy is another acceptable approach. Diuretics and glucocorticoids can be used for symptomatic treatment pending definitive therapy.

DON'T BE TRICKED

- Up to 16% of patients with SVC syndrome have a normal chest x-ray.

STUDY TABLE: Treatment for Superior Vena Cava Syndrome

Situation	Response
Syndrome caused by previously untreated SCLC, lymphoma, or germ cell tumor	Chemotherapy
Syndrome caused by previously treated SCLC, lymphoma, germ cell tumor, or chemoinsensitive malignancies	Radiation therapy alone or in combination with chemotherapy

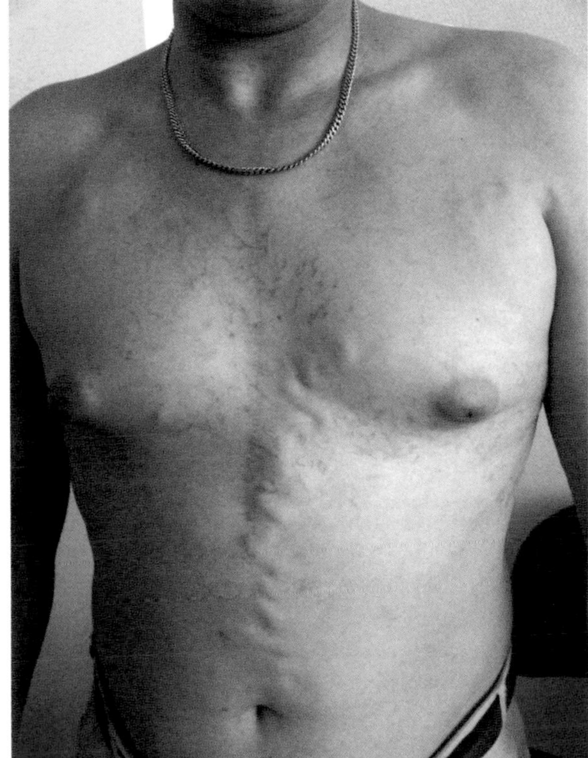

Superior Vena Cava Syndrome: Significantly dilated superficial veins transporting blood from the upper body to the lower caval vein herald the onset of SVC syndrome. By EMAHkempny - Own work, Public Domain, https://commons.wikimedia.org/wiki/File:Superior.vena.cava.syndrome.aak.jpg

Cardiac Tamponade

See also Cardiovascular Medicine, Cardiac Tamponade and Constrictive Pericarditis.

Diagnosis: Characteristic findings are:

- dyspnea, orthopnea, and clear lungs
- jugular venous distention and hepatic engorgement
- sinus tachycardia, hypotension, narrow pulse pressure, distant heart sounds, and pulsus paradoxus

Treatment: Life-threatening hemodynamic compromise is treated with immediate drainage of fluid by pericardiocentesis or pericardiotomy.

Pleural Effusion

See also Pulmonary and Critical Care Medicine, Pleural Effusion.

Diagnosis: Characteristic symptoms:

- dyspnea on exertion
- chest pain
- cough

Obtain chest x-ray or chest CT to establish a diagnosis, then perform thoracentesis for diagnosis.

Treatment: To reduce the incidence of recurrence, standard therapies include chest tube placement, prolonged drainage (over the course of a few to several days), and pleurodesis. Placement of indwelling pleural catheters is an option.

Tumor Lysis Syndrome

Diagnosis: Tumor lysis syndrome is the result of the rapid breakdown of malignant cells, resulting in dangerous increases in serum urate, potassium, and phosphate concentrations. Symptoms may include:

- nausea, vomiting, and diarrhea
- lethargy
- HF
- seizures, tetany, and syncope
- sudden death

Typically, tumor lysis syndrome occurs within 1 to 5 days of treatment and develops most commonly in patients with hematologic malignancies or other rapidly dividing tumors, such as acute leukemia and high-grade lymphoma. Risk factors include bulky disease, a high leukocyte count, high pretreatment levels of LDH or urate, compromised kidney function, and use of nephrotoxic agents. Spontaneous (pretreatment) tumor lysis syndrome occurs commonly in patients with leukemia and Burkitt lymphoma.

Prevention and treatment: Tumor lysis syndrome is prevented and managed by aggressive hydration and use of allopurinol or rasburicase. IV rasburicase is indicated for patients at high risk for tumor lysis syndrome or when rapid reduction of serum urate levels is indicated (e.g., emergently administered chemotherapy). Hyperkalemia is also aggressively treated. If acute kidney failure develops, hemodialysis may be indicated.

Febrile Neutropenia

Prevention

The prophylactic use of granulocyte colony-stimulating factor (G-CSF) or granulocyte-macrophage colony-stimulating factor (GM-CSF) reduces the risk of febrile neutropenia. Select as primary prophylaxis when the anticipated risk of neutropenic fever associated with chemotherapy is estimated to be 20% or greater or as secondary prophylaxis in patients with a previous episode of neutropenic fever.

Diagnosis

Fever is defined as a single oral temperature >38.3 °C (101.0 °F) or a temperature of >38.0 °C (100.4 °F) sustained over a 1-hour period. The first step in managing febrile neutropenia is identifying high- and low-risk patients.

- High risk is defined as neutropenia ≥7 days with an absolute neutrophil count ≤100/µL and/or significant comorbidities (e.g., hypotension, pneumonia, abdominal pain, neurologic changes).
- Low risk is defined as anticipated neutropenia <7 days and no or few comorbidities.

For all patients, obtain at least two sets of blood cultures drawn simultaneously from each central venous catheter lumen and peripheral site, and culture any obvious source of infection. Signs and symptoms guide imaging; no routine imaging tests exist.

Treatment

Management of high-risk febrile neutropenia:

- Admit all high-risk patients to the hospital for empiric IV antibiotics.
- Begin empiric monotherapy with an antipseudomonal β-lactam (e.g., cefepime), a carbapenem (e.g., imipenem-cilastin), or piperacillin-tazobactam.

Management of low-risk febrile neutropenia:

- Low-risk patients may be candidates for outpatient empiric antibiotic therapy.
- Begin oral or IV antibiotics in the clinic or hospital setting with transition to the outpatient setting if the patient remains stable during a 4- to 24-hour period of observation.
- Begin oral ciprofloxacin plus amoxicillin-clavulanate, except for patients already taking a fluoroquinolone.

Modify the initial therapy for patients at high risk for antibiotic-resistant organisms (e.g., patient unstable, early suggestive blood culture results):

- Add vancomycin, linezolid, or daptomycin for suspected MRSA infection.
- Add linezolid or daptomycin for suspected vancomycin-resistant enterococci.
- Begin empiric antifungal therapy for persistent fever despite 4 to 7 days of empiric antibiotics and anticipated neutropenia ≥7 days.

Continue antibiotics until the absolute neutrophil count is ≥500/µL or longer depending on clinical circumstances.

DON'T BE TRICKED

- Vancomycin is not recommended as standard initial therapy for febrile neutropenia.
- Do not use myeloid colony-stimulating factors for treatment of febrile neutropenia.
- Antiviral treatment is only indicated for clinical evidence of active viral infection.
- Typhlitis (necrotizing enterocolitis) should be suspected in patients with neutropenia and even minimal RLQ abdominal pain; obtain an abdominal CT scan.
- Diagnose angioinvasive aspergillosis in neutropenic patients with leukemia receiving prolonged antibiotic therapy.

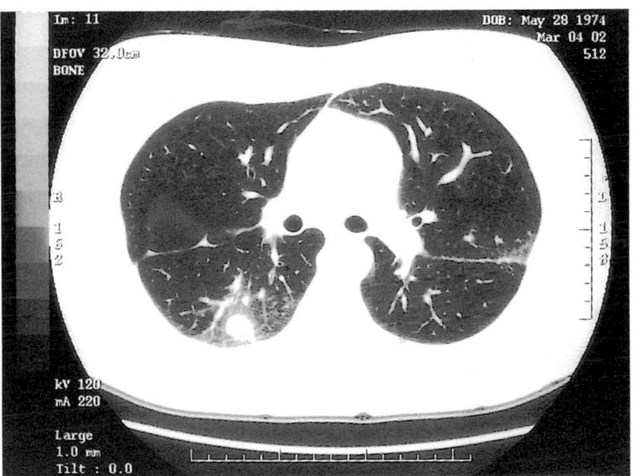

Invasive Aspergillosis: CT scan showing a dense infiltrate surrounded by a ground glass–appearing halo ("halo sign") suggestive, but not diagnostic, of invasive aspergillosis.

TEST YOURSELF

A 73-year-old man with AML develops febrile neutropenia on the eighth day of chemotherapy. Ceftazidime is begun, but after 5 days of therapy he remains febrile and neutropenic. Blood cultures are negative, and he has no localizing signs of infection.

ANSWER: For management, add amphotericin B or itraconazole.

Pulmonary and Critical Care Medicine

Pulmonary Function Tests

Indications

The four pulmonary function tests commonly used to measure static lung function are spirometry, flow-volume loops, lung volumes, and DLCO.

Key Tests and Patterns

Spirometry is used to diagnose airflow obstruction such as asthma, COPD, and bronchiectasis.

- $FEV_1/FVC < 0.7$ indicates airflow obstruction.
- A ≥12% increase in either FEV_1 or FVC and an increase ≥200 mL from baseline in either parameter with bronchodilator therapy indicates reversible airway obstruction.
- Equal reductions in FEV_1 and FVC suggest restrictive lung disease.

Flow-volume loops can help localize anatomic sites of airway obstruction. Refer to the "Flow-Volume Loops" figures and consider the following factors:

- a "scooped-out" pattern with a decreased slope on the expiratory curve that does not improve with bronchodilation indicates COPD
- a "scooped-out" pattern with a decreased slope on the expiratory curve that improves with bronchodilation indicates reversible obstructive airway disease (asthma)
- "flattening" in both inspiratory and expiratory curves and decreased airflow indicates fixed obstruction (e.g., tracheal stenosis)
- following attainment of peak flow, the flow rate declines linearly and proportionally to volume, producing a relatively straight slope characteristic of a normal flow-volume loop

Lung volumes aid in confirming findings on spirometry:

- TLC <80% indicates restrictive lung disease (fibrosis, neuromuscular disease, skeletal abnormalities)
- decreased vital capacity with increased residual volume indicates airflow obstruction

DLCO evaluates gas transport across the alveolar-capillary membrane.

STUDY TABLE: Interpreting DLCO

Finding	Interpretation
↓ DLCO and reduced lung volumes	Pulmonary fibrosis
↓ DLCO and normal lung volumes	Pulmonary vascular disease, anemia
↓ DLCO and airflow obstruction	COPD, bronchiectasis
↑ or normal DLCO and airflow obstruction	Asthma
↑ DLCO	Pulmonary hemorrhage, left-to-right shunt, polycythemia

DON'T BE TRICKED

- **In patients with low lung volumes, a normal DLCO suggests an extrapulmonary cause (e.g., obesity).**

STUDY TABLE: Understanding Important Pulmonary Tests	
Tests	**Considerations**
Pulse oximetry	Measures percentage of oxyhemoglobin; performed at rest or during exercise Use co-oximetry when carboxyhemoglobin is suspected (e.g., smoke inhalation, carbon monoxide poisoning)
Bronchial challenge testing	Challenges include cold air, exercise, histamine, and methacholine Airflow is measured before and after challenge Methacholine is commonly used for patients with a history suggestive of bronchospastic disease but normal spirometry
Cardiopulmonary exercise testing	Performed for unexplained dyspnea, symptoms disproportionate to the measured pulmonary function abnormality, and other exercise-related symptoms
6-Minute walk test	Useful to assess disability, need for supplemental oxygen, and prognosis in chronic lung conditions Simple oximetry and desaturation studies are performed at rest and with exertion
Exhaled nitric oxide test	Exhaled nitric oxide is increased in patients with airway inflammation, including asthma

DON'T BE TRICKED

- Pulse oximetry is normal in patients with carbon monoxide and cyanide poisoning.
- Pulse oximetry may be falsely low in patients with shock.

Normal

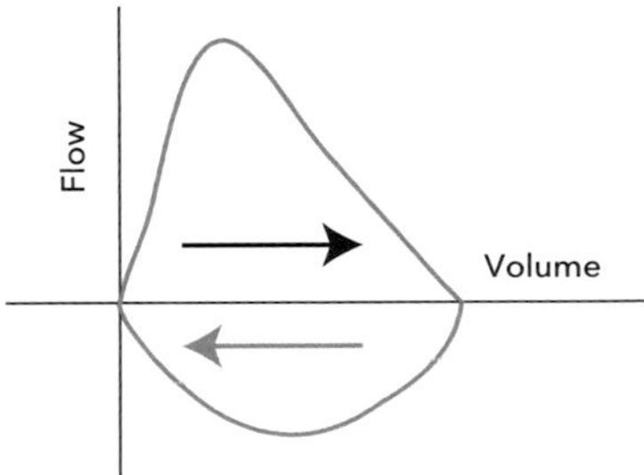

Obstructive

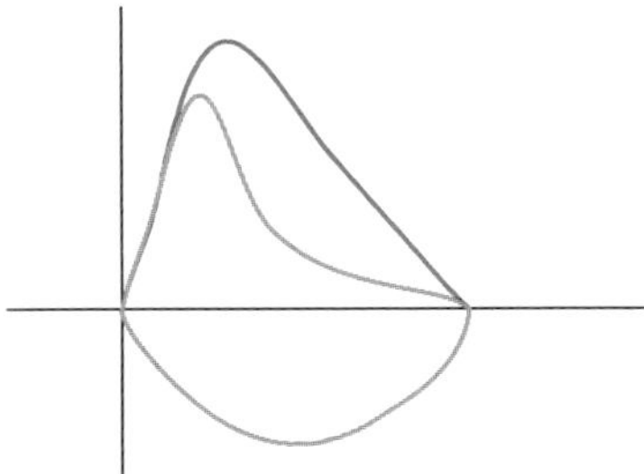

Restrictive

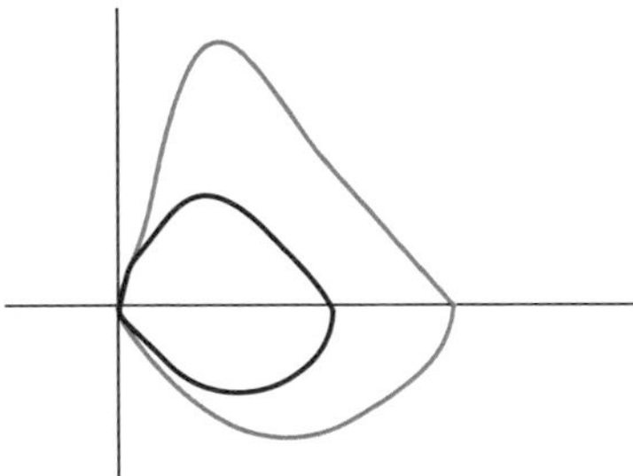

Upper Airway Obstruction

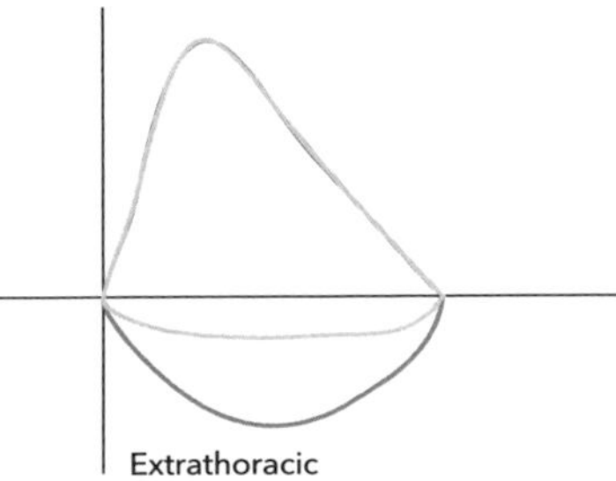

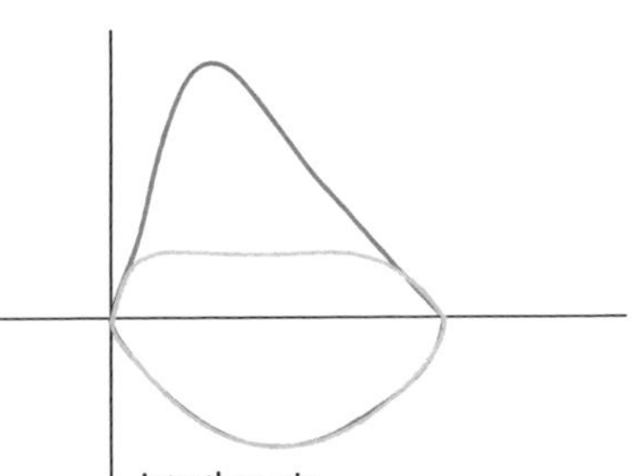

Flow-Volume Loops: Flow-volume loops plot flow (L/sec) as a function of volume.

Asthma

Diagnosis

The cardinal features of asthma are reversible airway obstruction, inflammation, and airway hyperresponsiveness.

Characteristic findings are wheezing and dyspnea; consider any cough that is nocturnal, seasonal, or related to a workplace or activity as possible asthma. Look for nasal polyps and aspirin sensitivity.

Testing

Diagnostic studies include spirometry before and after bronchodilator administration. In patients with atypical features, perform PFTs. The presence of airflow irreversibility, restrictive patterns, and significantly reduced vital capacity suggest other diseases.

Bronchoprovocation testing is indicated for patients with a suggestive clinical history for asthma but normal spirometry. Bronchoprovocation testing with exercise is indicated to diagnose exercise-induced asthma in patients who have dyspnea following exercise but normal spirometry.

DON'T BE TRICKED

- **Normal spirometry does not rule out asthma.**
- **A normal bronchoprovocation test rules out asthma; a positive test confirms airway hyperresponsiveness, of which asthma is one cause.**
- **Wheezing does not equal asthma; consider HF, COPD, vocal cord dysfunction, and upper airway obstruction.**

STUDY TABLE: Differential Diagnosis of Asthma

Disease	Characteristics
Chronic eosinophilic pneumonia	Chest x-ray shows "photographic-negative" pulmonary edema (peripheral pulmonary edema) Clinical findings: striking peripheral blood eosinophilia, fever, and weight loss in a long-term smoker Diagnose by bronchoscopy with biopsy or bronchoalveolar lavage showing a high eosinophil count
Allergic bronchopulmonary aspergillosis	Asthma manifests with eosinophilia, markedly high serum IgE levels, and intermittent pulmonary infiltrates Diagnose with positive skin test for *Aspergillus* and IgG and IgE antibodies to *Aspergillus,* characteristic radiographic opacities in the upper lobes This is often overlooked until onset of more advanced disease, including fixed obstruction and bronchiectasis
Eosinophilic granulomatosis with polyangiitis	Upper airway and sinus disease precedes difficult-to-treat asthma; look for flares associated with use of leukotriene inhibitors and glucocorticoid tapers Serum p-ANCA may be elevated Hallmark diagnostic finding is eosinophilic tissue infiltrates

Consider alternative diagnoses when asthma is difficult to control. Additional studies in these cases may include chest x-ray and echocardiography. Obtaining flow-volume loops and direct visualization of the larynx during an acute episode may be helpful in diagnosing tracheal obstruction and vocal cord dysfunction. Asthma may be an extraesophageal manifestation of GERD.

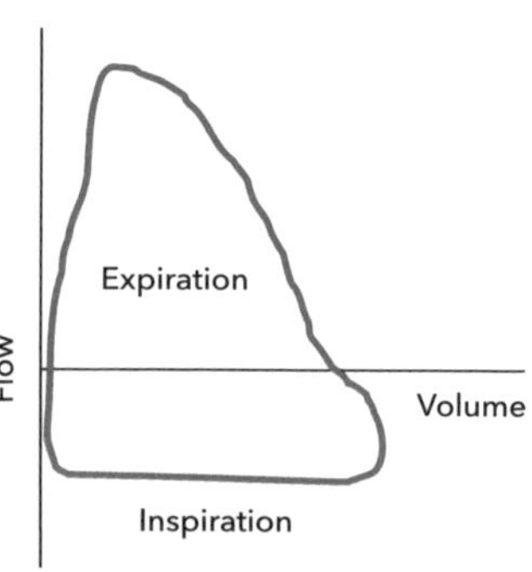

TEST YOURSELF

A 17-year-old man has difficult-to-control asthma associated with inspiratory tracheal sounds and minor wheezing. A flow-volume loop is shown.

ANSWER: For diagnosis, choose vocal cord dysfunction characterized by flattening of the inspiratory portion of the flow-volume loop.

Treatment

Asthma must be classified correctly to select proper therapy. Severity is based on the worst feature present.

STUDY TABLE: Step Classification of Asthma

Step Classification	Symptoms	Nocturnal Symptoms
Step 1: Intermittent	Symptoms ≤2 per week	≤2 per month Asymptomatic and normal PEF between exacerbations
Step 2: Mild persistent	Symptoms >2 per week but <1 per day	>2 per month
Step 3: Moderate persistent	Need for daily use of short-acting β-agonist	≥1 per week Acute exacerbations ≥2 per week
Step 4: Severe persistent	Continual symptoms that limit physical activity	Frequent

STUDY TABLE: Asthma Treatment

Step Classification	Treatment
Step 1: Intermittent	Select a short-acting β-agonist as needed
Step 2: Mild persistent	Add a low-dose inhaled glucocorticoid
Step 3: Moderate persistent	Add one of the following: 1. Low to medium doses of an inhaled glucocorticoid and a LABA (preferred) 2. Medium doses of an inhaled glucocorticoid 3. Low to medium doses of an inhaled glucocorticoid and a single long-term controller medication (leukotriene modifier or theophylline)
Step 4: Severe persistent	Add high doses of an inhaled glucocorticoid plus a LABA or LAMA and possibly oral glucocorticoids

If asthma is difficult to control, discontinue β-blockers (including ophthalmologic agents). If β-blockers must be continued, use selective β-blockers (metoprolol, atenolol). Also stop aspirin and NSAIDs if the patient is sensitive to these drugs.

Omalizumab is a monoclonal antibody directed at IgE for patients with moderate to severe persistent asthma with the following characteristics:

- inadequate control of symptoms with inhaled glucocorticoids
- evidence of allergies to perennial aeroallergen
- IgE levels between 30 and 700 kU/L

Anti-interleukin-5 monoclonal antibodies (mepolizumab, reslizumab) reduce symptoms, asthma exacerbations, and the need for oral glucocorticoids. Treatment is reserved for patients with an absolute eosinophil count >150 cells/µL and severe asthma not controlled with standard therapy.

Peak flow meters can be used at home for serial measurement of lung function and to assess the relationship of lung function to symptoms.

For all patients:

- annual influenza vaccination and pneumococcal vaccination for adults requiring controller medications
- instruction about proper inhaler technique
- evaluation for thrush, hoarseness, and osteopenia caused by inhaled glucocorticoids
- calcium and vitamin D supplements for patients taking chronic glucocorticoid treatment; early screening for osteoporosis with DEXA

DON'T BE TRICKED

- **Do not administer theophylline with fluoroquinolones or macrolides (may result in theophylline toxicity).**
- **Do not use LABAs as single agents in asthma (increased mortality rate).**

Treatment of exercise-induced asthma:

- For infrequent symptoms, treat with a SABA 15 to 30 minutes before exercise.
- For symptoms more than twice weekly, follow the Step Classification of Asthma Study Table (shown earlier).

Treatment of asthma in pregnancy:

- Control GERD.
- Step-care therapy for chronic asthma is the same for pregnant and nonpregnant patients.
- Early addition of glucocorticoids is indicated for rapid reversal of airway obstruction during an exacerbation.

Treatment of severe asthma exacerbation in the emergency department:

- Administer repeated doses of albuterol by continuous flow nebulizer or metered-dose inhaler with a spacer.
- Give early IV glucocorticoids when inhaled albuterol is ineffective.
- Inhaled ipratropium may be helpful.
- IV magnesium sulfate may be helpful for patients who have life-threatening exacerbations.
- Hospitalize patients who do not respond well after 4 to 6 hours.
- Intubate and mechanically ventilate patients with respiratory failure (see Invasive Mechanical Ventilation).
- Give oral glucocorticoids, inhaled glucocorticoids, an asthma action plan, and follow-up instructions to patients discharged home.

DON'T BE TRICKED

- **A normal arterial P_{CO_2} in a patient with severe symptomatic asthma indicates impending respiratory failure.**
- **Consider vocal cord dysfunction for patients with "asthma" that improves immediately with intubation.**

TEST YOURSELF

A 35-year-old woman with asthma has daily coughing and shortness of breath. She uses triamcinolone, 4 puffs twice daily, and albuterol, 2 puffs twice daily as needed. Her sleep is disturbed nightly by coughing. The chest examination shows soft bilateral expiratory wheezing. PEF is 60% of predicted.

ANSWER: For diagnosis, choose severe persistent asthma. For management, select adding a long-acting bronchodilator. The short-term addition of an oral glucocorticoid to the inhaled glucocorticoid and a long-acting bronchodilator would also be correct.

Chronic Obstructive Pulmonary Disease

Screening

Screening asymptomatic patients for COPD is not recommended.

Diagnosis

COPD is a heterogeneous disorder that includes emphysema, chronic bronchitis, obliterative bronchiolitis, and asthmatic bronchitis. Patients typically present with cough, sputum production, dyspnea, and decreased exercise tolerance and energy level. The features most predictive of COPD in a symptomatic patient are the combination of:

- smoking history
- wheezing on auscultation
- self-reported wheezing

Diagnose COPD when postbronchodilator spirometry shows an FEV_1/FVC ratio <0.70 associated with symptoms of chronic bronchitis, emphysema, or both.

Measure AAT level in patients with COPD <45 years who have a strong family history of COPD or without identifiable COPD risk factors (some guidelines recommend testing all patients).

STUDY TABLE: Mimics of COPD

Disease	Characteristics
Bronchiectasis	Often secondary to an inciting event, such as childhood pneumonia or TB; may be associated with foreign body, CF, immotile ciliary syndrome, nontuberculous mycobacteria, and aspergillus colonization Large-volume sputum production with purulent exacerbations; hemoptysis Chest x-ray showing "tram lines"; diagnose with HRCT
Cystic fibrosis	Obstructive pulmonary disease is most common presentation in adult patients; other symptoms may include recurrent respiratory infections, infertility Positive sweat chloride test result
Adult bronchiolitis	Found in current or former smokers; may be idiopathic or associated with other diseases such as RA Poorly responsive to bronchodilators; responds to smoking cessation and glucocorticoids
Bronchiolitis obliterans	Presents with dyspnea without improvement following bronchodilators, normal or hyperinflated lungs on chest x-ray; associated with injury to small airways; consider in patients after lung or stem cell transplantation
Upper airway obstruction	Stridor, which may be both inspiratory and expiratory Flow-volume loop shows expiratory or inspiratory flattening, or both

Treatment

Smoking cessation is essential in the management of all patients with COPD to reduce the rate of decline in lung function.

Treatment is determined by the frequency and severity of clinical symptoms and the exacerbation risk.

Strong evidence-based recommendations:

- For symptomatic patients with COPD and FEV_1 <60% of predicted, monotherapy using either long-acting anticholinergic agents (LAMAs or LABAs) is recommended.
- For symptomatic patients with an FEV_1 <50% of predicted, pulmonary rehabilitation is recommended.
- For patients with COPD who have severe resting hypoxemia (arterial Po_2 <55 mm Hg or O_2 saturation <88%), continuous oxygen therapy is recommended.

Weaker evidence-based recommendations:

- For stable patients with COPD with respiratory symptoms and FEV_1 between 60% and 80% of predicted, inhaled bronchodilators may be used.
- For symptomatic patients with stable COPD and FEV_1 <60% of predicted, combination inhaled therapies (LAMAs, LABAs, or inhaled glucocorticoids) may be considered.
- For symptomatic or exercise-limited patients with an FEV_1 >50% of predicted, pulmonary rehabilitation may be considered.

Additional indications for which long-term oxygen therapy should be considered:

- arterial blood Po_2 is 55 to 60 mm Hg with signs of tissue hypoxia (polycythemia, PH, right-sided HF)
- exercise arterial blood Po_2 is ≤55 mm Hg or O_2 saturation ≤88%

Other therapies for stable COPD:

- PDE-4 inhibitor (roflumilast) as add-on therapy for severe COPD
- long-term macrolide therapy (may reduce frequency of exacerbations when prescribed to patients with severe COPD and a history of frequent exacerbations)
- nocturnal noninvasive mechanical ventilation to improve oxygenation, improve sleep, and decrease daytime somnolence

- palliative use of oral or parenteral opioids in patients with severe COPD and unremitting dyspnea at end of life
- annual influenza and pneumococcal vaccination according to current guidelines
- consideration of lung volume reduction surgery for patients with upper lobe emphysema (heterogeneous disease) and low baseline exercise capacity to improve mortality, exercise capacity, and quality of life
- lung transplantation (can increase quality of life and functional capacity in select patients)
- augmentation therapy with IV human AAT for patients with severe AAT deficiency, AAT activity level <11 µm, and FEV_1 <65%

Antibiotics, glucocorticoids, oxygen supplementation, and noninvasive ventilation are indicated for exacerbations of COPD defined by increased sputum production, purulent sputum, and worsening dyspnea. Consider:

- tetracycline or trimethoprim-sulfamethoxazole for mild exacerbations
- β-lactam/β-lactamase inhibitor, extended-spectrum macrolides, second- or third-generation cephalosporins, or a fluoroquinolone for moderate or severe exacerbations
- IV or oral glucocorticoids
- short-acting bronchodilators (albuterol, ipratropium, or both)
- noninvasive ventilation (unless patient is obtunded, vomiting, or has excessive secretions)
- invasive mechanical ventilation if not responding or is not a candidate for noninvasive ventilation (see Invasive Mechanical Ventilation)
- pulmonary rehabilitation following hospital discharge

TEST YOURSELF

A 55-year-old man is evaluated for progressive dyspnea. He has a 40-pack-year cigarette smoking history. On spirometry, his FEV_1 is 54% of predicted. He is using an albuterol inhaler with increasing frequency. Therapy is prescribed.

ANSWER: For management, choose a LAMA or LABA.

DON'T BE TRICKED

- **Do not use short-acting and long-acting anticholinergic agents together.**
- **Short-term glucocorticoid use (<7 days) is as good as longer-term use.**
- **PDE-4 inhibitors are not indicated for acute bronchospasm.**
- **Clubbing is not a feature of COPD and suggests bronchiectasis, right-to-left cardiac shunts, or malignancy.**

Cystic Fibrosis

Diagnosis

Chronic airway inflammation and bacterial infection characterize CF-related pulmonary disease. Most adults with CF present with pulmonary disease. Characteristic findings are recurrent or persistent respiratory infections with *Pseudomonas aeruginosa*, *Staphylococcus aureus*, *Haemophilus influenzae*, or *Burkholderia cepacia*; bronchiectasis or hyperinflation; chronic sinusitis and nasal polyps; chronic or recurrent pancreatitis; clubbing; diabetes; inability to gain weight; infertility; and steatorrhea. The diagnosis is confirmed by a sweat chloride test followed by genetic testing.

DON'T BE TRICKED

- **In patients with CF and acute abdominal pain, consider intestinal intussusception.**

Treatment

All patients should receive pneumococcal conjugate and polysaccharide vaccines and influenza vaccine.

Select:

- antipseudomonal antibiotics for acute pulmonary exacerbations
- aerosolized tobramycin for suppression of chronic pulmonary infections
- aerosolized recombinant human DNase (dornase alfa) or hypertonic saline for persistent airway secretions
- inhaled bronchodilators and glucocorticoids for airway obstruction
- nighttime noninvasive mechanical ventilation for nocturnal hypoxemia or hypercarbia
- chest physiotherapy
- pancreatic enzyme replacement and fat soluble vitamin supplementation if indicated

Choose evaluation for transplantation for patients with advanced lung or liver disease.

TEST YOURSELF

A 34-year-old woman has had frequent episodes of bronchitis and three episodes of pneumonia in the past 5 years. Between episodes, she has a persistent cough producing yellow sputum. She also has been treated for multiple episodes of sinusitis. The patient is a lifelong nonsmoker. BMI is 18. The thorax is hyperresonant to percussion and has diminished air movement bilaterally. Digital clubbing is present.

ANSWER: For diagnosis, choose CF. For management, select sweat chloride testing followed by genetic testing.

Diffuse Parenchymal Lung Disease

Diagnosis

DPLD most commonly presents with dyspnea and cough, and imaging abnormalities are most often diffuse rather than focal. Consider DPLD as a cause of subacute or chronic progressive dyspnea after infection and HF have been excluded.

The diagnosis and differential of DPLD is aided by paying particular attention to the following:

- time course (typically months or years)
- active smoking history (suggests respiratory bronchiolitis-associated interstitial lung disease)
- occupation and environmental exposure history (e.g., automobile mechanics, ship builders, and asbestos exposure)
- rheumatologic disease review of symptoms
- exposure to drugs and/or radiation

Testing

Look for interstitial reticular or nodular infiltrates on chest x-ray; the type and pattern of the infiltrate correlate well with underlying pathology on lung biopsy.

Look for restrictive or combined restrictive/obstructive findings on pulmonary function tests.

Obtain chest HRCT, even if chest x-ray is normal, if clinical suspicion is high. Look for presence of hilar lymphadenopathy (sarcoidosis), pleural effusion (connective tissue-related DPLD), and pleural plaques (asbestosis).

STUDY TABLE: Distinguishing Features of Select Forms of DPLD	
Known Causes	
Drug induced	Examples: amiodarone, methotrexate, nitrofurantoin, chemotherapeutic agents
Smoking related	"Smokers" respiratory bronchiolitis characterized by gradual onset of persistent cough and dyspnea
	X-ray shows ground-glass opacities and thickened interstitium
Radiation	May occur 6 weeks to months after radiation therapy
Chronic aspiration	Aspiration is often subclinical
Pneumoconiosis	Asbestosis, silicosis, berylliosis
Connective tissue diseases	
Rheumatoid arthritis	May affect the pleura (pleuritis and pleural effusion), parenchyma, airways (bronchitis, bronchiectasis), and vasculature
	The parenchymal disease can range from nodules to organizing pneumonia to usual interstitial pneumonitis
Progressive SSc	Antibody to Scl-70 or PH portends a poor prognosis
Polymyositis/ dermatomyositis	Many different types of histology; poor prognosis
Hypersensitivity pneumonitis	Immune reaction to an inhaled low-molecular-weight antigen; may be acute, subacute, or chronic; ground-glass opacities on high resolution CT scan
Unknown Causes	
Idiopathic interstitial pneumonias	
Idiopathic pulmonary fibrosis	Chronic, insidious onset of cough and dyspnea, usually in a patient age >50 y; chest x-ray shows honeycombing, bibasilar infiltrates with fibrosis
	Diagnosis of exclusion (see Idiopathic Pulmonary Fibrosis)
Acute interstitial pneumonia	Dense bilateral acute lung injury similar to ARDS; 50% mortality rate
Cryptogenic organizing pneumonia	May be preceded by flulike illness; x-ray shows focal areas of consolidation that may migrate from one location to another
Sarcoidosis	Variable clinical presentation (see Sarcoidosis)
Rare DPLD with Well-Defined Features	
LAM	Affects women in their 30s and 40s; associated with spontaneous pneumothorax and chylous effusions
	Chest CT shows cystic disease
Chronic eosinophilic pneumonia	Chest x-ray shows "photographic negative" of HF, with peripheral alveolar infiltrates predominating
	Other findings may include peripheral blood eosinophilia and eosinophilia on bronchoalveolar lavage
Pulmonary alveolar proteinosis	Median age of 40 years, and males predominate among smokers but not in nonsmokers
	Diagnosed via bronchoalveolar lavage, which shows abundant protein in the airspaces; chest CT shows "crazy paving" pattern

DON'T BE TRICKED

- Patients with dyspnea for days or weeks (vs months) are more likely to have pneumonia or HF than DPLD.
- Plain radiography may be normal in 20% of patients with early DPLD; continue evaluation if suspicion remains high.
- Consider DPLD in patients with dyspnea and pulmonary crackles but no other findings of HF.

Treatment

When possible, treatment is directed toward the underlying cause (connective tissue disease), limiting exposure (drug discontinuation), and smoking cessation (respiratory bronchiolitis–associated interstitial lung disease). The evidence for glucocorticoid efficacy is weak.

Idiopathic Pulmonary Fibrosis

Diagnosis

IPF, the most common of the idiopathic interstitial pneumonias, is a fibrosing interstitial pneumonia. Characteristic findings are the gradual onset of a nonproductive cough and dyspnea over approximately 3 months in older adults. Physical examination findings include:

- normal temperature
- bibasilar crackles ("dry," end-inspiratory, and "Velcro-like" in quality)
- late phase cor pulmonale
- clubbing (25% of patients)

Testing

Chest x-ray shows peripheral reticular opacities and honeycomb changes at the lung bases. HRCT scan reveals subpleural cystic changes and traction bronchiectasis. A restrictive pattern is found on pulmonary function tests.

Serum ANA, rheumatoid factor, c-ANCA, and p-ANCA levels are negative or low. Video-assisted thoracoscopic lung biopsy is indicated for patients with atypical presentations.

Diagnosis is based on clinical and radiographic findings, absence of exposure to substances or drugs that can cause interstitial lung disease, and negative evaluation for rheumatologic disease.

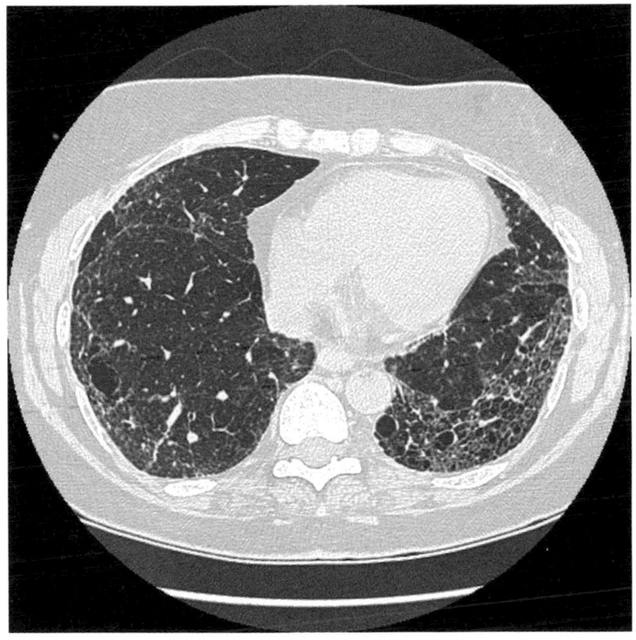

Idiopathic Pulmonary Fibrosis: High-resolution, thin-section chest CT scan showing extensive parenchymal involvement with fibrotic and honeycomb changes compatible with IPF.

Treatment

Lung transplantation may improve survival and quality of life. Pirfenidone and nintedanib have demonstrated benefit in slowing disease progression for select persons. Oxygen therapy is indicated for patients with hypoxemia.

DON'T BE TRICKED

- **Do not intubate and mechanically ventilate patients with respiratory failure caused by IPF.**

Sarcoidosis

Diagnosis

Sarcoidosis is a multisystem granulomatous inflammatory disease of unknown cause. Ninety percent of patients with sarcoidosis have pulmonary involvement, which may include a clinical presentation consistent with DPLD.

Characteristic findings include:

- fever, weight loss, and night sweats
- dry cough and dyspnea
- eye pain or burning and photosensitivity

- erythema nodosum
- violaceous or erythematous indurated papules, plaques, or nodules of the central face (lupus pernio); often associated with pulmonary disease
- a variety of papular, nodular, and plaque-like cutaneous lesions
- lymphadenopathy and hepatosplenomegaly
- asymmetric joint swelling
- Löfgren syndrome (fever, bilateral hilar lymphadenopathy, EN, and often ankle arthritis)
- uveoparotid fever (Heerfordt syndrome, featuring anterior uveitis, parotid gland enlargement, facial palsy, and fever)
- hypercalcemia (extrarenal production of calcitriol by granuloma cells) and kidney stones
- bilateral hilar lymphadenopathy, often with other enlarged mediastinal lymph nodes
- lymphadenopathy and lung parenchymal disease on chest x-ray

Testing

A definite diagnosis requires a compatible clinical picture, pathologic demonstration of noncaseating granulomas, and the exclusion of alternative explanations for the abnormalities (known causes of granulomatous inflammation such as infection). A diagnosis can be made without histologic studies in a patient with all features of Löfgren syndrome (95% diagnostic specificity).

Diagnostic studies include:

- PFT (sarcoidosis may cause obstruction, restriction, or both)
- fiberoptic bronchoscopy with transbronchial biopsy and bronchoalveolar lavage for interstitial lung disease or nodular lung involvement
- serum PTH level (low) for patients with hypercalcemia/hypercalciuria
- 1,25-dihydroxy vitamin D_3 level (high) in patients with kidney stones and hypercalcemia
- biopsy of suspicious skin lesions
- slit-lamp examination for all patients
- ECG to rule out heart block or other cardiac abnormalities in all patients

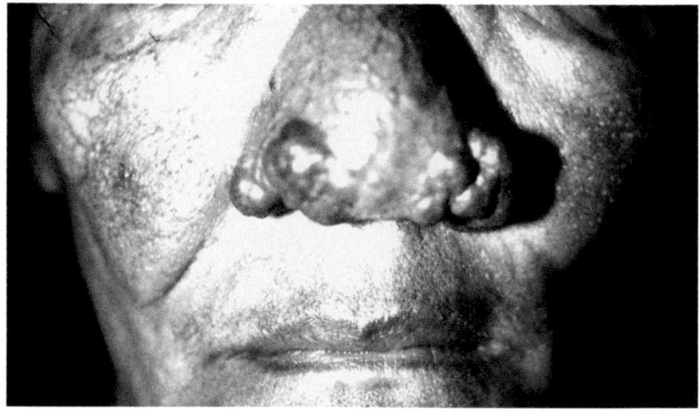

Waxy Papular Lesions: Waxy papular lesions on the nose consistent with sarcoidosis.

DON'T BE TRICKED

- **Always rule out TB and fungal infections by ordering appropriate stains and culture on tissue biopsy.**
- **Exposure to beryllium (often found in workers in light bulb or semiconductor factories) may cause a sarcoidosis-like clinical syndrome.**
- **Don't select a serum ACE level. It won't confirm the diagnosis or help in managing sarcoidosis.**

Treatment

Topical glucocorticoids are prescribed for skin lesions or anterior uveitis, and inhaled glucocorticoids are used for nasal polyps or airway disease. Oral glucocorticoids are indicated for progressive or symptomatic pulmonary sarcoidosis; hypercalcemia; or cardiac, ophthalmologic, or neurologic sarcoidosis. Patients with glucocorticoid-refractory disease are treated with immunosuppressive, cytotoxic, and antimalarial agents. Löfgren syndrome has a very high rate (80%) of spontaneous remission and resolution.

DON'T BE TRICKED

- Do not treat asymptomatic sarcoidosis.

TEST YOURSELF

A 66-year-old man is hospitalized because of azotemia and hypercalcemia. Laboratory studies show a normal serum PTH level and an elevated 1,25-dihydroxy vitamin D_3 level. A chest x-ray shows an interstitial infiltrate and an enlarged left paratracheal lymph node.

ANSWER: For diagnosis, choose sarcoidosis. For management, select transbronchial lung biopsy.

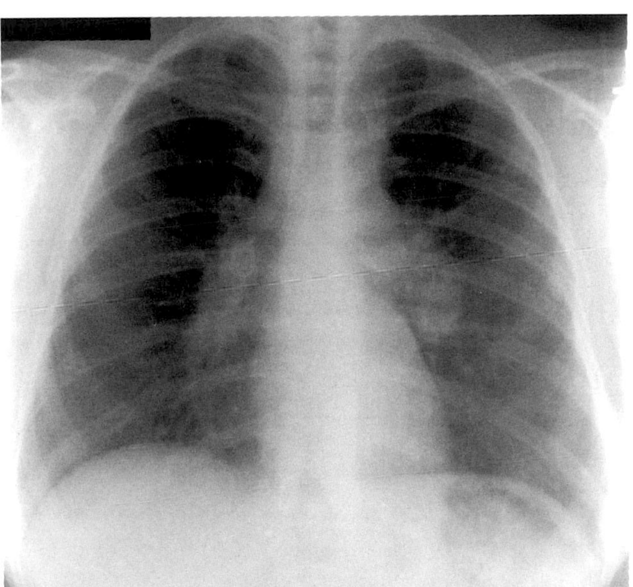

Sarcoidosis: X-ray shows bilateral hilar lymphadenopathy characteristic of sarcoidosis. Sarcoidosis can be associated with interstitial lung disease.

Occupational Lung Disease

Diagnosis

Clinical manifestations may include asthma, COPD, constrictive bronchiolitis, rhinitis, and restrictive diseases. Symptom onset following exposure can be acute (reactive airways disease/small airways dysfunction as occurs in acute chlorine gas exposure) as well as prolonged or subacute with a significant latent period (as with asbestosis).

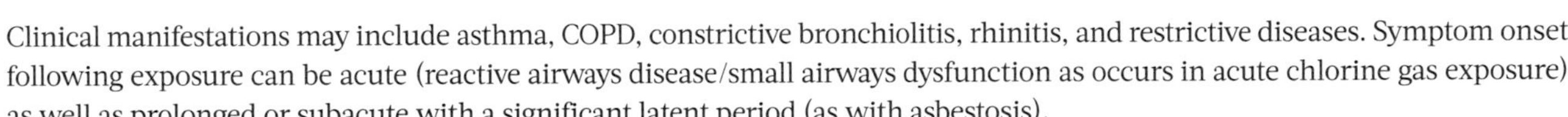

STUDY TABLE: Clues to Occupational Lung Disease
Relationship to clinical symptoms and work is temporal:
Symptoms worsen during or after work
Symptoms abate or improve with time off or away from the workplace
Work-related changes in FEV_1 or PEF
Coworkers are affected with similar symptoms
Workplace has known respiratory hazards (these can be identified by Material Safety Data Sheets from the workplace)
Symptoms fail to respond to initial therapy or are further exacerbated upon returning to work
Onset of a respiratory disorder without typical risk factors
Clustering of disease in one geographic area

A positive response to a specific inhalation challenge test is the "gold standard" for diagnosis, but not always necessary.

Treatment

The overriding principle is discontinuing the exposure. Occupational asthma and reactive airways dysfunction syndrome are treated with inhaled glucocorticoids.

DON'T BE TRICKED

- The incidence of TB is increased in those with silicosis and should be evaluated in patients with silicosis, fever, and cough.

TEST YOURSELF

A previously healthy 45-year-old man has a cough of 6 months' duration. He is a lifelong nonsmoker and works as an automobile spray painter. Physical examination discloses a few expiratory wheezes. FEV_1 is 0.65 and FEV_1/FVC ratio is 65% of predicted, and a 22% improvement occurs after bronchodilator administration.

ANSWER: For diagnosis, choose occupational asthma. For management, select spirometry or PEF measurement before and after work (or during vacation).

Asbestos-Associated Lung Diseases

Diagnosis

The most important risk factor for developing asbestos-related lung diseases is the cumulative exposure to the asbestos fiber. Occupations with the greatest exposure include those in the construction industry, the automotive servicing industry, and the shipbuilding and repair industry. The latent period for development of asbestosis and mesothelioma is 10 to 15 years. Exposure to asbestos increases the risk of lung cancer in cigarette smokers.

STUDY TABLE: Asbestos-Related Lung Syndromes

Condition	Characteristics
Pleural plaques (localized, often partially calcified)	Often an incidental finding; usually bilateral; most common manifestation of asbestos exposure Monitor patients for development of intrathoracic disease
Diffuse pleural thickening	Extensive pleural thickening extends into the visceral pleura and obliterates the costophrenic angles May cause hypercapnic respiratory failure secondary to impairment of ventilation
Rounded atelectasis	Presents as single or multiple masses caused by infolding of thickened visceral pleura with collapse of the adjacent peripheral lung The classic radiographic finding is a "comet tail" on chest CT scan extending from the hilum toward the base of the lung and then sweeping into the inferior pole of the lesion Can cause ventilatory failure
Benign pleural effusion	Exudative hemorrhagic or eosinophilic effusion; may be painful
Mesothelioma	Suggested by weight loss, fever, cough, dyspnea, chest pain, unilateral pleural abnormalities, and pleural effusion Tissue diagnosis required; cytologic diagnosis can be established by thoracentesis or closed pleural biopsy
Asbestosis	Manifests with bilateral interstitial fibrosis of the lung parenchyma, bibasilar inspiratory crackles, clubbing, restrictive physiology, and low DLCO
Lung cancer	Most asbestos-related cases occur in patients with asbestosis, but a diagnosis of asbestosis is not necessary to attribute lung cancer to asbestos exposure

Treatment

In patients with a history of asbestos exposure or asbestosis, the risk of lung cancer mortality can be decreased at any time with smoking cessation. Surgery is indicated for patients with localized mesothelioma, and radiation and chemotherapy are used to prevent recurrences. Most patients with mesothelioma have advanced disease and are treated symptomatically by controlling pleural effusions with thoracentesis.

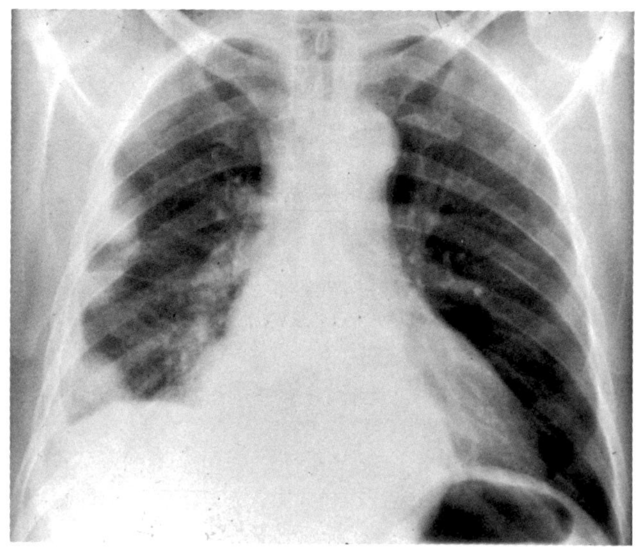

Mesothelioma: Frontal chest x-ray showing multiple pleural-based nodular infiltrates at the right chest wall and pleural thickening consistent with mesothelioma.

Pleural Effusion

Diagnosis

Most pleural effusions in the United States are the result of HF, pneumonia, or malignancy. A thoracentesis is indicated for any new unexplained effusion; however, observation and therapy without thoracentesis is reasonable in the setting of known HF, small parapneumonic effusions, or following CABG surgery.

Testing

Pleural fluid is characterized as transudative or exudative.

STUDY TABLE: Laboratory Tests for Identifying a Pleural Effusion as an Exudate

Test	Interpretation
Pleural fluid protein-serum protein ratio	>0.5
Pleural fluid LDH	>200 U/L (or >2/3 the upper limit of normal)
Pleural fluid LDH-serum LDH ratio	>0.6

An effusion is considered an exudate if any one of the above criteria are met. However, treatment (diuretics for HF), a dual diagnosis (HF and a concomitant parapneumonic effusion), or some specific diagnoses (e.g., chylothorax) can result in discordant exudates (an exudate by either the protein or LDH criterion but a transudate by the other criteria). A common cause of discordant findings is diuretic use. In the setting of ongoing diuresis, if the serum to pleural fluid albumin gradient is >1.2 g/dL, the fluid is most likely a transudate.

STUDY TABLE: Common Causes of Transudative and Exudative Pleural Effusions

Transudative Pleural Effusions	Exudative Pleural Effusions
Increased hydrostatic pressure (HF, constrictive pericarditis, SVC obstruction)	Infection
Decreased oncotic pressure (hypoalbuminemia, nephrotic syndrome, cirrhosis, malnutrition)	Neoplasm
	Autoimmune diseases
	Pulmonary infarction
	Hemothorax
	Benign asbestos effusion
	Post-coronary bypass
	Pancreatitis
	Yellow-nail syndrome (lymphatic disorders)

Pleural fluid cell counts and chemistries can further narrow the differential diagnosis.

STUDY TABLE: Pleural Fluid Cell Counts and Chemistries

If you see this...	Think this...
Bloody pleural fluid (RBC count 5000-10,000/µL)	Malignancy, pulmonary infarction, asbestos related
Nucleated cells >50,000/µL	Complicated parapneumonic effusions and empyema
Lymphocytosis >80%	TB, lymphoma, chronic rheumatoid pleuritis, sarcoidosis
pH <7.0	Complicated parapneumonic effusion, TB, rheumatoid and lupus pleuritis, esophageal rupture
Pleural fluid amylase to serum amylase ratio >1	Pancreatic disease, esophageal rupture, cancer
Glucose <60 mg/dL	Complicated parapneumonic effusion or empyema, cancer, TB, rheumatoid and lupus pleuritis, esophageal rupture

Other key points:

- Pleural fluid adenosine deaminase is elevated in most TB effusions.
- Pleural biopsy is most likely to yield a positive TB culture.
- The yield for positive malignant cytology is maximized after two samples.
- Thoracoscopy should be performed for an undiagnosed exudative effusion (two negative cytology examinations) when malignancy is suspected.

Treatment

Parapneumonic pleural effusion requires chest tube drainage when the pH is <7.2 or the pleural fluid glucose level is <60 mg/dL.

Anaerobes are cultured in up to 72% of empyemas; empiric antibiotic therapy should include anaerobic coverage.

For patients with malignant effusions, indwelling pleural catheters provide symptom relief, and up to 70% of patients achieve spontaneous obliteration of the pleural space (pleurodesis) after 6 weeks. Chemical pleurodesis with talc has a 90% success rate.

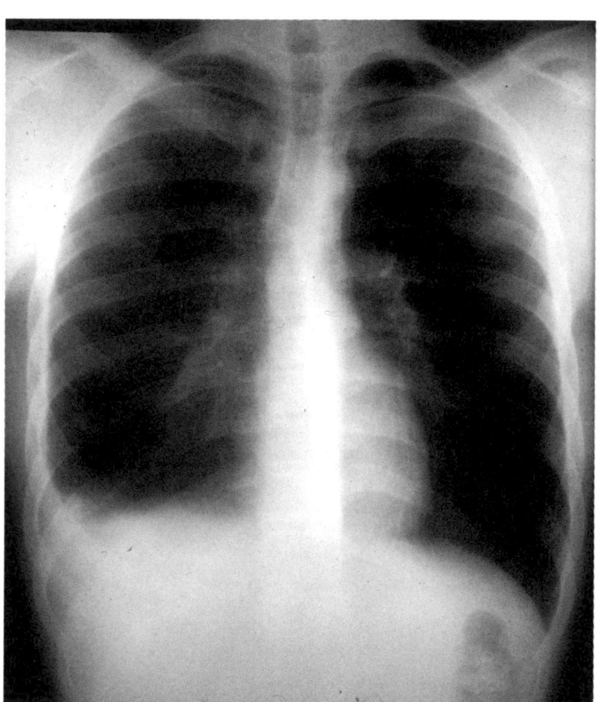

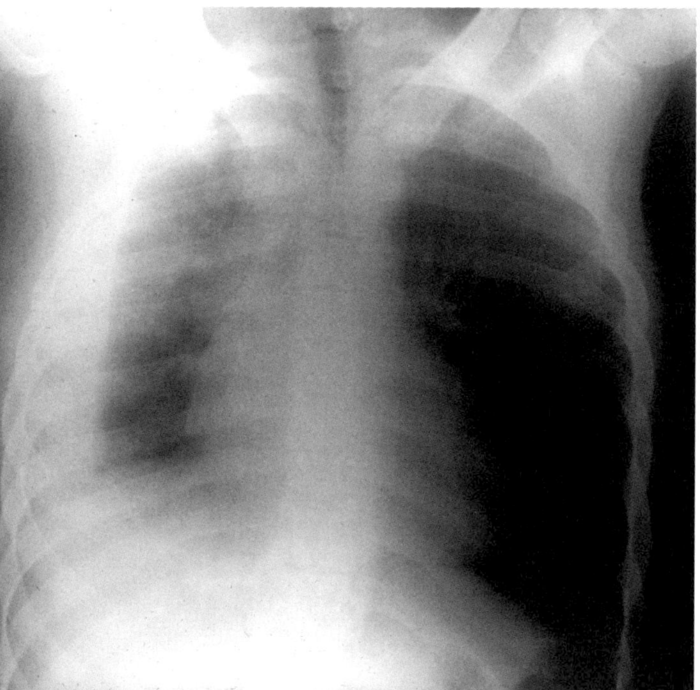

Pleural Effusion: Chest x-ray showing a right-sided pleural effusion (*left panel*) that layers out along the right thorax in the right lateral decubitus view (*right panel*).

DON'T BE TRICKED

- Always obtain thoracentesis for moderate to large effusions associated with pneumonia.
- Pleural effusions associated with nephrotic syndrome are common, but PE should be excluded in such patients because PE and renal vein thrombosis often occur in patients with nephrotic syndrome.
- Consider pulmonary LAM when chylothorax is diagnosed in a premenopausal woman.

TEST YOURSELF

A 65-year-old woman has a 2-week history of shortness of breath. A chest x-ray shows a large right-sided pleural effusion. Serum LDH is 190 U/L and total protein is 6.0 g/dL. On thoracentesis, pleural fluid protein is 2.8 g/dL and pleural fluid LDH is 110 U/L.

ANSWER: For diagnosis, choose a transudative pleural effusion.

Pneumothorax

Diagnosis

Characteristic symptoms are chest pain and dyspnea. Spontaneous pneumothorax is considered to be primary when the lung is overtly normal. Tall men who smoke are at risk. Other risk factors include cocaine use and Marfan syndrome. Subpleural blebs and bullae are commonly detected on CT scan and predispose to primary pneumothorax.

Secondary pneumothorax is associated with lung disease. Consider

- emphysema as the most common cause of secondary pneumothorax.
- pulmonary LAM in a premenopausal woman presenting with a spontaneous pneumothorax and lung disease.
- secondary pneumothorax in patients with HIV and *Pneumocystis jirovecii* pneumonia.
- tension pneumothorax with falling BP and oxygen saturation, tracheal deviation, and absence of breath sounds in one hemithorax.

Obtain an upright chest x-ray in patients with dyspnea, pleurisy, or both, even if the physical examination is normal.

Treatment

Treatment depends on the type of pneumothorax:

- observation and oxygen in asymptomatic patients with a small pneumothorax (rim of air <2 cm on chest x-ray)
- simple aspiration for symptomatic primary spontaneous pneumothorax of any size
- release of pressure with a large needle for tension pneumothorax followed by chest tube placement
- chest tube if a secondary pneumothorax measures >2 cm
- pleurodesis for a second primary spontaneous pneumothorax and after a first occurrence in secondary spontaneous pneumothorax

DON'T BE TRICKED

- Do not wait for chest x-ray results before treating suspected tension pneumothorax with needle decompression.

Pulmonary Hypertension

Screening

Patients with SSc (scleroderma) should be screened with TTE. Also screen the following patients: liver transplantation candidates with portal hypertension, first-degree relatives of patients with familial PAH, and patients with congenital heart disease with systemic-to-pulmonary shunts.

Diagnosis

PH is defined by a resting mean pulmonary arterial pressure of ≥25 mm Hg. The current classification system subdivides PH into five groups.

- Group 1 is distinguished by disease localized to small pulmonary arterioles resulting in high pulmonary vascular resistance and is referred to as PAH.
- Groups 2 through 5 refer to important secondary causes of PH and include left-sided heart disease, respiratory disorders (COPD, interstitial lung disease, and sleep-disordered breathing), and chronic venous thromboembolic disease.

Characteristic symptoms of PH include:

- unexplained dyspnea
- decreased exercise tolerance
- syncope and near-syncope
- chest pain
- lower extremity swelling

Physical examination findings indicating RV failure may include an RV heave, right-sided S_3, widely split S_2, increased P_2, increased jugular venous distention with a large *a* wave, and a murmur of TR.

Look for use of fenfluramine, amphetamines, and cocaine, as well as the presence of Raynaud phenomenon (suggesting SLE and SSc) and history of VTE.

Testing

Typical evaluation of Group 1 pulmonary hypertension (PAH) includes:

- echocardiography as the initial study; a systolic pulmonary artery pressure >40 mm Hg is suggestive of PH
- bubble contrast echocardiography or TEE is indicated to evaluate for intracardiac shunts (e.g., ASD)
- right heart catheterization to confirm the diagnosis and quantify the degree of PH
- left heart catheterization and coronary angiography exclude LV dysfunction as a cause of PH

If the diagnosis of PAH is confirmed, the next step is a vasoreactivity test using vasodilating agents to measure changes in pulmonary artery pressure with a right heart catheter in place.

Additional recommended tests to rule out other causes of PH include pulmonary function tests, liver function tests, polysomnography if clinically indicated, and serologic tests for HIV infection or connective tissue disease.

In some patients (<5%) after an acute PE, thromboemboli within the pulmonary arteries become remodeled into large occlusive scars, causing CTEPH and leading to right-sided HF.

Two diagnostic criteria for CTEPH:

- pulmonary arterial pressure ≥25 mm Hg in the absence of left-sided HF
- compatible imaging evidence of chronic thromboembolism by V/Q scanning

DON'T BE TRICKED

- **Most cases of PH are attributed to left-sided heart disease and hypoxic respiratory disorders.**
- **Do not select an HRCT scan to diagnose CTEPH. A V/Q scan is superior.**

Treatment

Therapy for PH groups 2 through 5 is typically directed at the underlying condition.

For Group 1 PH (PAH), vascular-targeted treatments provide symptomatic relief but are not curative.

- Calcium channel blockers are used for patients demonstrating a vasodilator response on right heart catheterization.
- Lung or heart-lung transplantation should be considered for patients in whom drug treatment is unsuccessful.
- Oxygen therapy is indicated for O_2 saturation ≤90%.

Life-long anticoagulant therapy is indicated in all patients with CTEPH. Pulmonary thromboendarterectomy is the only definitive therapy for CTEPH.

DON'T BE TRICKED

- **Do not select calcium channel blockers if pulmonary artery pressure is not decreased with a vasoreactivity test.**

Pulmonary Arteriovenous Malformation

Diagnosis and Testing

Pulmonary AVMs consist of abnormal communications between pulmonary arteries and veins. They are included in the differential diagnosis of hypoxemia, pulmonary nodules, and hemoptysis. The following suggest a pulmonary AVM:

- hemoptysis
- mucocutaneous telangiectasias
- evidence of right-to-left pulmonary shunts (hypoxemia, polycythemia, clubbing, cyanosis, stroke, brain abscess)

Chest CT is the initial diagnostic test.

Treatment

Symptomatic or large pulmonary AVMs (>2 cm) are treated with either embolotherapy or surgery.

TEST YOURSELF

A 46-year-old man is evaluated for a TIA. Telangiectasias are present on the lips. The lungs are clear, and cardiovascular and neurovascular examinations are normal. Laboratory evaluation reveals polycythemia and an arterial P_{O_2} of 68 mm Hg. Chest x-ray shows a 2-cm solitary pulmonary nodule.

ANSWER: For diagnosis, choose pulmonary AVM.

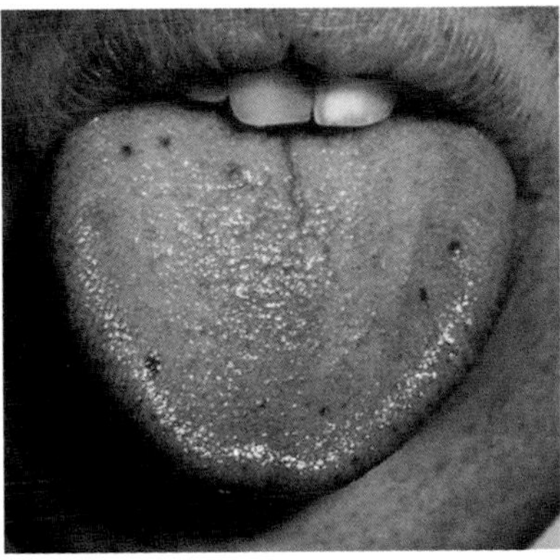

Telangiectasia: Telangiectasias on the tongue in a patient with hereditary hemorrhagic telangiectasia.

Lung Cancer Screening

In high-risk populations, lung cancer screening results in a 20% lung cancer mortality reduction. Screen patients between the ages of 55 and 74 to 79 years (guidelines vary) who have a 30-pack-year history of smoking and who are currently smoking or have quit within the last 15 years. Continue annual low-dose CT imaging until comorbidity limits survival or the patient reaches the age of 75 to 80 years. Stop screening in patients who have stopped smoking for 15 years.

DON'T BE TRICKED

- The risks of screening outweigh the benefit in patients at low risk for lung cancer.

Hemoptysis

Diagnosis

Bronchitis, bronchogenic carcinoma, and bronchiectasis are the most common causes of hemoptysis.

DON'T BE TRICKED

- Confirm that a patient has hemoptysis rather than epistaxis or GI bleeding; then check the platelet count and coagulation parameters.

STUDY TABLE: Diagnostic Tests for Hemoptysis

Test	Considerations
Chest x-ray	Crucial initial study, but normal findings do not exclude lung cancer
Fiberoptic bronchoscopy	For patients at high risk for lung cancer, even if chest x-ray is normal
Chest CT	Alternative test when fiberoptic bronchoscopy is contraindicated or when bleeding persists despite normal bronchoscopic findings

Treatment

Treatment is cause specific. The cause of death from massive hemoptysis is asphyxiation from airway obstruction. If the bleeding site can be localized to one lung, position the patient with the bleeding lung dependent. Intubation and mechanical ventilation are required when adequate gas exchange is threatened. Angiography can localize and treat bronchial artery lesions.

Solitary Pulmonary Nodule

Diagnosis

An SPN is a lesion of the lung parenchyma measuring ≤3 cm in diameter that is not associated with other lesions or lymphadenopathy and is not invading other structures. Approximately 35% of SPNs are bronchogenic carcinomas.

STUDY TABLE: Diagnostic Tests for a Pulmonary Nodule

Test	Considerations
Comparison with previous chest x-ray	Stability over time helps rule out malignancy
Contrast-enhanced CT	Most useful imaging method
Fiberoptic bronchoscopy with biopsy	Provides sufficient information in only 30% of lesions
Percutaneous transthoracic needle aspiration biopsy	Has a higher yield for malignant lesions but is not always diagnostic
PET scan	Positive in >90% of malignant solitary nodules >1 cm in diameter. Can demonstrate unsuspected mediastinal and/or distant disease.

The management of SPNs depends on the size and risk of malignancy. **Solid** SPNs <8 mm are managed differently than larger nodules and subsolid nodules. A **subsolid** nodule is less dense than a solid nodule, and normal lung structures such as blood vessels can be seen through the nodule. Subsolid nodules, either pure ground glass or with a solid component, often represent premalignant disease such as adenocarcinoma in situ.

STUDY TABLE: Fleischner Society Recommendations for Single Pulmonary Nodule Follow-Up

Risk Factors for Lung Cancer?	Size	Recommended Follow-Up
No (low-risk patient)	<6 mm	No follow-up
	6-8 mm	CT at 6-12 months, then consider CT at 18-24 months
	>8 mm	Consider CT at 3 months, PET/CT, or tissue sampling
Yes (high-risk patient)	<6 mm	Optional CT at 12 months
	6-8 mm	CT at 6-12 months, then CT at 18-24 months
	>8 mm	Consider CT at 3 months, PET/CT, or tissue sampling

Data from MacMahon H, Naidich DP, Goo JM, Lee KS, Leung ANC, Mayo JR, et al. Guidelines for management of incidental pulmonary nodules detected on CT images: from the Fleischner Society 2017. Radiology. 2017;284:228-243. [PMID: 28240562] doi:10.1148/radiol.2017161659.

STUDY TABLE: Fleischner Society Recommendations for Follow-Up of Solitary Subsolid Lung Nodule

Imaging Findings	Size	Recommended Follow-Up
Pure ground glass	<6 mm	No follow-up
	≥6 mm	CT at 6-12 months to confirm persistence, then CT every 2 years until 5 years
Part solid nodule	<6 mm	No follow-up
	≥6 mm	CT at 3-6 months to confirm persistence. If unchanged and solid component remains <6 mm, annual CT should be performed for 5 years

TEST YOURSELF

A 65-year-old man is incidentally found to have a 7 mm pulmonary nodule on chest x-ray obtained before an elective cholecystectomy. On chest CT, the nodule is subsolid, and no other nodules or lymphadenopathy is evident. He has a 50-pack year history of cigarette smoking.

ANSWER: For management, choose follow-up chest CT in 1 year.

Pulmonary mass, defined as >3 cm in diameter, is highly suspicious for malignancy in a patient with risk factors. Either a biopsy for tissue diagnosis (in the absence of suspected metastases) or surgical resection (if no evidence of metastatic disease) is typically the first step in the evaluation.

DON'T BE TRICKED

- Before ordering contrast CT, bronchoscopy, or PET scan, compare current image with previous image to determine stability over time.
- PET scans may be falsely negative in alveolar cell carcinoma or lesions <1 cm in diameter and falsely positive in various inflammatory lesions.
- A nonspecific negative result from fiberoptic bronchoscopy or transthoracic needle aspiration biopsy does not reliably exclude the presence of a malignant growth.

Mediastinal Masses

Diagnosis

The mediastinum can be divided into three separate compartments, which can help narrow the differential diagnosis of a mediastinal mass.

STUDY TABLE: Mediastinal Masses

Origin of Mass	Important Associations
Anterior Mediastinum	
Thymus	Most common tumor of anterior mediastinum; 40% have MG Other syndromes include pure red cell aplasia and acquired hypogammaglobulinemia
Teratoma/germ cell	Teratomas may contain fat, fluid, and bone discernable on CT imaging
Lymphoma	Second most common anterior mediastinal tumor; Hodgkin disease is the most common lymphoma
Thyroid	Often causes compressive symptoms (dyspnea, dysphagia)
Middle Mediastinum	
Lymph nodes	Lymphadenopathy is the most common cause of middle mediastinal masses
Cysts	Includes benign pericardial, bronchogenic, and esophageal cysts
Posterior Mediastinum	
Neurogenic tumors	Schwannomas are most common in adults

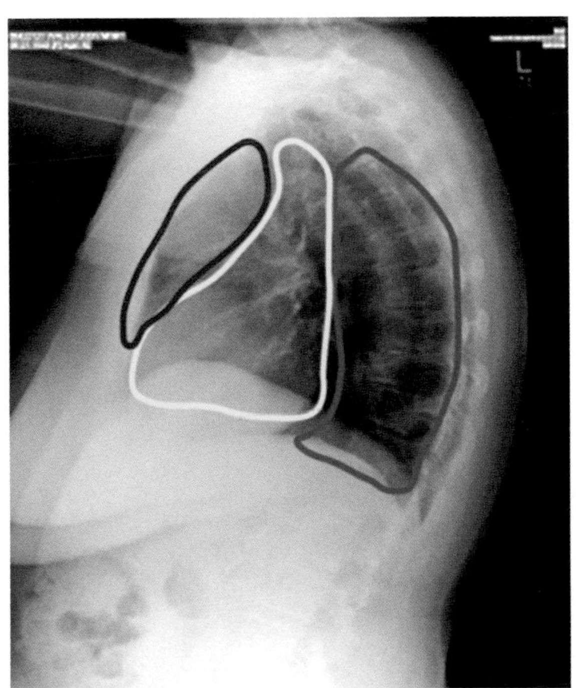

Mediastinum: A lateral chest x-ray demonstrates the anterior (red), middle (yellow), and posterior (blue) mediastinal compartments.

Obstructive Sleep Apnea

Diagnosis

OSAs are typically accompanied by oxyhemoglobin desaturations and are terminated by an awakening from sleep. The severity of OSA can be classified based on the number of apneas plus hypopneas per hour of sleep (apnea-hypopnea index [AHI]).

Characteristic findings of OSA include snoring, apnea, excessive daytime sleepiness, and obesity (determined by either BMI >30 or neck circumference >17 in) and an enlarged and elongated soft palate (crowded pharynx).

Occasionally, OSA first presents following a surgical procedure involving general anesthesia and/or narcotic analgesia, where repeated apneas, acute respiratory failure, and even death occur. Screening questionnaires (STOP-Bang) are available to identify OSA during preanesthesia evaluation.

Patients with untreated OSA have a greater likelihood of developing CAD, acute MI during sleep, systemic and PAH, HF, recurrent AF, stroke, insulin resistance, mood disorders, and parasomnias.

Diagnose OSA in patients with an AHI of >5/h during a sleep study. Other options include out-of-center sleep testing.

DON'T BE TRICKED

- Do not confuse obesity-hypoventilation syndrome with OSA. Obesity-hypoventilation syndrome is usually associated with COPD and always with elevated arterial P_{CO_2} levels when awake.
- Obesity-hypoventilation syndrome may coexist with OSA.
- Overnight oximetry has not been validated as a screening tool for OSA.

Treatment

Lifestyle changes, including weight loss, avoiding alcohol and sedatives before bedtime, and sleeping in the lateral position are always indicated. CPAP is the initial treatment of choice for OSA and has been shown to improve quality of life, cognitive function, and symptoms of daytime sleepiness.

BPAP therapy, in which inspiratory and expiratory pressures can be adjusted separately, may be useful in patients who have coexisting OSA and obesity-hypoventilation syndrome, who do not tolerate CPAP, have concurrent central sleep apneas, or have persistent oxygen desaturation because of hypoventilation despite CPAP therapy. Therapy may be required for up to 4 weeks before ABGs improve.

Oral appliances are an alternative to CPAP therapy for mild to moderate OSA. Oral appliances are not as effective as CPAP in reducing AHI.

DON'T BE TRICKED

- Supplemental oxygen is not recommended as a primary therapy for OSA.
- Upper airway surgery is not recommended as initial therapy for OSA.

High-Altitude–Related Illness

Diagnosis

HAI encompasses a number of disorders that can occur when a person residing at low altitude ascends to higher elevation. HAI is more common at elevations ≥2500 meters (approximately 8200 feet).

STUDY TABLE: High-Altitude Illnesses		
Disorder	**Pathophysiology**	**Clinical Findings**
High-altitude periodic breathing (HAPB)	Hypoxia-induced hyperventilation lowers Pco_2 toward the apneic threshold, decreasing respiratory rate, which raises Pco_2 and results in recurrent hyperventilation	Repetitive arousals from sleep, often with paroxysms of dyspnea
Acute mountain sickness (AMS)	Hypoxia and hypocarbia-induced alterations in cerebral blood flow	Headache, fatigue, nausea, and vomiting, in addition to disturbed sleep related to HAPB
High-altitude cerebral edema (HACE)	Brain edema at altitudes typically above 10,000-13,000 feet	Confusion, irritability, ataxia, coma, and death
High-altitude pulmonary edema (HAPE)	PH and pulmonary edema	Cough, dyspnea at rest, pink frothy sputum, hemoptysis, and pulmonary crackles

Prevention and Treatment

HAI can be prevented by gradually ascending. Acetazolamide accelerates the acclimatization. Acetazolamide, dexamethasone, and supplemental oxygen are used to treat AMS. Definitive treatment for HACE is immediate descent from altitude; dexamethasone, supplemental oxygen, and hyperbaric therapy may also be used. The HAPE treatment of choice is supplemental oxygen and rest.

DON'T BE TRICKED

- Do not treat HAPE with diuretics and nitrates.

Hypercapnic Respiratory (Ventilatory) Failure

Diagnosis

Hypercapnic respiratory (ventilatory) failure occurs when alveolar ventilation is inadequate and the level of CO_2 increases in the blood. Because oxygenation also depends on ventilation, patients are often hypoxic as well. However, hypoxia will often improve with supplemental oxygen. Chronic hypercapnic respiratory failure occurs most often in patients with:

- COPD
- neuromuscular disease (MG, ALS, MS)
- restrictive lung diseases (parenchymal lung disease, chest wall skeletal disorders, obesity)
- depressed respiratory drive (opioids and sedatives)

Testing

In patients with neuromuscular disease, pulmonary function tests show restriction on spirometry and lung volume measurement but normal diffusing capacity.

Patients with respiratory muscle weakness, obesity-hypoventilation syndrome, and disorders of ventilatory control first hypoventilate during REM sleep. Order polysomnography if nocturnal hypoventilation is suspected (daytime sleepiness, nocturnal awakenings, morning headaches).

TEST YOURSELF

A 36-year-old man with myotonic dystrophy awakens at night gasping for air and experiences increasing fatigue. Cardiopulmonary examination is normal. Neurologic examination shows 4+/5 strength in all muscle groups.

ANSWER: For diagnosis, choose nocturnal hypercapnic respiratory failure. For management, elect polysomnography.

Hypoxic Respiratory Failure

Hypoxic respiratory failure is caused by inadequate oxygenation of hemoglobin. The most common causes of hypoxic respiratory failure in the ICU are V/Q mismatch and shunt, which occurs when perfused areas of the lung are not ventilated.

Acute Respiratory Distress Syndrome

ARDS is a syndrome of hypoxemic respiratory failure presenting as noncardiogenic pulmonary edema. Precipitating causes of ARDS include pulmonary infection, hemorrhagic shock, pancreatitis, trauma, transfusions, and sepsis.

STUDY TABLE: Diagnosing and Classifying ARDS	
Features common to all cases of ARDS	Acute onset (<1 week), known clinical insults (ARDS risk factors)
	Bilateral lung opacities on imaging not fully explained by effusions, lobar/lung collapse or nodules
	Respiratory failure not explained by HF or volume overload (although ARDS can coexist with HF or fluid overload states)
Mild ARDS	Arterial Po_2/Fio_2 ratio of 201-300 mm Hg, measured with PEEP ≥5 cm H_2O
Moderate ARDS	Arterial Po_2/Fio_2 ratio of 101-200 mm Hg, measured with PEEP ≥5 cm H_2O
Severe ARDS	Arterial Po_2/Fio_2 ratio of ≤100 mm Hg, measured with PEEP ≥5 cm H_2O

STUDY TABLE: Mimics of ARDS

Disease	Characteristics
Cardiogenic pulmonary edema	History of cardiac disease, enlarged heart, S_3, chest x-ray showing an enlarged cardiac silhouette, pleural effusions, and Kerley B lines
	Rapid improvement with diuresis or afterload reduction
Diffuse alveolar hemorrhage	Acute kidney injury with microscopic or gross hematuria or other evidence of vasculitis present
	Associated with stem cell transplantation
	Hemosiderin-laden macrophages in bronchoalveolar lavage fluid
Acute eosinophilic pneumonia	Cough, fever, pleuritic chest pain, and myalgia; may be precipitated by initiation of smoking
	>15% eosinophils in bronchoalveolar lavage fluid
Hypersensitivity pneumonitis	Typically slower onset than ARDS (over weeks) with progressive course; however, may present in an advanced stage, mimicking ARDS
	Positive exposure history (farmers, bird fanciers, hot tub exposure)
Cryptogenic organizing pneumonia	May be precipitated by viral syndrome
	Slower onset than ARDS (>2 weeks) with progressive course; however, may present in an advanced stage, mimicking ARDS
Acute interstitial pneumonia	May be impossible to distinguish from ARDS
	Absence of typical inciting factors for ARDS
	May respond to glucocorticoid administration

Treatment

Optimal mechanical ventilation associated with the prevention of ventilator-associated lung injury includes:

- lung-protective ventilation using volume-controlled ventilation with a tidal volume of ≤6 mL/kg of ideal body weight (low tidal volume)
- plateau (end-inspiratory) pressure <30 cm H_2O (even if this results in "permissive" hypercapnia and acidosis)
- PEEP

Limiting IV fluids and using diuretics to keep CVP at lower targets has been associated with a more rapid improvement in lung function, shorter duration of mechanical ventilation, and shorter ICU length of stay but no effect on mortality.

Use of prone positioning in severe ARDS has a mortality benefit.

DON'T BE TRICKED

- Glucocorticoids are not indicated for the acute treatment of ARDS.

TEST YOURSELF

A 55-year-old woman with acute pancreatitis has increasingly severe shortness of breath for 12 hours. She has no history of cardiac disease. Pulse rate is 116/min, respiration rate is 40/min, and arterial O_2 saturation is 86% (on supplemental oxygen). Diffuse bilateral crackles are heard. Chest x-ray shows diffuse airspace disease. She is intubated and mechanically ventilated. With an FIO_2 of 1.0, her arterial PO_2 is 150 mm Hg.

ANSWER: For diagnosis, choose moderate ARDS. For management, select a tidal volume of 6 mL/kg of ideal body weight.

Noninvasive Positive-Pressure Ventilation

Indications in Critically Ill Patients

NPPV is the use of positive-pressure ventilation without the need for an invasive airway. NPPV may be used as the ventilatory mode of first choice in four conditions:

- COPD exacerbations (not stable COPD)
- cardiogenic pulmonary edema
- neuromuscular disease
- prevention of recurrent respiratory failure in recently extubated high-risk patients

The most common contraindications to NPPV include:

- respiratory arrest
- medical instability
- inability to protect airway and/or excessive nausea or vomiting
- uncooperative or agitated patient

Improvements in blood gas values and clinical condition should occur within 2 hours of starting NPPV. If not, intubation should be considered to avoid undue delay and prevent respiratory arrest.

Invasive Mechanical Ventilation

Indications

Patients may require invasive mechanical ventilatory support for hypoxic respiratory failure (low arterial PO_2) or impaired alveolar ventilation (increased arterial PCO_2). In general, if a patient cannot maintain an arterial PO_2 >60 mm Hg or an O_2 saturation >90% despite supplemental oxygen of 60% or higher, initiating mechanical ventilation is usually appropriate, regardless of the arterial PCO_2.

Management

In volume-targeted ventilation, set tidal volume first:

- the recommended range is 6 to 8 mL/kg of ideal body weight (≤6 mL/kg for ARDS)
- tidal volumes that are too high can result in barotrauma, respiratory alkalosis, and decreased cardiac output
- tidal volumes that are too low can result in atelectasis, hypoxemia, and hypoventilation

Set respiratory rate:

- the respiration rate is usually started at 8 to 14/min if the patient is otherwise clinically stable
- a respiratory rate that is too high can result in respiratory alkalosis and air trapping (auto-PEEP)
- a respiratory rate that is too low can result in hypoventilation, acidosis, hypoxemia, and patient discomfort

Set oxygen flow and PEEP to maintain arterial Po_2 >60 mm Hg.

Be alert for auto-PEEP.

- In the presence of increased airway resistance, a high demand for ventilation, or a short expiratory time, air flow may still occur at end exhalation, resulting in positive pressure in the alveoli at end exhalation.
- Suspect auto-PEEP if the flow tracing on the ventilator shows continuous expiratory flow until the start of inspiratory flow.

Common causes of auto-PEEP include COPD or acute asthma, ARDS (increased flow resistance), and a high minute ventilation (>12-15 L/min). Characteristic findings are wheezing and marked expiratory prolongation, drop in BP, and patient restlessness. Strategies to minimize auto-PEEP:

- treat airway obstruction (e.g., bronchodilators in COPD or asthma)
- decrease the respiratory rate or tidal volume
- increase the inspiratory flow rate (shorten inspiratory time)
- prolong the expiratory time
- allow permissive hypercapnia
- sedate and/or paralyze the patient

STUDY TABLE: Ventilator Management

If you would like to ...	... the intermediate step is ...	... make the ventilator do this by:	Notes:
Improve respiratory acidosis	↓ Arterial Pco_2	Increasing respiratory rate Increasing tidal volume: in volume control mode, directly choose the tidal volume; in pressure control mode, increase the inspiratory support pressure to increase tidal volume	Watch for auto-PEEP at high respiratory rates, which can cause hypotension by reducing preload Don't be tricked: If the patient has ARDS, respiratory acidosis (pH ~7.2) should generally be tolerated rather than raising the tidal volume >6 mL/kg
Improve respiratory alkalosis	↑ Arterial Pco_2	Decreasing respiratory rate Decreasing tidal volume	If the patient is breathing faster than the set ventilator rate, this strategy won't work Determine why respiratory alkalosis is present (sepsis, PE, liver disease, pain)
Improve tissue oxygenation	↑ O_2 saturation, arterial Po_2	Increasing Fio_2 Increasing PEEP	Occasionally, increasing PEEP will lower cardiac output by reducing preload; this can worsen oxygen delivery to tissues If no contraindications, attempt to increase preload with IV fluids

Difficult ventilation or complications of mechanical ventilation resulting from changes in airway resistance may first be manifested by an increase in the peak inspiratory pressure alone, resulting from:

- bronchospasm
- secretions in airways, endotracheal tube, or ventilator tubing
- obstructing mucus plug
- agitation with dyssynchrony with the ventilator

Difficult ventilation resulting from a change in lung compliance will be manifested by an increase in both peak inspiratory pressure and plateau pressure, resulting from:

- right mainstem intubation
- pneumothorax
- worsening airspace disease (ARDS, pneumonia, pulmonary edema)

Placing intubated patients in a semirecumbent position and using selective decontamination of the oropharynx (using topical gentamicin, colistin, or vancomycin) reduces the risk of VAP.

When a patient can maintain an arterial O_2 saturation >90% breathing FIO_2 ≤0.5, PEEP <5 cm H_2O, and pH >7.30, it is reasonable to consider extubation. Paired daily spontaneous awakening trials (withdrawal of sedatives) with daily spontaneous breathing trials result in a reduction in mechanical ventilation time, ICU and hospital length of stay, and 1-year mortality rates.

DON'T BE TRICKED

- **Do not select synchronized intermittent mandatory ventilation as a weaning mode because studies have demonstrated it actually takes longer to liberate patients from the ventilator.**

TEST YOURSELF

A 73-year-old woman who weighs 56 kg (123 lb) is admitted to the ICU with an exacerbation of severe COPD. Intubation and mechanical ventilation are required: FIO_2 of 0.4, tidal volume of 450 mL, and respiration rate of 16/min. Thirty minutes later, her BP has dropped to 82/60 mm Hg. She is restless and has diffuse wheezing with prolonged expiration.

ANSWER: For diagnosis, choose auto-PEEP. For management, select treatment of airway obstruction.

Sepsis

Diagnosis

Sepsis is life-threatening organ dysfunction caused by a dysregulated host response to infection. Septic shock is defined as a subset of sepsis in which profound circulatory, cellular, and metabolic abnormalities are associated with a greater risk of mortality than with sepsis alone.

Know the differential diagnosis of shock syndromes and their associated hemodynamic parameters.

STUDY TABLE: Shock Syndromes

Condition	Characteristics
Cardiogenic shock	Low cardiac output, elevated PCWP, and high SVR
Hypovolemic shock	Low cardiac output, low PCWP, and high SVR
Obstructive shock	Low cardiac output, variable PCWP, and high SVR Consider cardiac tamponade, PE, and tension pneumothorax
Anaphylactic shock	High cardiac output, normal PCWP, and low SVR Rash, urticaria, angioedema, and wheezing/stridor
Septic shock	High cardiac output (early) that can become depressed (late) and low SVR Fever and leukocytosis

SVR = systemic vascular resistance.

Treatment

STUDY TABLE: Treatment of Sepsis and Septic Shock

Treatment	Application
Fluid resuscitation	Balanced crystalloids 500-1000 mL boluses 2-4 L (30 mL/kg) in the first 6 h
Vasopressors	Norepinephrine, vasopressin (norepinephrine sparing agent) Indicated for persistent hypotension unresponsive to fluids Target MAP ≥65 mm Hg Target lactic acid ↓ by 10%-20% in first 6 h
Source identification and control	Blood cultures, cultures of potential sites of infection, chest x-ray, urinalysis
Antibiotic therapy	Initiate within 1 h of diagnosis Narrow coverage based on culture and sensitivity findings Reasonable choice for sepsis of unclear cause and low *Pseudomonas* risk: vancomycin plus one of the following: ceftriaxone or cefotaxime, piperacillin-tazobactam, or imipenem If high *Pseudomonas* risk: vancomycin plus two antipseudomonal agents (e.g., ceftazidime, cefepime, imipenem, piperacillin-tazobactam)
Hydrocortisone	200 mg/d IV for persistent hypotension despite fluids and vasopressors
Glucose control	Insulin therapy to maintain glucose between 140- 200 mg/dL
Mechanical ventilation	Tidal volume ≤6 mg/kg of ideal body weight if ARDS present

DON'T BE TRICKED

- Do not perform cortisol stimulation testing.
- Do not use noninvasive ventilation.

Nutritional Support During Critical Illness

Diagnosis

Nutrition is an essential part of management for patients in the ICU and can be given enterally or parenterally, with the enteral route preferred. Total parenteral nutrition is associated with GI mucosal atrophy and translocation of gut bacteria into the bloodstream, which predisposes patients to infection.

Treatment

Initiation of enteral nutrition is recommended at 24 to 48 hours following admission. Critically ill patients who cannot maintain volitional nutritional intake may be fed using a gastric tube, large-bore tube, small-bore tube, or postpyloric tube. The formula of 25 to 35 kcal/kg/d can be used to estimate caloric need in patients in the ICU. For patients who cannot tolerate enteral feeding, total parenteral nutrition should not be started before day 7 of an acute illness. However, parenteral nutrition should be started as soon as possible for severely malnourished patients and those at high risk of malnutrition when enteral nutrition is not possible.

ICU-Acquired Weakness

Diagnosis

ICU-acquired weakness includes critical illness polyneuropathy (with axonal nerve degeneration) and critical illness myopathy (with muscle myosin loss), resulting in profound weakness. ICU-acquired weakness may be first recognized when a patient is unable to be weaned from mechanical ventilation. Risk factors include hyperglycemia, sepsis, multiple organ dysfunction, and SIRS.

Therapy

Treatment is supportive and includes early mobility and ongoing physical and occupational therapy.

TEST YOURSELF

A 65-year-old woman with type 2 diabetes cannot be weaned from mechanical ventilation. She has required prolonged respiratory support because of ARDS secondary to septic shock and bacterial pneumonia. Her course was complicated by an episode of AKI. During spontaneous weaning trials, her tidal volume is low and respiratory rate is elevated. She has weakness of her extremities and hyporeflexia.

ANSWER: For diagnosis, choose ICU-acquired weakness. For management, select treatment with physical and occupational therapy.

Hyperthermic Emergencies

Severe hyperthermia is temperature >40.0 °C (104.0 °F) resulting from a failure of normal thermoregulation. Findings include loss of consciousness, muscle rigidity, seizures, and rhabdomyolysis with kidney failure, DIC, and ARDS.

STUDY TABLE: Severe Hyperthermia Causes and Therapy

Diagnosis	Suggestive History	Key Examination Findings	Treatment	Notes
Heat stroke (exertional)	Young athlete or soldier with environmental exposure	Encephalopathy and fever	Ice water immersion	Rapid response supports diagnosis
Nonexertional heat stroke	Age ≥70 years Use of anticholinergic, sympathomimetic, and diuretic drugs	Encephalopathy and fever	Evaporative, external cooling	Avoid ice water immersion
Malignant hyperthermia	Exposure to volatile anesthetic (halothane isoflurane, succinylcholine, or decamethonium)	Masseter muscle rigidity; ↑ arterial Pco_2	Stop the inciting drug Dantrolene	Monitor and treat; ↑ K^+ and ↑ arterial Pco_2
Neuroleptic malignant syndrome	Haloperidol, olanzapine, quetiapine, and risperidone or withdrawal from L-dopa; onset over days to weeks	Altered mentation, severe rigidity, ↑ HR, ↑ BP, no clonus, ↓ reflexes	Stop the inciting drug Dantrolene Bromocriptine	Resolves over days to weeks
Severe serotonin syndrome[a]	Onset within 24 h of initiation or increasing dose	Agitation, rigidity, clonus, ↑ reflexes	Stop the inciting drug Benzodiazepines Cyproheptadine	Resolves in 24 hours

[a]Not routinely considered a cause of severe hyperthermia but commonly confused with neuroleptic malignant syndrome

DON'T BE TRICKED

- Neuroleptic malignant syndrome may occur in patients who have abruptly discontinued L-dopa for Parkinson disease.
- The serotonin syndrome is often caused by the use of SSRIs and the addition of a second drug that increases serotonin release or blocks its uptake or metabolism.

TEST YOURSELF

A 45-year-old woman undergoes open cholecystectomy. At the conclusion of the operative procedure, her temperature has abruptly increased to 39.2 °C (102.5 °F).

ANSWER: For diagnosis, choose malignant hyperthermia caused by anesthesia. For management, select dantrolene initiation.

Hypertensive Emergency

Hospitalize a patient with hypertensive emergency (BP ≥180/120 mm Hg and symptoms or evidence of end-organ damage).

For a compelling condition (such as aortic dissection, severe preeclampsia or eclampsia, or pheochromocytoma crisis), SBP should be reduced to <140 mm Hg during the first hour and to <120 mm Hg in aortic dissection.

Without a compelling condition, SBP should be reduced by no more than 25% within the first hour; then, if stable, reduce to 160/100 mm Hg within the next 2 to 6 hours; finally, cautiously reduce to normal during the following 24 to 48 hours. See Neurology for treatment of hypertension associated with ischemic stroke and intracerebral hemorrhage.

For patients without a compelling indication, treatment consists of short-acting IV drugs administered in the ICU (e.g., nitroglycerin, nitroprusside, labetalol, nicardipine).

STUDY TABLE: IV Antihypertensive Drugs for Treatment of Hypertensive Emergencies in Patients with a Compelling Comorbidity

Comorbidity	Preferred Drugs
Acute aortic dissection	Esmolol, labetalol
Acute pulmonary edema	Nitroglycerin, nitroprusside β-Blockers contraindicated
ACS	Esmolol, nitroglycerin
AKI	Nicardipine
Eclampsia or preeclampsia	Hydralazine, labetalol, nicardipine ACE inhibitors, ARBs, renin inhibitors, nitroprusside contraindicated

DON'T BE TRICKED

- Do not select sublingual nifedipine for either hypertensive urgency or emergency.

Anaphylaxis

Diagnosis

Anaphylaxis is a life-threatening syndrome caused by the release of mediators from mast cells and basophils triggered by an IgE-allergen interaction (*anaphylactic reaction*) or by a non-antibody-antigen mechanism (*anaphylactoid reaction*). The most common causes are nut ingestion, insect stings, latex, and medications (penicillin, NSAIDs, aspirin).

Flushing, urticaria, conjunctival pruritus, bronchospasm, nausea, and vomiting usually develop within minutes to 1 hour if the antigen was injected or up to 2 hours if ingested.

Anaphylactic shock is caused by severe hypovolemia (fluid shifts owing to increased vascular permeability) and vasodilatation.

The diagnosis of anaphylaxis is made clinically. Death occurs from refractory bronchospasm, respiratory failure with upper airway obstruction, and cardiovascular collapse.

DON'T BE TRICKED

- **Consider latex allergy as cause of anaphylaxis during surgery or anaphylaxis in a woman during coitus.**

Treatment

Epinephrine is first-line therapy even if the only presenting signs are hives or pruritus. Use inhaled bronchodilators for bronchospasm and IV saline for shock or hypotension.

β-Blockers may blunt the effect of epinephrine, but epinephrine remains the drug of first choice; reserve glucagon for epinephrine-refractory anaphylaxis.

Patients with diffuse rash or anaphylaxis from hymenoptera sting (bee, yellow jacket, and wasp) should undergo venom skin testing and immunotherapy.

DON'T BE TRICKED

- **IM or subcutaneous epinephrine (0.3-0.5 mg of 1:1000) is first-line treatment for classic anaphylaxis. IV epinephrine (1:10,000) is reserved for anaphylactic shock or refractory symptoms.**
- **Red man syndrome seen with IV vancomycin infusion is not an allergic reaction.**

TEST YOURSELF

A 25-year-old woman has shortness of breath and wheezing after a bee sting 1 hour ago. Her BP is 80/50 mm Hg and HR is 110/min.

ANSWER: For diagnosis, choose anaphylaxis. For management, select epinephrine and IV fluids, observation for at least 12 hours, and self-administered epinephrine at discharge.

Angioedema

Diagnosis

Angioedema is characterized by a sudden, temporary edema, usually of the lips, face, hands, feet, penis, or scrotum. Abdominal pain may be present owing to bowel wall edema.

Mast cell-mediated angioedema is often associated with urticaria, bronchospasm, or hypotension. This can be the result of an allergic reaction (peanuts, shrimp, latex, insect stings) or to direct mast cell stimulation (NSAIDs, radiocontrast media, opiates).

Bradykinin-mediated angioedema is NOT associated with urticaria. In the setting of angioedema without urticaria, the differential is very limited.

STUDY TABLE: Differential Diagnosis of Bradykinin-Mediated Angioedema

Condition	Historical Clues/Disease Associations	Laboratory Studies
Hereditary angioedema	Family history of angioedema	Low C1 inhibitor and C4 levels
Acquired C1 inhibitor deficiency	Lymphoma, MGUS, or SLE	Low C1q levels (in addition to low C4 and C1 inhibitor levels)
ACE inhibitor effect	Medication history	Low C1 inhibitor and C4 levels

DON'T BE TRICKED

- In patients with urticaria and angioedema, do not diagnose hereditary angioedema.

Treatment

Select epinephrine, antihistamines, and glucocorticoids for acute episodes of mast cell–mediated (allergic) angioedema with airway compromise or hypotension. Patients should carry an epinephrine autoinjector. Use antihistamines alone in cases of allergic angioedema that is not part of an anaphylaxis syndrome (absent airway compromise or hemodynamic instability).

Select C1 inhibitor concentrate for acute episodes of bradykinin-mediated angioedema (hereditary or acquired angioedema); use FFP in an emergency. For long-term management of hereditary angioedema, select danazol and stanozolol to elevate hepatic synthesis of C1 esterase inhibitor protein.

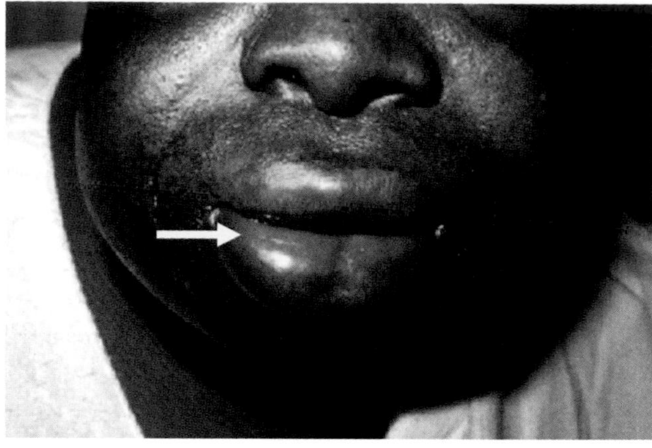

Angioedema: Angioedema differs from urticaria in that it covers a larger surface area and involves the dermis and subcutaneous tissues.

DON'T BE TRICKED

- **Epinephrine is not effective for hereditary angioedema.**

TEST YOURSELF

A 40-year-old man has a 1-year history of cramping abdominal pain and 2- to 3-day episodes of face and hand swelling that have not responded completely to epinephrine and antihistamines. His mother died suddenly of "suffocation."

ANSWER: For diagnosis, choose hereditary angioedema. For management, select serum C4 and C1 inhibitor levels (functional and antigenic) and treatment of severe acute episodes of swelling with C1 inhibitor concentrate.

Smoke Inhalation

Ensuring upper airway patency is the priority.

- Patients with a visibly damaged airway or stridor require immediate intubation.
- Assess carbon monoxide level.
- Cyanide exposure is common in house fires where cyanide is produced and aerosolized when vinyl burns. Cyanide is a common coexposure with carbon monoxide. A normal LDH level excludes cyanide poisoning. Treat cyanide poisoning with hydroxocobalamin.

DON'T BE TRICKED

- **Patients with inhalational injury involving the lower airways typically present with a clear chest x-ray; wheezing, cough, and dyspnea manifest 12 to 36 hours after exposure.**
- **Normal oxygen saturation does not exclude either carbon monoxide or cyanide poisoning.**

Poisoning with Therapeutic Agents

Key Considerations

STUDY TABLE: Poisoning with Common Therapeutic Agents

Toxin	Clinical Syndrome	Antidote/Intervention
Acetaminophen	Hepatotoxicity	*N*-acetylcysteine
Benzodiazepines	Sedative/hypnotic	Observation; flumazenil
β-Adrenergic blockers	Bradycardia, hypotension	Glucagon, calcium chloride, pacing
Calcium channel blockers	Bradycardia, hypotension	Atropine, calcium, glucagon, pacing
Digoxin	Dysrhythmias	Digoxin-immune fab
Heparin	Bleeding diathesis	Protamine sulfate
Narcotics	Narcotic effects	Naloxone
Salicylates	Metabolic acidosis/respiratory alkalosis	Urine alkalinization, hemodialysis
Tricyclic antidepressants	Anticholinergic effects	Blood alkalinization, α-agonist

Carbon Monoxide Poisoning

Diagnosis and Testing

Characteristic findings are unexplained flulike symptoms, frontal headache, lightheadedness, difficulty concentrating, confusion, delirium, coma, dyspnea, nausea, and chest pain that are often associated with use of a grill or burning heat source indoors. Order ABG studies and serum carboxyhemoglobin measurement for all patients with neurologic changes, dyspnea, chest pain, or smoke exposure. A carboxyhemoglobin level >25% in any patient is diagnostic of severe acute carbon monoxide poisoning.

DON'T BE TRICKED

- **Pulse oximetry data are unreliable because the oximeter is unable to differentiate carboxyhemoglobin from oxyhemoglobin.**

Treatment

Normobaric oxygen therapy is the treatment of choice. Hyperbaric oxygen therapy is indicated for patients with severe carbon monoxide poisoning (characterized by loss of consciousness and persistent neurologic deficits), pregnant patients, or patients with evidence of cardiac ischemia.

TEST YOURSELF

A 39-year-old man is found unconscious by his family. He had not been seen since late the previous evening. The outside temperature was below freezing overnight. He is unresponsive and deeply cyanotic. The patient is intubated and ventilated with 100% oxygen. Although the O_2 saturation is 100%, he remains comatose.

ANSWER: For diagnosis, choose carbon monoxide poisoning. For management, select carboxyhemoglobin level measurement.

Alcohol Poisoning

See the Nephrology chapter for discussion of alcohol poisoning.

Toxidromes

STUDY TABLE: Toxic Syndromes Manifestations and Treatments

Syndrome	Manifestations	Representative Drugs	Treatment
Sympathomimetic	Tachycardia Hypertension Diaphoresis Agitation Seizures Mydriasis	Cocaine Amphetamines Ephedrine Caffeine	Benzodiazepines for agitation Avoid β-blockers for hypertension Haloperidol may worsen hyperthermia
Cholinergic	"SLUDGE" Confusion Bronchorrhea Bradycardia Miosis	Organophosphates (insecticides, sarin) Carbamates Physostigmine Edrophonium Nicotine	Organophosphates poisoning requires external decontamination Atropine May require ventilatory support Add pralidoxime for CNS toxicity Benzodiazepines for convulsions
Anticholinergic	Hyperthermia Dry skin and mucous membranes Agitation, delirium Tachycardia, tachypnea Hypertension Mydriasis	Antihistamines Tricyclic antidepressants Antiparkinson agents Atropine Scopolamine	Physostigmine for those with peripheral and CNS symptoms Benzodiazepines for agitation May require ventilatory support
Opioids	Miosis Respiratory depression Lethargy, confusion Hypothermia Bradycardia Hypotension	Morphine and related drugs Heroin	Naloxone

SLUDGE = Salivation, Lacrimation, increased Urination and Defecation, Gastrointestinal upset, and Emesis.

Rheumatology

Approach to the Patient

Analyze joint disease using three parameters: acuity (acute or chronic), inflammation (inflammatory or noninflammatory), and number of joints involved (monoarticular, oligoarticular, or polyarticular).

STUDY TABLE: Features of Inflammatory vs. Noninflammatory Pain

Feature	Inflammatory Pain	Noninflammatory Pain
Physical examination findings	Erythema; warmth; soft-tissue swelling	No soft-tissue swelling; minimal or no warmth; bony enlargement and joint effusions may occur in OA
Morning stiffness	>60 min	<30 min
Constitutional symptoms	Fever; fatigue; malaise	Generally absent
Synovial fluid	Leukocyte count >2000/µL, neutrophils in acute inflammation, monocytes in chronic inflammation	Leukocyte count between 200/µL and 2000/µL, predominantly monocytes
Other laboratory findings	Elevated ESR, CRP; anemia of inflammation	Inflammatory markers usually normal or minimally elevated

STUDY TABLE: Synovial Fluid Characteristics

Characteristic	Normal	Noninflammatory[a]	Inflammatory[b]	Septic[c]
Leukocytes/µL	<200	200-2000	2000-100,000	>50,000 (usually >100,000)
PMN cells (%)	<25	<25	>50	>75

[a]Examples: OA, osteonecrosis, hemochromatosis, sickle cell disease.

[b]Examples: crystalline arthritis, RA, spondyloarthropathy, SLE.

[c]Infectious arthritis, including staphylococcal, gonococcal, and tuberculous.

Categorization of arthritis by number and distribution of involved joints narrows the differential diagnosis.

STUDY TABLE: Categories of Common Joint Disease

Acuity and Inflammation	Monoarticular	Oligoarticular (2-4 joints)	Polyarticular (≥5 joints)
Acute Inflammation[a]	Bacterial infection Crystal-induced	Disseminated gonococcal infection RF Lyme disease	Viral infections: hepatitis A and B, parvovirus, rubella, HIV
Chronic Inflammation	Infections related to fungi, mycobacteria, spirochetes (syphilis and Lyme disease)	Spondyloarthropathies	RA, SLE, psoriatic arthritis, crystalline arthritis
Chronic Without Inflammation	OA	OA	OA

[a]Acute is usually defined as symptoms for less than 6 weeks; chronic is symptoms lasting ≥6 weeks.

Serologic Studies in Rheumatologic Disorders

STUDY TABLE: Serologic Studies/Associations	
Test	**Association (does not establish diagnosis)**
ANA	SLE, SSc, Sjögren syndrome; titer does not correlate with disease activity
Anti-Sm	SLE; most specific for SLE but does not correlate with disease activity
Anti-U1 RNP	MCTD
Anticentromere pattern of ANA	CREST syndrome; SSc and PH
Anti-dsDNA antibody	SLE; correlates with disease activity, especially kidney disease
Anti-smooth muscle antibody	Autoimmune hepatitis
Anti-La/SSB antibody	Sjögren syndrome; neonatal SLE
Anti-Scl-70 antibody	SSc and pulmonary fibrosis/diffuse cutaneous SSc
Antihistone antibody	Drug-induced SLE
Anti-Ro/SSA antibody	Sjögren syndrome, neonatal heart block, subacute cutaneous lupus
c-ANCA (anti-PR3 antibody)	Granulomatosis with polyangiitis
p-ANCA (anti-MPO antibody)	Eosinophilic granulomatosis with polyangiitis and MPA
Anti-Jo-1 antibody	Polymyositis and antisynthetase syndrome
Anti-CCP antibody	Rheumatoid arthritis

CREST = calcinosis, Raynaud phenomenon, esophageal dysmotility, sclerodactyly, telangiectasia.

DON'T BE TRICKED

- **Do not test for ANA sub-serologies if ANA is negative unless subacute cutaneous lupus (anti-SSA) or polymyositis (anti-Jo-1) is suspected.**
- **Don't confuse anti-Sm antibodies (associated with SLE) and anti-smooth muscle antibodies (associated with autoimmune hepatitis).**

Rheumatoid Arthritis

Diagnosis

RA is a symmetric inflammatory polyarthritis that primarily involves the small joints of the hands and feet. Characteristic findings include:

- morning stiffness lasting >1 hour
- seven classic sites of symmetric joint pain (PIP, MCP, wrist, elbow, knee, ankle, and MTP joints)
- synovitis characterized by soft-tissue swelling or effusion
- subcutaneous nodules over bony prominences or extensor surfaces
- symptoms present for >6 weeks

Testing

Laboratory findings include:

- positive rheumatoid factor (sensitivity 80%; specificity 87%); 70% of RA patients have rheumatoid factor at time of diagnosis
- elevated ESR or CRP level
- normocytic anemia
- positive anti-CCP antibody assay (sensitivity 70%; specificity 95%); 70% of RA patients have anti-CCP antibody at time of diagnosis

X-ray: More than half of patients with untreated RA develop erosions within the first 2 years of disease if not appropriately treated; baseline and subsequent x-rays aid in the diagnosis and follow-up of therapy. Other findings include periarticular osteopenia and symmetric joint-space narrowing.

Ultrasonography is more sensitive than x-ray for identification of synovitis and erosions.

MRI is useful for detecting cervical spine subluxation or myelopathy.

DON'T BE TRICKED

- A negative rheumatoid factor does not exclude RA; anti-CCP antibody assay may be positive, or the patient may have seronegative RA.
- A positive rheumatoid factor alone is not diagnostic of RA.
- Fluctuations in rheumatoid factor do not mirror disease activity, and serial testing is not indicated.
- Not all symmetric arthritis is RA.

STUDY TABLE: Rheumatoid Arthritis Mimics

If you see symmetric arthritis and...	Diagnose this...
Skin rash and leukopenia	SLE
Psoriasis or pitted nails	Psoriatic arthritis
Day care worker or contact with small children	Parvovirus B19 infection (usually self-limited after 1-3 months)
2nd and/or 3rd MCP and PIP joint arthritis with hook-like osteophytes	Hemochromatosis
Raynaud phenomenon and sclerodactyly	SSc
Proximal muscle weakness	Polymyositis or dermatomyositis
Recent immunizations	Post-rubella immunization arthritis
Tophi with symmetric small joint involvement of the hands and feet	Chronic tophaceous gout

DON'T BE TRICKED

- Viral infections can cause short-lived inflammatory arthritis involving small joints; symmetric joint inflammation present >6 weeks strongly suggests RA.

STUDY TABLE: Extra-articular Manifestations of Rheumatoid Arthritis

If you see this in an RA patient...	Think this...
Arm paresthesias and hyperreflexia	C1-C2 subluxation (increased risk of cord compression with tracheal intubation)
Cough, fever, pulmonary infiltrates	Bronchiolitis obliterans organizing pneumonia (BOOP)
Foot drop or wrist drop	Mononeuritis multiplex (vasculitis)
Hoarseness	Cricoarytenoid involvement
Multiple basilar pulmonary nodules	Caplan syndrome (pneumoconiosis related to occupational dust; characterized by rapid development of multiple basilar nodules and mild airflow obstruction)
Dry eyes and/or mouth	Sjögren syndrome
Pleural effusion with low plasma glucose (<30 mg/dL)	Rheumatoid pleuritis
Pulmonary fibrosis	Rheumatoid interstitial lung disease
Skin ulcers, peripheral neuropathy	Rheumatoid vasculitis
Splenomegaly and granulocytopenia	Felty syndrome
Red, painful eye	Scleritis, uveitis
HF	Rheumatoid disease or anti-TNF therapy

Other complications include increased risk of pulmonary infections, CAD, and osteoporosis.

DON'T BE TRICKED

- **All RA patients undergoing general anesthesia should have cervical spine x-rays to assess for atlantoaxial subluxation.**

Treatment

"Treat to target," with the target being remission or low disease activity.

- Select NSAIDs and low-dose oral and intra-articular glucocorticoids for quick symptomatic relief; these agents do not alter the course of the disease.
- Methotrexate is the initial DMARD for most patients with RA and should be instituted immediately in patients with erosive disease. It is continued indefinitely and can be used in combination with other nonbiologic and biologic DMARDs. Leflunomide may be used with or as a substitute for methotrexate.
- Monotherapy with hydroxychloroquine or sulfasalazine or combination therapy with these agents is for early, mild, and nonerosive disease.
- Combination therapy with hydroxychloroquine, sulfasalazine, and methotrexate is more effective than monotherapy with methotrexate or sulfasalazine plus hydroxychloroquine.

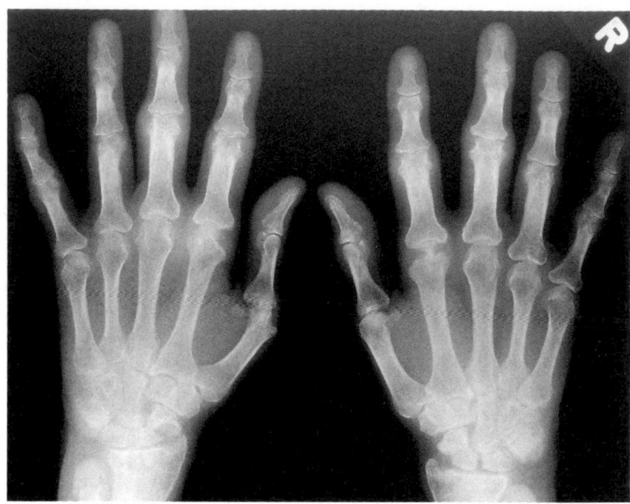

Hand X-ray, Rheumatoid Arthritis: Carpal, metacarpal, and PIP joints show periarticular osteopenia, joint-space narrowing, and marginal erosions, all characteristic of RA.

Biologic therapy: Indicated when disease control is not achieved with oral DMARDs. Initial therapy is a TNF-α inhibitor added to baseline methotrexate therapy. The TNF inhibitors include etanercept, infliximab, adalimumab, certolizumab, and golimumab. Tofacitinib is an oral biologic agent that may be effective in patients not responding to methotrexate.

- Screen for and treat latent TB before starting biologic therapy.
- Perform periodic TB screening during biologic therapy.

Common toxicities of TNF-α inhibitor therapy include pancytopenia, positive ANA associated with lupus-like syndromes, and demyelinating disorders. Combination therapy with multiple biologic therapies is not recommended.

Surgical intervention: Indications for surgical intervention include intractable pain, severe functional disability from joint destruction, or repair of ruptured tendons.

Other treatment considerations: Smoking may impair the response to therapy and exacerbate rheumatoid lung disease.

Manage secondary bone and cardiovascular disease, and prevent infection:

- DEXA scans to screen patients for osteoporosis
- calcium/vitamin D supplementation for all patients
- bisphosphonate therapy for osteoporosis
- evaluation and treatment of standard cardiovascular risk factors
- pneumococcal and yearly influenza vaccinations
- adjuvant physical and occupational therapy

DON'T BE TRICKED

- **Methotrexate and leflunomide are absolutely contraindicated in pregnancy and must be discontinued before conception.**
- **Hydroxychloroquine and sulfasalazine can be used during pregnancy.**

TEST YOURSELF

A 46-year-old man has a 3-month history of swelling of the PIP and MCP joints and 90 minutes of morning stiffness. Rheumatoid factor is negative.

ANSWER: For diagnosis, choose RA. For management, select anti-CCP antibody assay.

Sjögren Syndrome

Diagnosis

Sjögren syndrome may occur as a primary disease process or may be associated with another autoimmune disease, most commonly RA and SLE.

Sjögren syndrome is characterized by:

- keratoconjunctivitis sicca
- xerostomia
- salivary gland enlargement (occurs in nearly half of patients; most obviously in the parotid glands)

Testing

A cardinal feature is the presence of antibodies to Ro/SSA and La/SSB. A positive ANA, rheumatoid factor, and hypergammaglobulinemia are also frequently found. The presence of classic findings and anti-Ro/SSA and anti-La/SSB antibodies is sufficient to diagnose Sjögren syndrome; in unclear cases, a lip biopsy of minor salivary glands is the gold standard for diagnosis.

Follow-Up

Patients with Sjögren syndrome are up to 44 times more likely than the general population to have a B-cell lymphoma, with large B-cell and MALT lymphomas being the most common.

Be alert to the development of neonatal heart block in newborns of women with Sjögren syndrome because of the anti-Ro/SSA and anti-La/SSB antibodies.

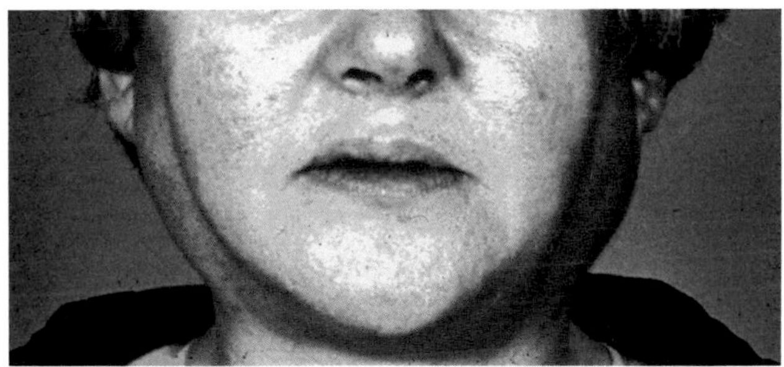

Parotid Gland Enlargement: Bilateral parotid gland enlargement in a patient with Sjögren syndrome.

Treatment

Treatment is symptomatic. Select artificial tear replacement and artificial saliva and mouth lubricants. Periodontal care every 6 months and fluoride treatments are advised.

Systemic immunosuppressive therapy is indicated only in patients with severe systemic manifestations.

Osteoarthritis

Osteoarthritis is the most common form of arthritis. It affects all tissues of the joint and is characterized by cartilage and meniscal degeneration.

Diagnosis

OA most often affects the lower cervical and lumbar spine; hips; knees; DIP, PIP, and first carpometacarpal joints.

Characteristic findings include:

- joint pain that is exacerbated by activity and relieved with rest; morning stiffness lasting <30 minutes
- reduced joint motion
- crepitus
- tenderness along the joint line
- bony enlargement (including Heberden and Bouchard nodes)
- involvement of the first carpometacarpal joint with "squaring" at the base of the thumb

In OA, an individual joint in the hand may be swollen or erythematous, but the presence of multiple swollen joints suggests concomitant CPP deposition or RA. OA is the probable cause if the DIP joints are involved, whereas RA (or psoriatic arthritis) is more likely if the MCP joints, wrists, or elbows are involved.

Two important variants are erosive OA of the hand and DISH.

Erosive inflammatory OA is characterized by pain and palpable swelling of the soft tissue in the PIP and DIP joints. This condition also may be associated with disease flares during which these joints become more swollen and painful. Compared with RA, erosive OA is common in the DIP joints, does not typically affect the wrists or elbows, and is not associated with rheumatoid factor, anti-CCP antibodies, or an elevated ESR or CRP level.

DISH is an often asymptomatic form of OA that causes flowing ossification along the anterolateral aspect of the vertebral bodies, particularly the anterior longitudinal ligament, in ≥4 contiguous vertebrae. However, neither disk-space narrowing nor syndesmophytes are visible as they are in lumbar spondylosis or ankylosing spondylitis, respectively. Common complications attributable to DISH include dysphagia, unstable spinal fractures, spinal stenosis, and myelopathy.

Secondary OA results from previous joint injury or metabolic diseases such as hemochromatosis. Consider metabolic causes when OA develops in atypical joints (e.g., MCP, shoulder, or wrist joints).

Testing

In most cases, laboratory studies are not indicated. An x-ray is not helpful in the diagnosis of hand OA (clinical examination is more specific) but is the gold standard for hip and knee OA, showing joint-space narrowing, subchondral sclerosis, and osteophytes. Synovial fluid is usually noninflammatory, with a leukocyte count <2000/µL. Ultrasonography is useful in the diagnosis of a Baker cyst.

DON'T BE TRICKED

- **In patients with typical OA radiographic changes, other diagnoses may be possible, including hemochromatosis, particularly if the 2nd and 3rd MCP joints are involved and have hook-like osteophytes.**
- **A ruptured Baker cyst (herniation of fluid-filled synovium of the posterior knee) or ruptured gastrocnemius muscle can mimic a DVT.**

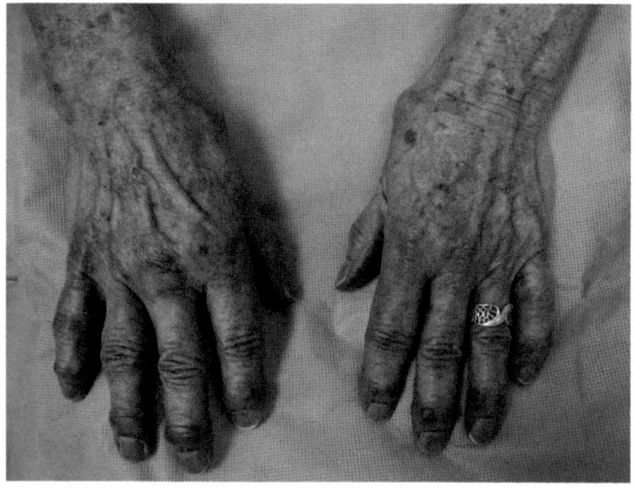

Hand Photograph, Osteoarthritis: Bony enlargement of the DIP joints and squaring of the first carpometacarpal joint characteristic of OA.

Treatment

Medical treatment includes:

- NSAIDs as initial therapy for hip and knee arthritis; topical NSAIDS for patients in whom oral NSAIDs are unsafe
- tramadol if NSAIDs are contraindicated or ineffective
- intra-articular glucocorticoids for acute exacerbations of knee OA
- quadriceps-strengthening exercises for knee OA
- weight loss for hip and knee OA

Joint arthroplasty of the hip or knee is indicated for pain that does not respond to nonsurgical treatment, especially when lifestyle or activities of daily living are affected.

A 2018 randomized trial demonstrated that treatment with opioids was not superior to treatment with nonopioid medications for improving pain-related function for chronic back pain or osteoarthritis-related hip or knee pain; pain intensity was significantly improved in the nonopioid group.

DON'T BE TRICKED

- **Patients with signs of inflammation should not undergo intra-articular glucocorticoid therapy until synovial fluid analysis excludes infection.**
- **Do not select arthroscopic lavage, debridement, or closed lavage for knee OA.**
- **Do not select hyaluronan intra-articular injection or oral supplements with glucosamine or chondroitin.**
- **Do not select oral NSAIDs for patients with CAD, HF, CKD, or ulcer disease.**

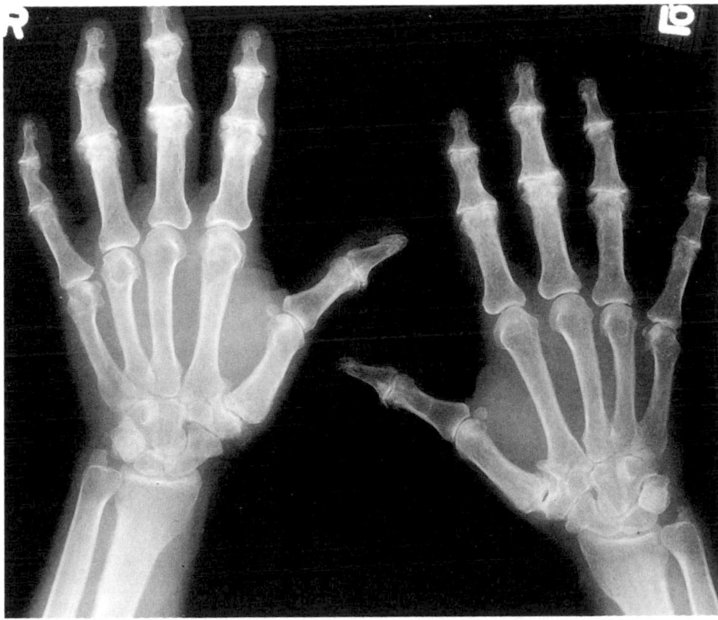

Hand X-ray, Osteoarthritis: Joint-space narrowing, sclerosis, and osteophyte formation are shown. Prominent involvement of the PIP and DIP joints indicates OA.

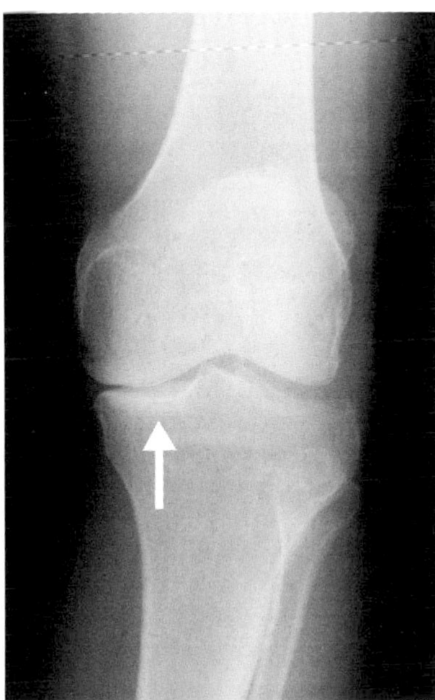

Knee X-ray, Osteoarthritis: Medial compartment joint space-narrowing and subchondral sclerosis consistent with OA are shown.

Hypertrophic Osteoarthropathy

Diagnosis

Hypertrophic osteoarthropathy causes a proliferation of skin and osseous tissue at the distal parts of the hands and feet. Characteristic findings are digital clubbing, painful periostosis of long bones, synovial effusions, and new periosteal bone formation.

Pain is generally alleviated by elevating the affected limbs. Associated disorders include lung cancer, chronic pulmonary infections, and right-to-left cardiac shunts.

TEST YOURSELF

A 64-year-old man has a 1-month history of bilateral ankle pain. Elevating his feet alleviates the discomfort. On physical examination, his lower legs are warm. Pitting edema begins 6 cm above the malleoli; this area is very tender to palpation. An x-ray shows new periosteal bone formation of the tibia above the ankle joints.

ANSWER: For diagnosis, choose hypertrophic osteoarthropathy. For management, select a chest x-ray to exclude lung cancer.

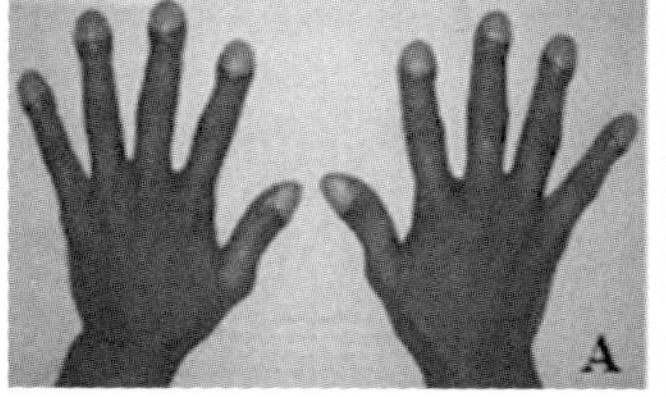

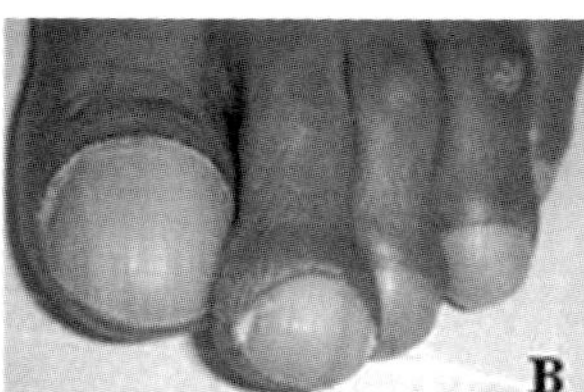

Hypertrophic Osteoarthropathy: Hypertrophic osteoarthropathy is characterized by clubbing and hypertrophic changes of the fingers and toes. Reprinted with permission from Shinjo SK, Levy-Neto M, Borba EF. Palindromic rheumatism associated with primary hypertrophic osteoarthropathy. Clinics (Sao Paulo). 2006 Dec;61(6):581-3. [PMID: 17187097]

Spondyloarthritis

Key Considerations

Spondyloarthritis comprises several systemic inflammatory joint disorders that share distinct clinical, radiographic, and genetic features. The spondyloarthritis disorders are:

- psoriatic arthritis
- reactive arthritis
- ankylosing spondylitis
- IBD-associated arthritis

Common characteristics include:

- inflammatory spine and sacroiliac disease
- asymmetric inflammation in ≤4 peripheral joints (typically large joints)
- inflammation at the sites of ligament and tendon insertion (enthesitis)
- the presence of HLA-B27
- extra-articular conditions, such as aortitis, colitis, urethritis, uveitis, and psoriasis
- absent rheumatoid factor and anti-CCP antibodies

DON'T BE TRICKED

- **HLA-B27 testing may support, but cannot independently confirm or exclude, a diagnosis of ankylosing spondylitis or other forms of spondyloarthritis.**

Psoriatic Arthritis

Characteristic findings are classic psoriasis and nail pitting in a patient with joint pain and stiffness. Skin involvement commonly precedes joint inflammation, although 15% of patients first develop joint inflammation.

The most common patterns of joint involvement are:

- asymmetric, lower extremity oligoarthritis (resembling reactive arthritis)
- symmetric polyarthritis (resembling RA) involving the DIP, PIP, and/or MCP joints

Less common presentations include:

- DIP involvement only
- chronic resorptive arthritis (arthritis mutilans) resulting in digital shortening with a "telescoping" appearance of the digits sometimes referred to as "pencil in a cup"
- spondylitis (spine or sacroiliac arthritis, usually asymmetric)

Sausage-shaped fingers or toes (dactylitis), often involving the DIP joints, are seen in psoriatic arthritis and help distinguish psoriatic arthritis from RA.

Testing: Patients with psoriatic arthritis tend to be seronegative for rheumatoid factor, but at least 15% are seropositive. Serum urate levels may be elevated because of rapid turnover of skin cells. Explosive onset or severe flare-up of psoriatic arthritis should prompt testing for HIV infection.

Treatment

- Select NSAIDs as initial therapy.
- Select methotrexate for peripheral joint disease and enthesitis not responding to NSAIDs; methotrexate will treat skin disease as well.
- A TNF-α inhibitor is indicated for axial disease unresponsive to NSAIDs, for methotrexate-resistant peripheral disease, or for skin disease.
- A TNF-α inhibitor is initially added to methotrexate, with discontinuation of methotrexate when benefit from the TNF-α inhibitor is demonstrated.
- The biologic agents ustekinumab (anti-IL-12/23 antibody) and secukinumab (anti-IL-17A antibody) have been approved for treating psoriasis and psoriatic arthritis and can improve dactylitis and enthesitis.
- NSAIDs, antimalarial drugs, and withdrawal from oral glucocorticoids may exacerbate psoriasis.

DON'T BE TRICKED

- **No relationship exists between the extent of skin and joint disease in patients with psoriatic arthritis.**
- **Although benefit can be demonstrated in control of skin disease and joint pain, methotrexate has not been shown to reduce progression of joint damage.**

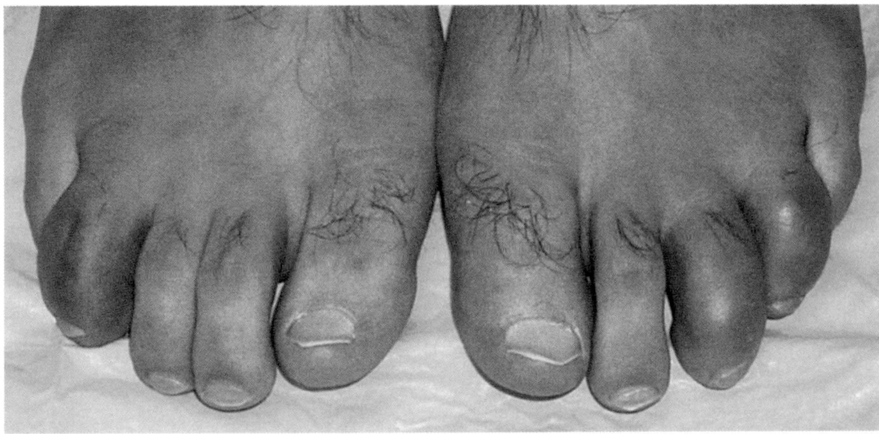

Dactylitis: Diffuse swelling of the left third and fourth toes and right fourth toe characteristic of dactylitis.

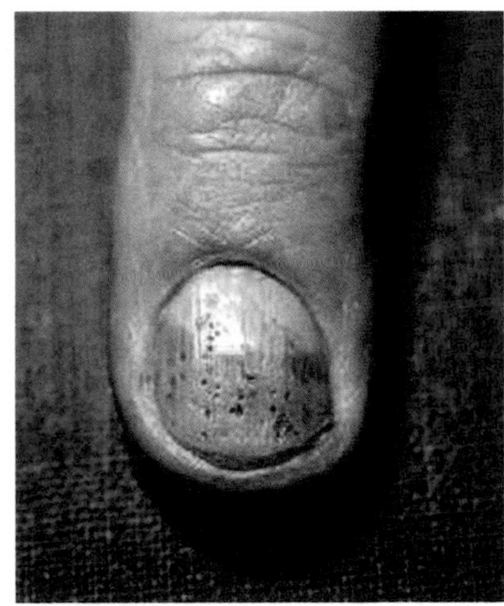

Psoriasis: Tiny pits scattered over the nail plate resulting from psoriatic involvement of the nail matrix.

Reactive Arthritis

Reactive arthritis is an acute aseptic inflammatory arthritis that occurs 1 to 3 weeks after an infectious event originating in the GU or GI tract. A high prevalence of HIV infection is found in patients with symptoms of reactive arthritis.

Characteristic findings include:

- monoarthritis or acute asymmetric oligoarthritis (usually in weight-bearing joints)
- dactylitis
- enthesopathy (especially of the Achilles tendon)
- sacroiliitis

Patients may also have keratoderma blennorrhagicum (a psoriasis-like lesion on the palms and soles) or circinate balanitis (shallow, moist, serpiginous ulcers with raised borders on the glans penis).

Testing/Treatment

- No diagnostic tests or radiographic changes are specific for reactive arthritis. Elevated acute phase reactants may be present, and x-rays may show a nonspecific inflammatory arthritis.
- Patients with a presentation suggesting reactive arthritis should be tested for HIV and GU infection (*Chlamydia*). Stool cultures for GI pathogens (*Salmonella, Shigella, Campylobacter,* and *Yersinia*) are recommended for patients with acute diarrhea; when the causative organism can be isolated, begin specific therapy.
- In the absence of an ongoing infection, reactive arthritis is usually self-limited, and symptoms resolve within 6 months; select symptomatic treatment with NSAIDs and glucocorticoid injections for these patients.

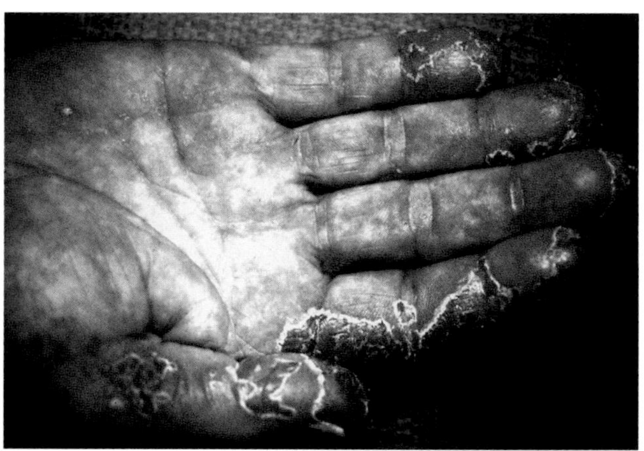

Keratoderma Blennorrhagicum: Keratoderma blennorrhagicum, a psoriasis-like lesion of the palms and soles, is associated with reactive arthritis.

DON'T BE TRICKED

- **The classic triad of arthritis, conjunctivitis, and urethritis (or cervicitis) is found in only one third of patients with reactive arthritis.**
- **Do not prescribe chronic antibiotic therapy for patients with reactive arthritis.**

TEST YOURSELF

A 33-year-old man has a 3-month history of left shoulder and right ankle pain and a left inflamed second toe. He had 4 days of bloody diarrhea 3 months ago.

ANSWER: For diagnosis, choose reactive arthritis, consistent with a previous enteric infection.

Ankylosing Spondylitis

Ankylosing spondylitis primarily affects the spine and sacroiliac joints. It also may involve the shoulders and hips. The small peripheral joints are not affected. Ankylosing spondylitis occurs most often in patients <40 years of age and presents as chronic inflammatory low back pain (more than 1 hour of morning stiffness). Characteristic symptoms are pain and stiffness that worsen at night and are relieved with physical activity or heat.

Physical examination findings include:

- decreased hyperextension, forward flexion, lateral flexion, and axial rotation
- diminished chest expansion
- asymmetric peripheral arthritis involving the large joints
- painful heels (enthesitis)

Extra-articular manifestations include acute anterior uveitis (most common), aortic valvular regurgitation, aortic aneurysm, cardiac conduction defects, apical pulmonary fibrosis and cavitation, and cauda equina syndrome.

A patient with ankylosing spondylitis with increased pain and mobility of the neck following a minor accident may have a fracture and requires an urgent CT of the cervical spine.

Laboratory testing: CRP and ESR may be normal or elevated; rheumatoid factor and other autoantibodies are absent.

Imaging: X-rays of the sacroiliac joints show sacroiliitis with erosions, pseudowidening of the joints, sclerosis, and ankylosis. X-rays of the spine show subchondral bony sclerosis, vertebral body squaring, and bony ankylosis ("bamboo spine").

When radiographic findings are equivocal or absent, MRI can detect the early changes of sacroiliitis.

DON'T BE TRICKED

- **Ankylosing spondylitis occurs in both men and women.**

Treatment: Select exercise to preserve range of motion and strengthen the spine extensor muscles to prevent kyphosis.

Drug therapy consists of:

- NSAIDs (not aspirin)–the mainstay of management
- glucocorticoid injections for recalcitrant enthesitis and persistent synovitis
- TNF-α inhibitors if inadequate response of axial disease to NSAIDs
- methotrexate, sulfasalazine, and hydroxychloroquine for peripheral joint disease
- calcium and vitamin D supplements for all patients
- bisphosphonate for osteopenia or osteoporosis

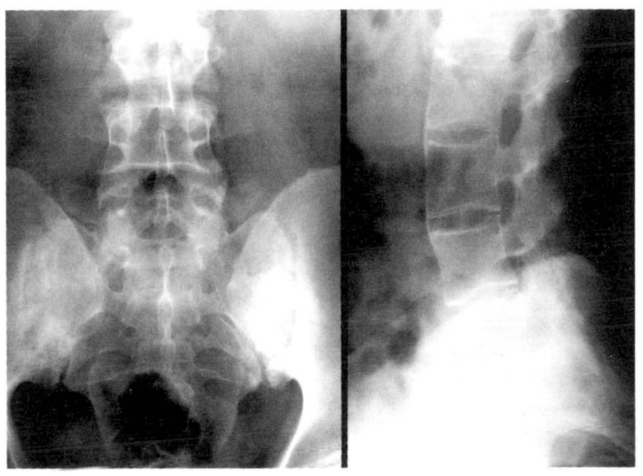

X-rays, Ankylosing Spondylitis: Sclerosis and erosions of sacroiliac joints and bridging of the intervertebral disks by syndesmophytes are characteristic of ankylosing spondylitis.

DON'T BE TRICKED

- **Do not prescribe methotrexate, sulfasalazine, or hydroxychloroquine for patients with axial disease because they are ineffective. Select a TNF-α inhibitor.**

TEST YOURSELF

A 40-year-old man with ankylosing spondylitis has increasing neck pain after a fall from the second rung of a ladder 5 days ago.

ANSWER: For diagnosis, choose acute cervical fracture. For management, select neck immobilization and emergent CT.

IBD-Associated Arthritis

IBD-associated arthritis can present in various ways:

- polyarticular arthritis resembling RA
- asymmetric oligoarthritis, predominantly of the lower extremities
- asymptomatic sacroiliac disease
- ankylosing spondylitis-like disease

Only the oligoarticular peripheral arthritis parallels IBD activity.

Treatment: Methotrexate and sulfasalazine alleviate IBD-associated arthritis symptoms and also treat the underlying bowel disease, but studies have not demonstrated that these drugs prevent joint disease progression. The TNF-α inhibitors infliximab and adalimumab are effective for IBD-associated arthritis.

DON'T BE TRICKED

- NSAIDs may result in worsening of associated IBD.

Systemic Lupus Erythematosus

Diagnosis

Approximately 90% of adult patients with SLE are women. Diagnosis is based on characteristic clinical features and laboratory studies.

Diagnose SLE when any four of the following are present:

- positive ANA
- malar ("butterfly") rash that spares the nasolabial folds and areas beneath the nose and lower lip
- discoid rash characterized by erythematous, raised patches with keratotic scaling and follicular plugging
- photosensitivity
- oral ulcers
- arthritis (joint pain is frequently the presenting symptom)
- serositis (pleural, pericardial, abdominal)
- kidney disorder (new-onset hypertension, proteinuria with or without hematuria)
- neurologic disorder (aseptic meningitis, cranial neuritis, encephalitis, mononeuritis multiplex, peripheral neuropathy, psychosis, seizures, stroke, transverse myelitis)
- hematologic disorder (autoimmune hemolytic anemia, leukopenia, lymphopenia, thrombocytopenia)
- immunologic disorder (APLA syndrome [venous and arterial thrombosis, recurrent fetal loss])

Additional SLE pearls:

- Subacute cutaneous lupus erythematosus is frequently drug induced (especially hydrochlorothiazide) and not related to systemic disease.
- Nonscarring alopecia is common in SLE.
- Periarticular inflammation can result in reducible subluxation of the digits, swan neck deformities, and ulnar deviation (Jaccoud [nonerosive] arthropathy).
- Pain or limitation of motion of the hips suggests osteonecrosis.
- Kidney disease is most common in patients with anti-dsDNA antibodies.
- Nephritis and a rising serum creatinine is an indication for urgent kidney biopsy.
- Autoantibodies that assist in the diagnosis of neuropsychiatric SLE include antineuronal, anti-NMDA receptor, antiribosomal P, and APLA/LAC.
- SLE parenchymal lung involvement is rare, and lung infiltrates are more likely to be infectious.
- Patients with quiescent SLE can have mild cytopenias that do not require intervention.
- Clinical manifestations of APLA/LAC include venous and arterial thrombosis, miscarriage, livedo reticularis, cytopenias, and cardiac valve thickening/vegetations.
- Newborns of mothers who are positive for anti-Ro/SSA or anti-La/SSB antibodies are at risk for developing neonatal lupus erythematosus, which may manifest as heart block.
- Drug-induced lupus is most often caused by hydralazine, procainamide, isoniazid, minocycline, or TNF-α inhibitors; symptoms are usually limited to arthritis, fever, and serositis.

DON'T BE TRICKED

- Do not diagnose SLE in a patient with a positive ANA and facial rash that involves the nasolabial folds; consider rosacea instead.

Testing

The ANA assay is sensitive but not specific for diagnosing SLE. Assays for anti-dsDNA and anti-Sm antibodies are highly specific. Anti-dsDNA antibodies correlate with disease activity.

Activation of the complement pathway, manifested by depressed serum C3 and C4 levels, often accompanies major flares of SLE.

In drug-induced lupus, ANA assays are positive, but anti-dsDNA and anti-Sm antibody assays are negative. Antihistone antibody assay may be positive.

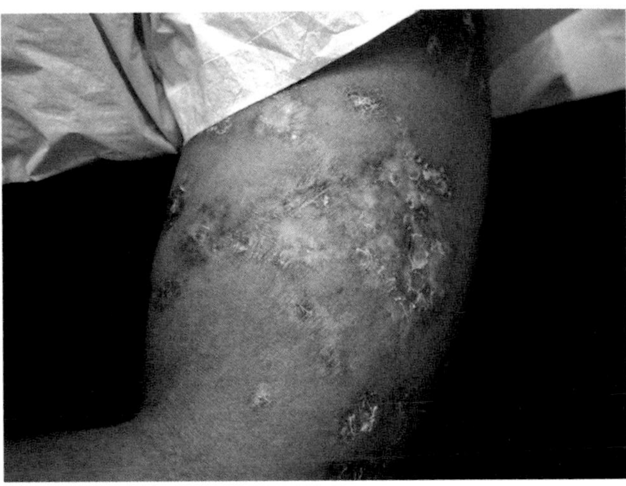

Rash in Systemic Lupus Erythematosus: The discoid rash of lupus erythematosus consists of chronic, slowly progressive, scaly, infiltrative papules and plaques or atrophic red plaques on sun-exposed skin surfaces. Discoid lupus can be present in the absence of any other clinical feature of SLE.

DON'T BE TRICKED

- An isolated low-titer ANA by immunofluorescence assay (1:40-1:80) is not likely to indicate systemic lupus.
- Myalgia, arthralgia, and fatigue are insufficient reasons by themselves to check an ANA panel.
- Monitoring serial ANA titers is not warranted because these values do not reflect disease activity.

Treatment

Major therapeutic points:

- Manage arthritis with NSAIDs and hydroxychloroquine; hydroxychloroquine should be continued indefinitely in most patients to help prevent flares of SLE, even in patients with quiescent disease.
- Manage photosensitive cutaneous lupus with sun block, topical glucocorticoids, and hydroxychloroquine.
- Manage life-threatening disease with high-dose glucocorticoids and (usually) cyclophosphamide or mycophenolate mofetil.
- Reduce atherosclerosis risk factors in all patients.
- Prescribe vitamin D and calcium supplements for all patients and bisphosphonates for those with osteoporosis and osteopenia.

DON'T BE TRICKED

- Patients taking hydroxychloroquine require annual routine ophthalmologic examinations.
- Medications that can be used in pregnant patients with SLE include hydroxychloroquine and prednisone.

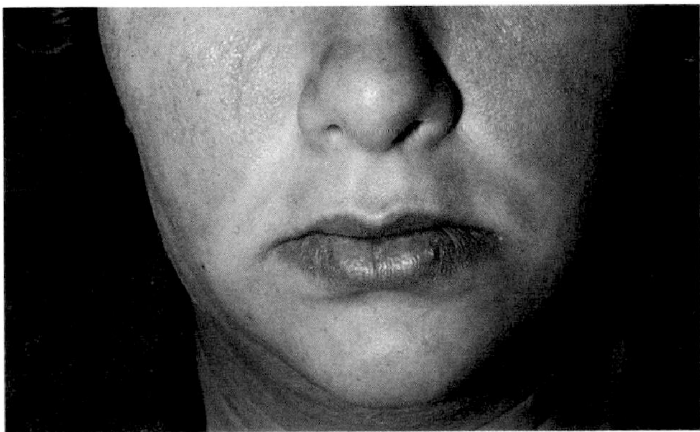

Malar Skin Rash: Bright red, sharply demarcated plaques in a butterfly pattern that spares the nasolabial folds and areas beneath the nose and lower lip are associated with SLE.

Systemic Sclerosis

Diagnosis

The presence of typical skin findings and one or more of the following features support a diagnosis:

- sclerodactyly
- digital pitting
- interstitial lung disease
- Raynaud phenomenon
- PH
- GERD and esophageal dysmotility
- pseudo-obstruction (small bowel)
- malabsorption owing to bacterial overgrowth
- calcinosis
- inflammatory arthritis, particularly in the DIP joints and wrists
- kidney disease

The primary cause of morbidity and mortality in patients with SSc is pulmonary disease.

Scleroderma renal crisis is characterized by hypertension with microangiopathic hemolytic anemia, thrombocytopenia, and acute kidney injury with mild proteinuria and bland urine.

Gastric antral vascular ectasia (GAVE or "watermelon stomach") can result in recurrent bleeding and chronic anemia.

SSc is classified according to the degree of skin involvement.

STUDY TABLE: Differentiating Diffuse from Limited Cutaneous Systemic Sclerosis

Findings	Diffuse Cutaneous SSc	Limited Cutaneous SSc
Skin findings	Skin thickening proximal to the elbows and knees, including chest and abdomen; may affect the face	Skin thickening distal to the elbows and knees; may affect the face
Antibodies	ANA and anti-Scl-70 antibodies	ANA and anticentromere antibodies
Pulmonary disease	Interstitial lung disease	PH
Scleroderma renal crisis	Present	Absent
CREST syndrome	Usually absent	Present

CREST = calcinosis, Raynaud phenomenon, esophageal dysmotility, sclerodactyly, telangiectasia.

DON'T BE TRICKED

- **Nailfold capillary destruction and dilated capillary loops distinguish early SSc with Raynaud phenomenon from primary Raynaud disease.**

Testing

Pulmonary disease: Screening tests for pulmonary diseases include HRCT and pulmonary function tests (including DLCO) for interstitial lung disease and echocardiography for PH. Baseline and annual monitoring of PAH is recommended in all patients with or without advanced interstitial lung disease.

Small bowel bacterial overgrowth: Hydrogen breath test can diagnose small bowel bacterial overgrowth.

Kidney disease: Up to 50% of patients have mild proteinuria, elevated plasma creatinine concentration, and/or hypertension, but most do not progress to AKI or CKD.

Several diseases present with scleroderma-like features:

STUDY TABLE: Scleroderma-like Conditions

Condition	Features	Considerations
Eosinophilic fasciitis	Edema of proximal extremities; sparing of hands and face; peripheral eosinophilia	Skin biopsy shows lymphocytes, plasma cells, and eosinophils Treat with glucocorticoids
Nephrogenic systemic fibrosis	Exposure to gadolinium in kidney disease; brawny, wood-like induration of extremities, sparing the digits	Changes in use and formulation of gadolinium have reduced incidence
Scleredema	Indurated plaques/patches on back, shoulder girdle, and neck	Seen in long-standing diabetes
Scleromyxedema	Waxy, yellow-red papules over thickened skin of face, upper trunk, neck, and arms	Associate with multiple myeloma or AL amyloidosis
Chronic GVHD	Lichen planus-like skin lesions or localized or generalized skin thickening	Occurs most commonly after HSCT

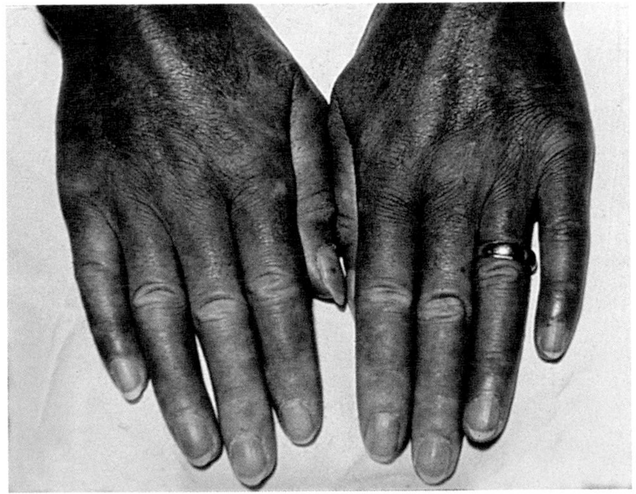

Sclerodactyly: Thickening and induration of the skin over the fingers and wrists is characteristic of scleroderma.

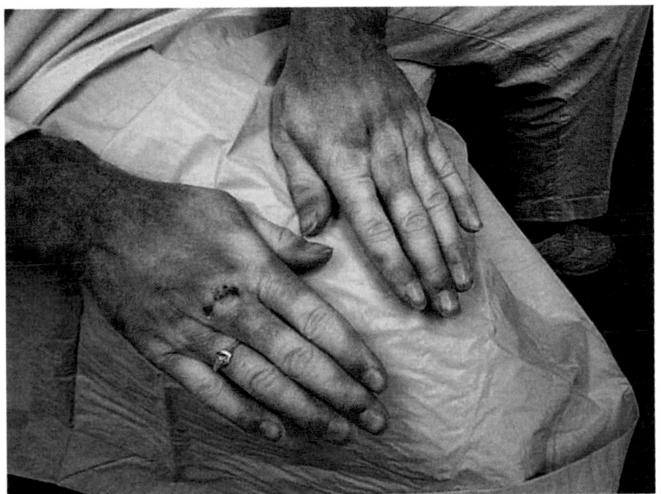

Raynaud Phenomenon: Areas of vasospastic skin blanching seen in a patient with Raynaud phenomenon.

DON'T BE TRICKED

- **Skin thickening or tightening without Raynaud phenomenon is not SSc but another scleroderma-like condition.**

Treatment

Treatment is for organ-specific manifestations; no overall disease-modifying therapy is available.

Raynaud phenomenon: Avoiding cold exposure and smoking reduce the risk of Raynaud episodes. Use amlodipine, felodipine, nifedipine, sildenafil, and nitroglycerin paste to manage symptoms.

Gastric and intestinal dysmotility: Prescribe PPIs for GERD and promotility agents (metoclopramide) for gastric and intestinal dysmotility.

Scleroderma renal crisis: Prescribe ACE inhibitors for scleroderma renal crisis regardless of the serum creatinine level; continue even in the setting of kidney failure.

Bacterial overgrowth: Prescribe broad-spectrum antibiotics for bacterial overgrowth.

Alveolitis: Treat active alveolitis or rapidly progressive interstitial lung disease with mycophenolate mofetil (preferred) or cyclophosphamide.

PAH: Treat PAH similarly to idiopathic PAH.

DON'T BE TRICKED

- **Glucocorticoid therapy is a risk factor for scleroderma renal crisis and may be associated with normotensive renal crisis (AKI in the absence of hypertension); do not use glucocorticoids to treat scleroderma.**

TEST YOURSELF

A 59-year-old woman has accelerated hypertension and CKD. She has a history of Raynaud phenomenon. BP is 160/122 mm Hg. Her fingers appear tapered with very smooth skin and ulcers on the fingertips. Serum creatinine level is 5.4 mg/dL.

ANSWER: For diagnosis, choose scleroderma renal crisis. For management, select an ACE inhibitor.

Mixed Connective Tissue Disease

MCTD is a specific syndrome that includes features of at least two of the following: SLE, SSc, and/or polymyositis in the presence of anti-U1-RNP antibodies.

Diagnosis

In addition to RNP antibodies, clinical features of MCTD may include:

- Raynaud phenomenon
- edema of the hands
- sclerodactyly
- synovitis
- myositis

The mortality of patients with MCTD is largely attributable to PH.

STUDY TABLE: Comparison of Mixed Connective Tissue Disease, Undifferentiated Connective Tissue Disease, and Overlap Syndrome

Condition	Typical Clinical Features	Diagnosis	Treatment
MCTD	Raynaud phenomenon; arthritis; puffy fingers; sclerodactyly; serositis; esophageal dysmotility; myositis; interstitial lung disease; PAH	Positive anti-U1-RNP antibodies Fulfills criteria for at least two of the following: SSc, polymyositis, and SLE	Disease/organ involvement specific Anti-inflammatories for symptoms; DMARDs, and/or immunosuppressives for arthritis or other major organ disease Vasodilators for PAH and Raynaud phenomenon PPI for esophageal disease
Undifferentiated connective tissue disease	Variable; most common include Raynaud phenomenon, arthralgia, skin rash, cytopenia, and serositis	Insufficient criteria for any specific connective tissue disease	Same as MCTD
Overlap syndrome	Variable; will have features satisfying two distinct autoimmune diseases (such as SLE, RA, polymyositis, and SSc)	Fulfills criteria for two distinct autoimmune diseases	Same as MCTD

DON'T BE TRICKED

- **Positive anti-Sm or anti-dsDNA antibodies supports the diagnosis of SLE, not MCTD.**

Fibromyalgia

Diagnosis

Diagnostic clues include:

- widespread pain ("hurt all over")
- waking unrefreshed ("always tired and fatigued")
- cognitive fatigue (forgets words or loses track of conversation mid sentence)
- exercise intolerance ("If I overdo it, I pay for it for several days.")
- lack of response to multiple medications
- diffuse tenderness to palpation
- Alternative diagnoses must be ruled out (hypothyroidism, adrenal insufficiency, depression)

Testing

Initial laboratory studies include a CBC, chemistry panel, TSH, and ESR or CRP, which are normal.

Treatment

Nonpharmacologic therapy such as regular aerobic exercise and cognitive behavioral therapy should be initiated in all patients.

Pregabalin, duloxetine, and milnacipran are FDA approved for fibromyalgia. Each provides a modest benefit over placebo.

DON'T BE TRICKED

- **Do not obtain ANA, rheumatoid factor, or anti-CCP antibodies in the evaluation of fibromyalgia.**
- **Do not diagnose fibromyalgia in the presence of red flags such as anemia, fever, synovitis, and weight loss.**
- **Do not use opioids or NSAIDS in the treatment of fibromyalgia.**

Gout

Diagnosis

Gout is caused by an inflammatory reaction to monosodium urate crystal deposition in synovial tissue, bursae, and tendon sheaths. Gout progresses through three stages:

- acute intermittent gout
- intercritical gout (the time between attacks of acute gout)
- chronic recurrent and tophaceous gout (characterized by persistent synovitis and possible formation of tophi)

Characteristic findings of acute intermittent gout include self-limited acute attacks of monoarticular arthritis (typically of the first MTP or tarsal joints) and hyperuricemia. If the disease presents with acute onset of pain at night at the first MTP joint (podagra), synovial fluid analysis is not required to make the diagnosis.

With time, attacks of gout may become more frequent and involve more joints. Patients may progress to have a chronic, smoldering arthritis. Tophi are yellowish nodular deposits of monosodium urate that develop on extensor surfaces of the extremities, on finger pads, and along tendons. Hydrochlorothiazide is a common drug-trigger of acute gout. Losartan, which has a modest uricosuric effect, is an effective antihypertensive in patients with gout. Transplantation-related gout is associated with the use of calcineurin antagonists (cyclosporine). Lead toxicity may present with gout, kidney disease, and abdominal pain.

Testing

Laboratory:

- Monosodium urate crystals (needle-shaped, negatively birefringent crystals) in the joint fluid and urate tophi are diagnostic. Crystals within synovial fluid neutrophils define acute gout, and extracellular crystals confirm chronic gout. Monosodium urate crystals may be visible on joint aspiration even when an acute flare is not occurring.
- The synovial fluid leukocyte count ranges from 2000 to 75,000/µL.
- In all patients suspected of having acute gout, synovial fluid Gram stain and cultures must be obtained to exclude infection.

Imaging: X-rays of patients with chronic gout show bone erosions with overhanging edges. Subcortical cysts and periarticular erosions may also be seen.

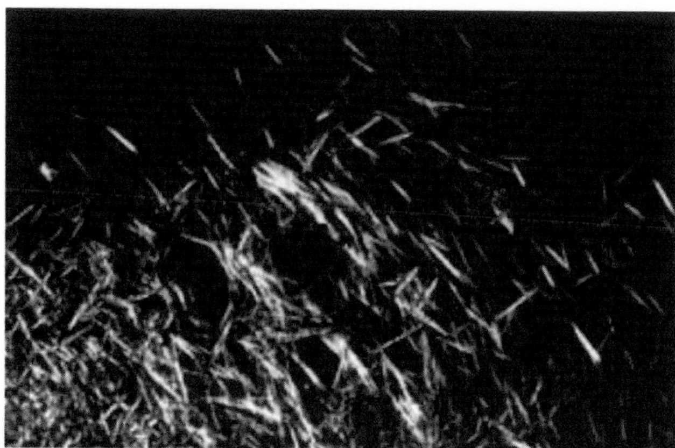

Monosodium Urate Crystals: Aspiration of a tophus showing monosodium urate crystals (needle-shaped, negatively birefringent crystals) as viewed with polarized microscopy.

DON'T BE TRICKED

- **An elevated serum urate level alone is not diagnostic of gout.**
- **A normal serum urate level at the time of an acute attack does not rule out gout.**
- **Synovial fluid leukocyte counts higher than 50,000/µL should raise suspicion for a concurrent bacterial joint infection, even when monosodium urate crystals have been identified.**

Treatment

Acute Gouty Flare

- Use NSAIDs, colchicine, and glucocorticoids as first-line therapies.
- Select oral glucocorticoids when NSAIDs are unsafe (in older adult or postoperative patients, patients requiring anticoagulation, and those with CKD or PUD)
- Prescribe intra-articular glucocorticoids for a single joint if other interventions are ineffective or contraindicated.

Recurrent Gout

- The ACP suggests a "treat to avoid symptoms" approach without specifically considering serum urate levels.
- The ACR and EULAR support a "treat-to-target" approach, reducing the serum urate level to less than 6.0 mg/dL in patients without tophi and less than 5.0 mg/dL in patients with tophi.
- The ACR and EULAR recommend urate-lowering therapy for patients with gout plus any of the following: (1) ≥stage 2 CKD; (2) ≥2 acute attacks per year; (3) one or more tophi; or (4) uric acid nephrolithiasis.
- Urate-lowering therapy (see following) can be initiated during an acute attack if adequate anti-inflammatory therapy is concurrently started.
- Medications that raise serum urate levels, such as thiazide diuretics, should be discontinued if possible.

Principles of treatment with a urate-lowering agent include:

- Treat most patients with allopurinol.
- Doses of allopurinol must be lowered for patients with kidney impairment. When starting allopurinol, also begin low-dose colchicine (or an NSAID) to prevent acute gout; colchicine (or NSAID) can be discontinued 3 to 6 months after the serum urate level stabilizes.
- Allopurinol should be avoided in high-risk populations (Han Chinese, Taiwanese, Korean patients with kidney disease) if positive for HLA-B*5801.

- Febuxostat is useful if patients cannot tolerate allopurinol and in patients with CKD.
- In chronic refractory gout or when standard urate-lowering therapy has been unsuccessful or not tolerated, select IV pegloticase. Pegloticase enzymatically converts urate to the more soluble compound allantoin.

Patients with kidney disease who are treated with allopurinol, especially those taking hydrochlorothiazide, have an increased risk for a rare but potentially fatal hypersensitivity syndrome characterized by severe dermatitis, fever, eosinophilia, hepatic necrosis, and acute nephritis. In patients with cardiovascular disease, febuxostat is associated with an increased risk of heart-related deaths and death from all causes, compared with allopurinol.

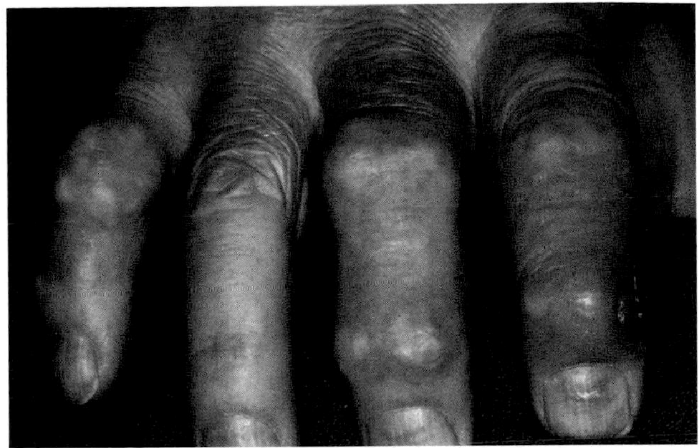

Chronic Tophaceous Gout: Swollen interphalangeal joints and multiple tophi characteristic of chronic tophaceous gout.

DON'T BE TRICKED

- Do not select NSAIDs for patients with gout who also have CKD or PUD.
- Urate-lowering therapy is of no benefit in the treatment of an acute gouty attack.
- Do not use allopurinol or febuxostat with azathioprine, because the combination can result in elevated azathioprine levels.
- Do not use uricosuric therapy (e.g., probenecid) in patients with a low estimated GFR who are at risk for nephrolithiasis or CKD.
- Do not prescribe colchicine for patients with kidney failure.

TEST YOURSELF

A 78-year-old man has a 6-hour history of an acutely painful and swollen left first MTP joint. Two days ago, he had an MI. His serum creatinine level is 1.7 mg/dL.

ANSWER: For diagnosis, select acute gout. For management, choose aspiration of the joint and treatment with an intra-articular glucocorticoid after infection is excluded.

Calcium Pyrophosphate Deposition

Diagnosis

The four clinical presentations of CPPD are:

- asymptomatic cartilage calcification (chondrocalcinosis)
- acute CPP crystal arthritis (pseudogout)
- chronic CPP crystal inflammatory arthritis
- OA with CPPD

Characteristic findings in acute CPP crystal arthritis (pseudogout) are:

- inflammation localized to one joint, affecting the knee, wrist, shoulder, or ankle
- acute onset of several painful joints following trauma, severe illness, or surgery
- rhomboid-shaped positively birefringent synovial fluid crystals

Characteristic findings in pyrophosphate arthropathy include:

- two distinct patterns: chronic CPP crystal inflammatory arthritis and OA with CPPD
- chronic CPP crystal inflammatory arthritis resembles RA
- OA with CPPD exhibits OA findings in atypical locations including wrist, MCP, or shoulder joints

Characteristic findings in cartilage calcification are:

- triangular fibrocartilage of the wrist joint (space between the carpal bones and distal ulna)
- menisci of the knee joint (appearing as a line in the cartilage)
- symphysis pubis

CPPD may be associated with underlying metabolic disorders. Screen patients with CPPD who are <50 years of age for:

- hemochromatosis
- hypomagnesemia
- hyperparathyroidism
- hypothyroidism

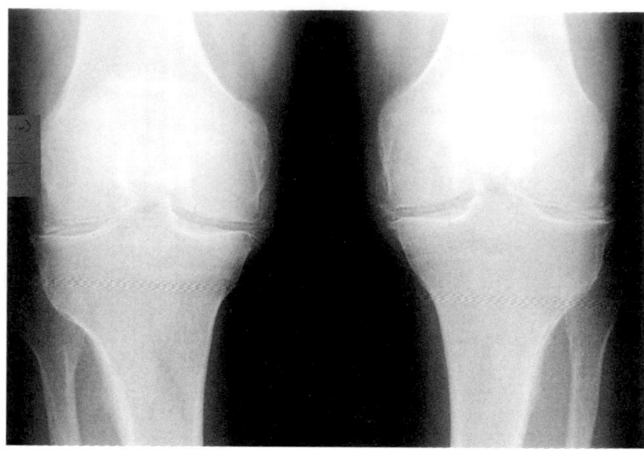

X-ray of Knees, Chondrocalcinosis: Linear calcifications of the meniscus and articular cartilage are characteristic of CPPD.

DON'T BE TRICKED

- The absence of chondrocalcinosis on x-ray does not rule out CPPD.

Treatment

Intra-articular glucocorticoids are indicated for acute pain in pseudogout involving one or two joints after infection is ruled out by arthrocentesis.

NSAIDs are appropriate as initial therapy for most patients with multiple joint involvement.

Prescribe colchicine for patients with any variant of CPPD that does not respond to NSAIDs or for patients with contraindications to NSAID therapy.

Prescribe systemic glucocorticoids for patients unable to take colchicine or NSAIDs.

Infectious Arthritis

Diagnosis

Infectious arthritis should be considered in any patient who presents with:

- sudden onset of monoarthritis
- acute worsening of chronic joint disease
- previously painless joint prosthesis that becomes painful
- radiographic loosening or migration of a cemented prosthetic device

The risk for infection is increased in persons with previously damaged joints (e.g., patients with RA), in older adults, and in immunosuppressed patients. In patients with underlying rheumatologic disorders, a sudden joint flare that is not accompanied by other features of the preexisting disorder and is unresponsive to usual therapy suggests a diagnosis of infectious arthritis.

The hallmark of an infected joint is pain that worsens with passive extension or when the joint is held in fixed flexion; an infected joint typically appears swollen and warm with overlying erythema.

Common organisms causing infectious arthritis:

- **Gram-positive organisms** are the most common causes of infectious arthritis in adults. *Staphylococcus aureus* is the most common offending organism, regardless of age or underlying risk factors.
- **Gonococcal arthritis** is the most common form of bacterial arthritis in young sexually active persons in the United States.

Disseminated gonococcal infection can produce two distinct syndromes: tenosynovitis, polyarthralgia, and dermatitis syndrome; and purulent gonococcal arthritis.

- Patients with the **tenosynovitis, polyarthralgia, and dermatitis syndrome** have cutaneous lesions that progress from papules or macules to pustules that are sterile on culture. Fever and chills are common.
- Patients with **purulent gonococcal arthritis** do not have systemic features or dermatitis. Synovial fluid cultures for *Neisseria gonorrhoeae* are positive in 50% of infected patients. Obtaining culture specimens from the pharynx, GU system, and rectum, in addition to synovial fluid cultures, increases the diagnostic yield.
- Evaluate for deficiencies in terminal complement components for patients with recurrent episodes of disseminated gonococcal infection.

Less common causes of infectious arthritis:

- **Gram-negative infections** are more common in older, immunosuppressed, and postoperative patients, and those with IV catheters.
- **Tuberculous arthritis** typically is an indolent, monoarticular arthritis involving the hip or knee; it does not cause systemic features, and is not associated with positive TST; Gram stain and culture of synovial fluid are negative. Diagnosis is made by synovial biopsy.
- **Fungal arthritis** typically manifests as subacute monoarthritis in patients with a systemic fungal infection.

A synovial fluid leukocyte count >50,000/µL is specific but not sensitive for infectious or crystalline arthropathy.

Always select arthrocentesis with Gram stain, polarized microscopy for crystals, cell count, and differential for an acutely swollen, painful joint (monoarthritis).

DON'T BE TRICKED

- Infectious arthritis can develop in patients with gout or pseudogout, and the presence of crystals in synovial fluid does not exclude a concomitant infection.
- X-rays are not helpful in the early diagnosis of acute native joint infection.

Treatment

Begin immediate empiric antibiotic therapy for suspected bacterial arthritis even if culture results are pending or negative.

STUDY TABLE: Empiric and Definitive Antibiotic Treatment for Septic Native Joint Arthritis

Likely or Identified Pathogen	First-Line Therapy	Second-Line Therapy	Comments
Gram-Positive Cocci			
If MRSA is a concern (risk factors or known MRSA carrier)	Vancomycin	Clindamycin; daptomycin; linezolid	—
MSSA	Nafcillin or cefazolin	—	Narrow treatment to MSSA coverage based on sensitivity data.
Gram-Negative Bacilli			
Enteric gram-negative bacilli	3rd generation cephalosporin (e.g., ceftriaxone or cefotaxime)	Fluoroquinolones	—

(Continued on the next page)

STUDY TABLE: Empiric and Definitive Antibiotic Treatment for Septic Native Joint Arthritis *(Continued)*			
Likely or Identified Pathogen	**First-Line Therapy**	**Second-Line Therapy**	**Comments**
Pseudomonas aeruginosa	Ceftazidime; cefepime; piperacillin-tazobactam	Carbapenems; aztreonam; fluoroquinolones	—
Gram-Negative Cocci			
Neisseria gonorrhoeae	IV ceftriaxone for at least 7 days plus 1 g of oral azithromycin × one dose	Fluoroquinolones (only if culture sensitivities confirm susceptibility)	In the absence of specific culture sensitivity data, "stepping down" to oral therapy is not recommended because of increasing resistance of *N. gonorrhoeae* to commonly used oral agents.
Gram Stain Unavailable or Inconclusive			
Likely pathogen depends on patient risk factors: consider MRSA, and gram-negative organism if immunocompromised, at risk for gonococcal infection, or with joint trauma; also consider community patterns of infection.	Vancomycin, or vancomycin + 3rd generation cephalosporin, or antipseudomonal antibiotic if pseudomonas suspected	—	Appropriate to start with broad antibiotic coverage and narrow coverage if culture data become available.
Borrelia burgdorferi (Lyme arthritis)	Oral doxycycline or amoxicillin × 28 days	—	If inadequate response or concurrent neurologic findings, IV ceftriaxone × 28 days.
Mycobacterium tuberculosis	3- to 4-drug treatment (e.g., isoniazid, pyrazinamide, rifampin, ethambutol, streptomycin)	—	Duration may vary from 6 months or longer
Fungal infections	Amphotericin B, echinocandin, or azoles depending on suspected organism or culture data	—	Prolonged treatment courses of several months

Use needle aspiration to drain reaccumulated purulent joint fluid. If this procedure fails, perform arthroscopy/arthrotomy drainage. Manage infected prosthetic joints with surgery plus antibiotics, usually for 6 weeks.

DON'T BE TRICKED

- **Suspect tubercular infectious arthritis if the appropriate empiric antibacterial therapy is unsuccessful.**

TEST YOURSELF

A 28-year-old woman has a 9-day history of arthritis, fever, and chills followed by pain and swelling of the second and third MCP joints. As swelling resolved, the right wrist became inflamed. As the wrist improved, the right knee became inflamed. She also has a 5-mm vesicle surrounded by erythema on the forearm.

ANSWER: For diagnosis, choose disseminated gonorrhea infection. For management, select ceftriaxone for gonorrhea and doxycycline for empiric treatment of chlamydia.

Inflammatory Myopathies

Diagnosis

The major inflammatory myopathies are polymyositis, dermatomyositis, and inclusion body myositis. Certain medications (glucocorticoids, statins) or alcohol may also cause a toxic myopathy.

The characteristic finding in polymyositis and dermatomyositis is the gradual onset of painless proximal muscle, pharyngeal, and respiratory muscle weakness.

Photosensitivity rashes are commonly associated with dermatomyositis. The presence of Gottron papules (scaly, purplish papules and plaques over the metacarpal and interphalangeal joints) and heliotrope rash (edematous lilac discoloration of periorbital tissue) is virtually diagnostic of dermatomyositis.

An antisynthetase syndrome is characterized by interstitial lung disease, inflammatory polyarthritis, fever, Raynaud phenomenon, "mechanic's hands" (scaly, rough, dry, cracked horizontal lines on the palmar and lateral aspects of the fingers), and increased risk of sudden death. It is seen in patients with polymyositis or dermatomyositis but not with inclusion body myositis.

Inclusion body myositis is characterized by the insidious onset of symptoms, which involve proximal and distal muscles, frequently with an asymmetric distribution. Quadriceps, wrist, and finger flexor muscle weakness is common.

Testing

ANA is present in 80% of patients with polymyositis or dermatomyositis and in <20% of patients with inclusion body myositis.

Autoantibodies to aminoacyl-transfer (t)RNA synthetase enzymes (e.g., anti–Jo-1 antibodies) are associated with the antisynthetase syndrome.

Diagnostic tests for inflammatory myositis include measurement of serum CK and aldolase levels and EMG. The characteristic triad of EMG findings is:

- short duration small, low-amplitude polyphasic potentials
- fibrillation potentials at rest
- bizarre, high frequency, repetitive discharges

Muscle biopsy is the definitive study. MRI of the proximal musculature, particularly the thighs, may assess the degree of muscle inflammation and damage and may be helpful when other diagnostic studies are equivocal or to identify the most promising biopsy site.

DON'T BE TRICKED

- **Serum AST and ALT levels may be elevated in myositis, mimicking liver disease.**
- **Muscle pain in patients with an inflammatory myopathy is atypical and, if present, is generally mild.**

STUDY TABLE: Mimics of Polymyositis

If you see this...	Diagnose this...
Muscle fasciculations	ALS
Oculomotor weakness with ptosis	Myasthenia gravis
Proximal muscle tenderness	Polymyalgia rheumatica
Muscle atrophy, hyporeflexia	Peripheral neuropathy
Goiter, delayed reflexes, weight gain	Hypothyroidism
Treatment with a statin	Statin myopathy
≥2 defined connective tissue diseases present	Overlap syndrome
Symptoms of ≥2 connective tissue diseases associated with high titers of anti-RNP antibodies	MCTD

If myositis is unresponsive to treatment, consider a diagnosis of inclusion body myositis.

Malignancy and Inflammatory Myopathies

The association of malignancy and with dermatomyositis and polymyositis is well established. The types of malignancies correlate with those that develop in an age-matched population, except that ovarian cancer is more common. Sex- and age-appropriate cancer screening should be performed at the time of diagnosis and at periodic intervals thereafter, and the index of suspicion should be high for malignancy if suggestive symptoms and signs develop.

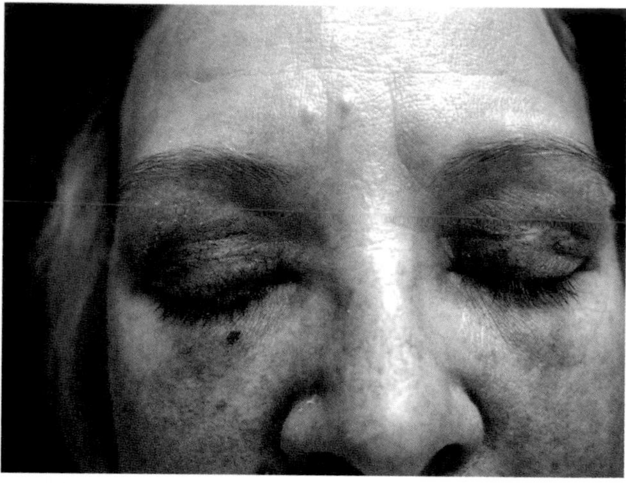

Heliotrope Rash: The heliotrope rash of dermatomyositis is a distinctive purple or lilac, symmetrical erythema of the eyelids that may be accompanied by slight edema, generally focused around the orbits.

Treatment

High-dose oral glucocorticoid therapy is first-line treatment for polymyositis and dermatomyositis.

Adding methotrexate and/or azathioprine may be indicated if disease is refractory to high-dose glucocorticoid therapy or if patients develop intolerable glucocorticoid-related side effects.

Rituximab is used for treatment of refractory polymyositis and dermatomyositis.

Hydroxychloroquine may help to treat cutaneous manifestations of dermatomyositis.

Baseline bone mineral density testing is indicated in patients who undergo long-term high-dose glucocorticoid therapy. Begin prophylactic therapy for osteoporosis with calcium and vitamin D supplementation and bisphosphonates.

DON'T BE TRICKED

- Suspect glucocorticoid-induced myopathy in patients with continued or new-onset worsening of proximal muscle weakness despite normalization of muscle enzyme levels.
- Always check TSH levels when evaluating myopathy.

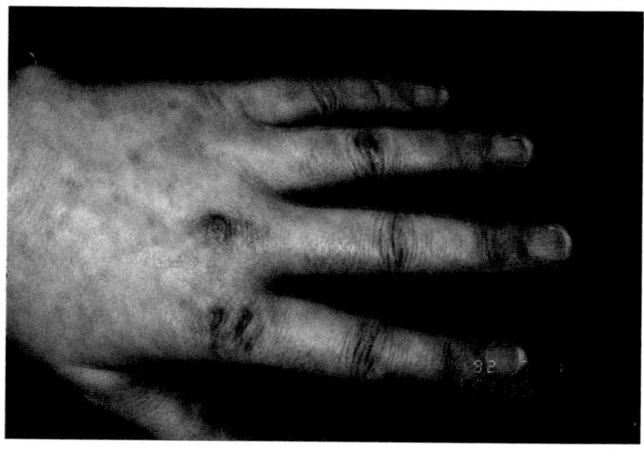

Gottron Papules: Red patches and plaques over the knuckles (Gottron papules) characteristic of dermatomyositis.

TEST YOURSELF

A 40-year-old man has a 6-week history of dyspnea, dry cough, fever, decreased appetite, and weight loss. He has progressive difficulty climbing stairs and reaching up to shampoo his hair. He has deep fissures and thickened skin on the palms of his hands.

ANSWER: For diagnosis, choose antisynthetase syndrome

Vasculitis

Diagnosis

Vasculitis is an inflammation of blood vessels that causes stenosis, obstruction, or attenuation with subsequent tissue ischemia, aneurysms, or hemorrhage. This condition may be secondary to an underlying process or occur as a primary disease of unknown cause. Primary vasculitides may be categorized based on the size of the blood vessel that is predominantly involved, the pattern of organ involvement, and the histopathology.

STUDY TABLE: Vasculitis Diagnosis		
Type	**Presentation**	**Testing**
Large-Vessel Vasculitis		
Giant cell arteritis	Older adults with fever, headaches, scalp tenderness, jaw claudication, and visual symptoms	ESR (>50 mm/h) and temporal artery biopsy
Polymyalgia rheumatica	Older adults with aching and morning stiffness in the proximal muscles of the shoulder and hip girdle Muscle strength and muscle enzymes are normal May develop in patients with giant cell arteritis or as a primary condition	ESR (usually >50 mm/h)
Takayasu arteritis	Young women with fever, malaise, weight loss, and arthralgia preceding arm/leg claudication, pulse deficits, vascular bruits, and asymmetric arm BP readings	Aortography
Medium-Vessel Vasculitis		
Polyarteritis nodosa	Nonglomerular kidney disease, hypertension, mononeuritis multiplex, and skin lesions (nodules, livedo reticularis, palpable purpura)	Hepatitis B serologic studies, biopsy of involved tissue (usually skin or testicle), and mesenteric or renal angiography (aneurysms and stenoses)
Primary angiitis of the CNS	Recurrent headaches, stroke, TIA, and progressive encephalopathy	LP, MRI, cerebral angiography, and brain biopsy (granulomatous vasculitis)
Small-Vessel Vasculitis		
Granulomatosis with polyangiitis	Recurrent middle ear infections, destructive rhinitis or sinusitis, saddle-nose deformity, tracheal collapse, pulmonary infiltrates/cavities/hemoptysis, and pauci-immune GN	C-ANCA and anti-PR3 antibody assay Biopsy skin or kidney
Microscopic polyangiitis	Pulmonary infiltrates, palpable purpura, and rapidly progressive pauci-immune GN	P-ANCA and anti-MPO antibody assay Biopsy skin, lung, or kidney
Eosinophilic granulomatosis with polyangiitis	Asthma, eosinophilia, elevated IgE, and pulmonary infiltrates/hemoptysis	P-ANCA and anti-MPO antibody assay and biopsy
Henoch-Schönlein purpura	Palpable purpura, joint, and gut involvement (abdominal pain), and GN	Skin biopsy (IgA immune complex deposition) or kidney biopsy (IgA nephropathy)
Hypersensitivity vasculitis (leukocytoclastic vasculitis)	Palpable purpura (lower legs), cutaneous vesicles, pustules, maculopapular lesions, urticaria, recent viral infection, drug exposure, or diagnosis of malignancy	Skin biopsy
Cryoglobulinemic vasculitis	Skin lesions (red macules, palpable purpura, nodules, or ulcers), GN, mononeuritis multiplex, and elevated serum aminotransferase levels	Serum cryoglobulins and hepatitis C serologic studies
Behçet syndrome	Oral and genital ulcers; uveitis; pathergy; nonerosive, asymmetric oligoarthritis; CNS or large artery vasculitis	Clinical diagnosis

DON'T BE TRICKED

- Aortic aneurysm and aortic dissection are potential complications of giant cell arteritis; aortic dissection may occur with or without preceding aneurysm formation.
- Polyarteritis nodosa kidney disease does not involve the glomerulus (no urine erythrocytes, casts, or proteinuria).
- Do not make a diagnosis of eosinophilic granulomatosis with polyangiitis in the absence of eosinophilia.

Treatment

STUDY TABLE: Treatment of Large-Vessel Vasculitis	
Disease	**Treatment**
Giant cell arteritis	Initial high-dose glucocorticoids; tocilizumab may be steroid sparing; low-dose aspirin; treat immediately to prevent blindness and obtain biopsy in <2 weeks
Polymyalgia rheumatica	Low-dose prednisone; relapse common and prolonged courses typical (1-3 years)
Takayasu arteritis	Prednisone

STUDY TABLE: Treatment of Medium-Vessel Vasculitis	
Disease	**Treatment**
Polyarteritis nodosa	Prednisone and cyclophosphamide for severe organ-threatening disease; treat concomitant HBV infection
Primary angiitis of the CNS	Prednisone and cyclophosphamide

STUDY TABLE: Treatment of Small-Vessel Vasculitis	
Disease	**Treatment**
Granulomatosis with polyangiitis	Prednisone and either cyclophosphamide or rituximab
Microscopic polyangiitis	Prednisone and either cyclophosphamide or rituximab
Eosinophilic granulomatosis with polyangiitis	Prednisone; cyclophosphamide added for severe, multiorgan disease
Henoch-Schönlein purpura	Typically self-limited; glucocorticoids or cyclophosphamide for severe, persistent GN
Hypersensitivity vasculitis	If drug-associated, withdraw offending drug
HCV-associated cryoglobulinemic vasculitis	Treat underlying HCV infection If organ dysfunction is severe, also treat with prednisone, cyclophosphamide, and plasmapheresis
Behçet syndrome	Prednisone; steroid-sparing agents may be required for major disease manifestations (uveitis, CNS, GI, or large artery involvement)

TEST YOURSELF

A 72-year-old woman has had a left temporal headache for the past 8 days with blurred and double vision that lasted 15 minutes this morning.

ANSWER: For diagnosis, choose giant cell arteritis. For management, select immediate prednisone, and arrange for temporal artery biopsy within 2 weeks.

A 32-year-old woman has a 6-month history of fever, myalgia, arthralgia, and weight loss. She is of Korean descent. Two days ago, she developed achy pain in her arms when working with her arms above her head.

ANSWER: For diagnosis, choose Takayasu arteritis. NOTE: When ethnicity is identified in a board question, it is an essential key to the diagnosis.

Relapsing Polychondritis

Diagnosis

Relapsing polychondritis is a systemic inflammatory connective tissue disease characterized by inflammation and destruction of cartilaginous structures. Characteristic findings are:

- red, hot, painful ears (most common presenting feature)
- respiratory stridor caused by tracheal collapse
- saddle nose deformity

Testing

Relapsing polychondritis is often a clinical diagnosis, and biopsy of affected cartilage is confirmatory. Saddle nose deformity can also occur in syphilis, cocaine use, leprosy, and granulomatosis with polyangiitis.

Treatment

NSAIDs, colchicine, or dapsone are used to treat minor disease manifestations.

Glucocorticoids and steroid-sparing agents are indicated for more severe disease.

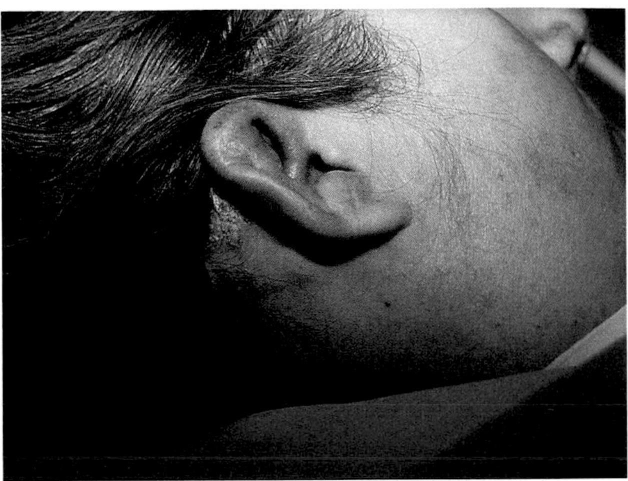

Polychondritis: Recurrent episodes of polychondritis involving the ear can permanently alter the structure of cartilage, resulting in a "cauliflower" appearance.

Familial Mediterranean Fever

Diagnosis

FMF occurs most often in persons from the Eastern Mediterranean basin. Characteristic findings are:

- recurrent, self-limited attacks of fever and serositis (abdominal or pleuritic pain)
- arthritis
- rashes that last 3 to 4 days

Testing

Laboratory findings include an elevated ESR and serum CRP concentration, positive serum amyloid A (AA) protein, proteinuria, and presence of the Mediterranean fever (*MEFV*) gene.

Treatment

Select colchicine for confirmed or suspected FMF to prevent symptomatic attacks and development of AA amyloidosis.

TEST YOURSELF

A 23-year-old woman has episodic fever and abdominal pain every 1 to 2 months, lasting 2 to 3 days per episode. She is well between episodes. She is Turkish. Physical examination and imaging studies are normal.

ANSWER: For diagnosis, choose FMF. For management, select colchicine.

Adult-Onset Still Disease

Diagnosis

The clinical features of AOSD include:

- quotidian fever in which the temperature usually spikes once daily and then returns to subnormal
- fatigue, malaise, arthralgia, and myalgia

- proteinuria
- serositis
- evanescent pink rash
- joint manifestations include a nonerosive inflammatory arthritis

Testing

Diagnosis is clinical, and other possible causes must be ruled out, including infection, malignancy, vasculitis, and drug reaction. Serum ferritin levels >2500 ng/mL are highly specific for this condition and reflect disease activity.

Treatment

NSAIDs are generally used as first-line agents in management; glucocorticoids may be useful in patients whose disease is refractory to NSAIDs.

In patients with refractory disease, therapy with methotrexate, a TNF-α inhibitor, or the interleukin-1 receptor antagonist anakinra may be helpful.

Complex Regional Pain Syndrome

Diagnosis

Complex regional pain syndrome is characterized by pain, swelling, limited range of motion, vasomotor instability, skin changes, and patchy bone demineralization of the extremities. It typically follows an injury, surgery, MI, or stroke. Look for onset of pain after injury, persistence of pain, and at least two associated symptoms or signs, including:

- neuropathic pain (allodynia, hyperalgesia, hyperpathia)
- autonomic dysfunction of the affected extremity (edema, color changes, sweating)
- swelling
- dystrophy (hair loss, skin thinning, ulcers)
- movement disorder (difficulty initiating movement, dystonia, tremor, weakness)

Testing

The finding of abnormal bone metabolism and osteoporosis by bone scan, bone densitometry, MRI, or plain x-ray supports the diagnosis.

Treatment

Physical therapy is essential to preserve joint mobility and prevent contractures and osteoporosis.

Glucocorticoids may abort the syndrome if started soon after symptom development.

Early sympathetic blockade is effective.

Gabapentin and tricyclic antidepressants are adjuvants for pain control. Bisphosphonates are effective treatment for pain, even in the absence of osteoporosis.

Abbreviations

3f-PCC	3-factor prothrombin complex concentrate
4f-PCC	4-factor prothrombin complex concentrate
5-ASA	5-aminosalicylic acid
5-FU	5-fluorouracil
5-HIAA	5-hydroxyindoleacetic acid
6-MP	6-mercaptopurine
A-a	alveolar-arterial oxygen gradient
AA	amyloid A
AAA	abdominal aortic aneurysm
AAT	α_1-antitrypsin
ABG	arterial blood gas
ABI	ankle-brachial index
ABIM	American Board of Internal Medicine
ABVD	doxorubicin (Adriamycin), bleomycin, vinblastine, dacarbazine
ACC	American College of Cardiology
ACE	angiotensin-converting enzyme
ACP	American College of Physicians
ACS	acute coronary syndrome
ACTH	adrenocorticotropic hormone
ADH	antidiuretic hormone
ADHD	attention-deficit/hyperactivity disorder
ADPKD	autosomal dominant polycystic kidney disease
ADT	androgen deprivation therapy
AED	antiepileptic drug
AF	atrial fibrillation
AFLP	acute fatty liver of pregnancy
AFP	α-fetoprotein
AGEP	acute generalized exanthematous pustulosis
AH	alcoholic hepatitis
AHA	American Heart Association
AHI	apnea-hypopnea index
AHR	abacavir hypersensitivity reaction
AIDS	acquired immunodeficiency syndrome
AIN	acute interstitial nephritis
AIP	autoimmune pancreatitis
AKI	acute kidney injury
ALL	acute lymphoblastic leukemia
ALS	amyotrophic lateral sclerosis
ALT	alanine aminotransferase
AMD	age-related macular degeneration
AMI	acute mesenteric ischemia
AML	acute myeloblastic leukemia
AMS	acute mountain sickness
ANA	antinuclear antibody
ANCA	antineutrophil cytoplasmic antibody
anti-CCP	anti-cyclic citrullinated peptide
anti-dsDNA	anti-double-stranded DNA
anti-HBc	antibodies to hepatitis B core antigen
anti-HBe	antibodies to hepatitis B e antigen
anti-HBs	antibodies to hepatitis B surface antigen
anti-MPO	anti-myeloperoxidase
anti-NMDA	anti-*N*-methyl-D-aspartate
anti-RNP	antiribonucleoprotein
anti-Sm	anti-Smith
anti-TNF	anti-tumor necrosis factor
AOSD	adult-onset Still disease
APLA	antiphospholipid antibody
aPTT	activated partial thromboplastin time
AR	aortic regurgitation; absolute risk
ARB	angiotensin receptor blocker
ARDS	acute respiratory distress syndrome
ARR	absolute risk reduction
ART	antiretroviral therapy
AS	aortic stenosis
ASCVD	atherosclerotic cardiovascular disease
ASD	atrial septal defect
ASH	alcoholic steatohepatitis
AST	aspartate aminotransferase
ATN	acute tubular necrosis
ATRA	all-*trans*-retinoic acid
ATS	American Thoracic Society
AUDIT-C	Alcohol Use Disorders Identification Test
AV	atrioventricular
AVM	arteriovenous malformation
AVNRT	atrioventricular nodal reentrant tachycardia
AVP	arginine vasopressin
AVRT	atrioventricular reciprocating tachycardia
β-hCG	beta-human chorionic gonadotropin
β_2-GPI	beta-2 glycoprotein I
BCC	basal cell carcinoma
BE	Barrett esophagus
BID	twice daily
BMI	body mass index
BNP	B-type natriuretic peptide
BP	blood pressure
BPAP	bilevel positive airway pressure
BPH	benign prostatic hyperplasia
BRCA	breast cancer susceptibility gene
BUN	blood urea nitrogen
CABG	coronary artery bypass graft
CAD	coronary artery disease
c-ANCA	cytoplasmic antineutrophil cytoplasmic antibody
CAP	community-acquired pneumonia
CAPOX	capecitabine plus oxaliplatin
CAUTI	catheter-associated urinary tract infection
CBC	complete blood count
CBT	cognitive behavioral therapy
CEA	carcinoembryonic antigen
CF	cystic fibrosis
CH_{50}	total hemolytic complement
CI	confidence interval
CK	creatine kinase
CKD	chronic kidney disease
CLL	chronic lymphocytic leukemia
CML	chronic myeloid leukemia
CMR	cardiac magnetic resonance (imaging)
CMV	cytomegalovirus
CNS	central nervous system
COPD	chronic obstructive pulmonary disease
CPAP	continuous positive airway pressure
CPP	calcium pyrophosphate
CPPD	calcium pyrophosphate deposition
CRAO	central retinal arterial occlusion

CRP	C-reactive protein
CRVO	central retinal vein occlusion
CSF	cerebrospinal fluid
CT	computed tomography
CTA	computed tomography angiography
CTEPH	chronic thromboembolic pulmonary hypertension
CUP	carcinoma of unknown primary
CVA	cerebrovascular accident
CVID	common variable immunodeficiency
CVP	central venous pressure
DASH	Dietary Approaches to Stop Hypertension
DAT	direct antiglobulin test
DBP	diastolic blood pressure
DCIS	ductal carcinoma in situ
DDAVP	1-deamino-8-D-arginine vasopressin
DEXA	dual energy x-ray absorptiometry
DHEAS	dehydroepiandrosterone sulfate
DI	diabetes insipidus
DIC	disseminated intravascular coagulation
DIP	distal interphalangeal
DISH	diffuse idiopathic skeletal hyperostosis
DKA	diabetic ketoacidosis
DLBCL	diffuse large B-cell lymphoma
DLCO	diffusing capacity of lung for carbon monoxide
DMARD	disease-modifying antirheumatic drug
DNA	deoxyribonucleic acid
DPLD	diffuse parenchymal lung disease
DRESS	drug reaction with eosinophilia and systemic symptoms
DVT	deep venous thrombosis
EBV	Epstein-Barr virus
ECG	electrocardiogram
EDTA	ethylenediaminetetraacetic acid
EE	eosinophilic esophagitis
EEG	electroencephalogram
EF	ejection fraction
EGD	esophagogastroduodenoscopy
EGFR	epidermal growth factor receptor
eGFR	estimated glomerular filtration rate
EHEC	enterohemorrhagic *Escherichia coli* O157:H7
EIA	enzyme immunoassay
ELISA	enzyme-linked immunosorbent assay
EM	erythema multiforme
EMG	electromyography
EN	erythema nodosum
ENT	ear, nose and throat
ERCP	endoscopic retrograde cholangiopancreatography
ESR	erythrocyte sedimentation rate
FDA	Food and Drug Administration
FE_{Na}	fractional excretion of sodium
FEPO4	fractional excretion of filtered phosphate
FEUrea	fractional excretion of urea
FEV_1	forced expiratory volume exhaled in 1 second
FFP	fresh frozen plasma
FIT	fecal immunochemical test
FMF	familial Mediterranean fever
FNAB	fine-needle aspiration biopsy
FOBT	fecal occult blood testing
FOLFIRI	5-fluorouracil, leucovorin, and irinotecan
FOLFIRINOX	5-fluorouracil, leucovorin, irinotecan, and oxaliplatin
FOLFOX	5-fluorouracil, leucovorin, and oxaliplatin
FSH	follicle-stimulating hormone
FTA-ABS	fluorescent treponemal antibody absorption test
FVC	forced vital capacity
G6PD	glucose 6-phosphate dehydrogenase
GAD65	glutamate decarboxylase antibody
GBM	glomerular basement membrane
GE	gastroesophageal
GERD	gastroesophageal reflux disease
GFR	glomerular filtration rate
GH	growth hormone
GI	gastrointestinal
GN	glomerulonephritis
GnRH	gonadotropin-releasing hormone
GP	glycoprotein
GU	genitourinary
GVHD	graft-versus-host disease
HACE	high-altitude cerebral edema
HAI	high-altitude illness
HAP	hospital-acquired pneumonia
HAPB	high-altitude periodic breathing
HAPE	high-altitude pulmonary edema
HAV	hepatitis A virus
HBeAg	hepatitis B e antigen
HBIG	hepatitis B immune globulin
HBsAg	hepatitis B surface antigen
HBV	hepatitis B virus
HCC	hepatocellular carcinoma
hCG	human chorionic gonadotropin
HCM	hypertrophic cardiomyopathy
HCV	hepatitis C virus
HELLP	hemolysis, elevated liver enzyme levels, and a low platelet count
HES	hypereosinophilic syndromes
HF	heart failure
HFpEF	heart failure with preserved ejection fraction
HFrEF	heart failure with reduced ejection fraction
HGA	human granculocytic anaplasmosis
HIDA	hepatobiliary iminodiacetic acid
HIPAA	Health Insurance Portability and Accountability Act
HIT	heparin-induced thrombocytopenia
HITT	heparin-induced thrombocytopenia with thrombosis
HIV	human immunodeficiency virus
HLA	human leukocyte antigens
HME	human monocytic ehrlichiosis
HNPCC	hereditary nonpolyposis colorectal cancer
HPA	human platelet antigen
HPV	human papillomavirus
HR	hazard ratio; heart rate
HRCT	high-resolution computed tomography
HSCT	hematopoietic stem cell transplantation
HSE	herpes simplex encephalitis
HSV	herpes simplex virus
HUS	hemolytic uremic syndrome
IA-2	islet antigen-2 antibody
IBD	inflammatory bowel disease
IBS	irritable bowel syndrome
IBS-C	irritable bowel syndrome with constipation
IBS-D	irritable bowel syndrome with diarrhea
IBS-M	mixed irritable bowel syndrome
ICD	implantable cardioverter defibrillator
ICH	intracerebral hemorrhage
ICU	intensive care unit
IDSA	Infectious Diseases Society of America
IE	infective endocarditis
IGF-1	insulin-like growth factor-1

IgM anti-HAV IgM antibodies to hepatitis A virus
IGRA interferon-γ release assay
IM intramuscular
INR international normalized ratio
IPF idiopathic pulmonary fibrosis
IPSS-R revised International Prognostic Scoring System
IRIS immune reconstitution inflammatory syndrome
ITP immune thrombocytopenic purpura
IV intravenous
IVC inferior vena cava
JVD jugular venous distention
KOH potassium hydroxide
LABA long-acting β_2-agonist
LAC lupus anticoagulant
LAM lymphanogioleiomyomatosis
LAMA long-acting muscarinic agent (also called long-acting anticholinergic agent)
LBBB left bundle branch block
LDH lactate dehydrogenase
LDL low-density lipoprotein
LES lower esophageal sphincter
LFT liver function test
LGI lower gastrointestinal
LH luteinizing hormone
LKM liver-kidney microsome
LLQ left lower quadrant
LMWH low-molecular-weight heparin
LN lupus nephritis
LP lumbar puncture
LR likelihood ratio
LTBI latent tuberculosis infection
LV left ventricular
LVAD left ventricular assist device
LVEF left ventricular ejection fraction
LVH left ventricular hypertrophy
MAC *Mycobacterium avium* complex
MAOI monoamine oxidase inhibitor
MALT mucosa-associated lymphoid tissue
MAP mean arterial pressure
MAT multifocal atrial tachycardia
MCI mild cognitive impairment
MCP metacarpophalangeal
MCTD mixed connective tissue disease
MCV mean corpuscular volume
MDS myelodysplastic syndromes
MEN1 multiple endocrine neoplasia type 1
MEN2 multiple endocrine neoplasia type 2
METs metabolic equivalents
MG myasthenia gravis
MGUS monoclonal gammopathy of undetermined significance
MHA-TP microhemagglutination assay for *Treponema pallidum*
MI myocardial infarction
MIBG metaiodobenzylguanidine
MMR measles, mumps, rubella
MPA microscopic polyangiitis
MPN myeloproliferative neoplasm
MPO myeloperoxidase
MR mitral regurgitation
MRA magnetic resonance angiography
MRCP magnetic resonance cholangiopancreatography
MRI magnetic resonance imaging
MRSA methicillin-resistant *Staphylococcus aureus*
MS multiple sclerosis
MSSA methicillin-sensitive *Staphylococcus aureus*
mTOR mammalian target of rapamycin
MTP metatarsophalangeal
MVP mitral valve prolapse
N/A not applicable
NAAT nucleic acid amplification testing
NAFLD nonalcoholic fatty liver disease
NASH nonalcoholic steatohepatitis
NCCN National Comprehensive Cancer Network
NET neuroendocrine tumor
NMO neuromyelitis optica
NNH number needed to harm
NNT number needed to treat
NOAC non–vitamin K antagonist oral anticoagulant
NPH intermediate-acting insulin or Lente
NPPV noninvasive positive-pressure ventilation
NSAIDs nonsteroidal anti-inflammatory drugs
NSCLC non–small cell lung cancer
NSTE-ACS non–ST-elevation acute coronary syndrome
NSTEMI non–ST-elevation myocardial infarction
NYHA New York Heart Association
OA osteoarthritis
OGTT oral glucose tolerance test
OSA obstructive sleep apnea
PAD peripheral arterial disease
PAH pulmonary arterial hypertension
p-ANCA perinuclear antineutrophil cytoplasmic antibodies
PCI percutaneous coronary intervention
PCNSL primary central nervous system lymphoma
PCOS polycystic ovary syndrome
PCR polymerase chain reaction
PCWP pulmonary capillary wedge pressure
PDA patent ductus arteriosus
PDE-4 phosphodiesterase type 4
PDE-5 phosphodiesterase type 5
PE pulmonary embolism
PEEP positive end-expiratory pressure
PEF peak expiratory flow
PEG polyethylene glycol
PET positron emission tomography
PF4 platelet factor 4
PFO patent foramen ovale
PFT pulmonary function test
PH pulmonary hypertension
PID pelvic inflammatory disease
PIP proximal interphalangeal
PMDD premenstrual dysphoric disorder
PMN polymorphonuclear
PMS premenstrual syndrome
PNES psychogenic nonepileptic seizures
PNH paroxysmal nocturnal hemoglobinuria
PO by mouth
PPI proton pump inhibitor
PR3 proteinase 3
PrEP pre-exposure prophylaxis
PSA prostate-specific antigen
PSC primary sclerosing cholangitis
PT prothrombin time
PTH parathyroid hormone
PTSD posttraumatic stress disorder
PUD peptic ulcer disease
PV polycythemia vera
PVC premature ventricular complex
RA rheumatoid arthritis
RANK receptor activator of nuclear factor kappa β

RAST	radioallergosorbent test
RBBB	right bundle branch block
RBC	red blood cell
R-CHOP	rituximab, cyclophosphamide, doxorubicin, vincristine, prednisolone
RCT	randomized controlled trial
REM	rapid eye movement
RF	rheumatic fever
rfVIIa	recombinant factor VIIa
RLQ	right lower quadrant
RNA	ribonucleic acid
RNP	ribonucleic protein
RPR	rapid plasma reagin
RR	relative risk
RRR	relative risk reduction
RTA	renal tubular acidosis
rtPA	recombinant tissue plasminogen activator
RUQ	right upper quadrant
RV	right ventricular
SAAG	serum-ascites albumin gradient
SABA	short-acting β_2-agonist
SAH	subarachnoid hemorrhage
SBP	systolic blood pressure
SCC	squamous cell carcinoma
SCLC	small cell lung cancer
SEID	systemic exertion intolerance disease
SGLT2	sodium-glucose transporter-2
SIADH	syndrome of inappropriate antidiuretic hormone secretion
SIBO	small intestinal bacterial overgrowth
SIRS	systemic inflammatory response syndrome
SJS	Stevens-Johnson syndrome
SLE	systemic lupus erythematosus
SNRI	serotonin-norepinephrine reuptake inhibitor
SPEP	serum protein electrophoresis
SPN	solitary pulmonary nodule
SSA	sulfosalicylic acid
SSc	systemic sclerosis
SSRI	selective serotonin reuptake inhibitor
STEMI	ST-elevation myocardial infarction
STI	sexually transmitted infection
SVC	superior vena cava
SVT	supraventricular tachycardia
T_4	free thyroxine
TAVR	transcatheter aortic valve replacement
TB	tuberculosis
TBI	traumatic brain injury
TBW	total body weight
Tdap	diphtheria and reduced tetanus toxoids and acellular pertussis vaccine
TEE	transesophageal echocardiography
TEN	toxic epidermal necrolysis
TIA	transient ischemic attack
TIBC	total iron-binding capacity
TIMI	Thrombolysis in Myocardial Infarction (risk score)
TIPS	transjugular intrahepatic portosystemic shunt
TLC	total lung capacity
TNF	tumor necrosis factor
TR	tricuspid regurgitation
TSH	thyroid-stimulating hormone
TSS	toxic shock syndrome
TST	tuberculin skin testing
TTE	transthoracic echocardiography
tTG	tissue transglutaminase
TTP	thrombotic thrombocytopenic purpura
UACS	upper airways cough syndrome
UAG	urine anion gap
UFH	unfractionated heparin
UGI	upper gastrointestinal
UPEP	urine protein electrophoresis
URI	upper respiratory infection
USPSTF	United States Preventive Services Task Force
UTI	urinary tract infection
VAP	ventilator-associated pneumonia
VDRL	Venereal Disease Research Laboratory
VEGF	vascular endothelial growth factor
VF	ventricular fibrillation
VKA	vitamin K antagonist
V/Q	ventilation/perfusion ratio
VSD	ventricular septal defect
VT	ventricular tachycardia
VTE	venous thromboembolism
vWD	von Willebrand disease
vWF	von Willebrand factor
VZV	varicella-zoster virus
WBC	white blood cell
WNND	West Nile neuroinvasive disease
WNV	West Nile virus
WPW	Wolff-Parkinson-White